MARONEY

THORACIC AND VISCERAL VASCULAR INTERVENTIONS

ZIV J. HASKAL, M.D., *EDITOR*
ASSISTANT PROFESSOR OF RADIOLOGY
UNIVERSITY OF PENNSYLVANIA SCHOOL OF MEDICINE
HOSPITAL OF THE UNIVERSITY OF PENNSYLVANIA
PHILADELPHIA, PENNSYLVANIA

ROBERT K. KERLAN, JR., M.D., *EDITOR*
ASSOCIATE CLINICAL PROFESSOR OF RADIOLOGY
UNIVERSITY OF CALIFORNIA, SAN FRANCISCO, SCHOOL OF MEDICINE
SAN FRANCISCO, CALIFORNIA

SCOTT O. TREROTOLA, M.D., *EDITOR IN CHIEF*
ASSOCIATE PROFESSOR OF RADIOLOGY
INDIANA UNIVERSITY SCHOOL OF MEDICINE
INDIANAPOLIS, INDIANA

Published by

The Society of Cardiovascular & Interventional Radiology

Library of Congress Catalog Card Number 96-069923

The Society of Cardiovascular & Interventional Radiology is accredited by the Accreditation Council for Continuing Medical Education to sponsor continuing medical education for physicians.

The Society of Cardiovascular & Interventional Radiology designates this continuing medical education activity for 20 credit hours in Category 1 of the Physicians Recognition Award of the American Medical Association.

FOREWORD

For several reasons it is a special pleasure to contribute this foreword to *Thoracic and Visceral Vascular Interventions*, the sixth in the SCVIR Syllabus/Videodisc Series.

The editors, Ziv Haskal and Bob Kerlan, are friends, and in a small way I feel a part of their careers. Bob Kerlan was a medical student when I was a radiology resident at the University of Southern California. He spent a lot of time in the department asking a million questions about radiology. Despite a ready-made opportunity in orthopedic surgery, he subsequently chose this career path and our field has been better off for it.

In 1992, although we barely knew each other, Ziv Haskal journeyed with me from California to the University of Pennsylvania and, to say the least, that has been a very productive and wonderful association.

Though Bob and Ziv practice on opposite sides of the country, it is pleasing to see yet another scholarly collaboration between fellow alumni from the University of California, San Francisco, a wellspring of interventional radiology and the birthplace of the videodisc and syllabus series. I was an SCVIR officer when the videodisc teaching series was conceived—though I take no credit for the idea or its execution—and from that vantage point, one fact is very clear: this project would have been nothing more than a pipe dream if not for the vision and drive of their UCSF colleague, Jeanne LaBerge.

The monograph is also a special treat because of the number and breadth of the contributors— over 60 radiologists of varying ages and from many different hospitals. This is the way education was meant to be—not a one-way street from academia to the community, but an interactive dialogue between practitioners from diverse practice settings.

I am delighted to see the Society take the lead in such an egalitarian role of continuing medical education. This model has naturally led to our next experiment: the on-line posting and discussion of cases that will premier with the 1996 Mortality and Morbidity Conference from Coeur D'Alene, Idaho. Internet access will permit everyone to "attend" the sessions. In the future, we anticipate that many different M&M cases and other educational materials will be contributed and discussed using this format. It doesn't take much imagination to see an enormous role for this technology in an image-driven, fast-breaking field such as ours.

I hope you enjoy reading this book and will consider contributing to the Society's new modes of communication and education.

Michael C. Pentecost, M.D.
Associate Professor of Radiology
University of Pennsylvania School of Medicine

PREFACE

The SCVIR Educational Materials Committee is pleased to release the sixth volume of the SCVIR Syllabus/Videodisc Series. Readers familiar with the SCVIR Syllabi will find this volume similar to previous volumes, with didactic tutorials, teaching file cases, and a CME quiz at the end. The discerning reader will notice a few subtle improvements, including expanded teaching file cases (both in number and content), as well as more in-depth coverage of several emerging areas in Interventional Radiology. In addition, two tutorials cover areas of "crossover" between Interventional and Neurointerventional Radiology. The reader is cautioned that some tutorials, particularly in these emerging areas, describe non-FDA approved ("off-label") use of devices, and that discussion of these procedures with the hospital's investigational review board is recommended before undertaking them.

Ziv Haskal and Bob Kerlan have done an outstanding job of assembling experts in this area and producing a comprehensive review of thoracic and visceral interventions. The SCVIR Educational Materials Committee is grateful to them for their dedication and hard work, as well as to Belinda Byrne and her production staff for their excellent work.

The continued success of the SCVIR Syllabus series is due to contributions from many individuals, but if not for the vision and hard work of Jeanne LaBerge, this series might never have come into existence. As we approach the completion of the series with upcoming volumes seven (Genitourinary interventions) and eight (Vascular diagnosis), the Educational Materials Committee continues to be indebted to Jeanne for laying the groundwork for this important project.

Scott O. Trerotola, M.D.
Editor in Chief
Chairman, SCVIR Educational Materials Committee

ACKNOWLEDGMENTS

The completion of this project required the diligent effort of the SCVIR production staff including Koreen Piazza, Teresa Lynn, Kevin Havener, and Paula Sinclair. We would like to thank them for their tireless work and outstanding effort in the creation of this book. We would also like to thank Christine Gralapp, the medical illustrator, for her art work, and Belinda Byrne, the project manager, for applying limitless pressure on us in order to meet deadlines, and never losing her smile.

As with the previous editors and authors, we would also like to acknowledge and thank Dr. Jeanne LaBerge for developing the concept of the SCVIR Syllabi. Largely through her individual effort, this series was created and has since benefited innumerable interventional radiologists.

On a personal note, we would like to thank our wives, Dina and Randi, for their patience and understanding.

Ziv J. Haskal, M.D.
and
Robert K. Kerlan, M.D.

CME INFORMATION

CME Essentials

The SCVIR Syllabus, *Thoracic and Visceral Vascular Interventions*, is part of a series of enduring materials planned and produced in accordance with the Accreditation Council for Continuing Medical Education Essentials. It has been developed for interventional radiologists, both practicing and in training, in both instructional text and computer-assisted formats.

Thoracic and Visceral Vascular Interventions constitutes a planned activity of continuing medical education with an estimated completion time of 20 hours. Topics covered for this CME activity are represented by the Table of Contents, Part One: Tutorials, on pages xiii and xiv of this volume, and principal faculty and their credentials can be found on pages ix–xii. An evaluation survey is provided as part of this CME activity to assess the value of these materials in meeting the educational needs of the end user.

Learning objectives addressed in this CME activity consist of the following:

1) Diagnose and direct appropriate management of complicated traumatic aortic injuries, aortic dissections, and aneurysms.
2) Be able to discuss embolization of pulmonary arteriovenous malformations, bronchial arteries, traumatic arterial injuries, and arteriovenous malformations.
3) Be able to discuss both basic and difficult chemoembolization treatments of hepatic malignancies and manage potential side effects of the agents delivered.
4) Direct appropriate invasive and noninvasive diagnosis and management of upper and lower gastrointestinal bleeding and mesenteric ischemia.

To become eligible for 20 hours of Category 1 CME credit, the user must submit the enclosed application form, an evaluation survey, and a completed quiz answer sheet, along with a $20 administrative fee, to:

SCVIR
Attention: CME Administrator
10201 Lee Highway, Suite 500
Fairfax, VA 20301

Financial Disclosure

The Society of Cardiovascular & Interventional Radiology has a policy requiring disclosure of the existence of any significant financial interest or other relationship that authors have to the manufacturer(s) of any commercial product(s) discussed in any SCVIR-sponsored educational activity.

Each contributor to the SCVIR Syllabus has indicated that he or she does not have any type of financial relationship with companies or organizations about whose products or services they are reporting.

SCVIR Syllabus, *Thoracic and Visceral Vascular Interventions*, date of release: September, 1996

CONTRIBUTORS

Sandra J. Althaus, M.D.
Assistant Professor of Radiology
Chief, Interventional Radiology
University of Washington Medical Center
Seattle, Washington

Michael A. Amygdalos, M.D.
Vascular and Interventional Radiologist
Saint Luke's Hospital
Bethlehem, Pennsylvania

James C. Andrews, M.D.
Associate Professor of Radiology
Mayo Clinic Rochester
Rochester, Minnesota

Linda J. Bagley, M.D.
Fellow, Neuroradiology
Hospital of the University of Pennsylvania
Philadelphia, Pennsylvania

Robert E. Barton, M.D.
Assistant Professor of Radiology
  and Interventional Therapy
Dotter Institute of Interventional Therapy
Oregon Health Sciences University
Portland, Oregon

Joseph Bonn, M.D.
Assistant Professor of Radiology
Jefferson Medical College
Thomas Jefferson University Hospital
Philadelphia, Pennsylvania

Timothy J. Carmody, M.D.
Fellow, Vascular and Interventional
  Radiology
Indiana University Medical Center
Indianapolis, Indiana

Patricia E. Cole, Ph.D., M.D.
Assistant Professor of Clinical Radiology
State University of New York at Stony Brook
Stony Brook, New York

Constantin Cope, M.D.
Professor of Radiology
Hospital of the University of Pennsylvania
Philadelphia, Pennsylvania

Michael D. Dake, M.D.
Assistant Professor of Radiology
  and Pulmonary Medicine
Stanford University Medical Center
Stanford, California

Michael D. Darcy, M.D.
Associate Professor of Radiology
Mallinckrodt Institute of Radiology
St. Louis, Missouri

Richard Duszak, Jr., M.D.
Vascular and Interventional Radiologist
The Reading Hospital and Medical Center
West Reading, Pennsylvania

Michael J. Flood, M.D.
Fellow, Interventional Radiology
Dotter Institute of Interventional Therapy
Oregon Health Sciences University
Portland, Oregon

Emily K. Folz, M.D.
Staff Radiologist
Wake Radiology Consultants
Raleigh, North Carolina

Roy L. Gordon, M.D.
Professor of Radiology
University of California, San Francisco
San Francisco, California

Jeffrey L. Groffsky, M.D.
Chief, Interventional Radiology
Saint Luke's Hospital
New Bedford, Massachusetts

Niki Harris, M.D.
Assistant Professor of Radiology
Indiana University Medical Center
Indianapolis, Indiana

Ziv J. Haskal, M.D.
Assistant Professor of Radiology
University of Pennsylvania School of Medicine
Hospital of the University of Pennsylvania
Philadelphia, Pennsylvania

CONTRIBUTORS

Keith M. Horton, M.D.
Clinical Assistant Professor of Radiology
F. Edward Hébèrt School of Medicine
Uniformed Services University
  of the Health Sciences
Bethesda, Maryland
Clinical Assistant Professor of Radiology
Howard University School of Medicine
Washington Hospital Center
Washington, D.C.

Robert W. Hurst, M.D.
Associate Professor of Radiology,
  Neurosurgery, and Neurology
Hospital of the University of Pennsylvania
Philadelphia, Pennsylvania

Erik K. Insko, M.D.
Hospital of the University of Pennsylvania
Philadelphia, Pennsylvania

Matthew S. Johnson, M.D.
Assistant Professor of Radiology
Indiana University Medical Center
Indianapolis, Indiana

John A. Kaufman, M.D.
Assistant Professor of Radiology
Harvard Medical School
Massachusetts General Hospital
Boston, Massachusetts

Robert K. Kerlan, Jr., M.D.
Associate Clinical Professor of Radiology
University of California, San Francisco
San Francisco, California

Joseph Krysl, M.D.
Assistant Professor of Radiology
University of Colorado
  Health Sciences Center
Denver, Colorado

Tom Livingston, M.D.
Fellow, Interventional Radiology
Baylor University Medical Center
Dallas, Texas

Shelley R. Marder, M.D.
Assistant Clinical Professor of Radiology
San Francisco General Hospital
University of California, San Francisco
San Francisco, California

Steven R. Maxfield, M.D.
Fellow, Interventional Radiology
Dotter Institute of Interventional Therapy
Oregon Health Sciences University
Portland, Oregon

Vincent G. McDermott, M.D.
Assistant Professor of Radiology
Duke University Medical Center
Durham, North Carolina

J. Mark McKinney, M.D.
Senior Associate Consultant
Mayo Clinic Jacksonville
Jacksonville, Florida

Donald L. Miller, M.D.
Professor of Radiology
F. Edward Hébèrt School of Medicine
Uniformed Services University
  of the Health Sciences
Bethesda, Maryland

Rendon C. Nelson, M.D.
Professor of Radiology
Director, Abdominal Imaging
Duke University Medical Center
Durham, North Carolina

Eric W. Olcott, M.D.
Assistant Professor of Radiology
Stanford University Medical Center
Stanford, California

Daniel Picus, M.D.
Professor of Radiology and Surgery
Chief, Vascular and Interventional Radiology
Mallinckrodt Institute of Radiology
St. Louis, Missouri

Jeffrey S. Pollak, M.D.
Associate Professor of Radiology
Yale University School of Medicine
New Haven, Connecticut

CONTRIBUTORS

Donald J. Ponec, M.D.
Vascular and Interventional Radiologist
Tri-City Medical Center
Oceanside, California

Robert Principato, D.O.
Clinical Instructor of Radiology
Cooper Hospital/University Medical Center
Camden, New Jersey

Richard D. Redvanly, M.D.
Assistant Professor of Radiology
Emory University Hospital
Atlanta, Georgia

Chet Rees, M.D.
Associate Attending Physician
Section Chief, Vascular and
  Interventional Radiology
Baylor University Medical Center
Dallas, Texas

Frank Rivera, M.D.
Associate Attending Physician
Director of Education, Vascular and
  Interventional Radiology
Baylor University Medical Center
Dallas, Texas

David Sacks, M.D.
Vascular and Interventional Radiologist
The Reading Hospital and Medical Center
West Reading, Pennsylvania

Jeet Sandhu, M.D.
Assistant Professor of Radiology
University of North Carolina Hospitals
Chapel Hill, North Carolina

Mark J. Sands, M.D.
Assistant Professor of Radiology
Case Western Reserve University
  School of Medicine
Cleveland, OH

Scott J. Savader, M.D.
Associate Professor of Radiology
  and Surgery
The Johns Hopkins Medical Institutions
Baltimore, Maryland

Rajiv Sawhney, M.D.
Assistant Professor of Radiology
University of California, San Francisco
Veterans Administration Medical Center
San Francisco, California

Richard R. Saxon, M.D.
Assistant Professor of Radiology
Dotter Institute of Interventional Therapy
Oregon Health Sciences University
Portland, Oregon

Donald E. Schwarten, M.D.
Saint Vincent Hospital
Indianapolis, Indiana

Charles P. Semba, M.D.
Assistant Professor of Radiology
Stanford University Medical Center
Stanford, California

Marcelle J. Shapiro, M.D.
Assistant Professor of Radiology
Jefferson Medical College
Thomas Jefferson University Hospital
Philadelphia, Pennsylvania

Richard D. Shlansky-Goldberg, M.D.
Assistant Professor of Radiology
Hospital of the University of Pennsylvania
Philadelphia, Pennsylvania

Harjit Singh, M.D.
Instructor, Cardiovascular
  and Interventional Radiology
The Johns Hopkins Medical Institutions
Baltimore, Maryland

Brian A. Solomon, M.D.
Hospital of the University of Pennsylvania
Philadelphia, Pennsylvania

CONTRIBUTORS

Michael C. Soulen, M.D.
Assistant Professor of Radiology
University of Pennsylvania Medical Center
Philadelphia, Pennsylvania

Ian A. Sproat, M.D., FRCP(C)
Associate Professor of Radiology
University of Wisconsin Hospitals and Clinics
Madison, Wisconsin

Kevin L. Sullivan, M.D.
Associate Professor of Radiology
Thomas Jefferson University Hospital
Jefferson Medical College
Philadelphia, Pennsylvania

Ian D. Timms, M.D.
Clinical Instructor of Radiology
Hospital of the University of Pennsylvania
Philadelphia, Pennsylvania

Scott O. Trerotola, M.D.
Associate Professor of Radiology
Director, Vascular and
    Interventional Radiology
Indiana University Medical Center
Indianapolis, Indiana

Anthony C. Venbrux, M.D.
Associate Professor of Radiology
    and Surgery
The Johns Hopkins Medical Institutions
Baltimore, Maryland

Anthony G. Verstandig, M.D.
Chief, Interventional Radiology
Hadassah University Hospital
Ein Kerem, Jerusalem
Israel

Susan D. Wall, M.D.
Professor of Radiology
University of California, San Francisco
Chief, Interventional Radiology
Veterans Administration Medical Center
San Francisco, California

Mark A. Westcott, M.D.
Assistant Professor
Beth Israel Medical Center
Albert Einstein College of Medicine
New York, New York

Robert I. White, Jr., M.D.
Professor of Radiology
Yale University School of Medicine
New Haven, Connecticut

David M. Williams, M.D.
Associate Professor of Radiology
University of Michigan Medical Center
Ann Arbor, Michigan

Mark W. Wilson, M.D.
Assistant Professor of Radiology
University of Michigan Medical Center
Ann Arbor, Michigan

Adam B. Winick, M.D.
Assistant Professor of Radiology
George Washington University Medical Center
Washington, D.C.

Wayne F. Yakes, M.D.
Director, Interventional Radiology and
    Interventional Neuroradiology
Radiology Imaging Associates, P.C.
Englewood, Colorado

CONTENTS

PART ONE: TUTORIALS

PART TWO: TEACHING FILE CASES

PART THREE: CME QUIZZES

TUTORIALS

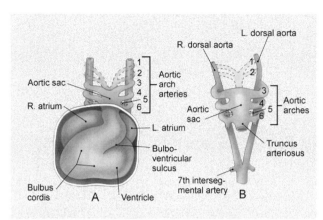

Figure 1. A. The primitive heart and aorta at approximately 6 weeks development. B. The dorsal aorta with the heart cut away. At 6 weeks, the 1st, 2nd, and 5th pairs of aortic arches have almost completely involuted during the transformation of the aortic arches into the adult vascular pattern.

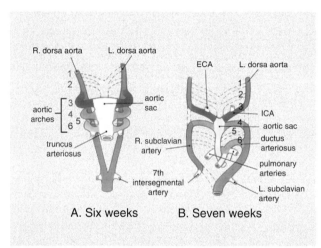

Figure 2. Development of the adult thoracic aorta. A. The aortic arches at 6 weeks with involution of the 1st, 2nd, and 5th arches. B. The aorta at 7 weeks. The different gray tones show the structures from which the developing vessels are derived.

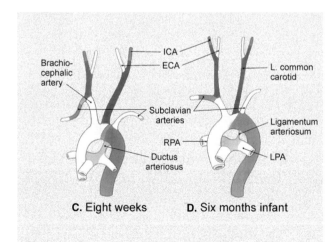

Figure 3. Development of the adult thoracic aorta. C. The configuration at 8 weeks development. D. The aorta at 6 months after birth.

TUTORIAL 1
ANATOMY OF THE THORACIC AORTA
Ian D. Timms, M.D., and
Richard D. Shlansky-Goldberg, M.D.

Introduction
The subjects addressed in this tutorial include:
1. Embryonic development of the thoracic aorta
2. Normal anatomy of the thoracic aorta
3. Variant anatomy of the thoracic aorta.

Embryology of the Thoracic Aorta—
The Primitive Aortic Arch Pattern
Early in embryonic development, there are two ventral aortas and two dorsal aortas. The two ventral aortas are fused at their origin from the truncus arteriosus, forming the aortic sac. The two dorsal aortas are located on either side of the midline and are fused at their caudal aspects, forming the descending aorta. Within each of the six branchial arches, arterial connections develop between the ventral aorta (the aortic sac) and the dorsal aorta on each side, resulting in six pairs of bridging vessels known as the aortic arches. In addition, several intersegmental arteries develop from the dorsal aortas. **Figure 1A** illustrates the primitive aortic pattern at about 6 weeks of development. **Figure 1B**, with the heart cut away, better demonstrates the dorsal aorta. By this time, the first, second, and fifth pairs of aortic arches have involuted almost completely.

Embryology of the Thoracic Aorta—
The Transformation into the Adult Pattern
During the sixth to eighth week of development, the primitive aortic arch pattern transforms into the familiar adult pattern by the involution of certain portions of the aortic arches and the persistence and growth of other portions **(Figs. 2, 3)**. Each aortic arch pair gives rise to the following vessels:

First pair—Portions of the maxillary and external carotid arteries.
Second pair—Portions of the stapedial arteries. Third pair—Common carotid arteries and portions of the internal carotid arteries.
Fourth pair—The left arch forms the segment of the aortic arch between the left common carotid and subclavian arteries. The right arch forms the proximal right subclavian artery.
Fifth pair—No derivatives.
Sixth pair—The left arch forms portions of the main and left pulmonary arteries and the ductus arteriosus. The right arch forms portions of the right pulmonary artery. Note that the left subclavian artery forms from the left seventh intersegmental artery.

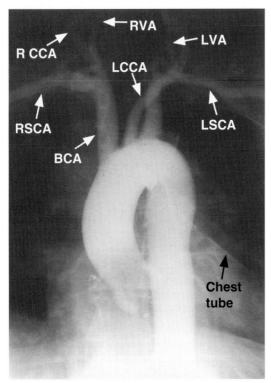

Figure 4. Normal thoracic aortogram, frontal projection. BCA=brachiocephalic artery; LCCA=left common carotid artery; LSCA=left subclavian artery; LVA=left vertebral artery; RCCA=right common carotid artery; RSCA=right subclavian artery; RVA=right vertebral artery.

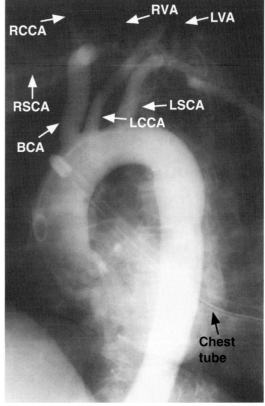

Figure 5. Normal thoracic aortogram, right posterior oblique projection. BCA=brachiocephalic artery; LCCA=left common carotid artery; LSCA=left subclavian artery; LVA=left vertebral artery; RCCA=right common carotid artery; RSCA=right subclavian artery; RVA=right vertebral artery.

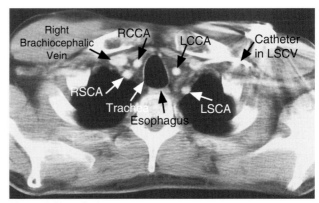

Figure 6. Near the lung apex.

"Normal" Anatomy of the Thoracic Aortic Arch
The familiar classic left aortic arch is present in approximately 70% of individuals. The first main branch is the brachiocephalic (innominate) artery (BCA) which is usually 3–4 cm in length and divides into the right subclavian artery (SCA) and the right common carotid artery (CCA). The second main branch is the left CCA, and the third, final main branch is the left SCA. The vertebral arteries (VA) arise from the SCA bilaterally. The intercostal arteries, the bronchial arteries, and the esophageal arteries arise as smaller direct branches from the descending thoracic aorta. **Figures 4** and **5** demonstrate a normal thoracic aortogram in a trauma patient. **Figures 6–12** demonstrate normal cross-sectional anatomy of the thoracic aorta.

Figures 6–12. Normal cross-sectional anatomy of the aorta and great vessels in a patient treated for lymphoma.

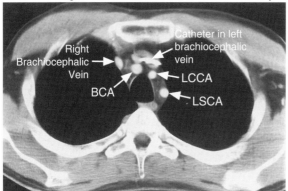

Figure 7. At the level of the left innominate vein crossing toward the superior vena cava.

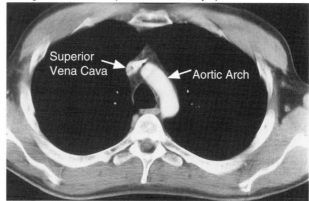

Figure 8. At the level at the top of the aortic arch.

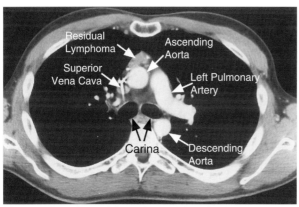

Figure 9. At the level of the carina and the left pulmonary artery.

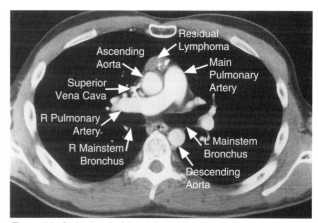

Figure 10. At the level of the right pulmonary artery. Note the mediastinal soft tissue mass representing the patient's treated lymphoma.

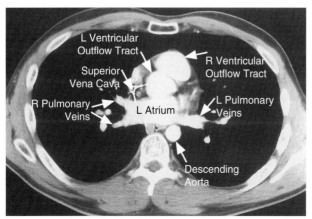

Figure 11. At the level of the left atrium.

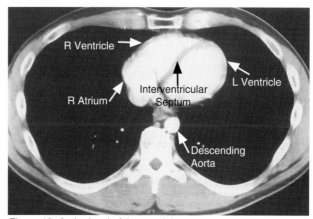

Figure 12. At the level of the ventricles.

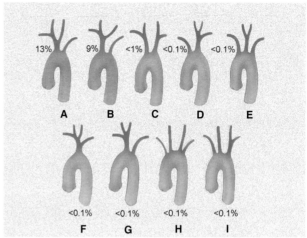

Figure 13. Variations in the branching pattern of the aortic arch which are seen in 23% of the population. The most frequent variation (A) is the common origin of the innominate and left common carotid arteries ("bovine arch").

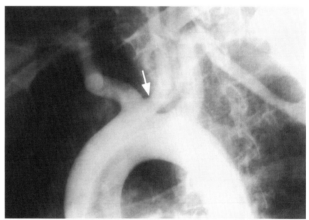

Figure 14. Proximal common origin of the brachiocephalic and left common carotid arteries (arrow).

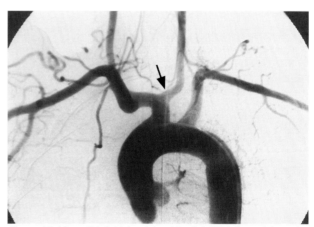

Figure 15. More distal, high origin of the left CCA (arrow) from the BCA.

Variant Anatomy of the Thoracic Aorta

Anomalies of the thoracic aorta are caused by a deviation from the normal pattern of persistence and involution of the aortic arches, with persistence of portions of the arches that are supposed to regress and/or regression of portions that are supposed to persist. **Figure 13** illustrates the variations in the branching pattern of the aortic arch, which are seen in 23% of the population. These are invariably asymptomatic, usually being discovered incidentally. The variations are as follows:

1. Common origin of the BCA and left CCA (13%), also known as a bovine arch **(Figs. 13A, 14)**
2. Left CCA originating from the BCA (9%) **(Figs. 13B, 15)**
3. Right and left brachiocephalic trunks (<1%) **(Fig. 13C)**
4. Left SCA originating from a bicarotid trunk (<0.1%) **(Fig. 13D)**
5. Bicarotid trunk (<0.1%) **(Fig. 13E)**
6. Common brachiocephalic trunk (<0.1%)**(Fig. 13F)**
7. Right SCA originating from a bicarotid trunk (<0.1%) **(Fig. 13G)**
8. No brachiocephalic trunk (<0.1%) **(Fig. 13H)**
9. Only a left brachiocephalic trunk (<0.1%) **(Fig. 13I)**.

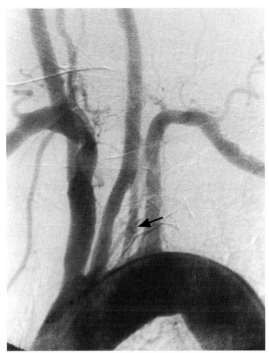

Figure 16. Discrete origin of the left vertebral artery from the aorta (arrow).

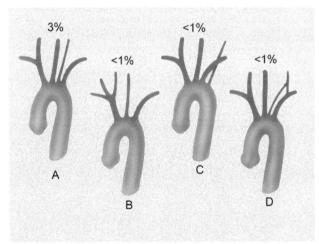

Figure 17. Variant origins of the left vertebral artery. The most common variation (A) is a separate origin of the vertebral artery from the aorta arising between the left CCA and the left SCA.

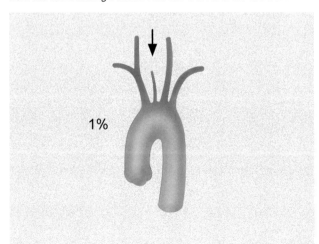

Figure 18. In approximately 1% of the population the thyroid ima artery arises directly from the aorta to supply the lower portion of the thyroid gland (arrow).

The Left Vertebral Artery as a Direct Branch from the Aortic Arch

In 4% of individuals, the left vertebral artery arises as a direct branch from the aortic arch instead of arising from the left SCA **(Figs. 16, 17)**. In this situation, the vertebral artery usually arises as the penultimate branch of the aortic arch, between the left CCA and the left SCA (3% of the population). Less commonly (1%), the vertebral artery is the last branch of the aortic arch. An anomalous origin of the left vertebral artery from the aortic arch can coexist with any of the previously discussed aortic arch branching variations, the most common association being with an aortic arch with the left CCA originating from the BCA (<1%). Rarely (<1%), the vertebral artery is formed from two separate limbs, one arising directly from the aorta as a penultimate branch and the other arising from the left SCA.

Thyroid Ima Artery as a Direct Branch from the Aortic Arch

The thyroid ima artery, also known as the lowest thyroid artery, is present in 6% of the population and supplies the isthmus of the thyroid gland. In approximately 1% of the population, the artery arises as a direct branch from the aortic arch, usually between the BCA and the left CCA **(Fig. 18)**. More commonly (3%), the artery arises from the BCA. The artery can also arise from the right CCA (1%), or more rarely from the subclavian, the internal mammary, or the inferior thyroid arteries.

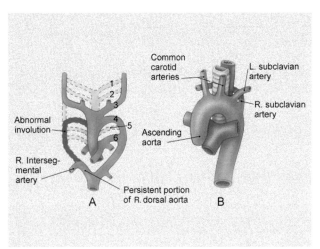

Figure 19. Left aortic arch with an aberrant right subclavian artery.
A. Embryology of the aberrant right subclavian artery. The right 4th
arch and a portion of the right dorsal aorta have involuted with the
7th intersegmental artery and the distal segment of the right dorsal
aorta forming the aberrant right subclavian artery. B. Adult
pattern. The artery courses behind the great vessels and usually
behind the esophagus.

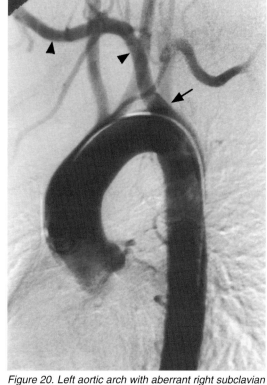

Figure 20. Left aortic arch with aberrant right subclavian
artery (arrowheads). The aberrant right subclavian
artery is the last great vessel off the aortic arch (arrow).

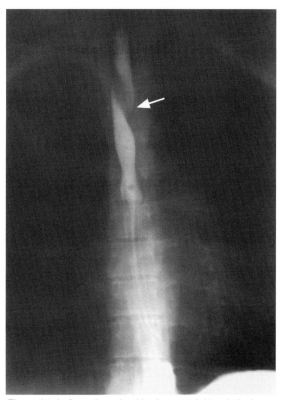

Figure 21. Left aortic arch with aberrant right subclavian
artery. An esophagogram demonstrates the impression
the aberrant vessel makes upon the esophagus (arrow).

Left Aortic Arch with an Aberrant Right Subclavian Artery

In 0.5% of the population, the right SCA is the last
branch of the left-sided aortic arch. This is the result
of abnormal involution of the right fourth aortic arch
and the right dorsal aorta, causing the right SCA to
form from the right seventh intersegmental artery
and the distal part of the right dorsal aorta **(Figs.
19A, 19B)**. The aberrant right SCA always turns to
the right behind the other great vessels **(Figs. 19,
20)**, and courses behind the esophagus **(Fig. 21)** in
the vast majority of cases. Although this anomaly
results in the formation of a vascular ring around the
trachea and/or esophagus, it rarely causes symptoms unless the artery is tortuous or aneurysmal
(dysphagia lusoria or dyspnea lusoria). Congenital
heart disease occurs in 10%–15% of these patients.
The aberrant SCA can arise from an aortic diverticulum. An aberrant right BCA is a rare anomaly
(<0.1%).

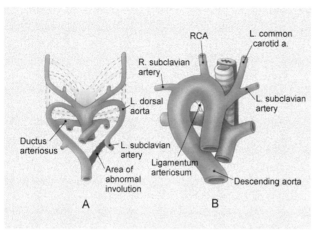

Figure 22. Right aortic arch with mirror-image branching. A. Embryology of the right aortic arch with mirror-image branching caused by abnormal involution of the left dorsal aorta and persistence of the right dorsal aorta and right 4th aortic arch. B. Post partum pattern of mirror-image branching of the aorta.

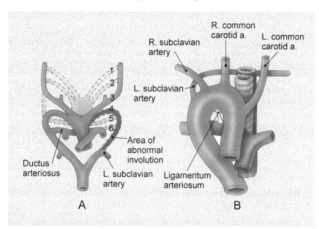

Figure 23. Right aortic arch with aberrant left subclavian artery. A. Embryologic involution of the left dorsal aorta proximal to the 7th intersegmental artery, and persistence of the right arch elements. B. Pattern of arterial branching of a right aortic arch and aberrant left subclavian artery.

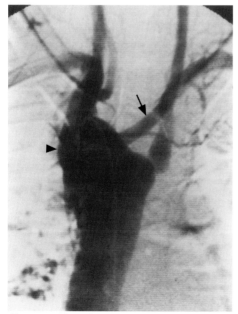

Figure 24. Frontal projection aortogram demonstrates a right aortic arch with an aberrant left subclavian artery (arrow) arising from an aortic diverticulum of Kommerell (arrowhead).

The Right Aortic Arch with Mirror-Image Branching

A right aortic arch results from the persistence of the entire right dorsal aorta and right fourth aortic arch with involution of the left dorsal aorta (Fig. 22A). This anomaly is rare, occurring in less than 0.1% of the population. Two branching patterns of the great vessels can occur with a right aortic arch (each with approximately equal frequency): 1) mirror-image branching; and 2) right aortic arch with an aberrant left SCA. With mirror-image branching (Fig. 22B), a left brachiocephalic trunk is the first branch, the right CCA is the second branch, and the right SCA is the last branch (a mirror image of the normal left aortic arch). This branching pattern has a high association (98%) with cyanotic congenital heart disease, the three most common types being tetralogy of Fallot, truncus arteriosus, and transposition of the great vessels. No vascular ring is formed with the mirror-image branching pattern.

The Right Aortic Arch with an Aberrant Left Subclavian Artery

The second type of branching pattern of the right aortic arch is characterized by an aberrant (usually retroesophageal) left SCA as the last branch from the aorta, preceded by (in order of branching) the left CCA, the right CCA, and the right SCA. This pattern results from the involution of the left dorsal aorta proximal to the left seventh intersegmental artery (which becomes the left subclavian artery) in addition to persistence of the right dorsal aorta and right fourth aortic arch (Fig. 23A). In contrast to the mirror-image type, this pattern is uncommonly (5%–12%) associated with congenital heart disease (Fig. 23B). The vascular ring around the trachea and esophagus is symptomatic in 5% of patients, usually due to a tight left ligamentum arteriosum completing the vascular ring or a large retroesophageal aortic diverticulum (of Kommerell) giving rise to the aberrant vessel (Fig. 24). An aberrant left BCA occurs with a similar frequency.

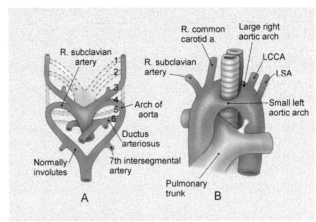

Figure 25. Double aortic arch. A. Embryology of the double aortic arch caused by failure of the right dorsal aorta to involute properly. B. Adult pattern of branching of a double aortic arch.

The Double Aortic Arch

This rare anomaly (<0.1%) represents persistence of the fetal double aortic arch system, caused by failure of the distal portion of the right dorsal aorta to involute **(Figs. 25A, 25B)**. The ascending aorta divides into two separate arches, with the right arch passing posterior to the esophagus and trachea and the left arch passing anterior to the esophagus and trachea **(Figs. 26–28)**. The two arches then reunite to form the aorta, which usually descends on the left side. This anomaly is the most common vascular ring requiring surgical correction. The relative size of each arch is variable but the right (posterior) arch is commonly large **(Figs. 29A–29C)**. Usually, the branches of the right (posterior) arch are the right SCA and right CCA, and those of the left (anterior) arch are the left CCA and left SCA, but if either arch is hypoplastic, the dominant arch tends to give rise to all of the vessels. Associated congenital heart disease is rare.

Coarctation of the Aorta

Coarctation is a congenital narrowing of the aorta. The embryologic basis is poorly understood, but coarctation is associated with Turner's syndrome, implicating genetic factors. There are two types: 1) post-ductal (adult or juxtaductal type); and 2) preductal (infantile, diffuse, or tubular hypoplasia type). The post-ductal type is characterized by a discrete, short-segment narrowing of the aorta located distal to the take-off of the left SCA at or just beyond the level of the ductus arteriosus **(Figs. 30A, 30B)**. These are usually asymptomatic, being discovered in childhood or early adulthood with upper extremity hypertension. The less common pre-ductal type is characterized by a narrowing (which often is severe and involves a long segment) proximal to the ductus arteriosus, which usually remains patent **(Figs. 31A, 31B)**. These are seen in the neonate or infant with congestive heart failure. Intra-cardiac defects occur in 50% of patients.

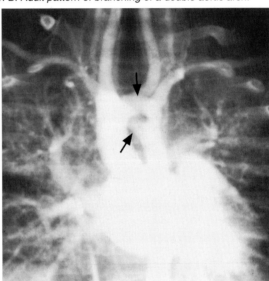

Figure 26. Thoracic aortogram of a double aortic arch (arrows) in a pediatric patient.

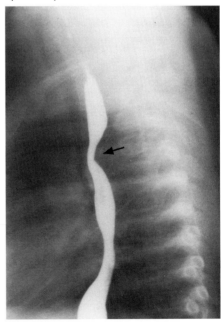

Figure 27. Lateral projection shows the impression the aortic ring makes upon the esophagus (arrow).

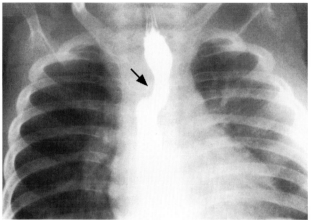

Figure 28. Frontal projection shows the impression the aortic ring makes upon the esophagus (arrow).

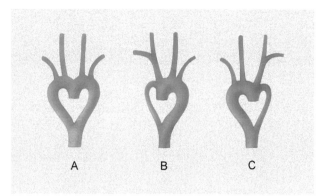

Figure 29. The variable relative sizes of the aortic arches. The right posterior arch is often large.

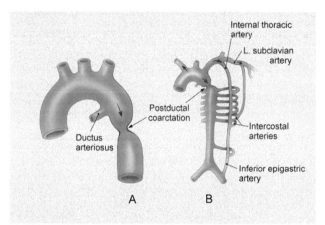

Figure 30. Post-ductal coarctation. A. The location of the narrowing is just distal to the left subclavian artery or ductus arteriosus. B. Routes for collateral filling of the post-coarctation aorta.

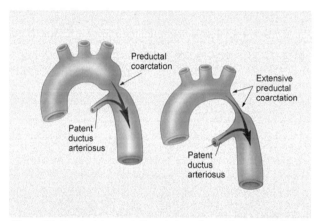

Figure 31. Preductal coarctation. A. Location of the coarctation, proximal to the ductus arteriosus. B. Long-segment coarctation is often associated with intracardiac defects.

The Cervical Aortic Arch

Rarely, the aortic arch is located in the low to mid neck region, above the level of the clavicle. This anomaly usually occurs in the setting of a right aortic arch. There is no association with congenital heart disease. A pulsatile mass in the neck is the usual clinical sign. The thoracic aortogram is diagnostic, showing the arch above the level of the clavicle.

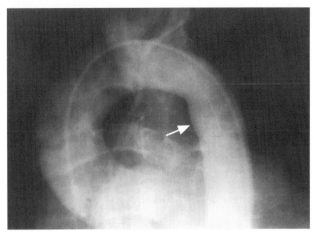

Figure 32. Normal ductus bump (arrow). The "bump" forms a smooth obtuse angle with the adjacent aorta.

The Ductus Diverticulum or Bump

The ductus diverticulum is a smooth luminal excrescence of the anteromedial portion of the proximal descending thoracic aorta which is commonly encountered at arteriography. This represents a remnant of the ductus arteriosus and is located just distal to the take-off of the left SCA. The angiographic appearance is varied; **Figures 32–34** demonstrate three examples. It is important to recognize the varied appearance of this anomaly so that it can be distinguished from a traumatic laceration of the aorta, which commonly occurs in a similar location, at the site of insertion of the ligamentum arteriosum.

Figures 35–38 illustrate four examples of traumatic lacerations of the proximal descending thoracic aorta. Distinguishing features suggesting a tear include large size, irregularity of contour, presence of a flap of disrupted tissue, and delayed washout or, very rarely, extravasation of contrast material.

Pseudocoarctation of the Aorta (Aortic Kinking)

This rare congenital anomaly results in kinking of the aorta, at the junction of the arch and the proximal descending thoracic aorta. The ascending aorta is abnormally elongated, causing the transverse aortic arch to be high and rendering the proximal descending aorta redundant. The kink in the aorta occurs where the aorta is tethered by the ligamentum arteriosum, and a congenitally short ligament may be a contributing factor. The proximal descending thoracic aorta attains the characteristic shape of the numeral three. There appears to be an association with aortic valve disease, including bicuspid aortic valve disease, but there is no association with other cardiac lesions. Pseudocoarctation can be distinguished from obstructive coarctation by the absence of clinical symptoms and the absence of a hemodynamically significant obstruction: there should be no rib notching (collaterals) and the gradient should be less than 10 mm Hg.

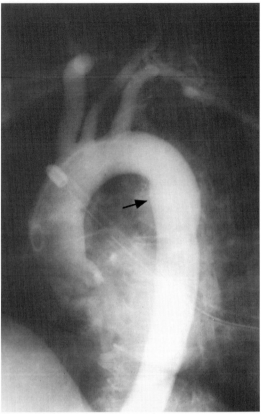

Figure 33. Normal ductus bump (arrow). The "bump" forms a smooth obtuse angle with the adjacent aorta.

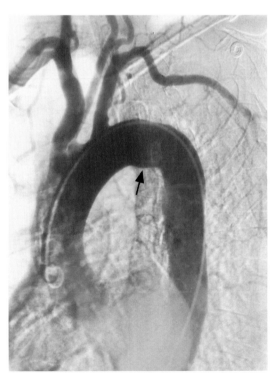

Figure 34. Normal ductus bump (arrow). The "bump" forms a smooth obtuse angle with the adjacent aorta.

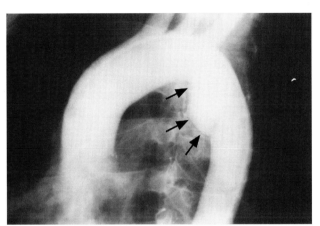

Figures 35–38. Traumatic aortic lacerations (arrows) that are not to be confused with a ductus bump.

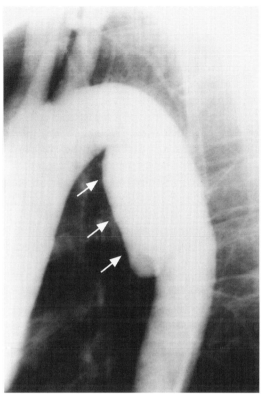

Figure 36.

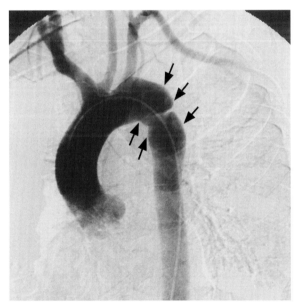

Figure 37.

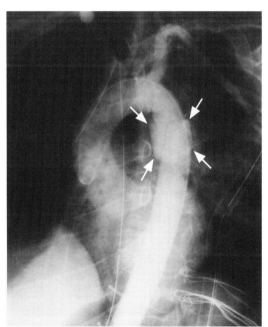

Figure 38.

Intercostal Arteries

The anterior intercostal arteries arise from the internal mammary (thoracic) artery on either side. There is considerable variation in the origins of the first three posterior intercostal arteries: 1) all three as direct branches from the aorta (5%); 2) all three arising from the superior intercostal artery (a branch of the costocervical trunk) (5%); 3) the first and second arising from the superior intercostal artery (60%); and 4) only the first arising from the superior intercostal artery (30%). The remainder of the posterior intercostal arteries arise as dorsal branches from the descending aorta. Usually, the right and left posterior intercostal arteries have separate origins from the aorta **(Fig. 39A)**. Common origins of the right and left can occur **(Fig. 39B)** as well as unilateral trunk formation, more common on the left **(Figs. 39C, 39D)**. The bronchial arteries often share a common origin with the intercostal arteries (intercostobronchial trunk).

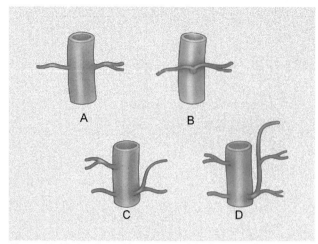

Figure 39. Variant branching pattern of the intercostal arteries.

The Radiculomedullary Arteries and the Arteria Radicularis Magna

The anterior spinal artery supplies approximately 80% of the spinal cord. Along its length, the anterior spinal artery receives branches from extraspinal arteries including the intercostal, bronchial, and lumbar arteries. Such branches are termed radiculomedullary branches. There are about four to nine such vessels located between the lower cervical and upper lumbar level which attain a diameter of about 1 mm **(Fig. 40)**. These vessels can be identified on arteriograms by their characteristic course: cephalad toward the spinal cord with a hairpin turn caudally when they reach the midline over the spinal column. Trauma to these vessels can result in neurological sequelae. The arteria radicularis magna (the artery of Adamkiewicz) is the largest radiculomedullary branch, providing blood supply to the lower two thirds of the spinal cord. It usually arises as a branch from a left lower posterior intercostal artery.

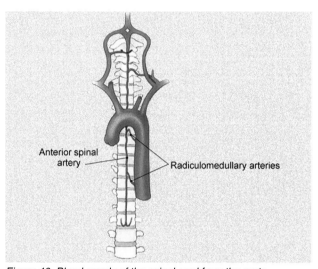

Figure 40. Blood supply of the spinal cord from the aorta.

For further information on this topic, please see Teaching File Cases 1, 2, and 3.

Selected Readings

Kadir S. Atlas of normal and variant angiographic anatomy. Philadelphia: W.B. Saunders Company, 1991.

Kadir S. Diagnostic angiography. Philadelphia: W.B. Saunders Company, 1986.

Lippert H, Pabst R. Arterial variations in man: classification and frequency. New York: Springer-Verlag, 1985.

Moore KL. The developing human: clinically oriented embryology. 3rd edition. Philadelphia: W.B. Saunders Company, 1982.

Strife JL, Bisset GS. Cardiovascular system. In: Kirks DR, ed. Practical pediatric imaging: diagnostic radiology of infants and children. 2nd edition. Boston: Little, Brown and Company, 1991.

End Notes

Figures 1, 2, 3, 19, 22, 23, 25, 30, and 31 from Moore KL. The developing human: clinically oriented embryology. 3rd edition. Philadelphia: W.B. Saunders Company, 1982; 307, 328, 330–333. Used with permission.

Figures 13, 39, and 40 from Kadir S. Atlas of normal and variant angiographic anatomy. Philadelphia: W.B. Saunders Company, 1991; 28, 45, 498. Used with permission.

Figures 17, 18, and 29 from Lippert H, Pabst R. Arterial variations in man: classification and frequency. New York: Springer-Verlag, 1985; 5, 6, and 7. Used with permission.

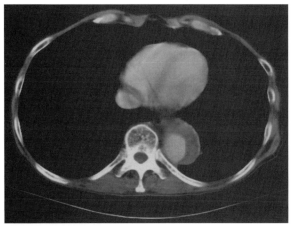

Figure 1. Axial section of a CT scan of a 67-year-old man with a thoracoabdominal aneurysm.

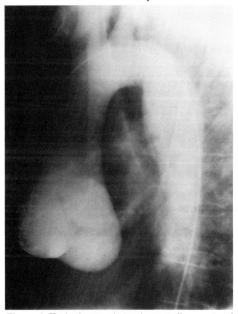

Figure 3. Typical pear-shaped ascending aorta of annuloaortic ectasia in a 42-year-old man.

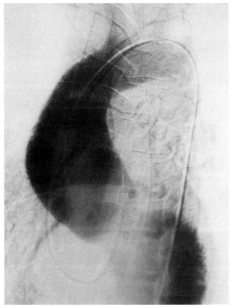

Figure 4. Ascending aortic aneurysm with a dissection flap at the aortic valve plane and acute aortic regurgitation in a 34-year-old man with Marfan's syndrome.

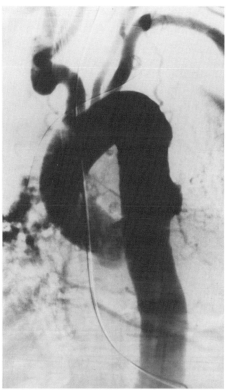

Figure 2. Subtraction right posterior oblique (RPO) arteriogram of a penetrating atherosclerotic ulcer of the descending thoracic aorta in an elderly man.

TUTORIAL 2
THORACIC ANEURYSMS
*Ian A. Sproat, M.D., FRCP(C), and
David M. Williams, M.D.*

Editor's Note: The important subject of thoracic aneurysms is dealt with in unusual depth because of the emerging therapeutic role of endovascular treatment in this area.

Introduction
The subjects addressed in this tutorial include:
1. The normal size ranges for the thoracic aorta; definition of aneurysm and suggested nomenclature for use with the term aneurysm
2. Atherosclerosis—its relationship to thoracoabdominal aneurysms **(Fig. 1)** and penetrating ulcer of the thoracic aorta **(Fig. 2)**
3. Diseases characterized by medial degeneration— annuloaortic ectasia **(Fig. 3)** and Marfan's syndrome **(Fig. 4)**
4. Miscellaneous lesions—Ehlers-Danlos syndrome.

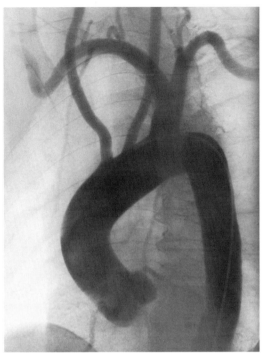

Figure 5. RPO subtraction aortography shows an aberrant right subclavian artery in a trauma victim with a focal aortic tear.

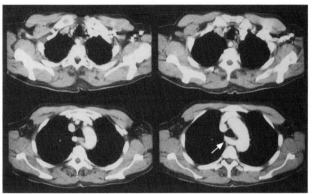

Figure 6. Thoracic CT scan depicting the retroesophageal path of an aberrant right subclavian artery (arrow) arising distal to the left subclavian artery.

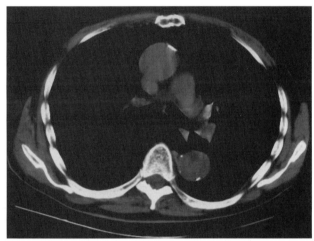

Figure 7. The thoracic CT section depicts mild enlargement of the ascending and descending aorta in an 80-year-old man. The relative diameters are maintained.

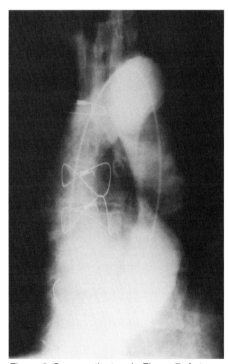

Figure 8. Same patient as in Figure 7. Anteroposterior (AP) thoracic aortogram shows tortuosity and mild dilatation with maintenance of parallelism between the aortic walls.

The Thoracic Aorta and Aneurysms

The normal thoracic aorta begins at the aortic root above the valve and has a diameter of 3.6–3.9 cm in the sinus portion. The tubular portion beginning at the sinotubular junction is 4–5 cm long and 2.8–3.5 cm in diameter. The arch is approximately 5 cm long, 2.5–3 cm in diameter, and gives rise to the brachiocephalic, left common carotid, and left subclavian arteries, in that order. Many variants of aortic arch and brachiocephalic arterial anatomy exist **(Figs. 5, 6)**. The descending thoracic aorta is widest (2.5–3 cm in diameter) at the isthmus (where the descending thoracic aorta communicates with the ductus) immediately beyond the left subclavian artery and tapers to 2.4–2.7 cm at the diaphragmatic hiatus. Diameters are, in general, 2 mm smaller in females. Aortic diameter increases with age **(Figs. 7, 8)**.

An aneurysm is present when a permanent segmental dilatation of an artery exists that is at least 1.5 times the expected diameter at that location **(Figs. 9, 10)**. Dilatation of a lesser degree is termed ectasia. These are morphologic definitions only and modifiers are needed to make the description complete. "True aneurysms" are bounded by at least some part of a thinned arterial wall; a "false aneurysm" implies a leak and is therefore bounded by hematoma and periaortic connective tissues.

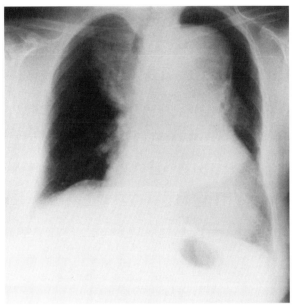

Figure 9. Posteroanterior (PA) chest radiograph in a 78-year-old woman with aneurysmal dilatation of the entire aorta.

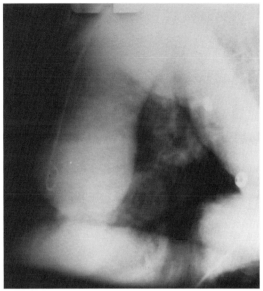

Figure 10. Lateral thoracic aortogram in a 78-year-old woman with aneurysmal dilatation of the entire aorta.

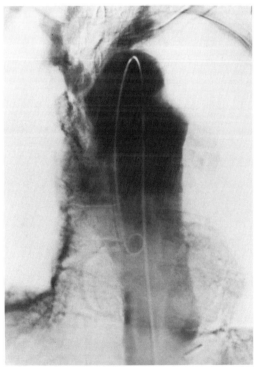

Figure 11. AP subtraction thoracic aortogram shows a cylindrical aneurysm of the descending thoracic aorta in an 81-year-old man.

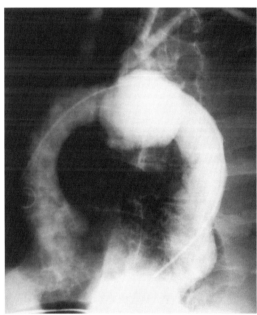

Figure 12. Saccular aneurysm at the aortic isthmus (actually a chronic contained rupture) with a fusiform thoracoabdominal aneurysm in a 70-year-old chronic alcoholic man.

Aneurysms may be fusiform, cylindrical (Fig. 11), or saccular (Fig. 12) in shape. They can be classified by etiology into congenital causes (eg, Ehlers-Danlos syndrome, Marfan's syndrome, post coarctation) or acquired (degenerative, post-traumatic, infectious, inflammatory, anastomotic). The site of an aneurysm is important with respect to its natural history and is an integral part of the description of the aneurysm.

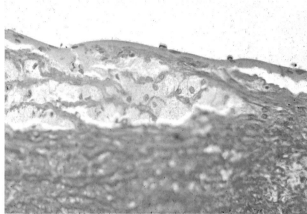

Figure 13. The intima is lifted off the media by the lipid-laden cells just under the endothelium. This is a fatty streak, the earliest lesion of atherosclerosis.

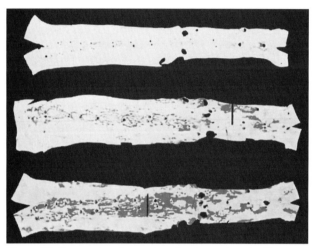

Figure 15. Progressive stages of aortic atherosclerosis. The aortas have been stained with sudan red to show fat. Even in early disease the darker-appearing plaque is aggregated around intercostal ostia and branch points.

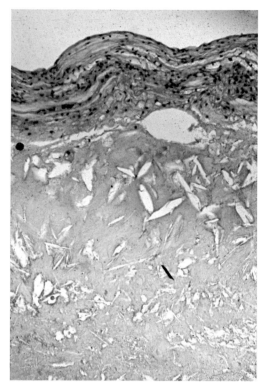

Figure 14. A typical fibro-fatty atherosclerotic plaque with "cholesterol clefts" (they look like shards of glass) under a fibrous cap.

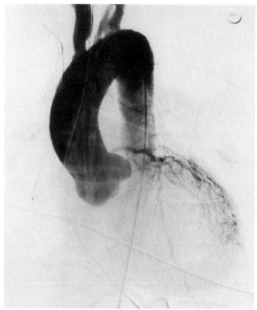

Figure 16. A 70-year-old man with occlusion of the right coronary artery and a smooth normal ascending aorta. The arch demonstrates minimal irregularity but there are stenoses at the brachiocephalic branch origins.

Atherosclerosis, Aging, and the Thoracic Aorta

In North America, atherosclerosis is a process that begins at birth. There is fairly clear evidence now that the fatty streak **(Fig. 13)** progresses to the typical fibrofatty atheroma or plaque **(Fig. 14)**. Similarly, epidemiologic studies have confirmed the roles of smoking, obesity, diabetes mellitus, hypertension, and hyperlipidemia, especially those types with a low high-density/low density lipoprotein-C ratio (HDL/LDL), in the development, progression, and severity of atherosclerosis. Other factors involved in the location of plaques include wall shear stress and the hemodynamics of flow around branch ostia and bifurcations **(Fig. 15)**. The ascending aorta is least affected by atherosclerosis, with the number and severity of plaques increasing with distance from the aortic valve **(Figs. 16–19)**. Atherosclerosis weakens the aortic wall by destroying the media and can lead to aneurysm formation. More typically, it leads to stenosis of branch orifices, intimal calcifications **(Fig. 20)**, thrombosis, and emboli.

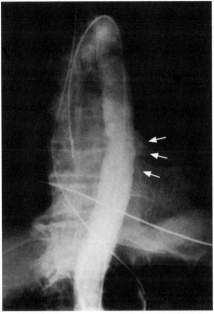

Figure 17. Same patient as in Figure 16. Note increasing atherosclerosis with wall irregularity, a shallow penetrating aortic ulcer, and intramedial hematoma (arrows) in the descending thoracic aorta.

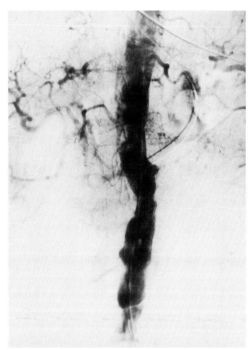

Figure 18. Same patient as in Figure 16. The abdominal aorta of this 70-year-old man is severely involved by large atherosclerotic plaques (worse than in the descending thoracic aorta), and there is occlusion of the left renal artery.

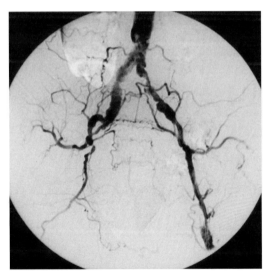

Figure 19. Same patient as in Figure 16. The atherosclerotic changes in the pelvis have resulted in severe iliac arterial stenoses and right external iliac artery occlusion.

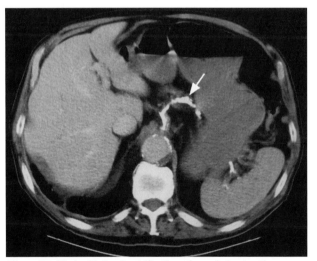

Figure 20. Marked intimal calcifications (arrow) due to atherosclerosis involving the celiac trunk and splenic artery in an 82-year-old man.

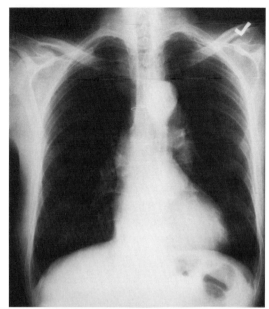

Figure 21. PA chest radiograph in an elderly man shows unfolding tortuosity and mild dilatation of the thoracic aorta.

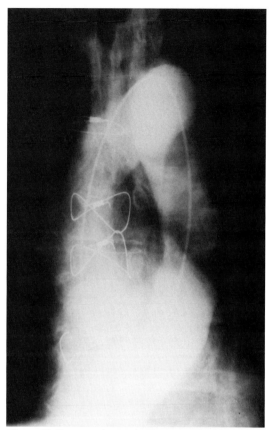

Figure 22. Same patient as in Figure 21. The AP thoracic aortogram shows unfolding and tortuosity in the thoracic aorta.

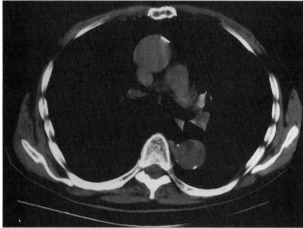

Figure 23. CT section shows maintenance of the relative diameters between the ascending and descending aorta (both are slightly dilated) in an elderly man.

Aging leads to a progressive reduction in the integrity of lamellar units in the thickest and middle layer of the aortic wall, the media. There is a reduction of smooth muscle cells, an increase in fibrous tissue, and thinning and fragmentation of elastic fibers. These changes decrease the elasticity of the aortic wall. Progressive thinning of the adventitial fibrous tissue leads to generalized widening of the aorta and elongation and unfolding with age **(Figs. 21–23)**. Hypertension alone can accelerate these age-related changes, but these alone do not disrupt the smooth profile of the wall of the aortic lumen as do uncomplicated atherosclerotic plaques, which lead to internal projections into the lumen, or, if the plaque is ulcerated **(Fig. 24)**, external projection of the lumen outside of the inner aortic wall.

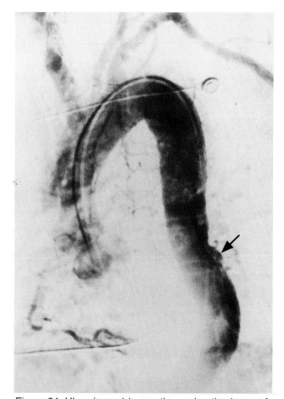

Figure 24. Ulcer (arrow) in an atherosclerotic plaque of the descending thoracic aorta in an elderly man, not unlike that which might be seen on a barium examination of the stomach.

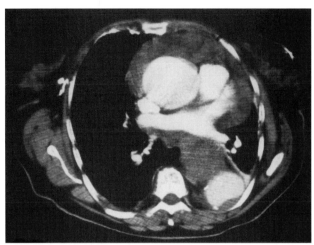

Figure 25. CT section shows a smooth round lumen without mural calcification in the ascending aortic aneurysm and an irregular lumen with mural calcification in the descending aortic aneurysm in a 78-year-old woman.

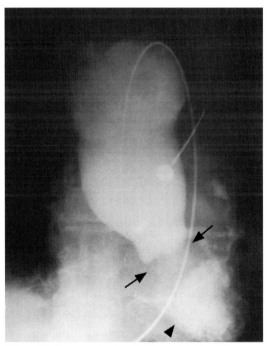

Figure 26. Same patient as in Figure 25. The AP aortogram shows smooth walls of the ascending aortic aneurysm. Note the aortic insufficiency (arrows) filling the left ventricle (arrowhead).

Thoracic and Thoracoabdominal Aneurysm
The etiological relationship between atherosclerosis and aneurysm formation in the thoracic aorta is unclear. In fact, aneurysms of the ascending aorta and arch usually have only minor degrees of atherosclerosis **(Figs. 25, 26)**; they are often only one grade (grade 0–3) worse on average than a normal aorta.

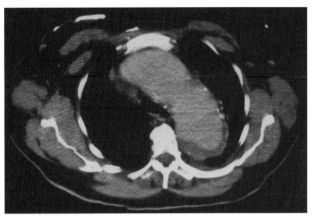

Figure 27. CT scan of an aneurysmal arch in a 78-year-old woman. Note that the intimal calcification and mural thrombus spares the proximal arch and increases distally.

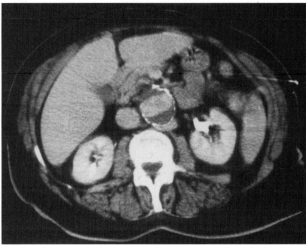

Figure 28. Abdominal CT scan of a small infrarenal aneurysm shows extensive calcified plaque and thrombus.

On the other hand, atherosclerotic changes are typically found within aneurysms of the descending thoracic aorta **(Fig. 27)** and abdominal aorta **(Figs. 28, 29)**, which are involved by grade 2–3 disease compared to grade 0–1 disease in age-matched controls without aneurysms. The proteases elastase and collagenase are elevated in infrarenal aortic aneurysms and normal in ascending aortic aneurysms. Collagenase only is elevated in descending aortic aneurysms. Increasing collagenase activity correlates with increasing aneurysm size and may be responsible for growth and rupture but not initiation of the aneurysm.

Aortic aneurysms can be ascribed to a progressive loss of resistance of the arterial wall to the constant hammering of the pulsatile aortic flow. Once dilatation has begun, LaPlace's law, $Tw=rP$ (where Tw is wall tension and r is the radius of the aneurysm), dictates continued expansion under the influence of systolic pressure with progressive thinning of the aortic wall **(Figs. 30–32)**. Therefore, the natural history of an aneurysm is eventual rupture **(Fig. 33)**. Abdominal aneurysms expand at a rate of up to 5 mm/year; expansion at a rate greater than this is considered a rapidly expanding aneurysm **(Figs. 34, 35)**. The risk of rupture over 5 years for aneurysms smaller than 5 cm in diameter is low but is 25% for aneurysms larger than 5 cm in diameter.

Similar data for thoracic aneurysms are unknown, although Pressler and McNamara found that 50% of patients with thoracic aortic aneurysms died of rupture over 10 years when not treated surgically.

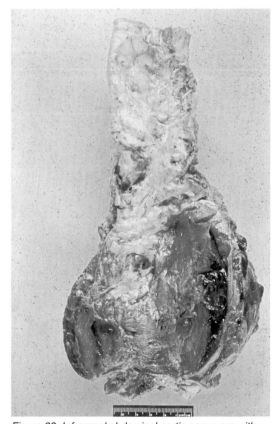

Figure 29. Infrarenal abdominal aortic aneurysm with mural thrombus. Note the extensive atherosclerotic disease in the abdominal aorta, including the aneurysm wall.

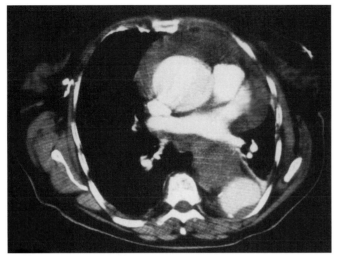

Figure 30. CT scan from 1990 shows a 6-cm aneurysm of the aortic root.

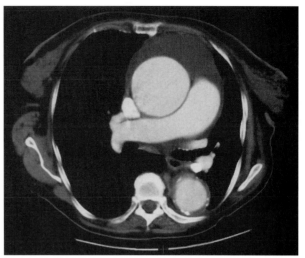

Figure 31. By 1991, the aortic root was 6.5 cm.

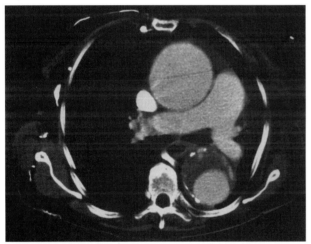

Figure 32. In 1993, the aortic root was 7–7.5 cm in diameter. Between 1991 and 1993 the descending thoracic component was repaired.

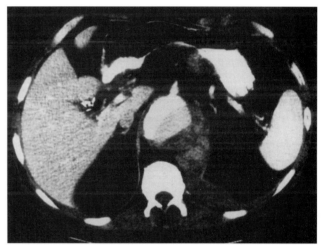

Figure 33. CT scan of a ruptured thoracoabdominal aneurysm at the diaphragmatic hiatus with contrast extravasation and a left hemothorax in a 62-year-old man.

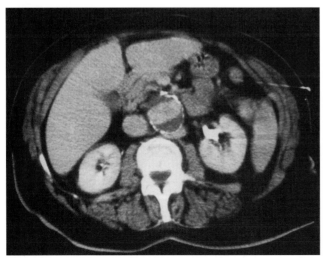

Figure 34. A rapidly expanding abdominal aortic aneurysm in a 78-year-old woman that was 4 cm in diameter in 1990.

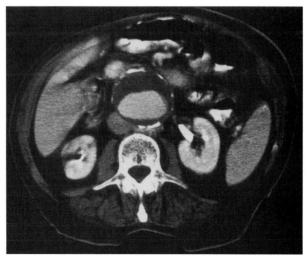

Figure 35. By 1993, the infrarenal abdominal aortic aneurysm had grown to 6 cm in diameter, a rate of almost 1 cm per year.

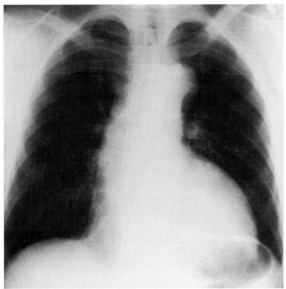

Figure 36. Curvilinear lateral displacement of the mid mediastinal contour on the right in a 38-year-old man who had replacement of a stenotic aortic valve due to a dilated ascending aorta.

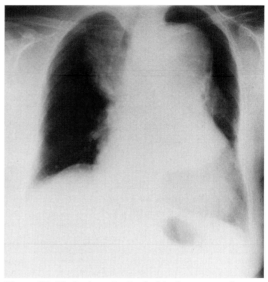

Figure 37. Marked mediastinal widening, a grossly enlarged aortic arch, and curvilinear calcification are seen in this 76-year-old patient with a huge thoracoabdominal aneurysm.

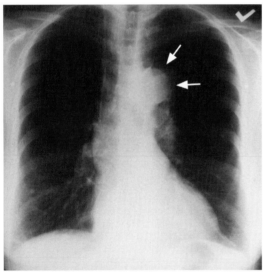

Figure 38. A prominent ascending aortic shadow and a focal bulge of the aortic knob (arrows) are seen in this 65-year-old woman with an unusual thrombosed focal arch aneurysm.

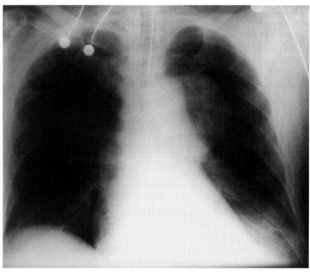

Figure 39. Aneurysm at the isthmus due to a chronic contained rupture of the aorta in a 70-year-old alcoholic man who sustained a motor vehicle trauma years ago.

Findings on Chest Radiographs

Aneurysms can affect any segment of the thoracic aorta and are usually first picked up on chest radiography. Findings include widening of the mediastinum or aortic knob **(Figs. 36, 37)**, mediastinal contour abnormalities **(Figs. 38–40)**, loss of parallelism of the aortic walls **(Figs. 41, 42)**, calcification in a fusiform or saccular aneurysm **(Fig. 43)**, filling in of the retrosternal space or retrotracheal triangle, lateral deviation of the aortic stripe, and displacement of adjacent structures or even erosion of the spine.

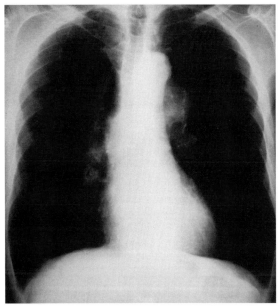

Figure 40. A ductus aneurysm in a 65-year-old man. Note the focal mediastinal bulge below the aortic knob.

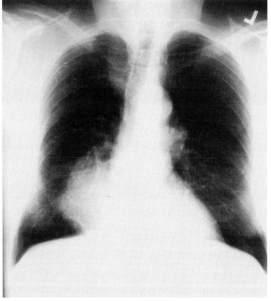

Figure 41. Note that the left lateral and right lateral aortic walls are divergent in this 72-year-old man with a thoracic aortic aneurysm.

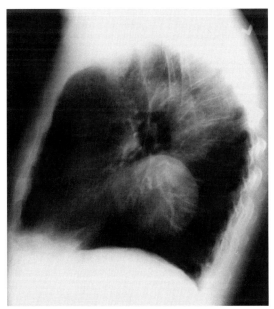

Figure 42. This aneurysm is displayed as a spherical retrocardiac mass on the lateral chest film of this 72-year-old man.

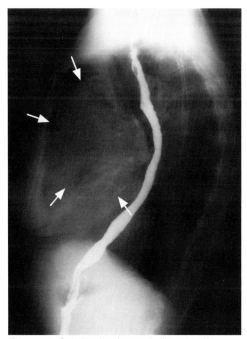

Figure 43. Calcification (arrows), filling in of the retrosternal space, and posterior displacement of the esophagus are seen in this 62-year-old woman with an ascending aortic aneurysm.

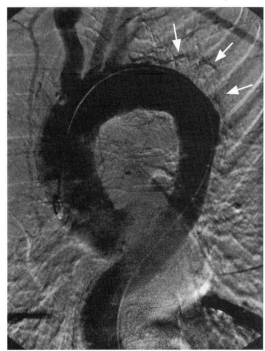

Figure 44. Same patient as in Figure 38. This digital subtraction RPO arch aortogram hints at the focal thrombosed aneurysm (arrows), but the lumen appears normal in size.

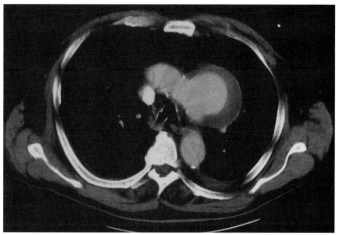

Figure 45. Because of the mural thrombus, the aortogram underestimates the true aneurysm diameter by over 2 cm.

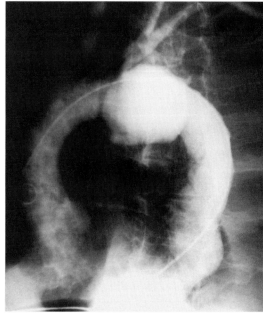

Figure 46. Same patient as in Figure 45. The RPO aortogram clearly underestimates the true aneurysm diameter.

Other Imaging Modalities

On computed tomography (CT) scanning, magnetic resonance (MR) imaging, and transesophageal echocardiography (TEE), the criteria for diagnosis of an aneurysm remain the same. Aneurysm size may be underestimated by aortography due to mural thrombus **(Figs. 44–46)**. CT scanning, MR imaging and sonography accurately depict the thrombus and the aortic wall. Additionally, CT and MR imaging better depict surrounding structures **(Figs. 47, 48)** and help detect thoracic fluid collections **(Figs. 49–51)** that may indicate a complicated or rupturing aneurysm. Spiral or even ultrafast CT scanning can suffer from artifact due to motion near the aortic valve or streak artifacts from calcium in the wall that can mimic dissection; therefore, these modalities cannot diagnose aortic insufficiency. MR imaging has multiplanar capability and does not require contrast material but it is slow and may not be readily available. Many patients cannot be scanned. TEE is fast and portable but has a limited field of view and is uncomfortable for the patient, necessitating sedation.

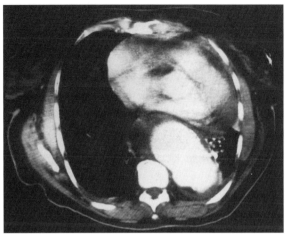

Figure 47. CT scan shows compression of the heart and left lower lobe of the lung by this large thoracoabdominal aneurysm.

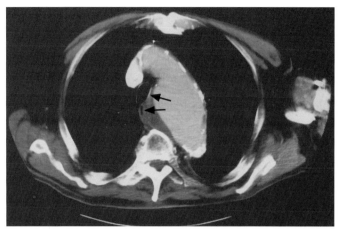

Figure 48. CT scan shows displacement of the trachea and esophagus (arrows) by an arch aneurysm whose walls are etched in calcium.

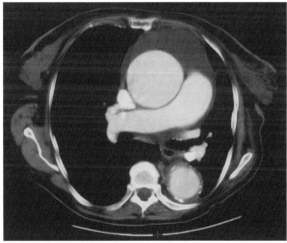

Figure 49. Pericardial effusion in this 79-year-old with a panthoracic aortic aneurysm.

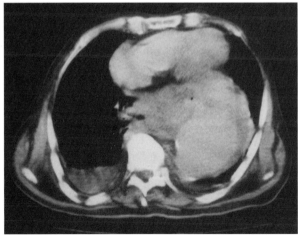

Figure 50. Ruptured thoracic aneurysm with extravasation and a hemothorax.

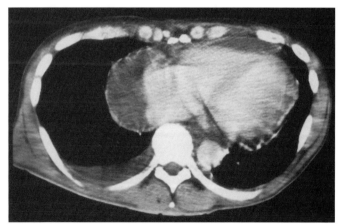

Figure 51. Dissection of the aorta complicated by pericardial and right pleural effusions in this 52-year-old man with Marfan's syndrome.

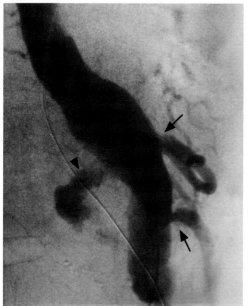

Figure 52. The lateral aortogram at the thoraco-abdominal junction shows the posterior location of the leak (arrowhead) in a ruptured thoracoabdominal aneurysm. The neck of the aneurysm both proximally and distally, and the celiac and superior mesenteric artery origins (arrows) are all clearly depicted. Although the image is subtracted, the spine is faintly seen.

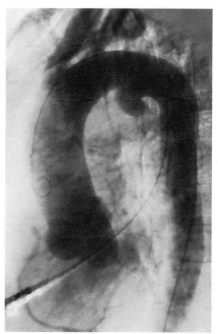

Figure 53. The relationship of the great vessels to the ductus aneurysm is clearly shown.

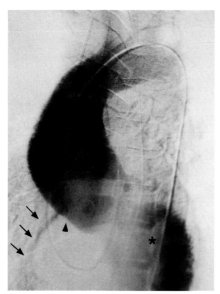

Figure 54. Note the right coronary artery (arrows) near the dissection flap (arrow-head), a dissecting ascending aneurysm, and aortic insufficiency (asterisk) in this 34-year-old man with Marfan's syndrome.

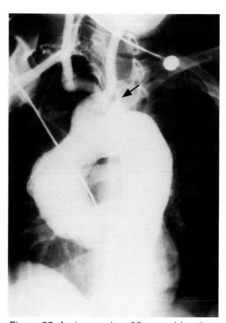

Figure 55. Aortogram in a 25-year-old patient with the aneurysmal form of Takayasu's aortitis with irregular aortic dilatation, a bovine origin of the right brachiocephalic and left common carotid arteries, and a tapered left subclavian artery occlusion (arrow).

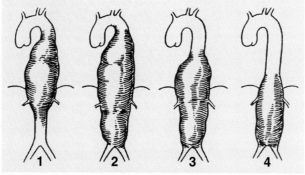

Figure 56. A pictorial depiction of Crawford's classification of thoracoabdominal aortic aneurysms.

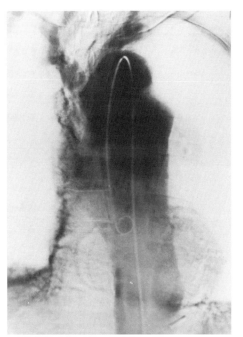

Figure 57. AP thoracic aortogram in an 81-year-old man with a Crawford type 1 thoracoabdominal aortic aneurysm (TAA).

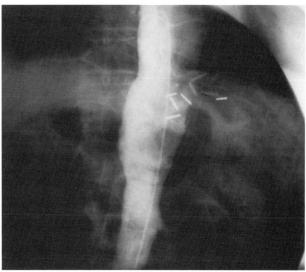

Figure 58. Abdominal aortogram in an 81-year-old man with a Crawford type 1 TAA.

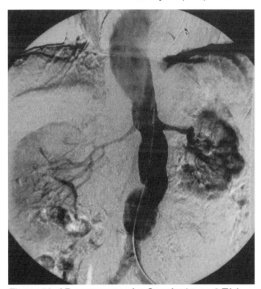

Figure 59. AP aortogram of a Crawford type 2 TAA (thoracic component not shown).

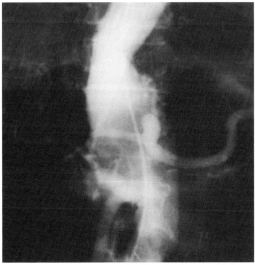

Figure 60. AP aortogram of a Crawford type 4 TAA (thoracic component not shown).

Aortography

Although the need for aortography in the evaluation of aneurysms is declining because of spiral CT scanning and the multiplanar capabilities of MR imaging, it is favored by surgeons who prefer its ability to provide more anatomical information **(Fig. 52)**. It is the best modality for determining the relationship of the aneurysm to the great vessels **(Fig. 53)**, coronary arteries **(Fig. 54)**, and aortic valve. It readily depicts aortic value insufficiency as well as pathology involving the branches of the aorta **(Fig. 55)**, something none of the other modalities do well. Aortography, like CT scanning, requires the administration of contrast material with its potential nephrotoxicity whereas TEE and MR imaging do not. It is invasive (and therefore costly) but has a low complication rate.

The Crawford classification of aneurysms involving the descending thoracic aorta is illustrated in **Figures 56–60**.

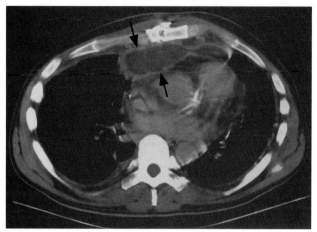

Figure 61. Infected substernal hematoma (arrows) after sternotomy for repair of an ascending aortic aneurysm. Note the disturbing streak artifacts.

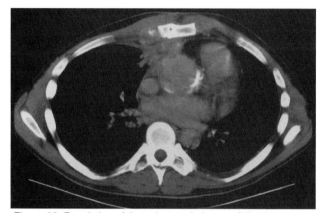

Figure 62. Resolution of the substernal abscess following percutaneous drainage.

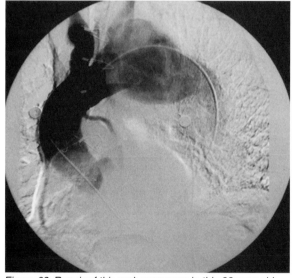

Figure 63. Repair of this arch aneurysm in this 83-year-old man may require combined sternotomy and thoracotomy. Prior sternotomy (note the wires and the aortocoronary vein graft) complicates the picture. Manipulation of the arch and great vessels increases the risk of stroke.

Treatment

The current standard treatment of thoracic aneurysms is surgery. Ascending aortic aneurysms require sternotomy **(Figs. 61, 62)**, hypothermia, and circulatory arrest. Arch aneurysms may require sternotomy and left thoracotomy **(Fig. 63)**.

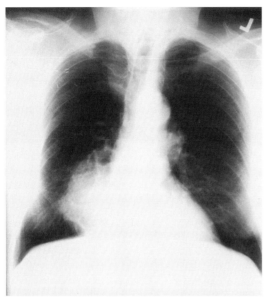

Figure 64. Large tortuous descending thoracic aneurysm in a 72-year-old man.

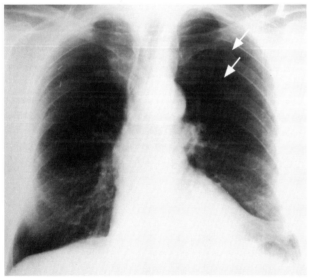

Figure 65. Evidence of prior left thoracotomy on this follow-up chest film showing healing where the left 5th and 6th ribs were cut (arrows).

Descending thoracic aneurysms are approached via left thoracotomy or thoracoabdominal incision **(Figs. 64, 65)**. All types of repair are complicated by perioperative myocardial infarction and renal failure. Repair of ascending and arch aneurysms carries the risk of stroke; descending aortic aneurysm repair can be complicated by paraplegia/paresis. Preoperative arteriographic localization of the spinal arterial supply has not been shown to reduce the rate of spinal cord injury. Acher et al reported a reduction in postoperative paraplegia by employing thiopental coma, core temperature cooling, cerebrospinal fluid drainage, and intravenous naloxone. In addition, intercostal, lumbar, or spinal arteries are not reimplanted; they are simply oversewn.

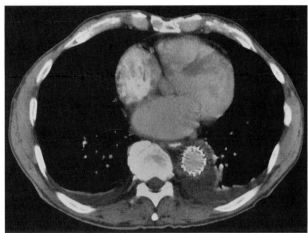

Figure 66. Self-expanding stent-graft with the metallic stents easily seen outlining the "new" lumen of the descending thoracic aorta.

Stent-Grafts

Although there are currently technical difficulties associated with interventional therapy for ascending and aortic arch aneurysms, there have been a number of descending thoracic and thoracoabdominal aneurysms recently treated successfully by deploying self-expanding endoluminal stent-grafts **(Fig. 66)**. These were placed either through a femoral artery cutdown or with an elephant trunk graft attached to the caudal aorta via a flank-splitting incision and retroperitoneal aortic approach. This intervention holds great promise for reducing surgical morbidity and mortality but paraplegia remains a complication. Current technology requires a 24-F introducer but investigation and design of smaller devices are underway.

Penetrating Atherosclerotic Ulcer of the Aorta

Unlike aneurysms, penetrating atherosclerotic ulcers **(Fig. 67)** of the aorta are intimately related to severe atherosclerotic disease of the aorta. Patients with this entity are generally elderly (mean age approximately 73 years), hypertensive, and have advanced aortic atherosclerosis. Whereas it may mimic aortic dissection clinically with acute chest pain that radiates to the back or a "tearing" sensation, it is pathologically distinct. Patients with dissection tend to be younger by a decade, and severe atherosclerosis may actually impede the progress of a dissection. An atherosclerotic plaque, typically located in the mid to distal descending thoracic aorta ulcerates and leaves a defect in the intima that may even extend into the media. This defect can lead to an intramedial hematoma **(Fig. 68)** with displacement of the intima, or it may even involve the entire wall thickness causing a pseudoaneurysm or frank rupture.

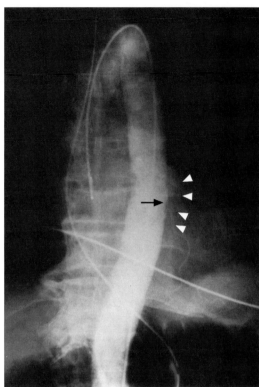

Figure 67. A shallow penetrating ulcer (arrow) of the mid descending thoracic aorta in this 70-year-old man. There is an intramedial hematoma (arrowheads) and severe atherosclerotic disease.

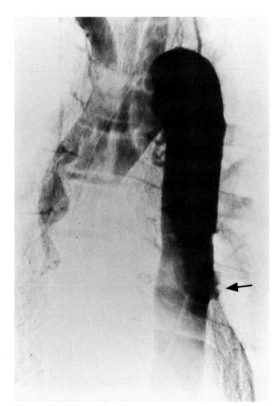

Figure 68. Subtraction thoracic aortogram shows the ulcer in the mid descending thoracic aorta (arrow). The straightening of the lateral wall is due to the intramedial hematoma associated with this ulcer.

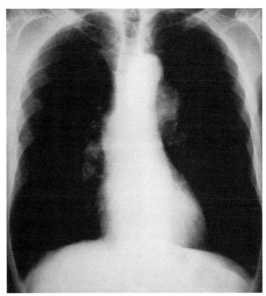

Figure 69. Focal enlargement of the aorta in a 65-year-old man. The aorta appears otherwise unremarkable.

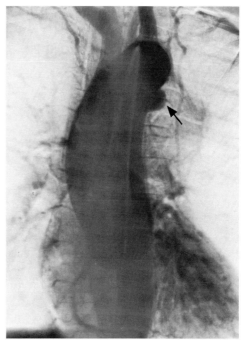

Figure 70. AP subtraction aortography shows the ulcer-like lumen of a largely thrombosed ductus aneurysm and not a penetrating ulcer (arrow). Notice the relative lack of aortic atherosclerotic disease.

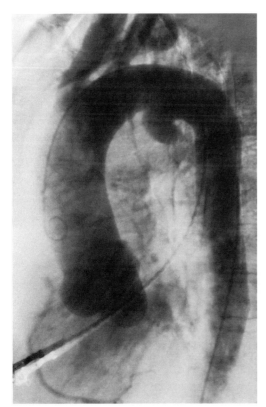

Figure 71. Lateral view subtraction aortography shows the ulcer-like lumen of a largely thrombosed ductus aneurysm and not a penetrating ulcer. Notice the relative lack of aortic atherosclerotic disease.

Penetrating Ulcers on Chest Radiography
On chest radiography, diffuse enlargement of the aorta is common; a focal enlargement is less likely **(Figs. 69–71)**. There may be mediastinal widening due to hematoma, or a pleural effusion, especially on the left.

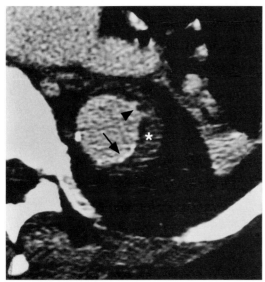

Figure 72. Detail of a thoracic CT scan at the level of the aortic ulcer. Note the shallow ulcer filled with contrast material (arrowhead), the elevated intima shown by calcification (arrow), and the intramedial hematoma (asterisk).

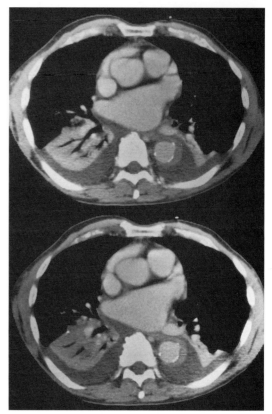

Figure 73. Same patient as in Figure 72.The CT scan shows calcification in the elevated intima, intramedial hematoma, and bilateral pleural effusions.

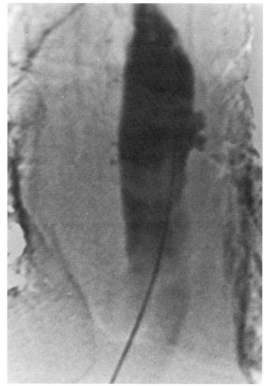

Figure 74. Same patient as in Figure 72. Early image from a digital subtraction arteriogram of the mid descending thoracic aortic penetrating ulcer.

On CT scanning, there is often an intramural hematoma with displaced intima and a shallow or deep ulcer crater filling with contrast material **(Fig. 72)** depending upon the degree of thrombus within the crater. The aortic wall may be thickened and may even be enhanced. Pleural or mediastinal fluid can be seen **(Figs. 73, 74)** and there may be frank pseudoaneurysm formation.

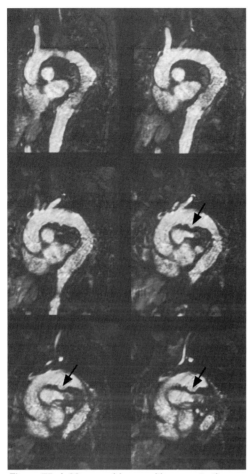

Figure 75. A 69-year-old man with a penetrating aortic ulcer, again in the region of the isthmus (arrow). There is atherosclerotic involvement and smaller ulcers with wall thickening in the descending aorta.

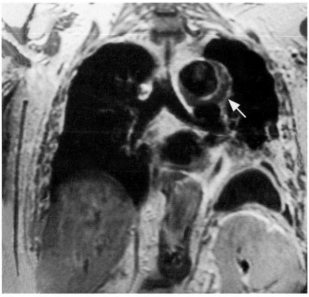

Figure 76. Coronal gated gadolinium-enhanced spin echo image shows the intramedial hematoma just distal to the ulcer, separated by the inner enhancing and elevated intima and the outer surrounding medioadventitial layer (arrow). There is compression of the left pulmonary artery.

MR imaging provides similar findings, but the equipment needed to monitor these patients may preclude the use of the magnet **(Figs. 75, 76)**. Transesophageal echocardiography is easy and fast and provides a good look at the descending aorta and can be used for follow-up of the lesion.

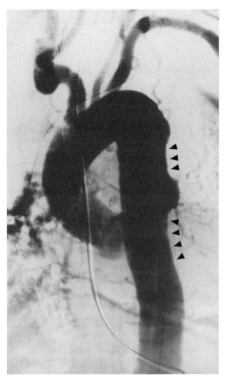

Figure 77. Proximal descending thoracic aortic penetrating ulcer, not unlike that seen on a barium examination of the stomach. Note the "heaped-up mucosa" on either side of the ulcer due to focal intramedial hematoma (arrowheads).

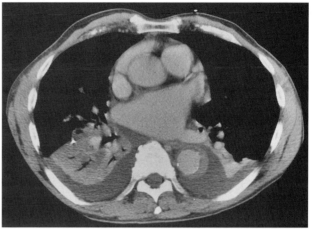

Figure 78. CT scan of a penetrating aortic ulcer at the level of the ulcer before treatment with a percutaneously placed stent-graft in the thoracic aorta.

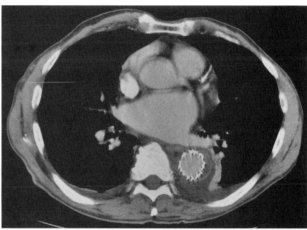

Figure 79. CT scan of a penetrating aortic ulcer at the level of the ulcer after treatment with a percutaneously placed stent-graft in the thoracic aorta. Note on the post-graft image that the intramedial hematoma is clearly delimited by the graft struts internally and the outer aortic wall externally. The effusions and pulmonary parenchymal changes have resolved.

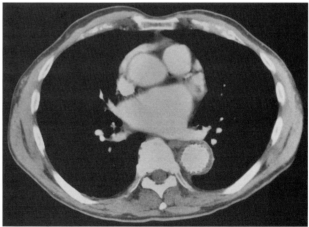

Figure 80. Follow-up CT scan 6 months after stent-graft placement.

Penetrating Ulcers on Aortography

On aortography, the ulcer is seen as a shallow or deep (**Fig. 77**), typically solitary lesion filling with contrast material like a gastric ulcer does on an upper gastrointestinal study. The aorta may be dilated, the wall may be thickened, or a pseudoaneurysm may be seen. The middle and distal thirds of the descending thoracic aorta are usually involved. Patients are initially treated as for a type B dissection, with blood pressure reduction and beta blockade. If patients are asymptomatic and there is no evidence of pseudoaneurysm or leak, conservative treatment may be tried, but close imaging follow-up is needed because the aorta may become aneurysmal or a pseudoaneurysm may develop. Persistent symptoms or complications, such as continued expansion of the intramural hematoma, necessitate surgery. Resection of the ulcer-bearing portion and the adjacent injured wall with interposition grafting (**Figs. 78–80**) may be needed.

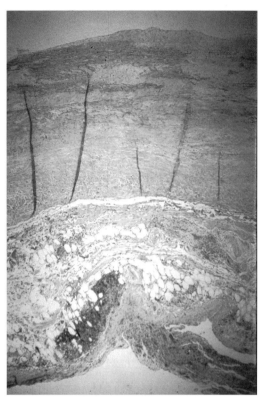

Figure 81. A small island of media with preserved elastic lamellae is all that remains in this patient with advanced medial degeneration, the remainder being replaced by a bland, pale ground substance. As is typical of this "disease," there are no inflammatory changes at all. The adventitial surface is at the bottom of the image.

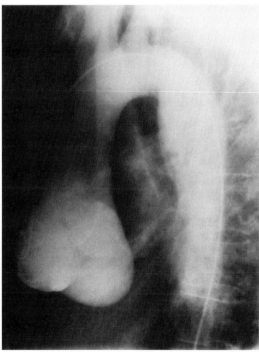

Figure 82. Lateral thoracic aortogram in a 42-year-old man shows an ascending aorta that really looks like a pear! This is annuloaortic ectasia.

Medial Degenerative Diseases

Erdheim's so-called cystic medial necrosis/degeneration is typified by elastic fiber fragmentation and loss associated with focal areas of destruction of the lamellae that are replaced by a bland ground substance **(Fig. 81)**, hence the term "cystic." The term is actually a misnomer since neither necrosis nor cysts are present. The syndrome leads to weakening of the media with resultant dilatation of the aorta typically involving the root and ascending portions and leading to the classic "pear-shaped" **(Fig. 82)** aorta of annuloaortic ectasia. In this condition, there may be total effacement of the sinotubular junction. The resultant root dilatation causes separation of the aortic valve commissures, which leads to aortic insufficiency that further aggravates the dilatation.

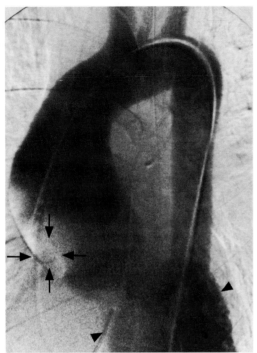

Figure 83. This 34-year-old man with Marfan's syndrome was being followed for asymptomatic progressive aortic root dilatation when aortic insufficiency developed (arrowheads). Compare the relative size of the pigtail catheter and the aortic root; the diameter of the pigtail (arrows) measures 1.5 cm.

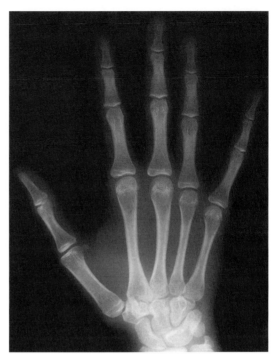

Figure 84. Right hand radiograph in a 15-year-old girl with Marfan's syndrome. The metacarpal index is 11.2.

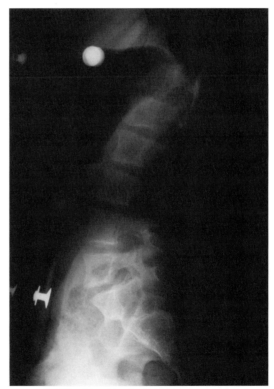

Figure 85. The lateral lumbosacral spine film shows posterior scalloping of the vertebral bodies and an enlarged spinal canal in this patient with Marfan's syndrome.

The aorta of patients with Marfan's syndrome **(Fig. 83)** looks identical but other stigmata of the disease are also present **(Figs. 84–88)**.

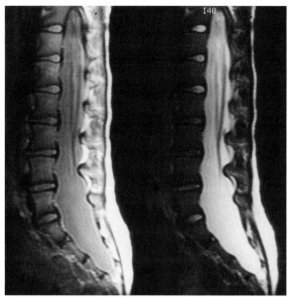

Figure 86. Proton density and T2-weighted sagittal MR images of the spine show dural ectasia in a 4-year-old girl with Marfan's syndrome.

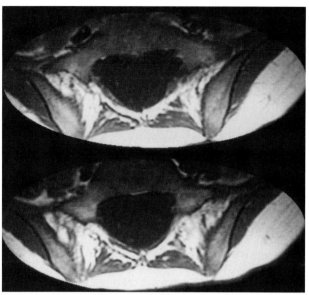

Figure 87. Same patient as in Figure 86. Axial T1-weighted MR images of the sacrum show dural ectasia.

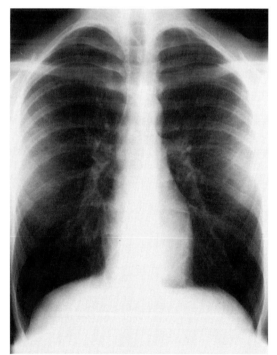

Figure 88. PA chest radiograph in an 18-year-old man with Marfan's syndrome who "fills the film."

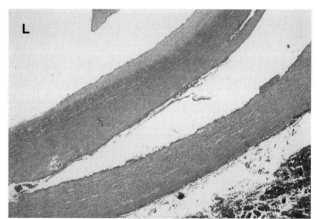

Figure 89. A large cleft due to dissection of the aorta is seen in the middle of the media in this young man who died from his Marfan's syndrome. The media, however, is normal without degenerative change. The lumen of the aorta is at the top. L=lumen.

Medial degeneration also occurs in the descending thoracic aorta. It has been implicated as a cause of aortic dissection, a common complication in Marfan's syndrome where the aorta is involved. However, medial degeneration is also a normal aging phenomenon in the aorta and is accelerated by hypertension, which is an undisputable risk factor for dissection and a common accompaniment in Marfan's syndrome. The degeneration may simply be a result of hemodynamic stress to the aortic wall. Some patients with Marfan's syndrome develop dissection in the absence of medial degeneration **(Fig. 89)**. Other connective tissue disorders may also manifest annuloaortic ectasia.

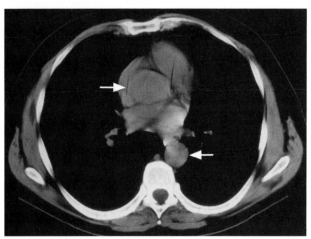

Figure 90. CT scan at the level of the aortic root in a 55-year-old man shows the aortic root diameter to be almost twice that of the descending aorta (arrows).

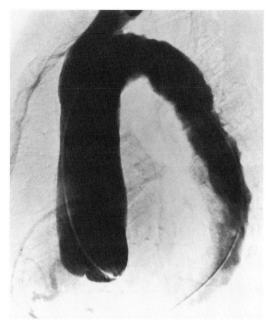

Figure 91. The subtracted lateral arch aortogram shows total effacement of the sinotubular junction of the aorta.

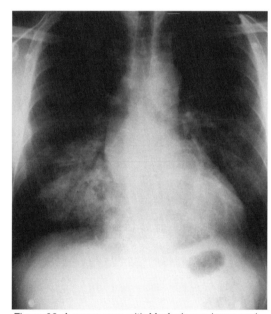

Figure 92. A young man with Marfan's syndrome and congestive heart failure due to acute aortic insufficiency, which is secondary to acute dissection of the ascending aorta resulting in a flail leaflet. Note that the left ventricle appears normal and the ascending aorta causes a bulge in the right border of the mediastinum.

If dissection has not supervened, annuloaortic ectasia has the appearance of a smooth-walled fusiform aneurysm **(Fig. 90)** with a broad base and tapering as it ascends the aorta from its root. The sinuses of Valsalva may be totally indistinct or at least partly effaced **(Fig. 91)**. If dilatation at the root is great enough, aortic insufficiency will be noted with dilatation of the left ventricle. The chest radiograph may manifest changes of congestive heart failure due to aortic valve insufficiency **(Fig. 92)**, and alteration in the right border of the mediastinum if the dilatation is great enough. In Marfan's syndrome, aneurysmal involvement may include the arch and descending aorta as well. CT and MR findings are simply those of an aneurysm. Patients with Marfan's syndrome present with aortic findings in their 3rd and 4th decades.

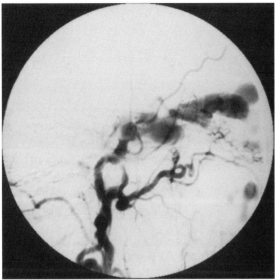

Figure 93. A 29-year-old woman with Ehlers-Danlos syndrome (type 4) who presented with a spontaneous carotid cavernous fistula and bilateral internal carotid artery dissection as shown on this lateral right common carotid arteriogram.

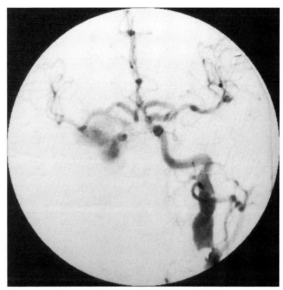

Figure 94. Same patient as in Figure 93. AP left common carotid arteriogram.

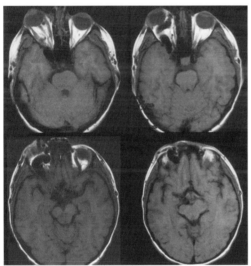

Figure 95. Same patient as in Figure 93. Axial T1-weighted MR scan of the head.

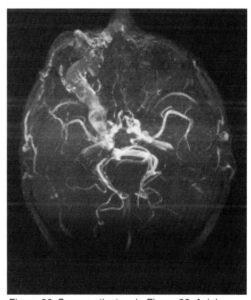

Figure 96. Same patient as in Figure 93. Axial phase contrast MR arteriogram of the head.

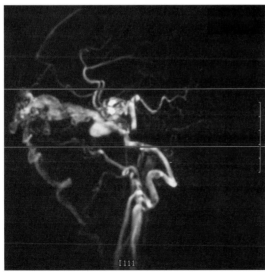

Figure 97. Same patient as in Figure 93. Sagittal phase contrast MR arteriogram of the right carotid system.

Miscellaneous Conditions—Ehlers-Danlos Syndrome
Ehlers-Danlos syndrome (type 4), occurs in auto-somal dominant or recessive forms that result in a deficiency of type 3 collagen. Although it is the most common hereditary dysplasia of connective tissue (besides Marfan's syndrome), it is still rare. Patients are typically young and present with arterial catastrophes **(Figs. 93–97)**. They manifest articular hypermobility and capillary fragility. Patients with Ehlers-Danlos type 4 do not have the bony, skull, ocular, and cardiac abnormalities of Marfan's syndrome. MR or CT arteriography should be favored over conventional arteriography in these patients because the arterial puncture site often develops a pseudoaneurysm that requires repair.

For further information on this topic, please see Teaching File Cases 3, 4, 7, 8, 9, and 23.

Selected Readings

Acher CW, Wynn MM, Hoch JR, Popic P, Archibald J, Turnipseed WD. Combined use of cerebral spinal fluid drainage and naloxone reduces the risk of paraplegia in thoracoabdominal aneurysm repair. J Vasc Surg 1994; 19:236–248.

Chen JT. Plain radiographic evaluation of the aorta. J Thorac Imaging 1990; 5:1–17.

Galloway AC, Colvin SB, LaMendola CL, et al. Ten-year operative experience with 165 aneurysms of the ascending aorta and aortic arch. Circulation 1989; 80:I249–I256.

Golden MA, Donaldson MC, Whittemore AD, Mannick JA. Evolving experience with thoracoabdominal aortic aneurysm repair at a single institution. J Vasc Surg 1991; 13:792–797.

Johnston KW, Rutherford RB, Tilson MD, Shah DM, Hollier L, Stanley JC. Suggested standards for reporting on arterial aneurysms. J Vasc Surg 1991; 13:452–458.

Kumar S, Subramanyan R, Mandalam KR, et al. Aneurysmal form of aortoarteritis (Takayasu's disease): analysis of 30 cases. Clin Radiol 1990; 42:342–347.

Lehnert B, Wadouh F, Dwenger A. Relationship between proteolytic enzymes and atherosclerosis in aortic aneurysms. Surgery 1991; 172:345–350.

Long A, Bruneval P, Laurian C, Cormier JM, Camilleri JP, Fiessinger JN. Takayasu's disease: diagnostic and therapeutic value of subclavian artery biopsy. Ann Vasc Surg 1990; 4:151–155.

Maeda S, Miyamoto T, Murata H, Yamashita K. Prevention of spinal cord ischemia by monitoring spinal cord perfusion pressure and somatosensory evoked potentials. J Cardiovasc Surg 1989; 30:565–571.

Mertens JC, van Dissel JT, Kibbelaar RE, Breedveld FC. The clinical spectrum of giant cell arteritis. Neth J Med 1993; 42:99–104.

Miller DL, Reinig JW, Volkman DJ. Vascular imaging with MRI: inadequacy in Takayasu's arteritis compared with angiography. AJR 1986; 146:949–954.

Movsowitz HD, David M, Movsowitz C, Kotler MN, Jacobs LE. Penetrating atherosclerotic aortic ulcers: the role of transesophageal echocardiography in diagnosis and clinical management. Am Heart J 1993; 126:745–747.

Ninet JP, Bachet P, Dumontet CM, Du Colombier PB, Stewart MD, Pasquier JH. Subclavian and axillary involvement in temporal arteritis and polymyalgia rheumatica. Am J Med 1990; 88:13–20.

Oskoui R, Davis WA, Gomes MN. Salmonella aortitis: a report of a successfully treated case with a comprehensive review of the literature. Arch Intern Med 1993; 153:517–525.

Pressler V, McNamara JJ. Aneurysm of the thoracic aorta: review of 260 cases. J Thorac Cardiovasc Surg 1985; 89:50–54.

Raider L, Landry BA, Brogdon BG. The retrotracheal triangle. Radiographics 1990; 10:1055–1079.

Rao SA, Mandalam KR, Rao VR, et al. Takayasu arteritis: initial and long-term follow-up in 16 patients after percutaneous transluminal angioplasty of the descending thoracic and abdominal aorta. Radiology 1993; 189:173–179.

Sarkar R, Coran AG, Cilley RE, Lindenauer SM, Stanley JC. Arterial aneurysms in children: clinicopathologic classification. J Vasc Surg 1991; 13:47–57.

Savader SJ, Williams GM, Trerotola SO, et al. Preoperative spinal artery localization and its relationship to postoperative neurologic complications. Radiology 1993; 189:165–171.

Seo JW, Park IA, Yoon DH, et al. Thoracic aortic aneurysm associated with aortitis: case reports and histological review. J Korean Med Sci 1991; 6:75–82.

Silver MD, ed. Cardiovascular pathology. 2nd edition. New York: Churchill Livingstone, 1991.

Stanson AW, Kazmier FJ, Hollier LH, et al. Penetrating atherosclerotic ulcers of the thoracic aorta: natural history and clinicopathologic correlations. Ann Vasc Surg 1986; 1:15–23.

Strong JP. Atherosclerotic lesions: natural history, risk factors, and topography. Arch Pathol Lab Med 1992; 116:1268–1275.

Subramanyan R, Joy J, Balakrishnan KG. Natural history of aortoarteritis (Takayasu's disease). Circulation 1989; 80:429–437.

Svensson LG, Crawford ES, Hess KR, Coselli JS, Safi HJ. Variables predictive of outcome in 832 patients undergoing repairs of the descending thoracic aorta. Chest 1993; 104:1248–1253.

Thompson BH, Stanford W. Utility of ultrafast computed tomography in the detection of thoracic aortic aneuryms and dissections. Semin Ultrasound CT MR 1993; 14:117–128.

Tyagi S, Kaul UA, Nair M, Sethi KK, Arora R, Khalilullah M. Balloon angioplasty of the aorta in Takayasu's arteritis: initial and long-term results. Am Heart J 1992; 124:876–882.

Valverde A, Tricot JF, de Crepy B, Bakdach H, Djabbari K. Innominate artery involvement in Type IV Ehlers-Danlos syndrome. Ann Vasc Surg 1991; 5:41–45.

Williams DM, Kirsh MM, Abrams GD. Penetrating atherosclerotic aortic ulcer with dissecting hematoma: control of bleeding with percutaneous embolization. Radiology 1991; 181:85–88.

Witteman JC, Kannel WB, Wolf PA, et al. Aortic calcified plaques and cardiovascular disease (the Framingham study). Am J Cardiol 1990; 66:1060–1064.

Yamada I, Shibuya H, Matsubara O, et al. Pulmonary artery disease in Takayasu's arteritis: angiographic findings. AJR 1992; 159:263–269.

Yamato M, Lecky JW, Hiramatsu K, Kohda E. Takayasu arteritis: radiographic and angiographic findings in 59 patients. Radiology 1986; 161:329–334.

End Note

Figure 56 from Golden MA, Donaldson MC, Whittemore AD, Mannick JA. Evolving experience with thoracoabdominal aortic aneurysm repair at a single institution. J Vasc Surg 1991; 13:793. Used with permission.

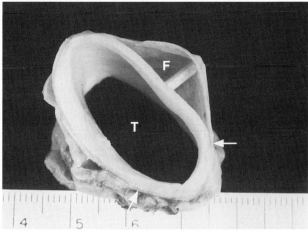

Figure 1. Cuff of the ascending aorta in type 1 dissection. Dissection spares the posterior aspect of the aorta (short arc between arrows). T=true lumen; F=false lumen.

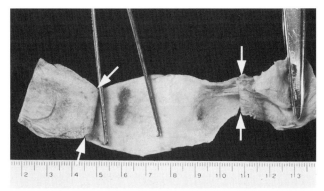

Figure 2. Cuff of the ascending aorta opened to expose the false lumen surface and lines of dissection (arrows).

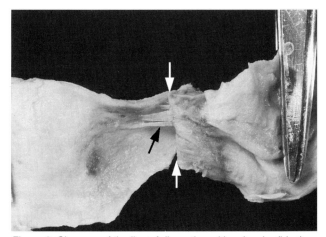

Figure 3. Close-up of the line of dissection with cobwebs (black arrow) bridging the line of dissection within the false lumen (white arrows).

TUTORIAL 3
AORTIC DISSECTION
David M. Williams, M.D., and
Ian A. Sproat, M.D., FRCP(C)

Editor's Note: The important subject of aortic dissection is dealt with in unusual depth because of the emerging therapeutic role of endovascular treatment in this area.

Introduction
The subjects addressed in this tutorial include:
1. Terminology related to aortic dissection
2. Classification of aortic dissection
3. Diagnosis of aortic dissection
4. Complications of aortic dissection
5. Percutaneous treatment of ischemic complications
6. Postoperative follow-up.

Medical Emergency
Acute aortic dissection is the most common aortic catastrophe, with an incidence of approximately 2,000 cases each year, which exceeds that of ruptured abdominal or thoracic aortic aneurysms. The mortality of acute dissection has been estimated at 1% per hour for the first 48 hours, with most deaths due to rupture of the false lumen into the pericardial or pleural space. Prompt diagnosis and treatment of acute dissection are clearly urgent goals of radiologist, cardiologist, and surgeon alike.

Terminology
Dissection
Aortic dissection consists of a hematoma within the aortic wall **(Figs. 1–5)**. The hematoma usually lies between the inner two thirds and outer one third of the media. A "classic dissection" is the double-barreled aorta **(Figs. 6–8)**. Two spiraling lines of dissection mark the junction of the true and false lumens, which are separated by the dissection flap (septal or mural flap). An atypical dissection is characterized by features such as a thrombosed false lumen or an unusual entry tear **(Figs. 9–13)**.

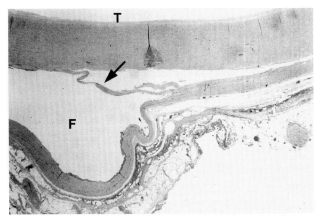

Figure 4. Hematoxylin and eosin stain of aortic dissection. Arrow marks the aortic cobweb. T=true lumen; F=false lumen.

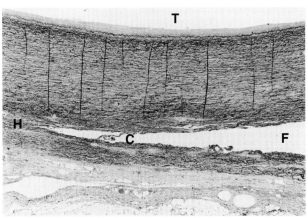

Figure 5. Elastin stain of aortic dissection. H marks the hematoma. C=cobweb within the false lumen (F); T=true lumen. (Vertical lines represent artifacts).

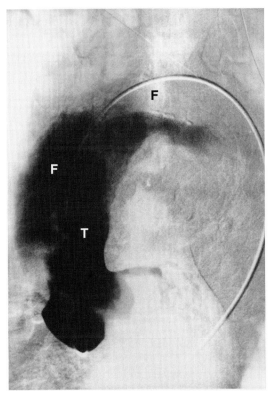

Figure 6. Double-barreled aorta in a DeBakey type 2 dissection. Injection in the ascending aorta. T=true lumen; F=false lumen.

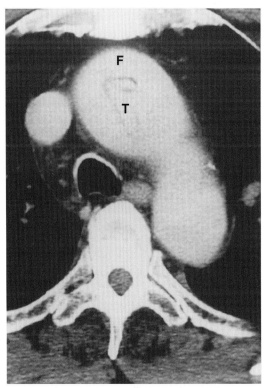

Figure 7. CT slice at the level of the aortic arch shows a double-barreled aorta. T=true lumen; F=false lumen.

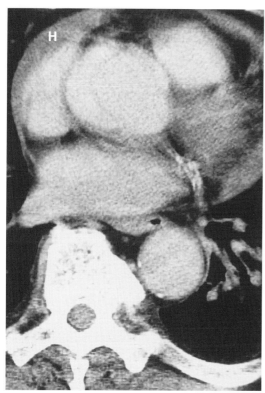

Figure 8. CT slice near the aortic root shows a double-barreled aorta. The descending aorta is intact. H=hemopericardium.

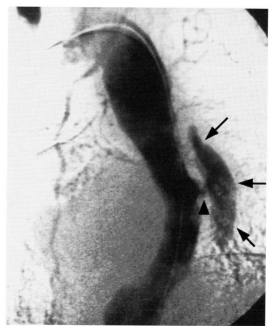

Figure 9. Penetrating ulcer (arrowhead) in the mid descending aorta with atypical, localized dissection (arrows).

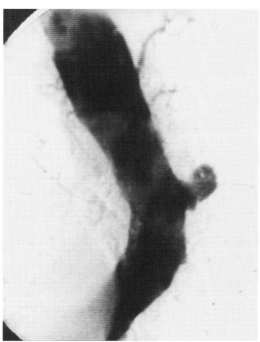

Figure 10. Same patient as in Figure 9. Follow-up aortogram 10 days later.

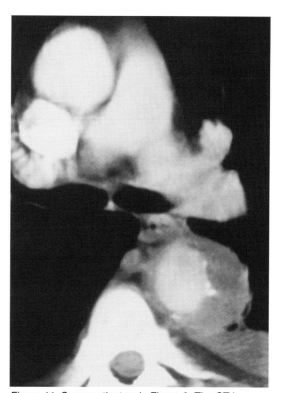

Figure 11. Same patient as in Figure 9. The CT image 5 days after the follow-up aortogram, just cephalad to the ulcer, shows atypical dissection.

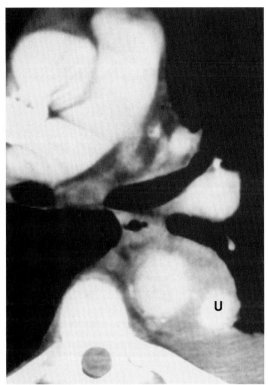

Figure 12. Same patient as in Figure 9. CT slice at the cephalic margin of the ulcer (U).

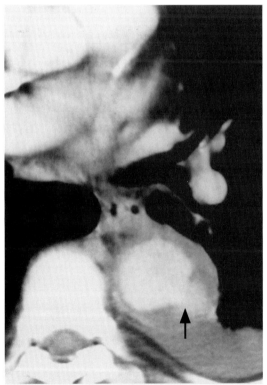

Figure 13. Same patient as in Figure 9. CT slice at the level of intimal disruption by the ulcer. Arrow indicates the ulcer crater.

Aneurysm

An aortic aneurysm is characterized by an increase in diameter of more than 50% from normal. Aortic ectasia is characterized by an increase of less than 50%. In both entities, the dilatation is contained by the aortic wall, or at least, by the adventitia. Unlike "dissection," which is a pathological definition, "ectasia" and "aneurysm" are morphological terms which require descriptive modifiers such as atherosclerotic, mycotic, syphilitic, etc.

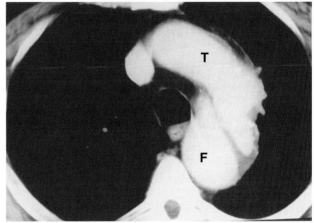

Figure 14. CT slice at the level of the arch and proximal descending aorta shows a chronic DeBakey type 3 dissection. T=true lumen; F=false lumen.

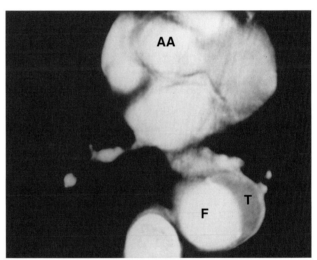

Figure 15. Same patient as in Figure 14. CT slice at the level of the aortic root shows an aneurysmal, opacified false lumen. The true lumen in the descending aorta is thrombosed (confirmed at autopsy). AA=ascending aorta; T=true lumen; F=false lumen.

Related Aortic Lesions

"Dissecting aneurysm" is a misleading phrase because it suggests a relationship between classic dissections and so-called atherosclerotic aneurysms. Aneurysms, except for the aneurysms of Marfan's syndrome and other medial degenerative diseases, are rarely complicated by classic dissections arising within them. However, if the false lumen of a dissection is large enough (so that the overall aortic diameter exceeds 1.5 times normal), the aorta is by definition aneurysmal **(Figs. 14–16)**.

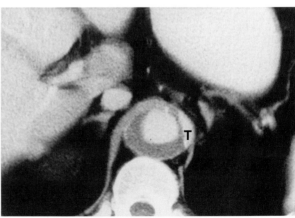

Figure 16. Same patient as in Figure 14. CT slice at the level of the upper abdominal aorta shows a narrow true lumen (T). The true lumen in the abdomen was reconstituted through the abrupted origin of the right renal artery (not shown).

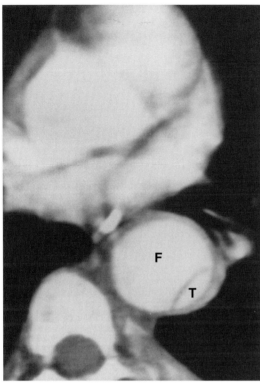

Figure 17. Chronic DeBakey type 3 dissection with aneurysmal false (F) and small true lumen (T).

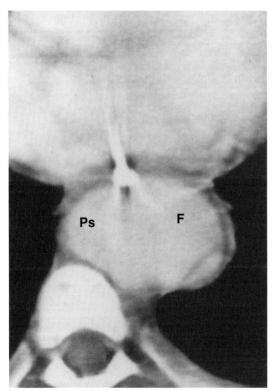

Figure 18. Same patient as in Figure 17. CT slice at a lower level shows medial extension of the false lumen (F) into a pseudoaneurysm (Ps) (confirmed at surgery).

A pseudoaneurysm is a hematoma which has breached the adventitia and is contained by periaortic soft tissues **(Figs. 17–20)**. A penetrating ulcer is a defect in the aortic wall involving the intima and media; the edge of the ulcer is intimately related to an atheroma **(Figs. 21–29)**. Seen in profile, ulcers have a variable appearance, at times resembling gastric ulcers.

Classification of Aortic Dissections

Aortic dissections are classified on the basis of the anatomic distribution of the dissection, not according to the location of the entry tear. The Stanford types A and B comprise dissections involving or sparing the ascending aorta, respectively. The DeBakey types 1 and 3 are equivalent to Stanford types A and B, respectively. The DeBakey type 2 dissection affects the ascending aorta but spares the descending aorta.

Patients with acute type A dissections are at risk for rupture of the false lumen into the pericardial sac, aortic valvular insufficiency, and coronary artery occlusion. There is wide consensus that aortic reconstruction constitutes a surgical emergency in these patients. In contrast, in many patients with type B dissections, aggressive medical therapy to lower mean blood pressure and pulse pressure can reduce the severity of symptoms, arrest propagation of the dissection, and lower the risk of rupture.

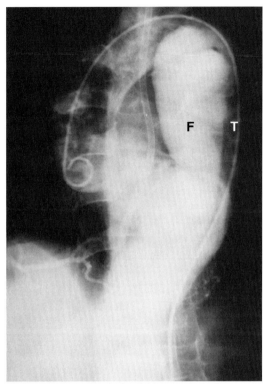

Figure 19. Aortogram in the right posterior oblique (RPO) projection shows a large false lumen (F) and a small (unopacified) true lumen (T).

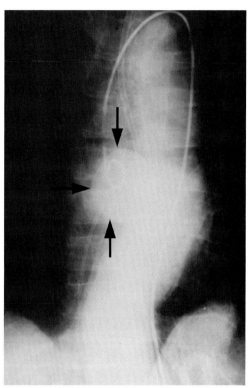

Figure 20. Same patient as in Figure 19. A late film from the aortogram in the anteroposterior (AP) projection shows a pseudoaneurysm (arrows).

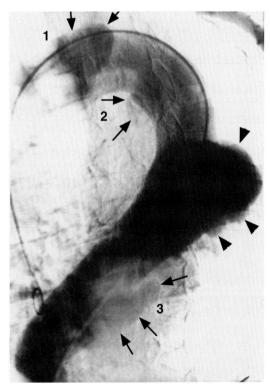

Figure 21. Aortogram in the RPO projection shows the aorta and multiple penetrating ulcers (arrows). The specimen corresponding to the large ulcer (arrowheads) caused hemoptysis and is shown in Figure 24. Ulcers 1 and 2 are seen in cross-section in Figure 25.

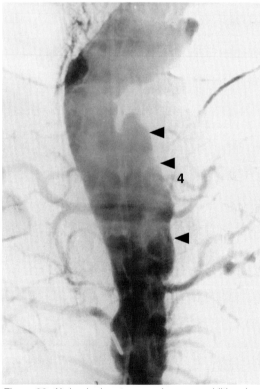

Figure 22. Abdominal aortogram shows an additional ulcer (arrowheads) at the level of the celiac artery.

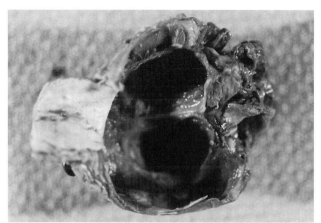

Figure 23. Surgical specimen of the large ulcer from Figure 21 at the base of the mid descending aortic pseudoaneurysm. This was a source of aortopulmonary-bronchial fistula.

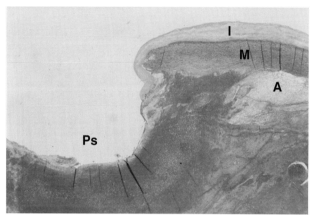

Figure 24. Elastin stain, longitudinal section, through the edge of the large ulcer shown in Figure 23. Ps=pseudoaneurysm; I=intima; M=media; A=adventitia.

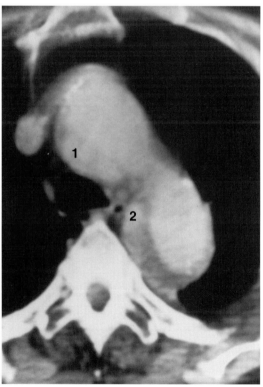

Figure 25. The baseline CT scan at the level just below the arch, shows ulcers 1 and 2 from Figure 21.

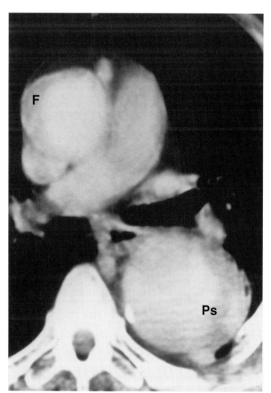

Figure 26. Baseline CT scan at the level of the large penetrating ulcer and pseudoaneurysm (Ps). Thrombosed false lumen of the atypical ascending aortic dissection (F) was contiguous with ulcer 1 from Figures 21 and 25.

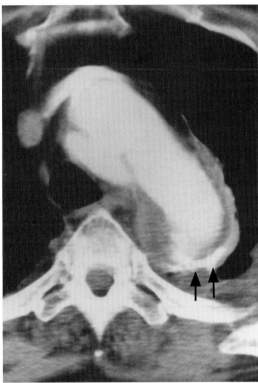

Figure 27. CT scan 1 week later, after resection of the large ulcer. Ulcer 2 has thrombosed (compare with Figure 25). A felt wrap at the upper anastomosis is partly visible (arrows).

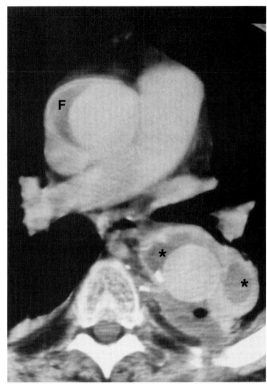

Figure 28. CT slice at the level caudal to Figure 27. The thrombosed false lumen (F) in the ascending aorta is clearly seen. Postoperative changes surround the Dacron graft (asterisks).

Goals of Imaging

The primary goal of imaging is to establish or exclude involvement of the ascending aorta. This issue is crucial and must be settled as expeditiously as possible, since it determines whether or not the patient undergoes emergent reconstruction of the ascending aorta. After ascending aortic involvement is confirmed, whether to proceed further with imaging to document the location of the entry tear and evaluate the rest of the aorta depends on the preferences of the thoracic surgeon. Many surgeons will operate on type A dissections solely on the basis of findings on transesophageal echocardiography (TEE).

When clinically indicated, a second goal of imaging is to document which lumen supplies which vessel and to measure the perfusion pressure available to compromised branches. Pressures can be measured at angiography by cannulating the true and false lumens and, when necessary, the branch arteries. Imaging can also be performed in order to establish baseline size of the false lumen and the extent of dissection.

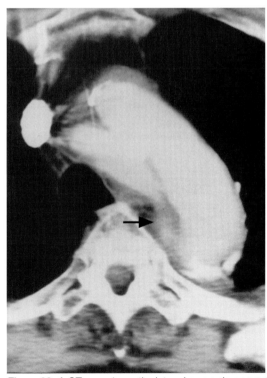

Figure 29. A CT scan 4 months later shows enlargement of ulcer 1 and reopening of ulcer 2 (arrow). Compare with Figures 21, 25, and 27.

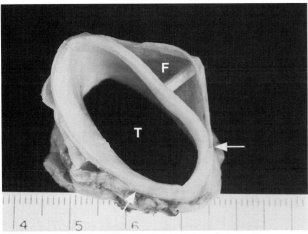

Figure 30. Cuff of the ascending aorta in type 1 dissection. Dissection spares the posterior aspect of the aorta (short arc between arrows). T=true lumen; F=false lumen.

Choosing an Imaging Study

The choice of an imaging study depends not only on the intrinsic strengths and limitations of the study, but on the expertise and availability of the radiologist and cardiologist and on the preferences of the thoracic surgeon. The sensitivities of magnetic resonance (MR) imaging, TEE, and computed tomography (CT) scanning for detecting aortic dissection have been reported to be 98%, 98%, and 94%, respectively. The specificities were reported to be 98%, 87%, and 77%, respectively. The lower specificity of TEE was primarily due to false positives in the ascending aorta. Portable TEE equipment allows convenient screening for dissection in the emergency department or intensive care unit. Diagnostic uncertainties can be clarified with MR imaging or spiral CT scanning. In institutions with strong TEE, MR imaging, and spiral CT scanning facilities, the role of angiography in classic dissection is limited to evaluation and treatment of ischemic syndromes due to branch vessel compromise.

Classic Aortic Dissection— Pathological Features

Classic aortic dissection has the following features:
1. Double-barreled aorta which contains the true and false lumens, with the intervening wall, or dissection septum, constituting the mural flap **(Fig. 30)**.

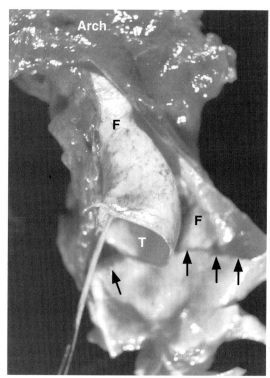

Figure 31. Autopsy specimen of an acute type 1 dissection. There is a circumferential entry tear (arrows). T=true lumen; F=false lumen.

2. The typical entry tear is a laceration oriented transversely to the long axis of the aorta, several centimeters long, occurring on a background of undistinctive and relatively featureless intima **(Figs. 31–33)**.

3. The false lumen propagates and develops a re-entry tear into the true lumen, or ruptures externally.

4. The false lumen usually supports longitudinal flow; that is, it provides blood transport to one or more aortic branch arteries.

Classic Aortic Dissection—
Chest Radiograph Features

The chest radiograph features are nonspecific; the findings depend upon the location of the dissection and its complications. The aorta is often enlarged and typically tortuous. There may be displacement of intimal calcification of greater than 4 mm from the wall, particularly in the transverse arch, where, on the posteroanterior (PA) view, one is looking nearly end-on at the lumen. If acute aortic valve insufficiency occurs, the chest radiograph will often manifest acute pulmonary edema. Pleural effusions may be present. The trachea and esophagus may be deviated to the right by the descending aorta, or to the left by the ascending aorta.

Classic Aortic Dissection—
Imaging Features

The classic aortic dissection has the following imaging features:

1. Two channels within the aorta can be demonstrated by aortography, MR imaging, CT scanning, or TEE, with an intervening line or plane representing the mural flap **(Figs. 34–36)**.

2. The entry tear is seen as a break in the mural flap (CT, MR, TEE), or its location is inferred from the presence of a jet of contrast material or flow signal from one lumen into the other. The entry tear is in the ascending aorta approximately two thirds of the time and just distal to the left subclavian artery approximately one third of the time **(Fig. 37)**.

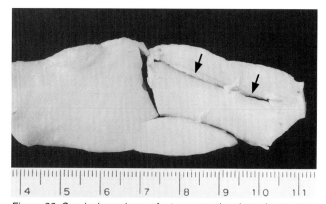

Figure 32. Surgical specimen of a transversely oriented entry tear in an acute type 1 dissection (arrows), viewed from the intimal surface.

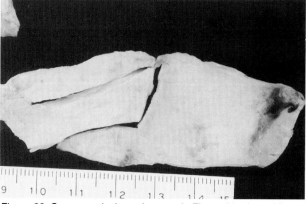

Figure 33. Same surgical specimen as in Figure 32, viewed from the nonintimal (false lumen) surface.

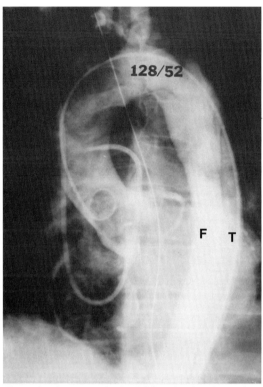

Figure 34. Aortogram in the RPO projection shows the double-barreled appearance of the aorta following blunt chest trauma.

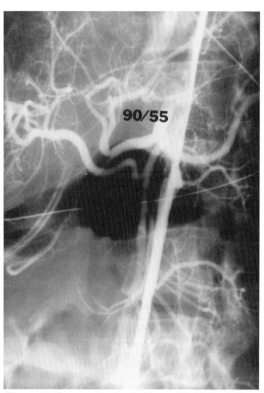

Figure 35. Same patient as in Figure 34. Abdominal aortogram shows compromise of the visceral arteries and a blood pressure deficit below the diaphragm (BP=90/55 mm Hg). Infarcted bowel was resected.

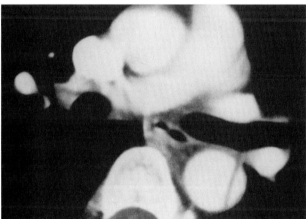

Figure 36. Same patient as in Figure 34. Traumatic type 3 dissection. A CT slice at the level of the right pulmonary artery shows a double-barreled aorta.

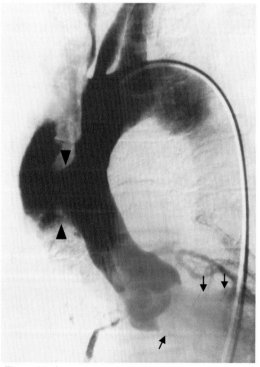

Figure 37. Acute type 1 dissection with compromise of the innominate artery and a large entry tear (arrowheads) just proximal to the innominate origin. Aortic insufficiency (arrows) and right coronary artery compromise are present.

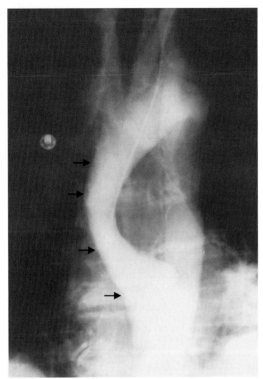

Figure 38. Acute type 1 dissection with deformed and scalloped true lumen (arrows) and nonopacified false lumen.

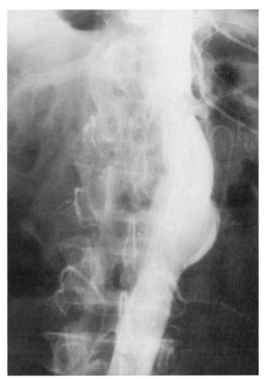

Figure 39. Same patient as in Figure 38. The false lumen in the abdomen fills the intercostal and lumbar arteries.

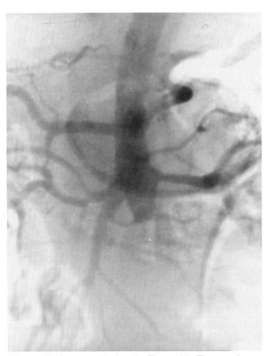

Figure 40. Same patient as in Figure 38. The true lumen in the abdomen is occluded below the renal arteries.

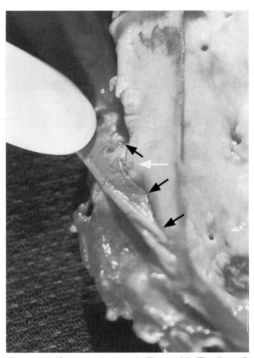

Figure 41. Same patient as in Figure 38. The line of dissection (black arrows) skirts the celiac artery origin (white arrow). An infrarenal aortic aneurysm was present.

3. Re-entry tears have the same imaging appearance as entry tears and form near medial structures that resist extension of a dissection, such as aortic branch arteries **(Figs. 38–41)**.

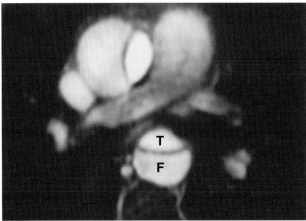

Figure 42. MR arteriogram shows differential flow in the true (T) and false (F) lumens.

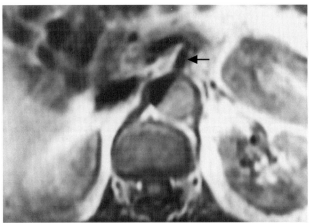

Figure 43. MR arteriogram shows differential flow in the true and false lumens. The low signal intensity of the superior mesenteric artery (SMA) flow matches that of the true lumen (arrow).

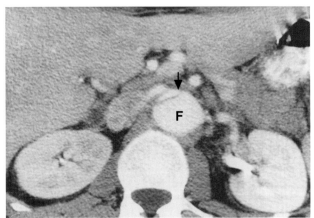

Figure 44. Spiral CT scan demonstrates a lag in true lumen (arrow) perfusion of the right kidney compared with earlier false lumen (F) flow to the left kidney. See also Figure 69.

4. Differential blood flow in the lumens causes differential opacification of the lumens on contrast studies and flow artifacts on nonenhanced MR and TEE studies **(Figs. 42–44)**.

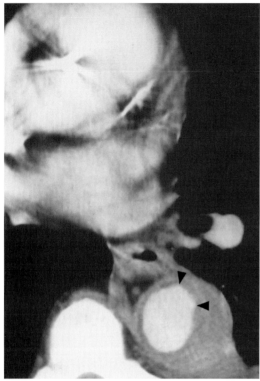

Figure 45. Same patient as in Figures 9–13. Atypical dissection with thrombosed false lumen; the entry tear is a penetrating ulcer (arrowheads).

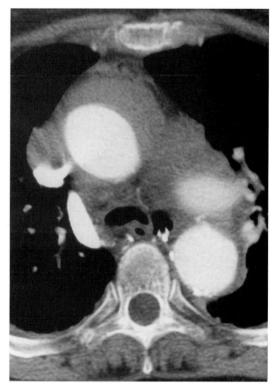

Figure 46. Atypical dissection (incipient classic type 1 dissection). The CT scan shows a periadventitial hematoma surrounding the ascending aorta and pulmonary artery. Intramural hemorrhage in the ascending aorta is also present.

Atypical Aortic Dissection— Pathological Features

Some aortic dissections escape the conventional classifications. Although some authors favor classifying as type B all dissections which are not type A, the relative rarity of atypical dissections even in large reported series of dissections precludes sweeping statements on proper treatment. The atypical dissection has one or both of the following features:

1. The false lumen is thrombosed, except that a patent blind channel or small cavity may be present at the entry tear **(Fig. 45)** with a localized turbulent vortex of "flow." In dissections with a thrombosed false lumen, there is no or, at most, a small re-entry tear (we have not observed one) and, by definition, no sustained longitudinal flow.

2. The entry tear is atypical in location (eg, in the distal descending or abdominal aorta) or morphology (eg, a short transverse tear, a cavity resembling a gastric ulcer, or a longitudinal laceration) **(Figs. 46–51)**.

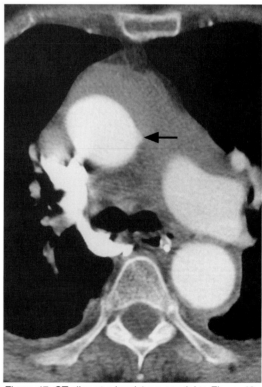

Figure 47. CT slice at a level 1 cm caudal to Figure 46 shows an ulcer-like entry tear (arrow).

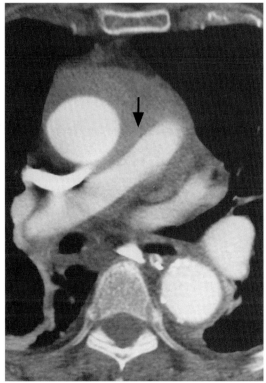

Figure 48. CT slice at a level 3 cm lower than Figure 46 shows a hematoma (arrow) compressing the pulmonary artery.

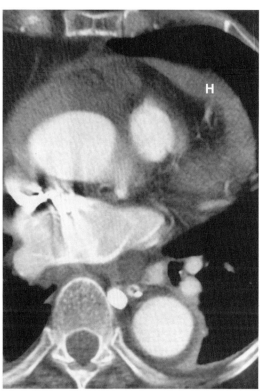

Figure 49. CT slice at a level 6 cm lower than Figure 46 shows hemopericardium (H).

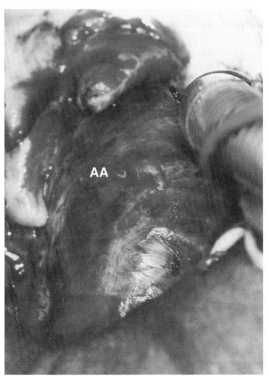

Figure 50. Surgical view of the ascending aorta (AA), viewed from the patient's head, with hemopericardium and periadventitial hematoma.

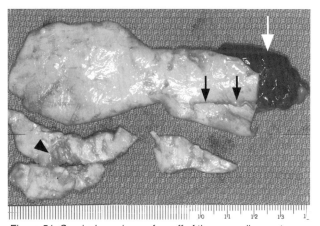

Figure 51. Surgical specimen of a cuff of the ascending aorta contains a 2-cm transverse entry tear (black arrows) on a featureless intimal surface; erosive atheromas are present (arrowhead). Thrombus in the false lumen is also present (white arrow).

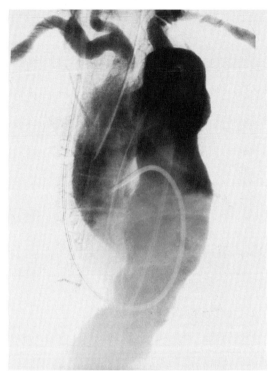

Figure 52. Leaking thoracic aortic aneurysm with atypical dissection (intramural hemorrhage) at the site of rupture. No leak is appreciated on the thoracic aortogram.

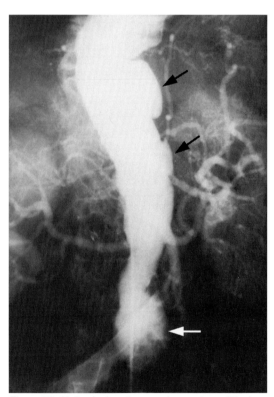

Figure 53. Abdominal aortogram shows ulcers (black arrows) and an infrarenal aneurysm (white arrow).

Atypical Aortic Dissection—Etiologies
1. Ruptured aneurysms are sometimes accompanied by localized intramural (intramedial) hemorrhage near the site of rupture (**Figs. 52–57**).

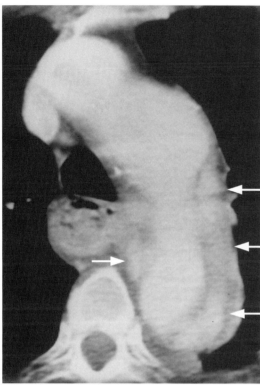

Figure 54. CT slice at the level of the aortic arch shows contrast material outside the aortic lumen (arrows).

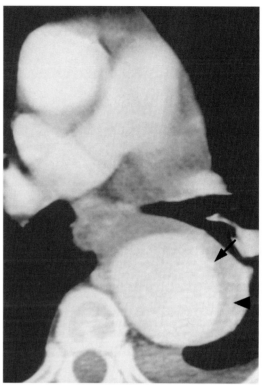

Figure 55. CT slice at a level 4 cm caudal to Figure 54 shows a low-attenuation crescentic wedge of intramural hematoma between the intimal calcium (arrow) and the enhancing aortic wall (arrowhead).

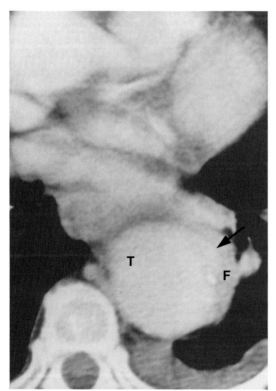

Figure 56. CT slice at a level 6 cm below Figure 54 shows contrast material in the largely thrombosed false lumen (arrow). T=true lumen; F=false lumen.

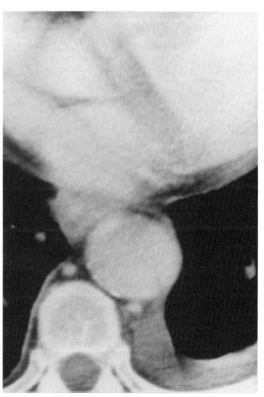

Figure 57. CT slice at a level 8 cm below Figure 54 shows an uncomplicated aneurysm.

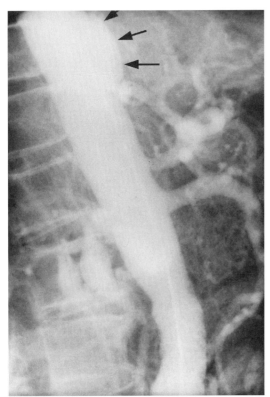

Figure 58. Lateral abdominal aortogram shows a penetrating ulcer on the anterior surface of the thoracoabdominal aorta (arrows).

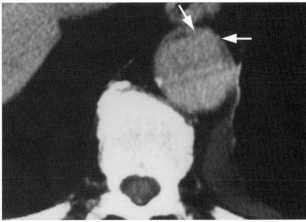

Figure 59. CT slice in the lower thoracic aorta shows the ulcer as a subtle anterior bulge in the aortic lumen (arrows).

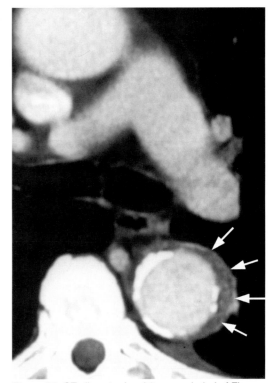

Figure 60. CT slice at a level 8 cm cephalad of Figure 59 shows retrograde extension of atypical dissection (intramural hemorrhage, arrows).

2. Penetrating ulcers by definition extend into the media. Some of these result in intramural hemorrhage which can propagate for great distances (Figs. 58–60).

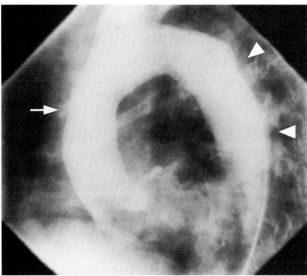

Figure 61. Incipient classic type 1 dissection. The ciné thoracic aortogram shows contrast material pooling outside the ascending aorta with flattening of the surrounding anterior wall (arrow). The wall of the descending aorta is thickened (arrowheads). The entry tear was a 5-mm transverse tear in the featureless intimal surface.

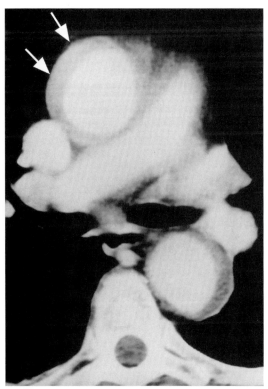

Figure 62. CT slice through the ascending aorta shows high-attenuation thrombus in the false lumen (arrows); no intimal tear was seen. The descending aorta is also involved.

3. With incipient classic dissection, the entry tear is short, transverse, and set in a background of relatively featureless intima. Perhaps because the tear is so short and flow across it is so slow, blood in the false lumen is thrombosed **(Figs. 61, 62)**.

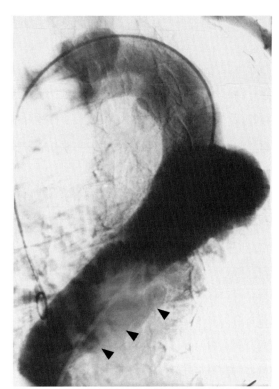

Figure 63. Same patient as in Figures 21–29. The thoracic aorta was transected through this lower ulcer (arrowheads) to accommodate the interposition graft.

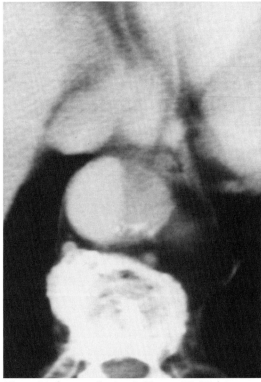

Figure 64. Same patient as in Figures 21–29. Intramural hemorrhage due to a penetrating aortic ulcer.

4. Entry tear in the lower thoracic or abdominal aorta. Many of these lesions, as described in numerous case reports, appear to be due to penetrating ulcers **(Figs. 63, 64)**.

5. Spontaneous intramural hemorrhage is a hypothetical lesion in which intramural hemorrhage develops without an intimal tear. We have not seen a convincing case.

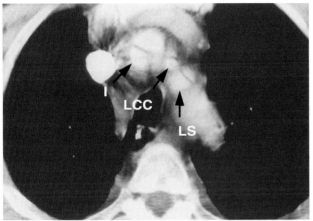

Figure 65. CT slice through the brachiocephalic arteries in an acute type 1 dissection. All three vessels are involved. I=innominate artery; LCC=left carotid artery; LS=left subclavian artery. The same patient is shown in Figures 66–73.

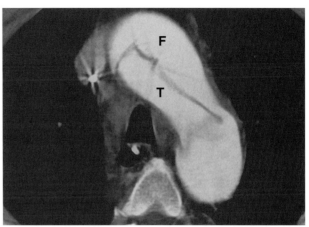

Figure 66. CT slice 2 cm below Figure 65 shows the true and false lumens. T=true lumen; F=false lumen.

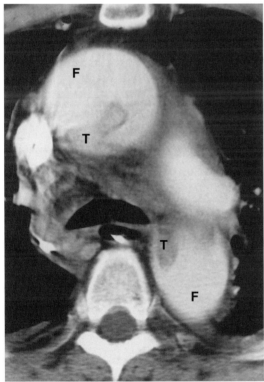

Figure 67. CT slice 4 cm below Figure 65 shows a small true lumen.

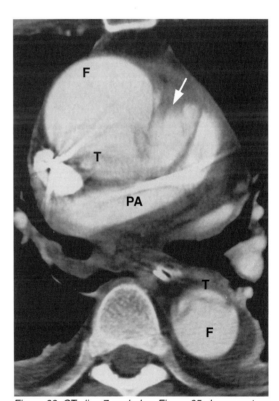

Figure 68. CT slice 7 cm below Figure 65 shows rupture of the false lumen (arrow) compressing the pulmonary artery (PA). T=true lumen; F=false lumen.

Complications of Dissection
1. Expansion or rupture of the false lumen **(Figs. 65–73)** causing pain, hypotension, or death by cardiac tamponade or exsanguination.
2. Obstruction or occlusion of major aortic branches **(Figs. 74–82)** resulting in myocardial infarction, stroke, renal or mesenteric ischemia, spinal cord infarction, or lower extremity ischemia.

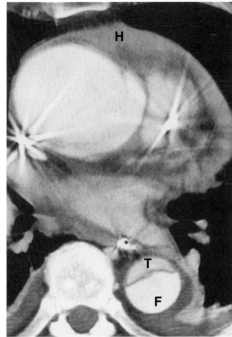

Figure 69. CT slice 10 cm below Figure 65 shows hemopericardium (H). Differential opacification of the true and false lumens is due to differential flow in the two lumens. See also Figures 42–44.

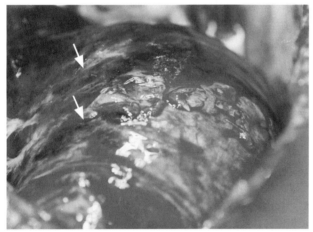

Figure 71. Surgical view of the heart and ascending aorta, seen from the patient's head, shows hemopericardium (arrows).

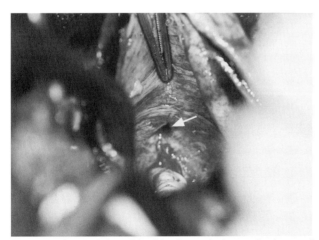

Figure 73. Surgical view of the false lumen in the proximal ascending aorta shows the right coronary artery origin (arrow).

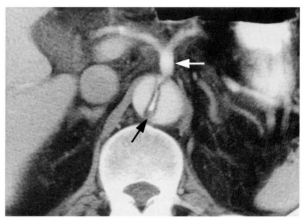

Figure 70. CT slice at the level of the celiac artery origin (white arrow). The true lumen is a narrow slit (black arrow).

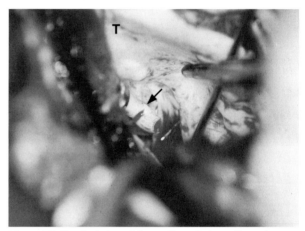

Figure 72. Surgical view of the aortic root shows the pale endothelialized surface of the true lumen (T) in the proximal ascending aorta. The force of the dissection abrupted and everted the right coronary artery 8 mm from its origin (arrow).

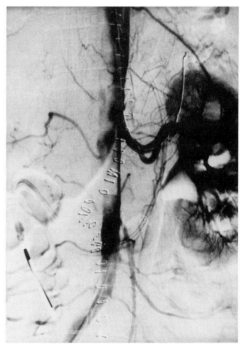

Figure 74. Abdominal aortogram in a woman with traumatic aortic dissection and right leg ischemia shows the left renal and right common iliac arteries arising from the true lumen. The right renal artery did not fill during false lumen injection.

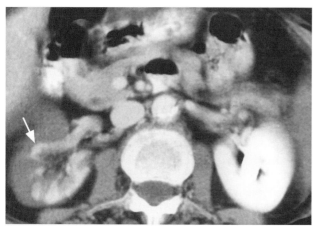

Figure 75. Same patient as in Figure 74. The CT slice at the level of the renal arteries shows compromised perfusion to the right kidney (arrow), which led to infarction and atrophy. The aortic true lumen is compressed posteriorly.

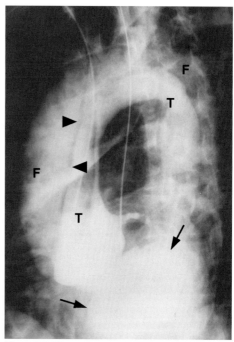

Figure 76. Thoracic aortogram in a man with bilateral lower extremity ischemia and acute type 1 dissection shows a narrow true lumen (T), a large false lumen (F), aortic insufficiency (arrows), and a mural flap (arrowheads).

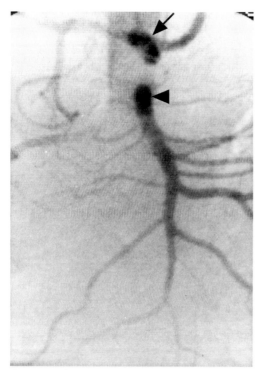

Figure 77. Same patient as in Figure 76. The true lumen fills the celiac artery (arrow) and the superior mesenteric artery (arrowhead) but is occluded distally.

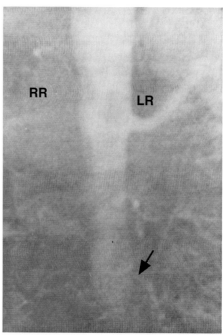

Figure 78. Same patient as in Figure 76. The false lumen fills the left and right renal arteries and the inferior mesenteric arteries (arrow). The iliac arteries did not opacify on either injection. LR=left renal artery; RR=right renal artery.

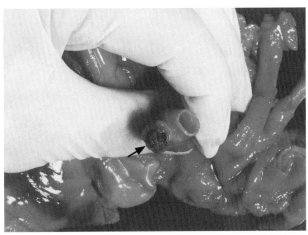

Figure 79. Acute type 1 dissection related to cocaine toxicity in a young man presenting in status epilepticus. There is thrombus in the false lumen of the right subclavian artery (arrow).

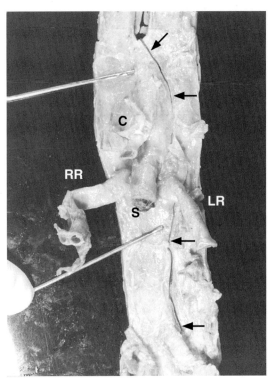

Figure 80. Thrombus is also present in the false lumen of the superior mesenteric artery (S). The curved line (arrows) through the adventitia provided access to the false lumen. C=celiac artery; LR=left renal artery; RR=right renal artery.

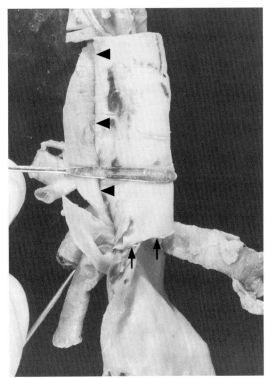

Figure 81. The line of dissection (arrowheads) skirts the celiac and superior mesenteric artery origins and re-enters the abdominal aorta through a transverse re-entry tear at the left renal artery origin (arrows).

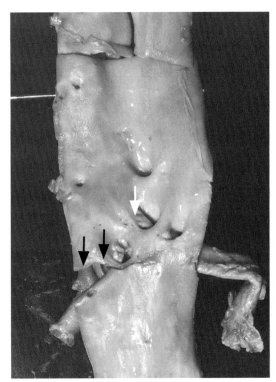

Figure 82. Hematoma in the false lumen deforms the SMA origin (white arrow). A left renal artery re-entry tear is visible (black arrows).

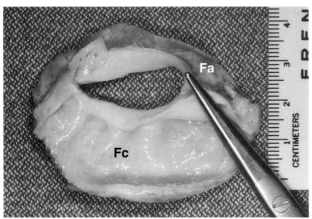

Figure 83. Surgical specimen of a cuff of the ascending aorta shows an acute type 1 dissection (Fa) complicating a chronic type 1 dissection (Fc). The true lumen is in the center of the specimen.

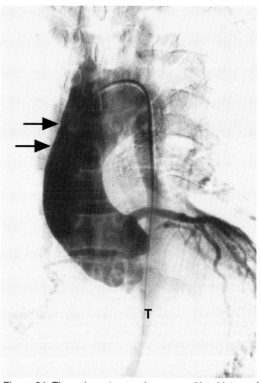

Figure 84. Thoracic aortogram in a man with a history of chronic type 3 dissection shows flattening of the contour of the distal ascending aorta (arrows). T=true lumen. The same patient is shown in Figures 84–101.

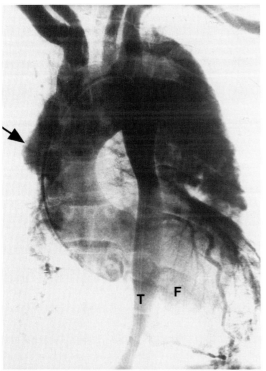

Figure 85. The late arterial phase of the thoracic aortogram shows false lumen extending from the proximal ascending aorta (arrow) into the distal descending aorta. T=true lumen; F=false lumen.

3. Extension of the dissection or de novo dissection elsewhere in the aorta **(Fig. 83)**. A type 3 dissection may dissect retrograde into the ascending aorta **(Figs. 84–88)**.

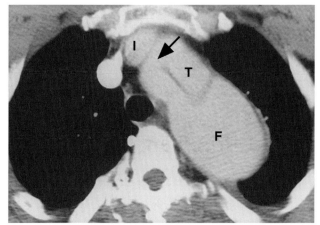

Figure 86. CT slice through the arch and the proximal descending aorta shows the entry tear (arrow). I=innominate artery; T=true lumen; F=false lumen.

Branch Vessel Obstruction–Introduction

As a consequence of the relative obstruction of the true lumen beginning at the entry tear, false lumen pressure is greater than or equal to true lumen pressure in classic dissections. More specifically, because the false lumen constitutes an ectatic channel in wide continuity with the aortic root, false lumen pressure matches aortic root pressure. Consequently, aortic branches which have been sheared off the true lumen and are supplied exclusively by the false lumen are seldom compromised; we have not encountered such a case. Compromised branches are almost invariably supplied by the true lumen or by both lumens. When a branch is sheared off the true lumen, a hole is left in the mural flap corresponding to its native origin. Whether this hole can act as a hemodynamically significant re-entry tear to help perfuse the true lumen depends on where it lies in the final configuration of the mural flap.

A second consideration in acute classic dissection is that the true lumen collapses even if no gradient between the two lumens is present. This happens because the portion of the aortic wall which constitutes the dissection septum is no longer subject to any significant transmural pressure. If a significant gradient between the false and true lumens is present, the true lumen is compressed as well as collapsed. Although this collapse and compression can be reversed focally with deployment of an uncovered stent, adjacent segments of the true lumen may remain collapsed.

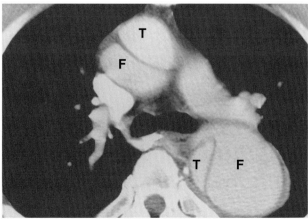

Figure 87. CT slice 3.5 cm below Figure 86 shows false lumen in the distal ascending aorta.

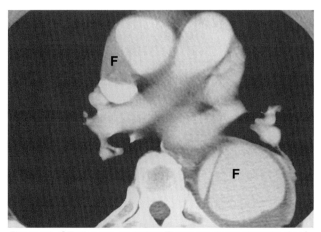

Figure 88. CT slice 6.0 cm below Figure 87 shows thrombosis of the proximal aspect of the false lumen (F).

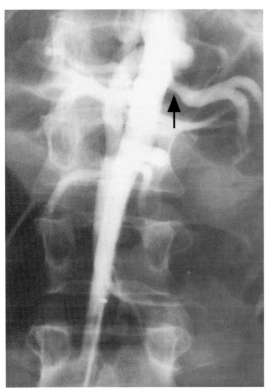

Figure 89. Film 1 of 4 sequential films from the abdominal aortogram of the case illustrated in Figures 84–88. There is phasic filling of the left renal artery from the opacified true lumen followed by unopacified blood from the false lumen. The left renal artery is opacified from true lumen contrast material (arrow).

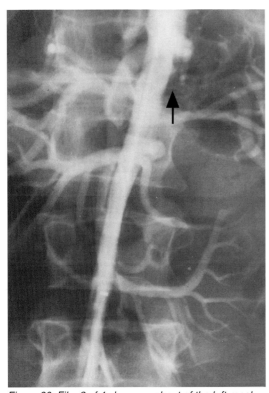

Figure 90. Film 2 of 4 shows washout of the left renal artery due to filling from the unopacified false lumen (arrow).

Diagnosis of Branch Vessel Obstruction

A branch may be compromised either because the true lumen supplies inadequate flow or pressure into it, or the hematoma dissects into it and narrows its lumen **(Figs. 89–101)**, or both. Frequently, the true lumen is a compressed C-shaped envelope extending from the entry tear to the re-entry tear(s) in the abdomen or pelvis. The dissection flap may cover a branch origin like a curtain, even though the line of dissection spares the branch.

Demonstration by CT or MR scanning that the true lumen is not a compressed envelope, and that the line of dissection spares a particular branch origin, probably rules out ongoing ischemia due to dissection in that vascular territory. If CT or MR findings and clinical symptoms suggest an ischemia syndrome, then arteriography with manometry in both lumens may be necessary for confirmation.

In type A dissections, repair of the ascending aorta usually takes precedence over direct treatment of ischemic complications. Institution of total heart bypass from the groin directly perfuses the true lumen distal to the entry tear and relieves most infradiaphragmatic ischemic complications. This relief is maintained when unobstructed antegrade flow in the true lumen is restored after resection of the entry tear and aortic reconstruction.

In unusual cases of type A dissection, such as when ischemic bowel and bacteremia are present, the surgeon may be reluctant to place a synthetic graft, and the management of the ischemic syndrome takes precedence. Most infradiaphragmatic ischemic complications of dissection can be managed percutaneously; therefore, when aortic reconstruction does not take precedence, the patient should be referred to Interventional Radiology for angiographic diagnosis and treatment.

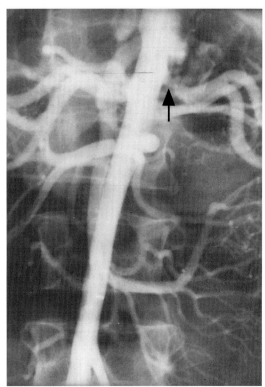

Figure 91. Film 3 of 4 shows true lumen re-opacification of the left renal artery (arrow).

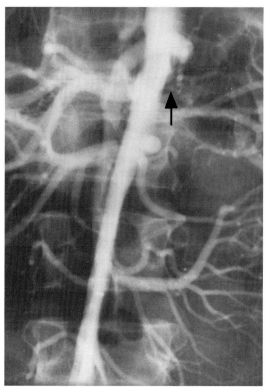

Figure 92. Film 4 of 4 shows washout by blood from the unopacified false lumen (arrow).

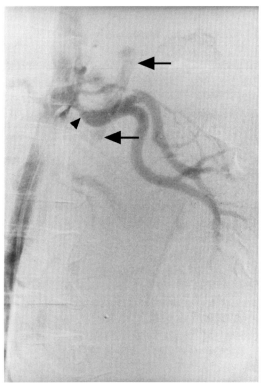

Figure 93. Selective left renal arteriogram (arrowhead) from a true lumen injection. The false lumen is faintly opacified (arrows).

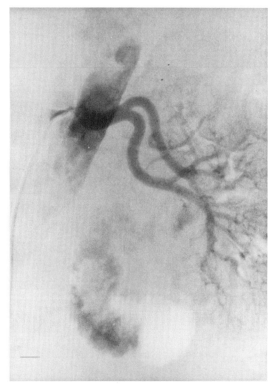

Figure 94. Selective left renal arteriogram from within the false lumen fills the left renal artery through the re-entry tear.

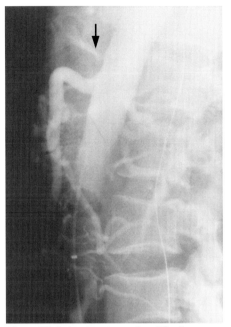

Figure 95. Lateral aortography of the true lumen shows narrowing of the celiac artery origin (arrow). This was principally perfused from the false lumen.

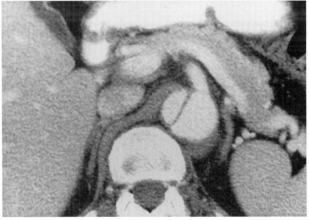

Figure 97. CT slice through the superior mesenteric origin shows the artery's apparent origin from the false lumen despite brisk filling during true lumen injection (see Figure 95).

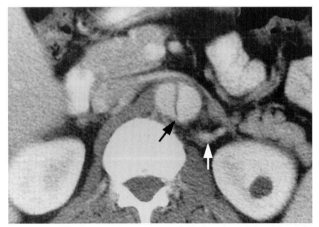

Figure 98. CT slice at a level just cephalad to the origin of the left renal artery (white arrow) shows a re-entry tear posteriorly (black arrow).

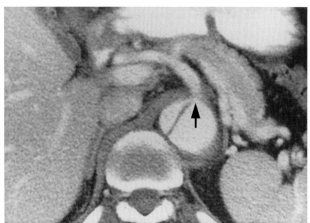

Figure 96. CT slice at the level of the celiac artery shows a gap in the mural flap that indicates a re-entry tear at the celiac origin (arrow).

Branch Vessel Obstruction— Percutaneous Treatment

Percutaneous treatment options include balloon fenestration of the dissection septum, stenting of the true lumen of the aorta, and stenting of compromised aortic branches.

Fenestration is indicated to establish local blood flow between the two lumens, and is useful when a significant pressure gradient between the lumens accounts for compromised flow to critical branches. In the usual case, fenestration raises true lumen pressure and leaves false lumen pressure (which follows the aortic root) unchanged.

After fenestration, the true lumen may remain collapsed and critical visceral branches may remain isolated from physiological flow. In these cases, an intravascular stent may be deployed in the true lumen of the aorta to buttress it open. The optimal location for the stent is within the true lumen between the site of fenestration and the critical branch origin.

When the dissecting hematoma (which by definition is part of the false lumen) extends into a branch origin, fenestration of the dissection septum will not relieve the branch vessel stenosis, since fenestration does not lower the pressure in, or decompress, the false lumen. In this case, stenting of the branch origin is indicated. The endpoint of percutaneous intervention is the achievement of good inflow and prompt washout and elimination of significant pressure gradients between the false and true lumens as well as across major aortic branch origins.

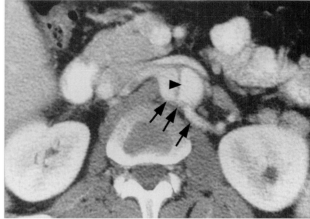

Figure 99. The left renal artery (arrows) passes posterior to the false lumen (arrowhead).

Fenestration—Procedure

The procedure of fenestration is "experimental" in nature and its benefits have not been validated in large patient series. The goals of fenestration are to create a tear in the dissection septum at a chosen level, and to allow local blood flow and pressure equilibration between the true and false lumens. The dissection septum is punctured at the desired level using a Rösch-Uchida needle set (Cook, Bloomington, IN), or equivalent. It is theoretically safer to puncture the septum beginning in the smaller (generally the true) lumen and passing into the more capacious (generally the false) lumen.

The fenestration should be performed close to the level of the compromised vessels. The principal reason for choosing this level is that the true lumen may remain collapsed/compressed even after fenestration elevates true lumen pressure to the false lumen pressure level.

Choice of Puncture Site

A femoral artery with a weak pulse generally communicates with the true lumen of the aorta. We use this true-lumen access for the fenestration needle. A femoral artery with a strong pulse generally communicates with the false lumen through a large re-entry tear at the aortic or iliac bifurcation; we use this false-lumen access for intravascular ultrasound (IVUS) monitoring of the procedure.

Access to the abdominal true lumen from a false-lumen access can generally be obtained by searching for re-entry tears at the bifurcations, especially where the guide wire momentarily snags, or near the origins of visceral arteries. CT scanning, MR imaging, biplane aortography, or IVUS show the spatial relationship of the two lumens. The needle should be directed perpendicular to the septum, from the smaller to the larger lumen, using IVUS and/or fluoroscopic guidance.

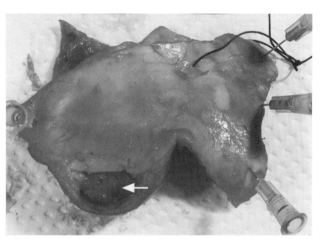

Figure 100. Surgical specimen of the distal ascending aorta shows the intimal surface of the true lumen (opened). Thrombus in the false lumen is visible (arrow) where the aorta was transected proximally to accept the graft.

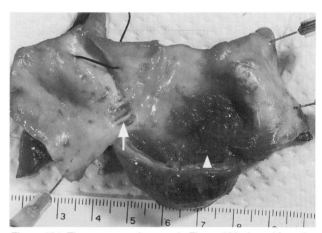

Figure 101. The same specimen as in Figure 100 viewed from the opened false lumen surface shows thrombus in the blind sac of the retrograde dissection (arrowhead) and cobwebs bridging the line of dissection (arrow).

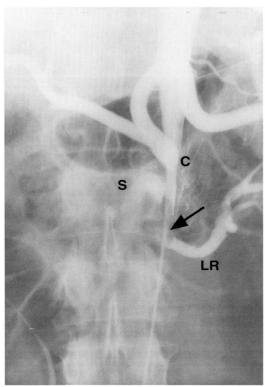

Figure 102. True lumen injection in the upper abdomen fills the celiac (C), superior mesenteric (S), and left renal (LR) arteries. There is a filling defect at the left renal artery origin (arrow).

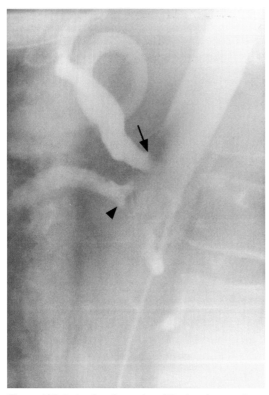

Figure 103. Lateral aortography of the true lumen shows filling of the celiac (arrow) and superior mesenteric arteries (arrowhead), with proximal luminal compromise similar to that affecting the renal artery.

Fenestration—Step by Step

1. Survey the hemodynamics of the dissection with use of CT scanning, MR imaging, aortography with manometry, and IVUS imaging, as necessary, to define the relation of the true and false lumens and determine the vascular supply to critical organs and limbs, and to document perfusion pressure deficits.

2. Choose puncture sites, determine the appropriate level of fenestration, insert the Rösch-Uchida needle, and aim the needle using IVUS and/or fluoroscopic guidance.

3. Advance a 5-F catheter with a needle; remove the needle; slowly retract the catheter while gently injecting contrast material until washout indicates that the catheter tip is intravascularly located.

4. Repeat step 3 if the catheter tip is in the true lumen. If it is in the false lumen, exchange the catheter for a 12-mm percutaneous transluminal angioplasty (PTA) catheter, center the balloon at the site of needle perforation, and dilate. The mural flap tears easily, and little or no resistance is felt while the balloon is being dilated. IVUS imaging can be used to confirm that the balloon crosses the septum separating the lumens, as in the case reported below. As the IVUS is slowly retracted from above to below the fenestration site, the balloon is seen to pass from the false into the true lumen.

5. Reassess anatomy and hemodynamics. If the true lumen of the aorta near a critical branch artery remains collapsed, stents can be deployed in the aortic true lumen as necessary.

6. If stenoses of critical branches are present due to dissecting hematoma, stents can be deployed as necessary. The most common indication for this procedure is iliac artery stenosis.

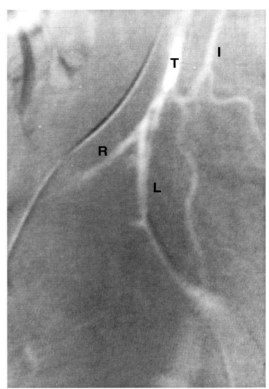

Figure 104. Injection of the true lumen (T) just distal to the level of the renal artery shows marked compression of the true lumen and compromised flow in the inferior mesenteric (I) and left (L) and right (R) common iliac arteries.

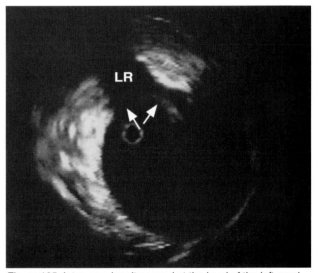

Figure 105. Intravascular ultrasound at the level of the left renal artery demonstrates that the arteriographic filling defect is due to the dissection flap (arrows) which intermittently prolapses into the hypoechoic left renal artery orifice (LR).

Case Report of Aortic Fenestration and Stent Placement

A 60-year-old man with hypertension awoke with left-sided chest pain that felt like a "stake in my chest." A CT scan showed a type B dissection. On the following morning, he had increased chest pain. Femoral pulses were strong. Emergent aortography showed that the false lumen supplied the right renal artery and both iliac arteries, and that the true lumen supplied compromised celiac, superior and inferior mesenteric, and left renal arteries **(Figs. 102–104)**. IVUS imaging showed that the dissection septum blocked the left renal artery origin like a curtain, and even prolapsed into the artery during systole **(Fig. 105)**.

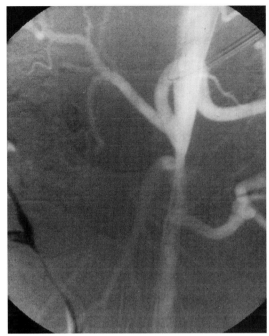

Figure 106. Injection of the true lumen after fenestration at the level of the left renal artery. Aortic flow is visibly improved.

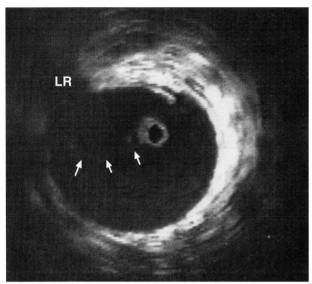

Figure 107. IVUS at the level of the left renal artery shows re-expansion of the true lumen; the dissection flap (faintly visible, arrows) no longer prolapses into the left renal artery (LR).

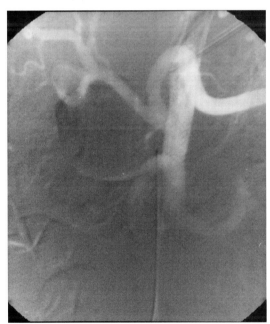

Figure 108. True lumen injection after deployment of a Palmaz 308 stent within the infraceliac aorta (dilated to 14 mm). The hourglass narrowing below the celiac artery has been eliminated.

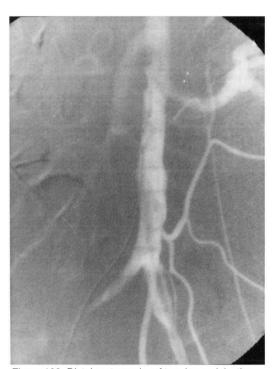

Figure 109. Distal aortography of true lumen injection after stent deployment demonstrates marked improvement in the true lumen caliber and inferior mesenteric artery filling. The iliac arteries are adequately filled by the false lumen.

The right, but not the left, renal collecting system was visualized with the use of fluoroscopy. Fenestration at the level of the left renal artery expanded the distal aorta and improved left renal flow **(Figs. 106, 107)**. Persistent narrowing of the true lumen near the SMA responded to a 308 Palmaz stent (Johnson & Johnson Interventional Systems, Warren, NJ) dilated to 14 mm **(Figs. 108, 109).**

Follow-up of Surgically Treated Dissections

The complications of aortic dissection have been described above. Complications of surgical repair which directly affect the aorta include anastomotic pseudoaneurysm or dissection, aortoenteric or aortobronchial fistula, aortic insufficiency, ring abscess, and infected graft and/or prosthetic valve. Aortic valve function and perivalvular complications are best followed by TEE. MR and CT imaging provide good comprehensive views of the chest or abdomen and are ordinarily repeated once per year, unless remaining disease or a known complication of surgical repair indicates more frequent follow-up. The presence of stainless steel stents in the aorta or branches degrades MR images of all structures in the vicinity of the stents, and in this clinical circumstance CT scanning is the preferred follow-up study. A history of iodinated contrast material allergy or renal failure favors MR imaging for follow-up.

For further information on this topic, please see Teaching File Cases 11, 12, and 24.

Selected Readings

Cigarroa JE, Isselbacher EM, DeSanctis RW, Eagle KA. Diagnostic imaging in the evaluation of suspected aortic dissection. New Engl J Med 1993; 328:35–43.

Nienaber CA, von Kodolitsch Y, Nicolas V, et al. The diagnosis of thoracic aortic dissection by noninvasive imaging procedures. New Engl J Med 1993; 328:1–9.

Nienaber CA, Spielmann RP, von Kodolitsch Y, et al. Diagnosis of thoracic aortic dissection: magnetic resonance imaging versus transesophageal echocardiography. Circulation 1992; 85:434–447.

Petasnick JP. Radiologic evaluation of aortic dissection. Radiology 1991; 180:297–305.

Yamada T, Tada S, Harada J. Aortic dissection without intimal rupture: diagnosis with MR imaging and CT. Radiology 1988; 168:347–352.

Williams DM, Joshi A, Dake MD, Deeb GM, Miller DC, Abrams GD. Aortic cobwebs, an anatomic marker identifying the false lumen in aortic dissection: imaging and pathologic correlation. Radiology 1994; 190:167–174.

End Note

The authors thank Gerald D. Abrams, M.D., for microphotographs of histological sections; G. Michael Deeb, M.D., for surgical specimens; and Dasika Narasimham, M.D., and Do Yun Lee, M.D., for a critical reading of the manuscript.

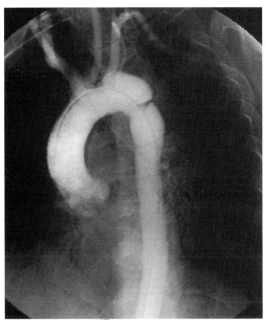

Figure 1. Thoracic aortogram demonstrates a traumatic aortic pseudoaneurysm distal to the left subclavian artery.

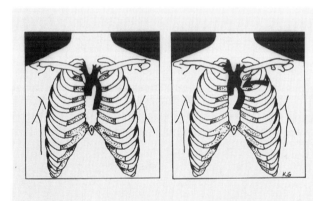

Figure 2. Diagram of the thoracic aorta. Normal appearance on the left and a site of "osseous pinch" on the right (arrow).

TUTORIAL 4
THORACIC AORTIC TRAUMA
Mark A. Westcott, M.D., and
Marcelle J. Shapiro, M.D.

Introduction
The subjects addressed in this tutorial include:
1. The mechanism of thoracic aortic injury
2. The clinical indications for radiographic analysis
3. Plain film findings
4. The role of noninvasive imaging
5. Angiographic technique, findings, and pitfalls
6. The types of thoracic aorta and great vessel injury.

With the advent of high-speed vehicular travel, the incidence of blunt chest and thoracic aortic trauma has increased dramatically. Aortic rupture is a cause of death in 16% of patients involved in motor vehicle accidents and other accidents involving rapid deceleration. The importance of its early diagnosis and treatment was first documented by Parmley in 1958: only 15% of patients with aortic rupture survive long enough to be hospitalized; if undiagnosed, aortic rupture carries a 30% mortality rate at 6 hours, 50% at 24 hours, and 90% within 4 months. Three to five percent of patients with undiagnosed injuries go on to develop a chronic pseudoaneurysm, which has an ever-present risk of rupture. These statistics demand a prompt and thorough clinical and radiologic evaluation of any patient surviving a rapid deceleration injury **(Fig. 1)**.

Mechanism
It was initially believed that traumatic aortic rupture was caused by a combination of traction, torsion, and hydrostatic forces acting primarily at points of attachment: the aortic root, isthmus, and diaphragmatic hiatus. However, more recent investigations on cadavers have shown that the mechanism of aortic injury is compressive forces on the manubrium, first rib, and medial clavicles that cause them to rotate posteriorly and impact upon the thoracic spine, thereby shearing interposed vascular structures ("osseous pinch"). The subsequent disruption of the intima and media may be contained by the adventitia and/or periadventitial structures, leading to pseudoaneurysm formation **(Fig. 2)**.

Clinical Presentation
Patients with thoracic aorta or great vessel injury often present with nonspecific symptoms and signs including chest and back pain, dysphagia, dyspnea, and/or a mid scapular systolic murmur. A rare but more specific sign is elevation of the blood pressure and pulse amplitude in the upper extremities with a decrease in the lower extremities suggesting an acute post-traumatic coarctation syndrome. Paralysis due to an interruption in blood supply to the spinal cord is a rare complication of thoracic aortic rupture.

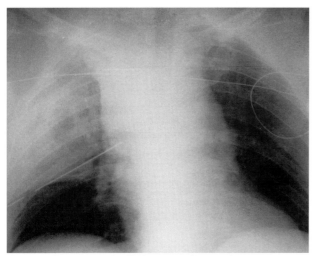

Figure 3. Posteroanterior (PA) chest radiograph from a 46-year-old woman involved in a motor vehicle accident (MVA). There is marked widening of the superior mediastinum with obscuration of the normal aortic arch contour, along with a right upper lobe density representing pulmonary contusion.

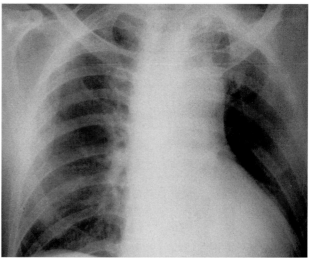

Figure 4. PA chest radiograph from a 45-year-old unrestrained driver involved in an MVA with direct blunt trauma to the chest from the steering wheel. There is marked mediastinal widening and loss of aortic arch contour.

Plain Film Findings

While many plain film findings have been associated with thoracic aortic injury, few are specific for aortic disruption. Most findings represent changes from mediastinal hemorrhage, which is usually produced by disruption of small vessels and not the aorta. The index of suspicion for an aortic injury rises in the presence of mediastinal hemorrhage because the forces which create both are similar. The most frequently identified radiographic abnormalities are:

1) Mediastinal widening—A mediastinum that measures greater than or equal to 8 centimeters at the T4 level in the absence of a vertebral fracture is the most common finding with mediastinal hemorrhage **(Fig. 3)**. Some authors have touted a mediastinal width to chest width ratio of greater than 0.25–0.38 as a more reliable indicator of aortic rupture. Supine chest radiographs with poor inspiratory effort tend to overestimate the width of the mediastinum, thereby limiting the value of these measurements. Therefore, all efforts to obtain an erect, posteroanterior chest radiograph should be made in order to adequately exclude mediastinal widening.

2) Loss of aortic knob contour—This finding has the highest sensitivity for aortic rupture, especially in combination with mediastinal widening, but the specificity is low **(Fig. 4)**.

3) Deviation of the nasogastric tube to the right of midline at T4.

4) Deviation of the trachea to the right **(Fig. 5)**.

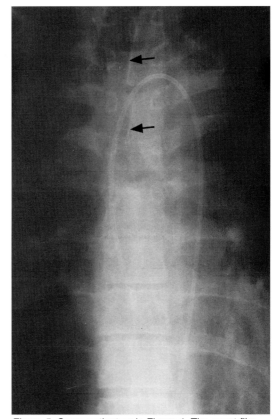

Figure 5. Same patient as in Figure 4. The scout film from the anteroposterior aortogram shows deviation of the trachea to the right side of the spine (arrows) with associated increased soft tissue density in the superior mediastinum.

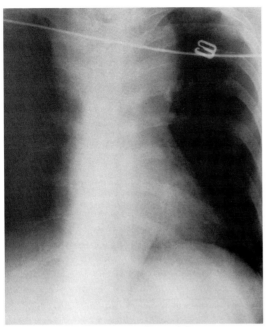

Figure 6. The supine chest radiograph from an unrestrained driver involved in an MVA shows marked widening of the superior mediastinum with obscuration of the aortic arch and descending aorta.

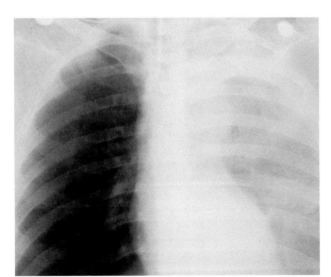

Figure 7. Supine chest radiograph from a young man involved in an MVA with confirmed thoracic aortic transection. There is a left hemothorax along with obscuration of the aortic arch.

5) Depression of the left mainstem bronchus—Depression greater than 40 degrees from the horizontal on an inspiratory erect film.

6) Apical pleural cap—This is usually on the left, associated with other plain film findings, and is indicative of hemothorax.

7) Abnormal contour of the aorta with enlargement and/or obscuration of the descending aorta (Fig. 6).

8) Left hemothorax (Fig. 7).

9) Widening of paraspinal lines in the absence of sternal or vertebral fracture.

10) Less common signs—These include displacement of the superior vena cava or aortic intimal calcification and enlargement of the cardiac silhouette secondary to hemopericardium.

Despite this list, there is no single sensitive or specific plain film finding which confirms aortic rupture. A normal-appearing mediastinum on a technically adequate erect chest radiograph tends to exclude the diagnosis, and some investigators would therefore argue that a period of observation is sufficient. With any clinical or radiographic suspicion in a patient who experienced a severe deceleration injury, further diagnostic studies are warranted.

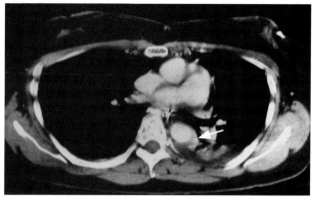

Figure 8. Axial CT scan from a woman involved in a "head on" collision. The physical exam showed a sternal fracture and multiple rib fractures. There is a high-attenuation area surrounding the descending aorta (arrow) representing a mediastinal hematoma, in addition to atelectasis and pleural effusion.

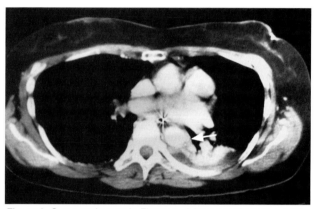

Figure 9. Same patient as in Figure 8. A lower cut from the axial CT scan shows streak artifacts running across the mediastinum, partially obscuring the aortic contour abnormality in the proximal descending aorta (arrow). A tear was confirmed on a subsequent aortogram.

Computed Tomography

Computed tomography (CT) scanning is a less invasive, less expensive, potentially more expedient examination which requires less technical expertise and fewer support staff than arteriography. However, the utility of CT scanning in this clinical setting has been debated, mainly because of its greater ability to identify secondary signs of aortic disruption rather than primary signs. The most common finding on CT examination is mediastinal hemorrhage, a secondary sign frequently caused by disruption of small and medium sized arteries or veins **(Fig. 8)**. Primary (direct) CT findings include abrupt changes in aortic caliber, irregularity of the arch contour, and/or the presence of an intimal flap. Unfortunately, these findings can easily be obscured by patient or cardio-vascular motion and/or volume averaging on conventional axial imaging **(Fig. 9)**.

Studies performed to date also have not accurately determined the false negative rate of CT scanning. Most authors of large series have assumed that a CT examination that depicted a normal mediastinum effectively excluded aortic injury and that such patients could be observed clinically. However, there have been reports of confirmed aortic rupture in patients who had a normal initial CT examination. Based upon extensive experience at the University of Maryland Shock Trauma Center, Mirvis et al believe that if properly performed and interpreted, CT scanning can *reduce* the number of negative arteriograms obtained. However, CT scanning cannot completely eliminate the need for arteriography.

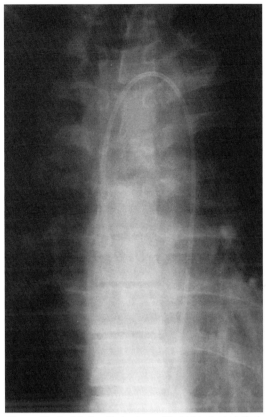

Figure 10. A pigtail catheter is positioned just cephalad of the aortic valve cusps for diagnostic aortography.

The advent of spiral CT technology has afforded a previously unavailable opportunity to evaluate the aorta directly, raising the possibility of a completely noninvasive screening evaluation in cases of blunt trauma. Data regarding the utility of spiral CT scanning in this setting has been limited to a recent series by Gavant et al. These authors used spiral scanning to screen over 1,500 patients with non-trivial blunt chest trauma. The authors reported 100% sensitivity and 81.7% specificity in detecting aortic injuries. They therefore concluded that a normal-appearing aorta on spiral CT scanning, even in the face of a mediastinal hematoma, is sufficient to exclude a significant aortic injury. However, with indeterminate findings or an inadequate study of the aorta, emergency aortography is still required. Unfortunately, the statistics of this study are based on the assumption that a normal-appearing mediastinum (ie, no evidence of hematoma) effectively excludes any aortic injury. Once again, the predictive value of a negative CT scan has not been delineated. The use of spiral CT as a screening study to exclude aortic injury appears promising. However, adoption of spiral CT alone as a screening tool must await a larger, multicenter series where all patients are studied by both CT and arteriography.

Arteriography
Currently arteriography remains the gold standard for the evaluation of thoracic aortic and great vessel trauma. When performed by an experienced angiographer, thoracic aortography is a safe, expedient, sensitive, and specific examination.

Technique
Using standard Seldinger technique and transfemoral approach, a pigtail catheter is advanced into the ascending thoracic aorta above the valve cusps **(Fig. 10)** to ensure opacification of both the aortic root and great vessels. While leading with a floppy-tipped guide wire, any resistance to passage of the catheter should prompt a gentle hand injection of contrast material to insure intraluminal passage. Occasionally a selective catheter may be needed to negotiate a stenotic segment. Difficulty in passage of a guide wire or catheter may warrant use of an alternate vascular route such as a transaxillary/transbrachial arterial approach or an intravenous digital subtraction angiogram. The latter does not provide the line-pair resolution necessary to exclude a subtle aortic tear, but it can demonstrate a large disruption that prevents easy passage of catheters from standard arterial approaches.

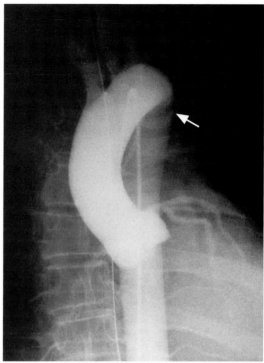

Figure 11. Same patient as in Figure 8. The PA projection from the thoracic aortogram shows a subtle crescentic double density visible in the proximal descending aorta at the level of the isthmus (arrow), confirmed to be aortic transection.

At least two views of the aorta should be obtained, extending from the root to the diaphragmatic hiatus and including the proximal great vessels. Standard views include the right posterior oblique (RPO) (~45 degrees), and PA projections **(Figs. 11, 12)**. In patients with a right aortic arch or suspicion of an anterior injury, a right anterior oblique (RAO) projection may be helpful **(Figs. 13, 14)**. Either conventional or digital subtraction arteriography (DSA) may be performed. DSA is often faster, requires less contrast material and smaller catheters, and saves on film costs. Some angiographers contend that small intimal injuries may be missed on DSA and that at least one view should be performed with conventional imaging. Conventional arteriography usually requires an injection of 60–80 mL of 76% contrast material during a 2-second-long injection, while DSA requires approximately half of this volume. Regardless of technique, rapid filming is necessary to insure adequate visualization. If an injury is identified, a cardiothoracic surgeon should be notified immediately. An arterial sheath may be left in place to avoid any operative delay and to provide continuous arterial access.

Angiographic Findings—Acute Injury
The most common angiographic finding is a pseudoaneurysm at the level of the aortic isthmus just distal to the left subclavian artery (90%). The false aneurysm is identified as a collection of contrast material that extends beyond the expected contour of the aorta, involving a portion or the entire circumference **(Figs. 15, 16)**, and which persists into the venous phase. Most pseudoaneurysms are contained by adventitia and/or periadventitial tissues; free extravasation is rarely seen. Occasionally, a linear lucency representing the lacerated intimal and medial layers of the aortic wall may be identified within the pseudoaneurysm.

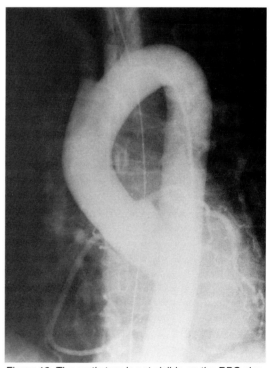

Figure 12. The aortic tear is not visible on the RPO view.

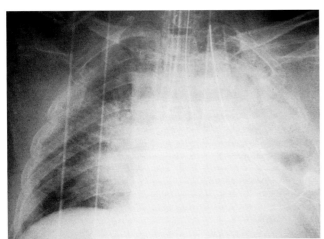

Figure 13. Supine chest radiograph from a woman struck "head on" at high speed. There is mediastinal widening, obscuration of the aortic arch and descending aorta, opacification of the left hemithorax representing both pulmonary contusion and hemothorax, and multiple rib fractures. Aortography was performed, but conventional projections failed to reveal a tear.

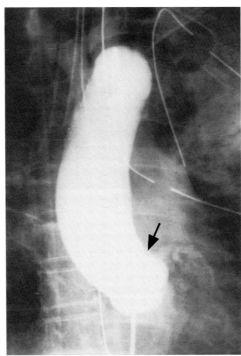

Figure 14. Same patient as in Figure 13. Because of a high index of suspicion, an RAO arteriogram was obtained. There is a small intimal defect immediately above the aortic valve along the anterior aortic wall (arrow). Surgery confirmed a nontransmural tear, which was primarily repaired.

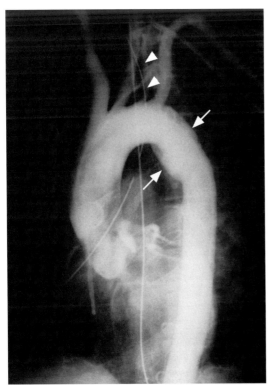

Figure 15. RPO projection from the thoracic aortogram of an unrestrained driver involved in a high-speed MVA. Complete aortic transection just distal to the left subclavian artery is represented by the extraluminal, circumferential collection of contrast material (arrows). This was surgically confirmed and successfully repaired. There is also variant anatomy with the left vertebral artery originating directly from the arch between the left common carotid and subclavian arteries (arrowheads).

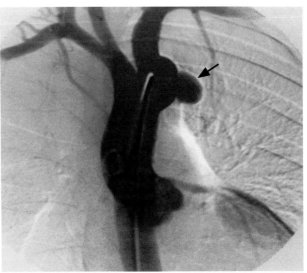

Figure 16. A patient with a severe deceleration injury in which she was thrown from a bicycle. There is a 1.5-cm traumatic pseudoaneurysm originating from the inferolateral portion of the aorta distal to the left subclavian artery (arrow).

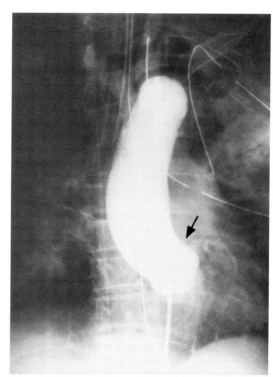

Figure 17. Same patient as in Figure 13. There is a subtle intimal defect along the anterior aortic wall representing a surgically proven nontransmural traumatic tear (arrow).

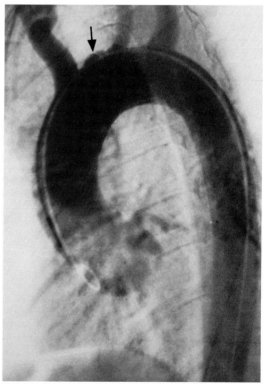

Figure 18. RPO thoracic aortogram in a driver who hit a telephone pole, sustaining a C3–4 vertebral fracture-dislocation and sternal fracture. The focal extraluminal collection of contrast material between the innominate and left common carotid arteries (arrow) is associated with a small intimal defect. This traumatic aortic transection was successfully surgically repaired.

Injury may occur at other sites including the ascending aorta/aortic root (5%) **(Fig. 17)** and, rarely, the descending thoracic aorta at the diaphragmatic hiatus (1%), as well as any site along the aortic arch **(Fig. 18)**. The true incidence of ascending aortic tears is higher than that identified by angiography (22% in autopsy series), because a greater percentage of these patients die before receiving medical attention. Three to four percent of patients have multiple sites of injury **(Figs. 19, 20)**. Occasionally, an intimal flap, identified as a lucency within the contrast-filled aorta, may be the only finding and may be best seen on subtraction images **(Figs. 21, 22)**.

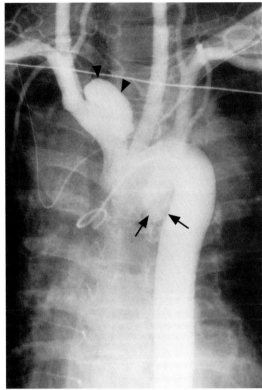

Figure 19. RPO thoracic aortogram of an automobile driver involved in a high-speed MVA. A large pseudoaneurysm originates from the innominate artery (arrowheads). A pseudoaneurysm is present at the level of the isthmus in the proximal descending thoracic aorta (arrows).

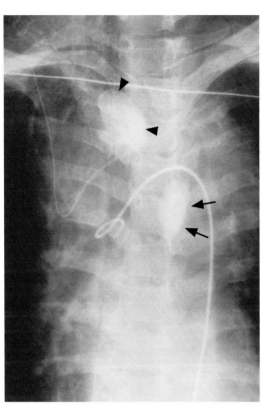

Figure 20. Same patient as in Figure 19. A delayed image from the aortogram shows persistent collections of contrast material at sites of traumatic tears in the innominate artery (arrowheads) and proximal descending aorta (arrows).

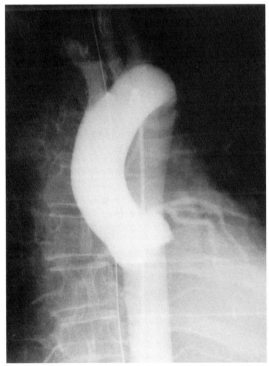

Figure 21. Same patient as in Figure 11. The thoracic aortogram shows a crescentic, extraluminal double density in the proximal descending aorta.

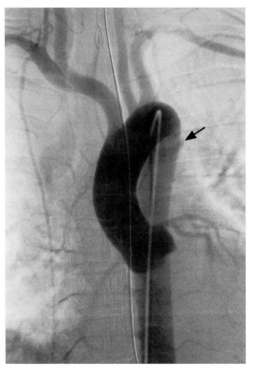

Figure 22. Optical subtraction image from the same patient as in Figure 11. The extraluminal double density is more readily identified on the subtraction image (arrow). This was a surgically confirmed aortic transection.

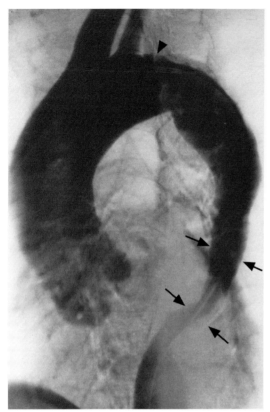

Figure 23. RPO projection, subtraction image, from a thoracic aortogram of a young woman who had been thrown from a building as a result of a bomb blast in World War II. A chest radiograph revealed a calcified pseudoaneurysm (not shown). The thoracic aortogram shows an occluded left subclavian artery (arrowhead) and marked narrowing of the descending aorta (arrows) felt to represent a traumatic coarctation.

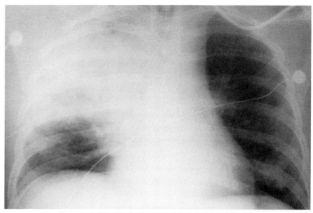

Figure 24. Chest radiograph from a young man involved in an MVA shows a large right pulmonary contusion, subpleural hematoma, and rib fractures. There is also associated obscuration of the aortic arch and widening of the mediastinum. On aortography, the aortic arch proved normal.

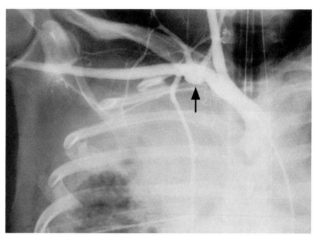

Figure 25. Selective innominate arteriography shows a traumatic pseudoaneurysm (arrow) of the right subclavian artery in the region of the right vertebral, costocervical, and internal mammary arteries.

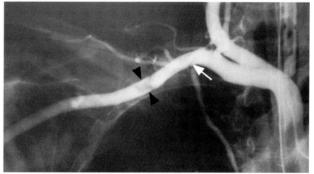

Figure 26. Selective innominate arteriography shows an intimal defect (arrow) and associated clot in the right subclavian artery (arrowheads). This was associated with multiple rib fractures and a right clavicular fracture.

Acute Post-Traumatic Aortic Coarctation Syndrome

Acute post-traumatic aortic coarctation syndrome is a rare entity caused by partial occlusion of the aorta by an intimal flap and/or compression by an adjacent pseudoaneurysm **(Fig. 23)**. Clinically this syndrome may be recognized as an increase in blood pressure and pulse amplitude in the upper extremities with a concomitant decrease in the lower extremities.

Brachiocephalic Artery Injuries

Brachiocephalic artery injuries occur more frequently in combination with aortic or other brachiocephalic lacerations. The innominate artery is the second most common site of vascular injury in cases of blunt chest trauma. The common carotid and subclavian arteries should also be assessed, although injuries to these vessels are rarely seen **(Figs. 24, 25)**. The potential for a great vessel injury demands caution when thoracic aortography is performed from a transbrachial approach **(Fig. 26)**.

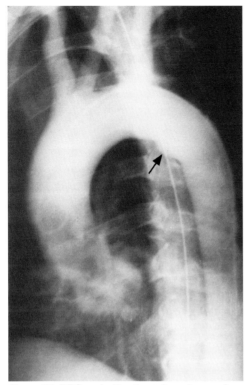

Figure 27. RPO projection thoracic aortogram from a young patient involved in an MVA. The focal convexity along the ventromedial wall of the aorta (arrow) represents a typical "ductus bump" and not an aortic transection.

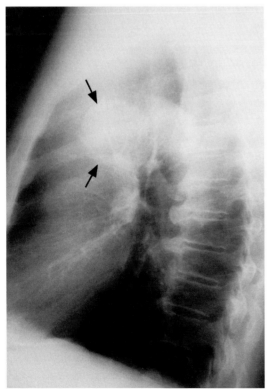

Figure 29. Same patient as in Figure 28. The lateral chest radiograph shows the mediastinal mass (arrows).

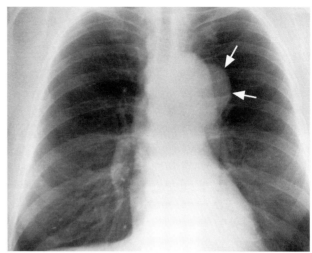

Figure 28. PA chest radiograph from a 54-year-old man who fell from a ladder 2 years earlier. There is a mediastinal mass filling the aortopulmonary window (arrows).

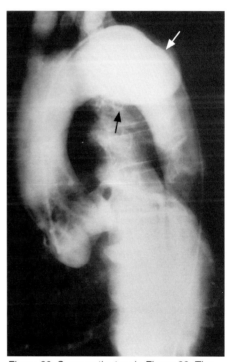

Figure 30. Same patient as in Figure 28. The thoracic aortogram confirms a traumatic pseudoaneurysm immediately distal to the left subclavian artery (arrows).

Angiographic Pitfalls

Anatomic variants and abnormalities that are not life-threatening may mimic a pseudoaneurysm at angiography. The ductus diverticulum ("bump") represents the remaining distal portion of the embryonic right arch and is seen angiographically in 9%–26% of patients as a focal convexity of the proximal descending thoracic aorta along the ventromedial wall **(Fig. 27)**. It forms obtuse angles with the aortic wall; however, the superior angle may occasionally be acute. A pseudoaneurysm will usually form an acute angle with the aorta, involve the entire circumference, and show delayed washout of contrast material **(Figs. 28–30)**.

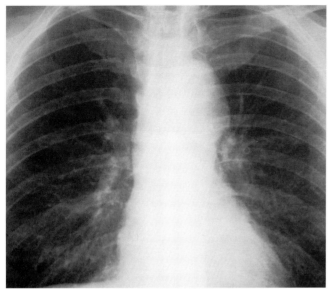

Figure 31. A 48-year-old man with a history of melanoma was noted to have a progressively widening mediastinal mass in the aortopulmonary window on a chest radiograph performed to rule out metastases.

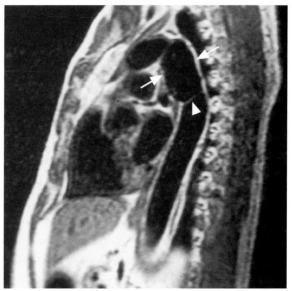

Figure 32. Sagittal T1-weighted MR image shows enlargement of the proximal descending aorta (arrows) with an intimal flap indicating a pseudoaneurysm (arrowhead).

Chronic Injury

Approximately 2%–3% of patients with traumatic aorta ruptures are not diagnosed at the time of injury and eventually develop chronic pseudoaneurysms. These pseudoaneurysms are typically saccular and involve the medial wall of the aorta immediately distal to the left subclavian artery. Patients often survive injury at this location because multiple mediastinal structures including the trachea, pulmonary artery, left mainstem bronchus, and aortic arch aid in containing the rupture. The diagnosis is often made years after the initial injury, either during evaluation for an unrelated condition **(Fig. 31)** or for symptoms related to the pseudoaneurysm such as hoarseness, dyspnea, and cough which have developed in the interim. The chest radiograph usually shows a mediastinal mass in the aorto-pulmonary window often with a calcified rim, and CT scanning, MR imaging, and/or angiography confirm the presence of a pseudoaneurysm **(Figs. 32–35)**. Surgical excision with placement of an interposition graft is recommended soon after the diagnosis is made, because the risk of rupture remains even years following the initial event. Although the procedure is still in its infancy, endovascular stent-graft placement across a traumatic aortic tear may prove in the future to be a viable treatment alternative.

For further information on this topic, please see Teaching File Cases 4, 5, and 6.

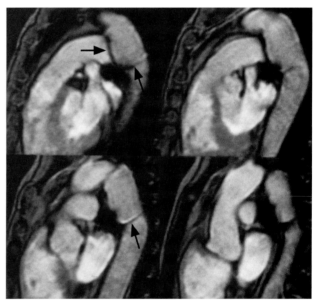

Figure 33. Cine loop MR image confirms the presence of blood flow into the pseudoaneurysm. There are intimal defects both proximally and distally (arrows).

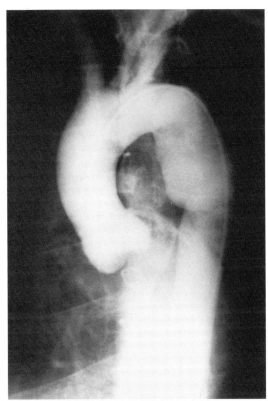

Figure 34. An early image from the thoracic aortogram confirms the presence of a traumatic pseudoaneurysm in the proximal descending aorta. This was surgically repaired.

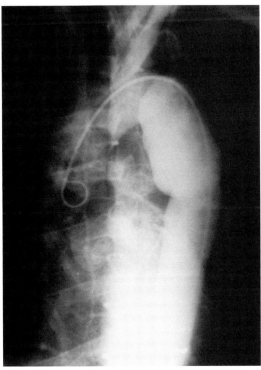

Figure 35. A later image from the thoracic aortogram shows the traumatic pseudoaneurysm in the proximal descending aorta.

Selected Readings

Ben-Menachem Y. Rupture of the thoracic aorta by broadside impacts in road traffic and other collisions: further angiographic observations and preliminary autopsy findings. J Trauma 1993; 35:363–367.

Cohen AM, Crass JR, Thomas HA, Fisher RG, Jacobs DG. CT evidence for the "osseous pinch" mechanism of traumatic aortic injury. AJR 1992; 159:271–274.

Cohen AM, Crass JR. Traumatic aortic injuries: current concepts. Semin Ultrasound CT MR 1993; 14:71–84.

Crass JR, Cohen AM, Motta AO, Tomashefski JF Jr, Wiesen EJ. A proposed new mechanism of traumatic aortic rupture: the osseous pinch. Radiology 1990; 176:645–649.

Dennis LN. Superior mediastinal widening from spine fractures mimicking aortic rupture on chest radiographs. AJR 1989; 152:27–30.

Fisher RG, Chasen MH, Lamki N. Diagnosis of injuries of the aorta and brachiocephalic arteries caused by blunt chest trauma: CT vs aortography. AJR 1994; 162:1047–1052.

Fisher RG, Hadlock F. Laceration of the thoracic aorta and brachiocephalic arteries by blunt trauma. Report of 54 cases and review of the literature. Radiol Clin North Am 1981; 19:91–110.

Gavant ML, Menke PG, Fabian T, Flick PA, Graney MJ, Gold RE. Blunt traumatic aortic rupture: detection with helical CT of the chest. Radiology 1995; 197:125–133.

Gundry SR, Williams S, Burney RE, Cho KJ, Mackenzie JR. Indications for aortography in blunt thoracic trauma: a reassessment. J Trauma 1982; 22:664–671.

Hilgenberg AD, Logan DL, Akins CW, et al. Blunt injuries of the thoracic aorta. Ann Thorac Surg 1992; 53:233–239.

Madayag MA, Kirshenbaum KJ, Nadimpalli SR, Fantus RJ, Cavallino RP, Crystal GJ. Thoracic aortic trauma: role of dynamic CT. Radiology 1991; 179:853–855.

Marnocha KE, Maglinte DD. Plain film criteria for excluding aortic rupture in blunt chest trauma. AJR 1985; 144:19–21.

McLoud TC, Isler RJ, Novelline RA, Putman CE, Simeone J, Stark P. The apical cap. AJR 1981; 137:299–306.

Mirvis SE, Bidwell JK, Buddemeyer EU, Diaconis JN, Pais SO, Whitley JE. Imaging diagnosis of traumatic aortic rupture: a review and experience at a major trauma center. Invest Radiol 1987; 22:187–196.

Mirvis SE, Bidwell JK, Buddemeyer EU, et al. Value of chest radiography in excluding traumatic aortic rupture. Radiology 1987; 163:487–493.

Mirvis SE, Pais SO, Gens DR. Thoracic aortic rupture: advantages of intraarterial digital subtraction angiography. AJR 1986; 146:987–991.

Morgan PW, Goodman LR, Aprahamian C, Foley WD, Lipchik EO. Evaluation of traumatic aortic injury: does contrast-enhanced CT play a role? Radiology 1992; 182:661–666.

Morse SS, Glickman MG, Greenwood LH. Traumatic aortic rupture: false-positive aortographic diagnosis due to a typical ductus diverticulum. AJR 1988; 150:793–796.

Rabinsky I, Sidhu GS, Wagner RB. Mid descending aortic traumatic aneurysms. Ann Thorac Surg 1990; 50:155–160.

Raptopoulos V, Sheiman RG, Phillips DA, Davidoff A, Silva WE. Traumatic aortic tear: screening with chest CT. Radiology 1992; 182:667–673.

Sefczek DM, Sefczek RJ, Deeb ZL. Radiographic signs of acute traumatic rupture of the thoracic aorta. AJR 1983; 141:1259–1262.

Shively BK. Transesophageal echocardiography in the diagnosis of aortic disease. Semin Ultrasound CT MR 1993; 14:106–116.

Simeone JF, Deren MM, Cagle F. The value of the left apical cap in the diagnosis of aortic rupture: a prospective and retrospective study. Radiology 1981; 139:35–37.

Tomiak MM, Rosenblum JD, Messersmith RN, Zarins CK. Use of CT for diagnosis of traumatic rupture of the thoracic aorta. Ann Vasc Surg 1993; 7:130–139.

Trerotola SO. Can helical CT replace aortography in thoracic trauma? Radiology 1995; 197:13–15.

Williams DM, Dake MR, Bolling SF, Deeb GM. The role of intravascular ultrasound in acute traumatic aortic rupture. Semin Ultrasound CT MR 1993; 14:85–90.

Woodring JH, Fried AM, Hatfield DR, Stevens RK, Todd EP. Fractures of first and second ribs: predictive value for arterial and bronchial injury. AJR 1982; 138:211–215.

Woodring JH, King JG. The potential effects of radiographic criteria to exclude aortography in patients with blunt chest trauma. Results of a study of 32 patients with proved aortic or brachiocephalic arterial injury. J Thorac Cardiovasc Surg 1989; 97:456–460.

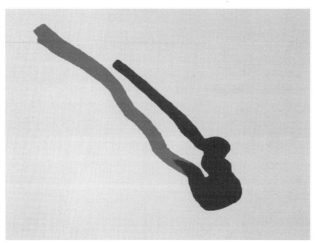

Figure 1. Schematic of a simple pulmonary arteriovenous malformation.

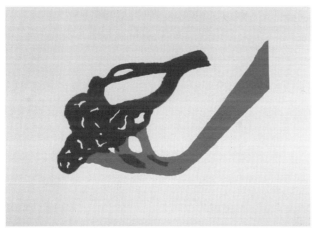

Figure 2. Schematic of a complex pulmonary arteriovenous malformation.

TUTORIAL 5
PULMONARY ARTERIOVENOUS MALFORMATIONS

Jeffrey S. Pollak, M.D., and
Robert I. White, Jr., M.D.

Introduction
The subjects addressed in this tutorial include: 1. Pathology of pulmonary arteriovenous malformation 2. Background 3. Pathophysiology and clinical manifestations 4. Diagnostic evaluation 5. Treatment 6. Follow-up 7. Related disorders: acquired fistula and pulmonary artery aneurysm.

Pathology of Pulmonary Arteriovenous Malformation
A pulmonary arteriovenous malformation (PAVM) consists of the abnormal connection of a pulmonary artery directly to a pulmonary vein, bypassing the capillary bed. The usual appearance is that of a single artery, a single draining vein, and a thin-walled, aneurysmal connection **(Fig. 1)**. Less commonly, numerous arteries and veins may be seen. When this occurs, the communication is generally a complex intervening network of vessels, similar to the nidus of a high-flow systemic or cerebral arteriovenous malformation **(Fig. 2)**. Between 33% and 50% of patients with PAVMs have multiple lesions, and in 8%–42% of patients, the PAVMs are bilateral. The lesions are frequently located just beneath the pleura.

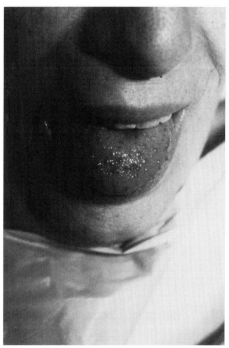

Figure 3. Lingual and facial telangiectasia.

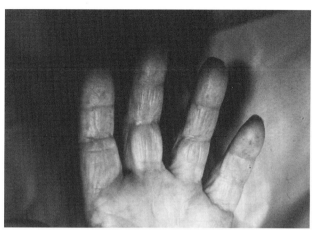

Figure 4. Finger telangiectasia.

Hereditary Hemorrhagic Telangiectasia (Osler-Weber-Rendu Syndrome)	
Primary Organ Involvement	**Manifestations**
• Skin	• Telangiectasia, bleeding
• Nose	• Epistaxis (90%)
• Lung	• PAVM (15%)
• CNS	• Stroke, abscess, vascular malformations
• Gastrointestinal tract	• GI bleeding (20%)

Figure 5. Table of HHT manifestations.

Background

In our experience, over 80% of PAVMs occur in patients with hereditary hemorrhagic telangiectasia (HHT) (Osler-Weber-Rendu syndrome). This disorder has the classic triad of epistaxis, mucocutaneous telangiectasia (face and tongue in **Figure 3**, and fingers in **Figure 4**), and autosomal dominant inheritance. While its prevalence is reported to be 2 to 3 per 100,000, we believe that careful family screening will uncover many undiagnosed patients. In the setting of HHT, there is roughly a 15% risk of PAVM, although the risk is even higher when a family member has PAVM. In fact, HHT appears to be a genetically heterogeneous disorder. The specific gene for HHT associated with PAVM has recently been identified as endoglin; it lies on chromosome 9 and produces an endothelial cell receptor for transforming growth factor ß. The manifestations of HHT are listed in **Figure 5**. Sporadic cases account for the remainder of PAVMs.

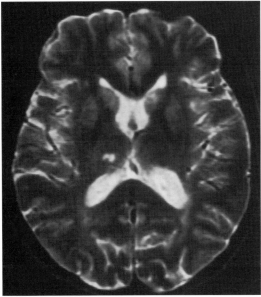

Figure 6. T2-weighted magnetic resonance scan shows a right thalamic infarct.

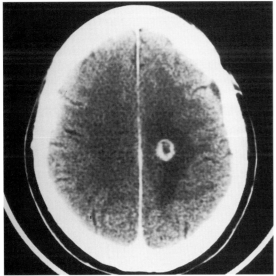

Figure 7. CT scan shows a ring-enhancing left parietal brain abscess.

Diagnostic Evaluation for Suspected PAVM: Potential Modalities

- History and physical—evidence of PAVM or HHT
- Chest radiographs
- Arterial blood gases and oxygen saturation
— On room air and 100% O_2, to assess for shunt
— Supine and erect
- Contrast echocardiography
- Radionuclide shunt studies
- CT scanning—conventional, spiral, and 3-D
- Pulmonary arteriography

Figure 8.

Pathophysiology and Clinical Manifestations

Right-to-left shunting of blood results in arterial hypoxemia and permits paradoxical emboli. Additionally, these thin-walled lesions may rupture. Clinical manifestations of PAVM include dyspnea (70%), fatigue, cyanosis, clubbing, polycythemia, stroke or transient ischemic attacks (55%), brain abscess (9%), and hemoptysis and hemothorax (9%). High-output cardiac failure is rare, although it has been described in neonates. In our experience, the central nervous system sequelae of stroke **(Fig. 6)**, transient ischemic attack, and abscess **(Fig. 7)** are more common modes of presentation than are cyanosis and dyspnea. Polycythemia is unusual, probably due to epistaxis and gastrointestinal bleeding in patients with HHT.

Diagnostic Evaluation

In addition to evaluating patients with manifestations suspicious for PAVM, it is important to assess asymptomatic patients with HHT **(Fig. 8)**. The goal is not just to determine if a PAVM is present, but also whether it is of sufficient size to require treatment. Our approach is to obtain chest radiographs and arterial blood gases on room air and 100% oxygen. A low resting PaO_2 (less than 90 mm Hg) or insufficient rise on 100% O_2 (less than 600 mm Hg) is suggestive of a significant PAVM. In addition, these serve as pretherapy baseline measurements.

Other investigators have suggested that supine and erect oxygen saturation measurements by pulse oximetry provide an easier, less invasive diagnostic method. A drop in arterial oxygen when the patient is standing erect is frequent and is caused by the predilection of PAVMs for the lower lobes. Radionuclide shunt studies have also been described as a method to quantitate the right-to-left shunt.

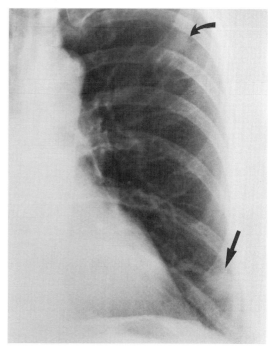

Figure 9. Plain chest radiograph shows PAVMs in the left lower lobe (straight arrow) and in the left upper lobe (curved arrow).

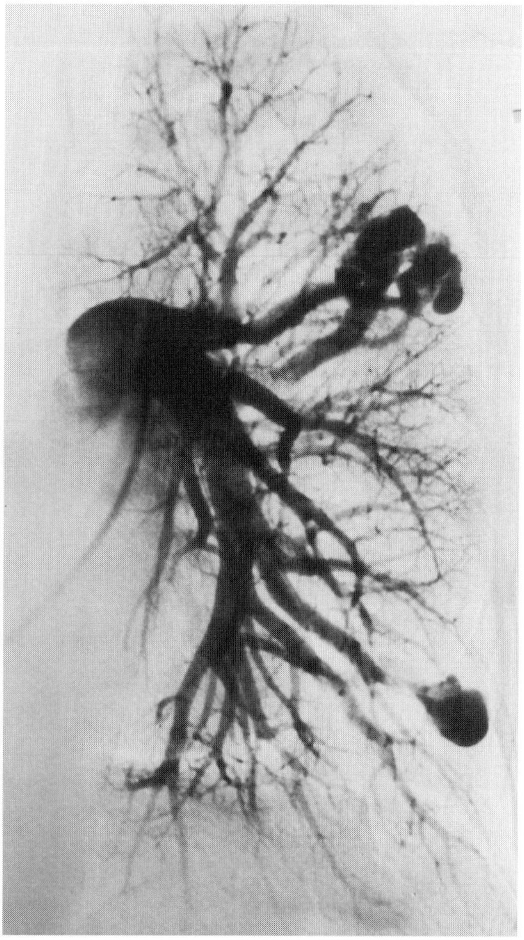

Chest Radiography

Chest radiographs may show a lobular soft tissue mass representing the aneurysm or nidus **(Fig. 9)**, with feeding and draining vessels. The aneurysm of simple lesions is generally well defined, but identification of the arterial channel emanating from the hilum and the venous channel leading to the left atrium is often difficult. Complex malformations **(Fig. 9)** may appear multilobulated and may have less well-defined margins. **Figure 10** is the arteriogram for the patient shown in **Figure 9**. A negative chest radiograph should not be relied upon alone for excluding the presence of PAVM. Lesions hidden by the diaphragms represent one pitfall of plain films.

Figure 10. Pulmonary arteriogram corresponding to the chest radiograph shown in Figure 9. The upper lobe lesion is a complex PAVM while the lower lobe lesion is a simple PAVM.

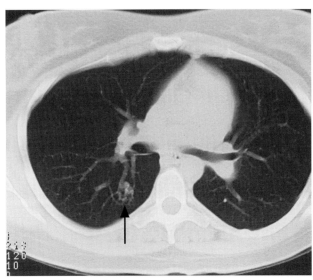

Figure 11. CT scan of a complex PAVM in the superior segment of the right lower lobe (arrow).

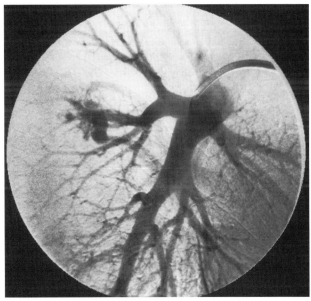

Figure 12. Corresponding pulmonary arteriogram to Figure 11.

Computed Tomography (CT) Scanning
CT scanning appears to be highly sensitive for diagnosing PAVM and localizing the involved lung segment. Criteria for diagnosis are a noncalcified nodule or serpiginous mass with feeding and draining vessels **(Figs. 11, 12)** which enhance. False positive studies (eg, vascular metastases) have been reported.

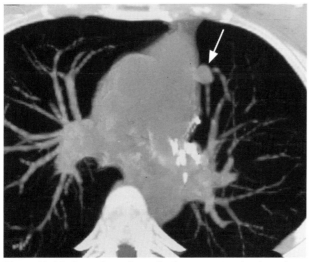

Figure 13. Maximum intensity projection reconstruction from the CT scan of a simple PAVM (arrow).

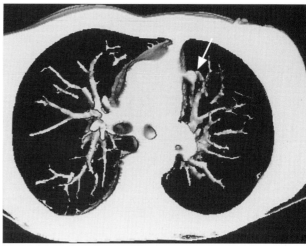

Figure 14. Cephalad view of the shaded-surface reconstruction from the CT scan of the simple PAVM shown in Figure 13 (arrow).

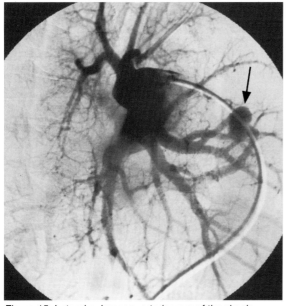

Figure 15. Lateral pulmonary arteriogram of the simple PAVM shown in Figures 13 and 14 (arrow).

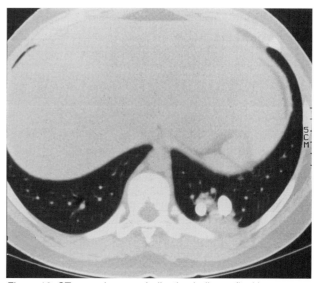

Figure 16. CT scan shows embolization balloons flanking a persistent PAVM.

Spiral CT scanning with three-dimensional techniques appears to enhance the ability to characterize a lesion as simple or complex **(Figs. 13–15)**. While it appears that aneurysms can be accurately measured by CT, it is less clear if the minimum size of the feeding arteries can be accurately determined, a key factor in deciding whether to treat asymptomatic patients. CT scanning may be especially valuable after therapy, showing persistence of a lesion **(Fig. 16)** and new or enlarging lesions.

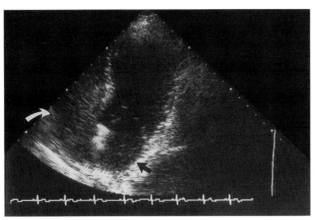

Figure 17. The apical four-chamber view from a transthoracic contrast echocardiogram shows left atrial echoes (black arrow) appearing 4 seconds after right chamber echoes, which are still present (white arrow).

Contrast Echocardiography

Ten mL of agitated saline injected intravenously normally produces echogenic microbubbles only in right cardiac chambers, since they are filtered by the pulmonary capillary bed. Detection of echoes in left-sided chambers is highly sensitive for right-to-left shunts. Careful assessment for intracardiac defects (eg, septal defects or patent foramen ovale) and the delayed appearance of left atrial echoes compared to right-sided enhancement (usually by three to four heart beats) increases specificity for PAVM. **Figure 17** is an apical four-chamber view from a transthoracic study showing left atrial echoes appearing 4 seconds after right chamber echoes, which are still present. The major limitation of echocardiography is its inability to predict the size, number, or location of malformations, all of which are critical in determining not only how to treat a patient, but also whether a patient should be treated.

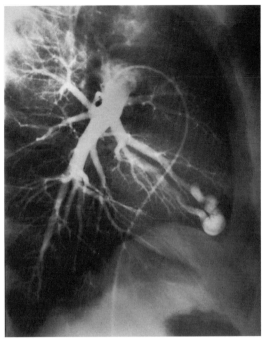

Figure 18. Lateral right pulmonary arteriogram shows a single simple PAVM in the middle lobe.

Figure 19. Frontal left pulmonary arteriogram shows a complex PAVM in the lower lobe.

Pulmonary Arteriography

Pulmonary arteriography is the definitive diagnostic study. Both lungs must be thoroughly studied because of the prevalence of multiple lesions. Frontal and oblique projections are generally obtained. More than 70% of PAVMs will show the single feeding artery, connecting aneurysm, and early, single draining vein of the simple variety **(Fig. 18)**. Twenty percent of PAVMs are complex, with numerous feeding and draining vessels and an intervening nidus **(Fig. 19)**. Uncommonly, a diffuse pattern is present, with numerous PAVMs of varying sizes involving one or more segments of the lung **(Fig. 20)**. Lesions can be quite small, and, indeed, in patients with underlying HHT, the presence of multiple tiny PAVMs must be assumed even if not evident on the arteriogram. While superimposed pulmonary vessels may occasionally mask a PAVM, it would likely be too small to warrant therapy.

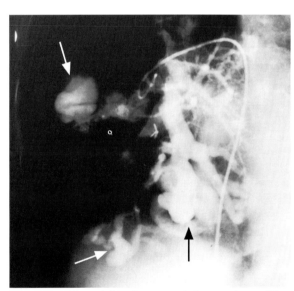

Figure 20. Oblique right pulmonary arteriogram shows diffuse involvement with numerous lesions of various sizes (arrows).

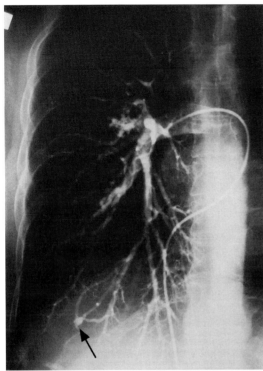

Figure 21. Simple right lower lobe PAVM (arrow) that is too small to embolize for prophylaxis against major paradoxical embolism.

Surgical Therapy for PAVM

Methods	*Disadvantages*
• Arterial ligation • Local excision • Segmentectomy • Lobectomy • Pneumonectomy	• Discomfort • Long recuperation • Sacrifice of normal lung tissue • Bilateral thoracotomies • Repeat thoracotomy for growing lesions • Surgical morbidity/mortality

Figure 22.

Preparation for Embolotherapy

• Diagnostic pulmonary arteriogram
—Identify proper approach & obliquity for each lesion
• Anticoagulation: heparin 3,000–5,000 units
• Avoid intravenous clots and air bubbles
— Avoid multiple punctures of the same vessel
— Phlebotomy for polycythemia
• Monitoring
— Electrocardiography
— Blood pressure
— Pulse oximetry

Figure 23.

Treatment—Indications

Treatment of PAVMs is indicated to alleviate symptoms of hypoxemia and reduce the risks of paradoxical embolization and rupture. Conservative therapy has unacceptably high rates of morbidity and mortality, reaching as high as 33% and 29%, respectively. A reasonable goal is the occlusion of all malformations having a feeding artery of at least 3 mm in diameter. Shunts smaller than this **(Fig. 21)** are unlikely to place the patient at significant risk for a major bland embolus; therefore, unless there are numerous, closely positioned lesions, we do not treat asymptomatic PAVMs smaller than 3 mm. It should be remembered that bacterial embolus resulting in brain abscess remains a potential source of morbidity for a malformation of any size.

Surgery

Surgical approaches include local excision of the PAVM, segmentectomy, and lobectomy. Simple ligation of feeding vessels is difficult to perform and runs the risk of missing feeding arteries. Limitations of surgery **(Fig. 22)** include the need for thoracotomy with its attendant morbidity and mortality (up to 6% mortality in some series), the sacrifice of some normal lung tissue, and the problems created by multiple lesions, bilateral lesions, and subsequently enlarging lesions elsewhere in the lung.

Embolotherapy—Preparation

Embolization should only be performed after a complete diagnostic arteriogram of each lung has been obtained. This permits identification of all abnormalities and helps determine the proper route of approach. An 8-F sheath is placed in the femoral vein and 3,000–5,000 units of heparin infused. Care must be taken to avoid introducing air or clots through intravenous lines, since these could result in paradoxical emboli. If the patient has polycythemia, phlebotomy should be performed to reduce the risk of deep venous thrombosis. Additionally, if multiple, closely-timed catheterizations are required, the femoral veins on either side should be used alternately to further reduce this risk. **Figure 23** summarizes preparatory measures.

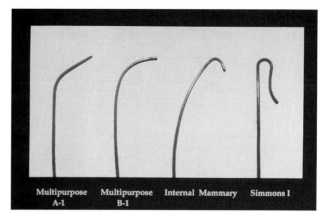

Figure 24. Catheters used for vessel selection during embolotherapy.

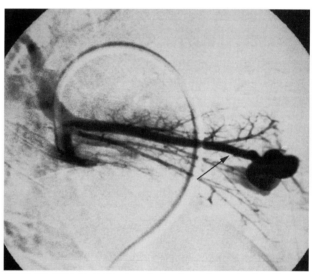

Figure 25. Proposed site of occlusion (arrow), proximal to the aneurysm but beyond significant lung branches.

Embolotherapy—Methods of Selective Catheterization

A 7-F multipurpose catheter and Bentson-type wire are useful for selecting branches supplying malformations in most areas of the lung, although occasionally internal mammary and Simmons-shaped catheters are helpful **(Fig. 24)**. Arteriography confirms proper selection and permits determination of the precise site for occlusion; however, contrast material should never be injected if backflow is not achieved, because of the risk of paradoxical air embolism. Respiratory motion occasionally poses a problem in maintaining catheter position; to mitigate this, patients can be asked to hold their breath at a certain level.

Principles of Embolization

The optimal site for occlusion is at the narrowest segment of an artery feeding a PAVM that is also beyond any substantial branches to normal lung tissue **(Fig. 25)**. The aneurysm itself does not need to be embolized, and attempting to do so may result in rupture or migration of the embolic device. Similarly, the "nidus" of complex lesions does not need to be embolized. Unlike systemic arteriovenous malformations, occlusion of all feeding arteries is generally feasible and therefore sufficient to alleviate the symptoms and risks related to PAVMs. Either detachable balloons or embolization coils can be used to provide occlusion.

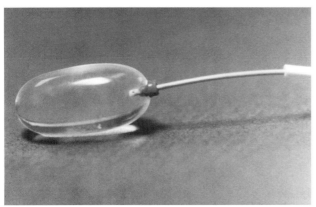

Figure 26. Interventional Therapeutics Corporation Detachable Silicone Balloon.

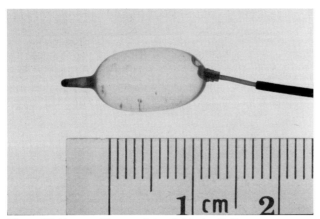

Figure 27. Nycomed-Ingenor latex Goldvalve Balloon.

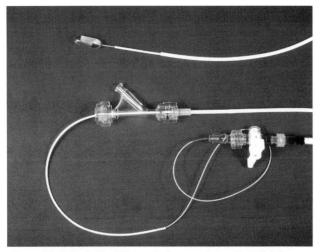

Figure 28. Detachable Silicone Balloon system with 2-F delivery catheter, 4-F coaxial detachment catheter, and 8-F introducer catheter with Y-adapter.

Detachable Balloons—Material

Currently, no detachable balloons are approved by the Food and Drug Administration for any indication. The two best known devices are the Detachable Silicone Balloon (Interventional Therapeutics Corporation, South San Francisco, CA) **(Fig. 26)** and the latex Goldvalve balloon (Nycomed-Ingenor Laboratoires, Paris, France) **(Fig. 27)**. Both come in a variety of sizes with maximum inflation diameters ranging from 4 to 14 mm. They have self-sealing valves that permit insertion of a thin, flexible catheter used for delivery and inflation which has a coaxial detachment catheter. A wide-lumen 8-F or larger introducer catheter is usually required for delivery **(Fig. 28)** with an attached Y-adapter to permit injections of contrast material.

Characteristics of Detachable Balloons

The Detachable Silicone Balloon (DSB) is made of silicone and is semipermeable. Consequently, it must be inflated with isotonic fluid to prevent swelling and rupture. Iohexol 140 (Winthrop Pharmaceuticals, New York, NY) at 273 mosm/L is an acceptable agent. Latex is not osmotically active, so the Goldvalve balloon has no such requirement. Both balloons have expansion ratios on the order of 4–7:1 **(Fig. 29)**. Vascular occlusion is the consequence of cross-sectional obstruction of blood flow. Long-term occlusion is assured if the detachable balloon remains inflated at least 3 weeks, by which time organized thrombus and vessel obliteration about the detachable balloon should have developed.

Delivery of Detachable Balloons

Once the multipurpose catheter is in the desired location, a 260-cm Rosen wire (Cook, Bloomington, IN) is used to exchange for the 8-F introducer (this usually comes with a smaller inner catheter to provide support and a taper). The balloon is advanced by manually feeding the coaxial delivery-detachment catheter system through the introducer. The Y-adapter permits contrast material injections to confirm appropriate balloon positioning both before and after it is test inflated **(Fig. 30)**. If its location and stability are acceptable, the detachment catheter is advanced to the hub of the detachable balloon and the delivery catheter is retracted.

Coil Emboli—Material

Coil emboli are familiar to most interventionalists. Briefly, these consist of short lengths of wrapped wire with multiple polyester fibers caught between the turns. The wire is shaped into helices of predetermined diameters (conventionally available up to 15 mm now), although more complex shapes are made as well. **Figure 31** shows an 8-mm-diameter x 5-cm-long embolization coil in stretched and relaxed states. The stretched coils come in gauges permitting their introduction through 0.038-, 0.035-, 0.025-, and 0.018-inch lumen catheters, although only the first two sizes are usually needed in the pulmonary circulation. Vascular occlusion is principally due to the induction of thrombus and, to a lesser extent, physical obstruction of blood flow.

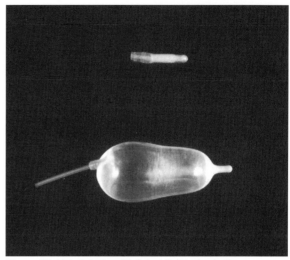

Figure 29. Uninflated and inflated Goldvalve balloons.

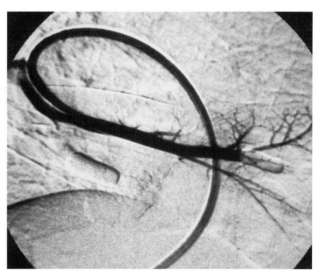

Figure 30. Arteriogram of a test inflation of a DSB in the feeding artery to the PAVM shown in Figure 25.

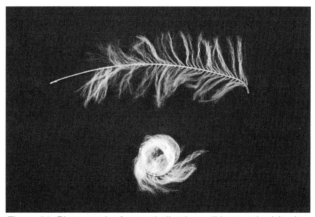

Figure 31. Photograph of an embolization coil in stretched (top) and relaxed (bottom) states.

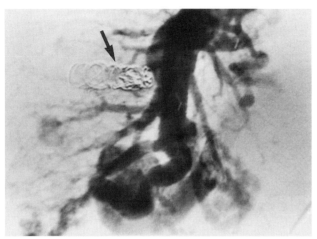

Figure 32. Same patient as in Figure 20. Nested coils (arrow) occluding one large PAVM in this patient with numerous lesions.

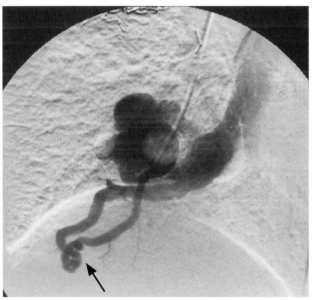

Figure 33. Occlusion balloon in the artery feeding the large malformation in the lower lobe seen in Figure 32. A smaller PAVM is also being supplied by this artery, inferiorly and laterally (arrow).

Delivery of Coil Emboli
Once an end-hole-only catheter is in appropriate position, the coils can be delivered through it using a Newton straight wire (Cook). Since the arteries feeding PAVMs are frequently relatively large, multiple coils that are progressively smaller in diameter are often needed to produce occlusion **(Fig. 32)**. The initial coils should be slightly larger than the vessel diameter to ensure stability, but not so large as to back the catheter out. With short feeding arteries, an occlusion balloon catheter can be used to maintain position during coil delivery. This catheter is also helpful for a more controlled embolization of large, high-flow PAVMs. **Figure 33** shows an occlusion balloon in the artery feeding the large lower lobe malformation seen in **Figure 32**. A smaller PAVM is also being supplied by this artery, inferiorly and laterally.

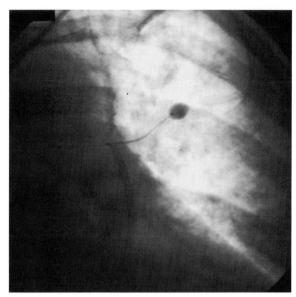

Figure 34. Detachable balloon floated into a left upper lobe branch that could not be catheterized.

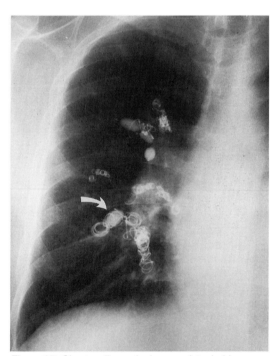

Figure 35. Chest radiograph shows a detachable balloon within a preliminary framework of coils (arrow).

Choice of Embolic Agent

Detachable balloons have several advantages. Flow directionality is possible to a limited degree, which is helpful when a feeding artery cannot be catheterized easily **(Fig. 34)**. Test occlusion is possible, permitting deflation and repositioning, and reducing the risk of paradoxical embolization. Furthermore, detachable balloons do not rely on clot formation. However, they are more cumbersome to use than coils, requiring greater preparation time and special catheters; they can rarely release prematurely or deflate; they have poor stability in markedly tapered vessels (which tend to protrude them); and they are more expensive than coils. This last disadvantage is tempered by the need for multiple coils when treating large lesions. Effective occlusion can also be achieved by placing a detachable balloon within a preliminary framework of coils that permits a more stable balloon position **(Fig. 35)**.

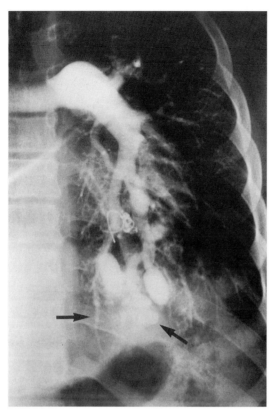

Figure 36. Growth of two branches (arrows) to a complex PAVM 30 months after embolization with detachable balloons and coils.

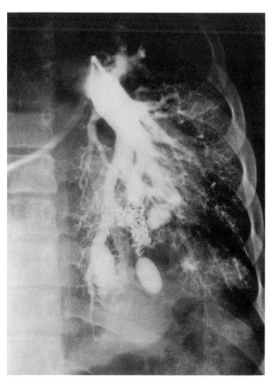

Figure 37. The second branch in Figure 36 is well seen only after coil embolization of the larger lateral branch.

Results of Embolotherapy

Complete occlusion can be achieved in nearly all lesions. Difficulties arise when diffuse lesions are located where unacceptably large volumes of lung would need to be sacrificed. Additionally, complex PAVMs with multiple feeding arteries may have an unrecognized nonembolized branch. This should be searched for on a final, nonselective arteriogram. Nevertheless, small accessory branches may escape detection and grow with time in up to 10% of patients. **Figure 36** shows growth of two branches to a complex PAVM 30 months after embolization with detachable balloons and coils; the second branch is only well seen after embolization of the larger lateral one **(Fig. 37)**. Clinically, hypoxemia improves, with improved respiratory symptoms and exercise capacity. Paradoxical migration of bland emboli and stroke remains a risk if patients have residual PAVMs with arteries exceeding 3 mm in diameter.

Procedural Complications of Embolotherapy

Paradoxical air embolization has occurred in 5% of cases. This has been well tolerated but can cause transient angina and bradycardia if it passes into the nondependent right coronary artery. Nitroglycerin and atropine should be on hand to treat this complication. Migration of embolic devices, either elsewhere in the lung or paradoxically, is rare, occurring in less than 1% of cases. Depending on location, retrieval may be necessary. **Figure 38** shows a snare retrieving an 8-mm coil that had migrated into an adjacent branch. Paradoxical thromboembolism has not been seen in our experience, arguing against the residual aneurysm acting as a source for emboli. PAVM rupture is rare and should be managed with continued embolization and prevented by avoiding intraaneurysmal embolization. We have seen deep venous thrombosis in a single patient due to repeated catheterization of the same vein. No major clinically significant complications have occurred in our experience.

Postprocedural Complications of Embolotherapy

Transient pleurisy, presumably due to infarction of normal lung parenchyma included in the embolized territory, occurs in approximately 20%–33% of cases, starting within several days of embolization and lasting for a few days. Incentive spirometry is routinely prescribed to avoid atelectasis, and a nonsteroidal anti-inflammatory agent can ameliorate the chest pain and fever. Late deflation of silicone detachable balloons is uncommon. We noted this in only 6% of cases in a series of PAVMs treated with the Detachable Silicone Balloon, although only one of the four resulted in recanalization, and this had deflated before 3 weeks. Late deflation may be more likely when the balloon is adjacent to a coil. Paradoxical embolization did not occur but recurrent dyspnea and hypoxemia prompted re-embolization. We have seen recanalization through coils as well **(Fig. 39)**. No serious late complications have been seen.

Advantages of Embolotherapy

Embolotherapy provides effective relief of symptoms and protection against future sequelae of PAVM with minimal risk, minimal discomfort, and minimal loss of normal lung parenchyma **(Fig. 40)**. Additionally, it requires only a short hospitalization and permits easy treatment of multiple and bilateral lesions as well as new, persistent, or enlarging lesions at a later date.

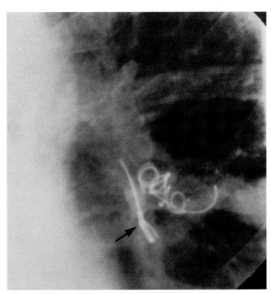

Figure 38. A coil that had migrated into an adjacent pulmonary artery was retrieved with a snare (arrow).

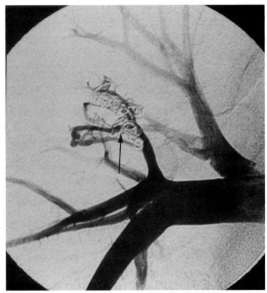

Figure 39. Recanalization through coils (arrow).

Advantages of Embolotherapy for PAVM

- Effective relief of symptoms and risks of PAVM
- Minimal procedural risk:
  — No mortality
  — Low morbidity
- Minimal discomfort during and after procedure
- Minimal loss of normal lung parenchyma
- Easy to treat multiple lesions
- Easy to repeat for new or enlarging PAVMs
- Lower cost than surgery

Figure 40.

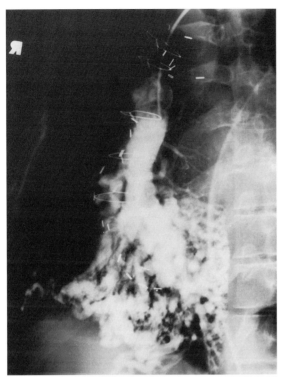

Figure 42. Numerous right basilar pulmonary arteriovenous fistulas in a patient several decades after placement of a Glenn shunt.

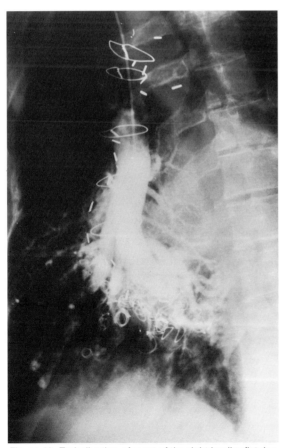

Figure 43. Embolization of most of the right basilar fistulas seen in Figure 42.

Follow-up After Embolotherapy

• Repeat chest radiographs and arterial blood gases at 1 day, 1 month, 1 year, and every 3–5 years thereafter.
• Concern if there is:
—Recurrent hypoxemia
—Early deflation of detachable balloon (less than 30 days)
—New lesions or persistence of an aneurysm for longer than 1 year
• Prophylactic antibiotics prior to "dirty" procedures, such as dental work
—All patients with HHT until screened negative for PAVM
—Other patients with known residual PAVMs

Figure 41.

Postprocedure Care

Follow-up **(Fig. 41)** has consisted of repeat blood gases and chest radiographs at 24 hours, 1 month, 1 year, and then every 3–5 years, as well as corresponding clinical evaluations. Spiral CT scanning will likely play an important role in future follow-up evaluations. It is important to determine whether late recanalization of a lesion has occurred, accessory vessels to complex lesions have grown, or other small lesions have grown to a significant level. All patients with HHT should be assumed to have residual small PAVMs. These patients, as well as patients with sporadic PAVM but known residual disease, should take prophylactic antibiotics prior to undergoing procedures that may produce bacteremia (eg, dental work) for the remainder of their lives. While this will not protect against paradoxical bacterial embolization, it should prevent progression to abscess.

Acquired Pulmonary Arteriovenous Fistula

Other abnormalities of the pulmonary circulation may be treated by embolization. While uncommon, acquired pulmonary arteriovenous fistula (PAVF) can result from trauma, cirrhosis (hepatopulmonary syndrome), prior Glenn or Fontan shunts for cyanotic congenital heart disease (superior vena cava or right atrium to pulmonary artery connections), metastatic carcinoma (primarily thyroid), infections (schistosomiasis, actinomycosis), and amyloidosis. When sufficiently large and numerous, PAVF can give symptoms and signs similar to those of PAVM. **Figure 42** shows numerous right basilar fistulas in a patient several decades after a Glenn shunt had been placed. His oxygen saturation rose from 54% to 84% after embolization of most of these lesions **(Fig. 43)**. Embolotherapy principles and techniques used to treat PAVF are similar to those used to treat PAVM.

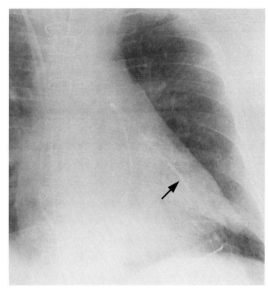

Figure 44. The chest radiograph shows the inappropriately peripheral position of a Swan-Ganz catheter in the left lung (arrow).

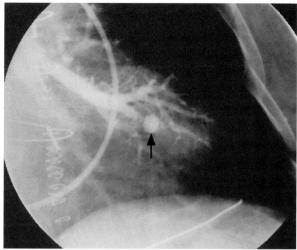

Figure 45. Same patient as in Figure 44. Peripheral false aneurysm due to the Swan-Ganz catheter (arrow).

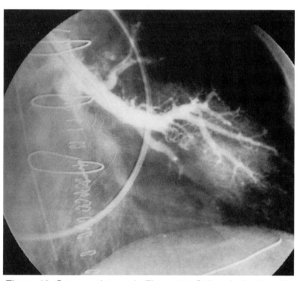

Figure 46. Same patient as in Figure 44. Coil embolization of the branch with the pseudoaneurysm.

Pulmonary Artery Aneurysm

True and false pulmonary artery aneurysm, without PAVF, are serious conditions, with significant risks of rupture and death. When the aneurysm is centrally located, surgical methods to repair the artery yet preserve flow are preferred; when the aneurysm is peripheral, embolization is effective, as occlusion can usually be accomplished with minimal sacrifice of normal lung. Etiologies of pulmonary artery aneurysm include pneumonitis with secondary vascular erosion (eg, Rasmussen aneurysm of tuberculosis), septic arterial seeding, vasculitis (eg, Behçet's syndrome), degenerative processes, lesions associated with congenital heart disease, and trauma. A Swan-Ganz catheter injury should be considered when an intensive care unit patient develops hemoptysis or a new infiltrate or mass. **Figure 44** shows a Swan-Ganz catheter in the peripheral left lung which was inadvertently inflated, resulting in 250 mL of hemoptysis. A pseudoaneurysm was discovered and embolized **(Figs. 45, 46)**.

For further information on this topic, please see Teaching File Case 21.

Selected Readings

Bartter T, Irwin RS, Nash G. Aneurysms of the pulmonary arteries. Chest 1988; 94:1065–1075.

Barzilai B, Waggoner AD, Spessert C, Picus D, Goodenberger D. Two-dimensional contrast echocardiography in the detection and follow-up of congenital pulmonary arteriovenous malformations. Am J Cardiol 1991; 68:1507–1510.

Burke CM, Safai C, Nelson DP, Raffin TA. Pulmonary arteriovenous malformations: a critical update. Am Rev Respir Dis 1986; 134:334–339.

Chilvers ER, Peters AM, George P, Hughes JM, Allison DJ. Quantification of right-to-left shunt through pulmonary arteriovenous malformations using 99-Tc albumin microspheres. Clin Radiol 1988; 39:611–614.

Chilvers ER, Whyte MK, Jackson JE, Allison DJ, Hughes JM. Effect of percutaneous transcatheter embolization on pulmonary function, right-to-left shunt, and arterial oxygenation in patients with pulmonary arteriovenous malformations. Am Rev Respir Dis 1990; 142:420–425.

Dines DE, Seward JB, Bernatz PE. Pulmonary arteriovenous fistulas. Mayo Clin Proc 1983; 58:176–181.

Ference BA, Shannon TM, White RI Jr, Zawin M, Burdge CM. Life-threatening pulmonary hemorrhage with pulmonary arteriovenous malformations and hereditary hemorrhagic telangiectasia. Chest 1994; 106:1387–1390.

McAllister KA, Grogg KM, Johnson DW, et al. Endoglin, a TGF-ß binding protein of endothelial cells, is the gene for hereditary haemorrhagic telangiectasia type 1. Nat Genet 1994; 8:345–351.

Peery WH. Clinical spectrum of hereditary hemorrhagic telangiectasia (Osler-Weber-Rendu disease). Am J Med 1987; 82:989–997.

Pollak JS, Egglin TK, Rosenblatt MM, Dickey KW, White RI Jr. Clinical results of transvenous systemic embolotherapy with a neuroradiologic detachable balloon. Radiology 1994; 191:477–482.

Remy J, Remy-Jardin M, Giraud F, Wattinne L. Angioarchitecture of pulmonary arteriovenous malformations: clinical utility of three-dimensional helical CT. Radiology 1994; 191:657–664.

Remy J, Remy-Jardin M, Wattinne L, Deffontaines C. Pulmonary arteriovenous malformations: evaluation with CT of the chest before and after treatment. Radiology 1992; 182:809–816.

Remy-Jardin M, Wattine L, Remy J. Transcatheter occlusion of pulmonary arterial circulation and collateral supply: failures, incidents, and complications. Radiology 1991; 180:699–705.

White RI Jr, Lynch-Nyhan A, Terry P, et al. Pulmonary arteriovenous malformations: techniques and long-term outcome of embolotherapy. Radiology 1988; 169:663–669.

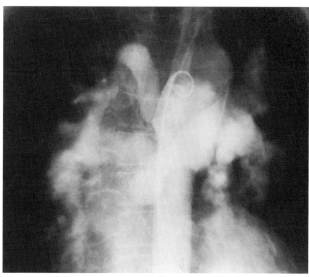

Figure 1. Pulmonary atresia—early phase of injection.

TUTORIAL 6
BRONCHIAL ARTERY
EMBOLIZATION
Robert E. Barton, M.D.

Introduction
The subjects addressed in this tutorial include:
1. Indications for embolization
2. Anatomy, angiographic technique, and findings
3. Embolization technique.

Indications
Bronchial artery embolization is most commonly indicated for the treatment of severe hemoptysis. Massive hemoptysis, defined as the expectoration of at least 300 mL of blood in less than 24 hours, is associated with a very high mortality when treated medically. Prompt surgical intervention improves the survival rate significantly but is often not feasible in patients with severe pulmonary disease. When surgery is not appropriate, embolization of the bleeding arteries can be life-saving. Embolization is usually not considered for recurrent hemoptysis that is not life-threatening. In patients with cystic fibrosis, however, recurrent minor hemoptysis interferes with postural drainage and physiotherapy. Embolization is appropriate in these patients as well.

Bronchial embolization can also be used to treat systemic to pulmonary artery collaterals due to congenital heart disease. Collaterals from the bronchial and other systemic arteries develop in response to the restriction of pulmonary artery blood flow seen in pulmonary atresia **(Figs. 1, 2)**, tetralogy of Fallot, and transposition of the great vessels. In addition to causing hemoptysis, these collaterals can produce congestive heart failure if flow is excessive. These collaterals are frequently ligated when the underlying cardiac anomaly is repaired surgically, but embolization can prove helpful in selected cases.

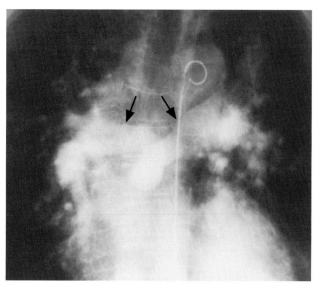

Figure 2. Pulmonary atresia—late phase of injection. Systemic to pulmonary artery collaterals (arrows).

Causes of Massive Hemoptysis from Systemic Arteries
• Tuberculosis
• Aspergillosis
• Bronchiectasis
• Cystic fibrosis
• Lung abscess
• Pulmonary atresia or stenosis
• Chronic pulmonary embolism
• Lung cancer

Figure 3.

Classification of Bronchial Artery Anatomy by Cauldwell		
I	41%	2 left bronchial arteries and 1 right ICBT
II	21%	1 left bronchial artery and 1 right ICBT
III	21%	1 left bronchial artery, 1 common bronchial trunk, and 1 right ICBT
IV	10%	2 left bronchial arteries, 1 right bronchial artery, and 1 right ICBT

Figure 4.

Classification of Bronchial Artery Anatomy by Botenga		
I	28%	2 left bronchial arteries and 1 right ICBT
II	17%	1 left bronchial artery and 1 right ICBT
III	17%	1 left bronchial artery, 1 common bronchial trunk, and 1 right ICBT
IV	11%	2 left bronchial arteries, 1 right bronchial artery, and 1 right ICBT
V	8.5%	1 left bronchial artery, 1 right bronchial artery, and 1 right ICBT
VI	8.5%	1 common bronchial trunk, and 1 right ICBT
VII	4.3%	1 common bronchial trunk

Figure 5.

Causes of Massive Hemoptysis

Pulmonary arteries are rarely the source of significant hemorrhage. Massive hemoptysis almost always arises from systemic arteries which become enlarged in response to a variety of diseases **(Fig. 3)**. Benign inflammatory conditions such as tuberculosis, aspergillosis, and bronchiectasis account for the majority of cases. Cystic fibrosis is becoming a more frequent cause of hemoptysis as patients with this disease live longer. Cancer is responsible for massive hemoptysis in relatively few patients.

Anatomy

Bronchial artery anatomy is extremely variable as is shown by classifications reported by Cauldwell **(Fig. 4)** and Botenga **(Fig. 5)**. Arteries usually arise from the descending thoracic aorta anywhere between T4 and T7. In most cases, there are either one or two bronchial arteries on each side. On the right, a bronchial artery arises from an intercostal artery, the intercostobronchial trunk (ICBT), in over 90% of patients. This vessel originates from the right lateral or posterolateral aortic wall. **Figure 6** shows an enlarged bronchial artery arising from the ICBT. **Figure 7** shows the same ICBT after occlusion of the bronchial artery.

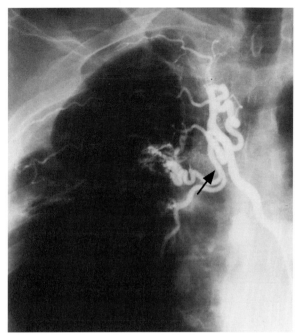

Figure 6. ICBT (arrow) before embolization.

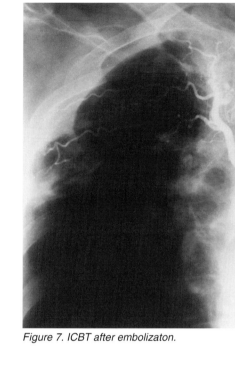

Figure 7. ICBT after embolizaton.

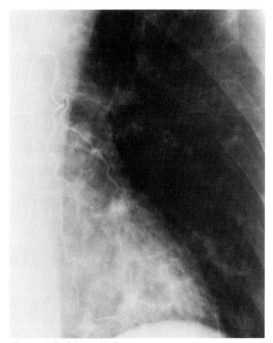

Figure 8. Left bronchial artery.

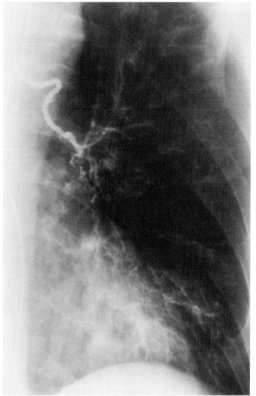

Figure 9. Same patient as in Figure 8. Second left bronchial artery.

Left bronchial arteries usually arise directly from the anterior wall of the aorta and are multiple in 70% of cases. **Figures 8** and **9** show two left bronchial arteries in the same patient.

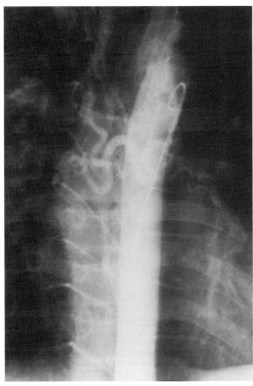

Figure 10. Aortogram shows a common bronchial trunk.

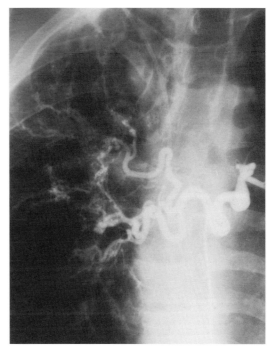

Figure 11. Common bronchial trunk—selective injection.

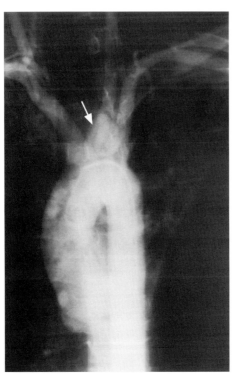

Figure 12. Bronchial artery arising from the aortic arch (arrow).

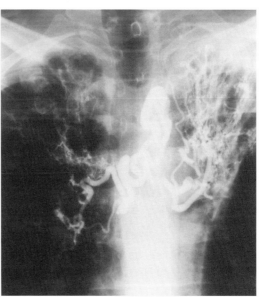

Figure 13. Bronchial artery arising from the aortic arch—selective injection.

Occasionally, right and left bronchial arteries arise from a common trunk **(Figs. 10, 11)**. Bronchial arteries occasionally arise from the aortic arch **(Figs. 12, 13)** and rarely from subclavian artery branches.

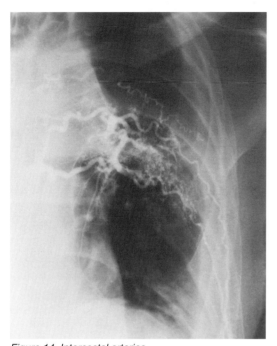

Figure 14. Intercostal arteries.

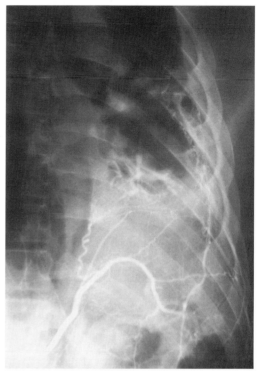

Figure 15. Inferior phrenic artery.

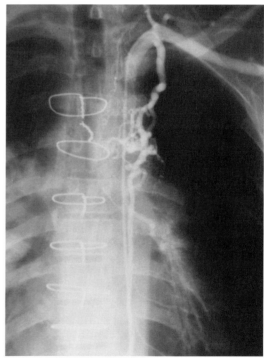

Figure 16. Internal mammary artery.

Anastomotic channels normally exist between bronchial and other mediastinal arteries which can become enlarged in pathologic conditions. In addition, transpleural collaterals can also develop, particularly with aspergillosis. These nonbronchial collateral arteries can cause hemoptysis and must be addressed when bronchial artery injection fails to demonstrate a likely source of hemorrhage. The intercostal **(Fig. 14)**, inferior phrenic **(Fig. 15)**, internal mammary **(Fig. 16)**, and thyrocervical arteries as well as other subclavian branches are commonly involved.

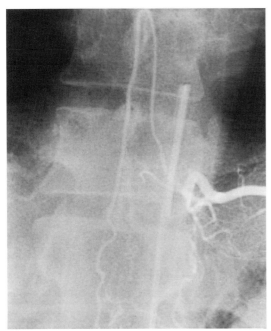

Figure 17. Spinal artery.

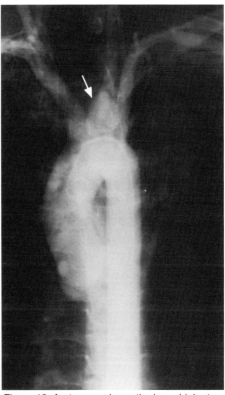

Figure 18. Aortogram shows the bronchial artery arising from the aortic arch (arrow).

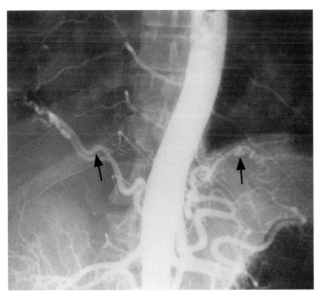

Figure 19. Aortogram shows inferior phrenic arteries (arrows).

Some arteries studied during bronchial arteriography may supply the spinal cord. The most important artery, the artery of Adamkiewicz, arises from an intercostal or lumbar artery, usually between T8 and L2. It is located on the left about 80% of the time and has a distinctive appearance, ascending just lateral of the midline before making a hairpin turn to descend in the midline **(Fig. 17)**. Branches to the thoracic spinal cord can arise from other arteries, most notably the right intercostobronchial trunk. Left bronchial arteries, which come directly from the aorta, usually do not supply the cord. The thyrocervical and costocervical arteries may also supply the cord.

Arteriographic Technique

We begin most examinations with a descending thoracic aortogram, although many interventionalists perform an aortogram only if difficulty is encountered in catheterizing the bronchial arteries. Although normal bronchial arteries are usually not seen on aortic injections, abnormal bronchial arteries are commonly visible. The aortogram may reveal bronchial arteries with unusual origins that would be missed on selective catheterizations. This artery arising from the aortic arch is an example **(Fig. 18)**. In addition, nonbronchial systemic arteries that contribute to hemoptysis, such as the intercostal or inferior phrenic arteries **(Fig. 19)**, may also be demonstrated.

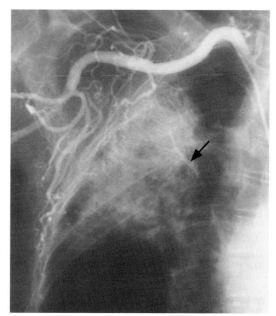

Figure 20. Subclavian arteriogram shows a pulmonary artery shunt (arrow).

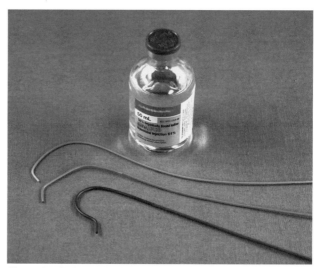

Figure 21. Catheters for bronchial arteriography.

When the site of bleeding is in the upper lobe of a lung, a subclavian arteriogram is performed on the affected side. **Figure 20** is a subclavian injection in a patient with cancer in the right upper lobe. Note the shunting to the pulmonary artery.

Selective arteriography of the bronchial arteries and other collateral vessels is then carried out using appropriately shaped 4–5-F catheters **(Fig. 21)**. Low osmolar contrast material is used for all selective injections. Injection rates vary tremendously depending on the size of the vessel studied and the amount of shunting. The appropriate rate must be determined by a test injection. Wedged injections should be avoided. Although most of the images shown in this tutorial are cut film, we now prefer digital subtraction arteriography in most cases.

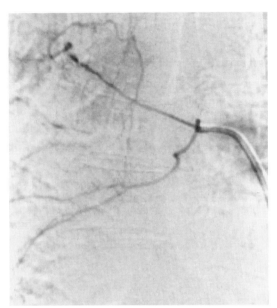

Figure 22. Normal bronchial artery.

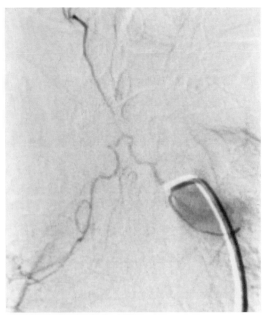

Figure 23. Normal bronchial artery.

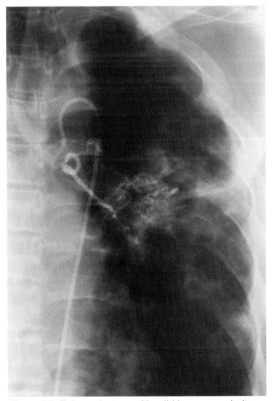

Figure 24. Enlarged artery with mild hypervascularity.

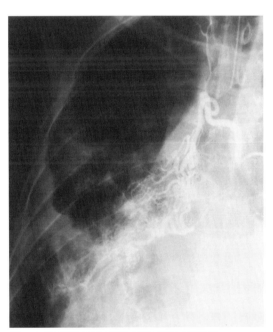

Figure 25. Enlarged artery with more extreme hypervascularity.

Arteriographic Findings in Hemoptysis

Normal bronchial arteries **(Figs. 22, 23)** are small and are usually not seen on the aortogram. With chronic lung disease, the bronchial arteries enlarge significantly. The abnormalities most commonly seen with hemoptysis are enlargement and tortuosity of the feeding arteries and hypervascularity of the involved area. **Figure 24** is a selective left bronchial artery injection which shows mild enlargement of the artery with abnormal hypervascularity in the central portion of the lung. More extreme hypervascularity is seen in **Figure 25**.

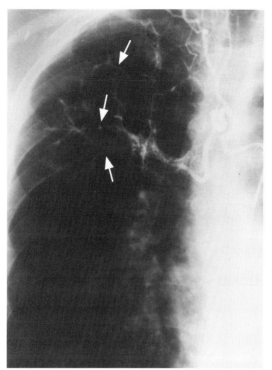

Figure 26. Shunting to the peripheral pulmonary arteries (arrow) from an intercostobronchial arterial trunk injection.

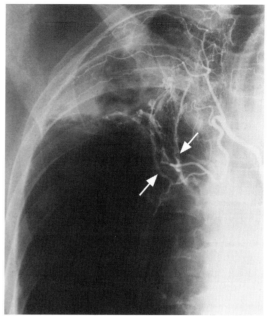

Figure 27. Shunting to the peripheral pulmonary arteries (arrow) from a bronchial injection.

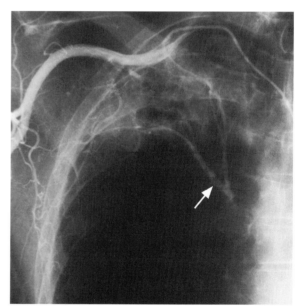

Figure 28. Shunting to the peripheral pulmonary arteries (arrow) from a subclavian artery injection.

Another common arteriographic finding is shunting from systemic to pulmonary arteries which can be seen on injection of bronchial arteries or non-bronchial collateral vessels. **Figure 26** demonstrates shunting to peripheral pulmonary arteries on injection of an intercostobronchial trunk. In another patient shunting is seen on both bronchial **(Fig. 27)** and subclavian arteriograms **(Fig. 28)**.

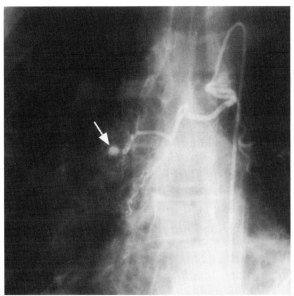
Figure 29. Peripheral bronchial artery aneurysm (arrow).

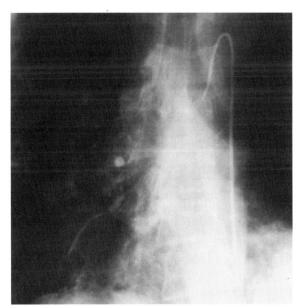
Figure 30. Extravasation of contrast material into a lower lobe bronchus.

The abnormalities on bronchial arteriography which are most specific and which reliably indicate the site of bleeding are aneurysms of bronchial arteries and extravasation of contrast material. These findings are relatively uncommon, however. **Figure 29** demonstrates a peripheral bronchial artery aneurysm. Later films from the same injection show extravasation of contrast material into a lower lobe bronchus **(Fig. 30)**.

Choice of Embolic Agent
The embolic agents most commonly used for bronchial embolization are Gelfoam sponge (Upjohn, Kalamazoo, MI) cut into 2-mm pledgets and polyvinyl alcohol (PVA) particles 250–500 microns in size. Particles of this size permit a relatively distal embolization with little risk of tissue necrosis.

Absolute ethanol and polymerizing agents such as cyanoacrylate have been used in the past but are now considered inappropriate because of the risk of tissue necrosis. Coil springs should be avoided because they produce a permanent proximal occlusion which permits the development of collaterals which may be very difficult to treat should bleeding recur.

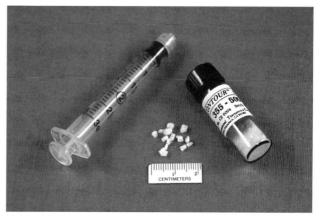

Figure 31. Gelfoam pledgets and PVA.

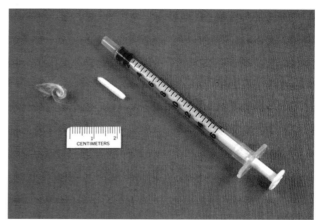

Figure 32. Gelfoam torpedo.

Embolization Technique

We embolize only those arteries supplying the area of the lung that is suspected of bleeding based on clinical information and the angiographic appearance. The vessel to be occluded is catheterized as selectively as possible so that the catheter tip is beyond normal branches such as intercostal arteries that arise together with the bronchial arteries. A coaxial 3-F microcatheter may be necessary to achieve a good catheter position. Some consider the presence of a spinal artery to be an absolute contraindication to embolization, but others will perform the embolization if the catheter can be advanced well beyond the origin of the spinal artery.

Once an acceptable catheter position has been achieved, small Gelfoam pledgets or PVA particles **(Fig. 31)** suspended in contrast material are injected slowly, with care being taken to avoid reflux. Frequent test injections are performed to assess progress. Once flow in the vessel being embolized has slowed, a spinal branch that did not fill earlier may be seen. When flow in the vessel being embolized is nearly stagnant, we usually occlude the vessel with a Gelfoam "torpedo" **(Fig. 32)**. Although the use of coils is generally avoided, they may be needed to occlude very large bronchial arteries.

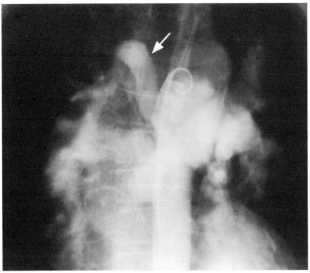

Figure 33. Aortic injection demonstrates systemic to pulmonary artery collaterals (arrow).

Figure 34. Pulmonary arteries are opacified through the collaterals.

Immediate Control of Hemoptysis			
	No. of Patients	*No. Controlled*	*% Controlled*
Rabkin	306	278	91%
Uflacker	64	49	77%
Remy	49	41	84%
Fellows	13	12	92%

Figure 35.

Recurrent Hemoptysis after Embolization			
	No. of Patients	*No. Recurred*	*% Recurred*
Rabkin	158	36	23%
Uflacker	56	12	21%
Remy	41	6	15%

Figure 36.

Complications

Bronchial embolization is relatively safe when performed properly. The most feared complication, transverse myelitis due to embolization of the spinal artery, has proven to be extremely rare. Bronchial injury has been reported with the use of alcohol and cyanoacrylate, so these agents are now generally avoided. Pulmonary infarction can occur if the bronchial artery is the only source of blood flow to the lung, as is the case with congenital heart disease **(Figs. 33, 34)** or pulmonary embolism. The most common complication is chest pain, occasionally associated with dysphagia. These symptoms are usually self-limited and resolve in a few days.

Results

Bronchial embolization has proven effective in controlling acute hemoptysis with success rates of 77%–91% **(Fig. 35)**. Rabkin et al reported failure to control hemoptysis in only 28 of 306 patients who underwent bronchial embolization. In 26 of these 28 patients, the pulmonary arteries were ultimately shown to be the source of bleeding.

Hemorrhage recurs in about 20% of patients **(Fig. 36)** and can frequently be managed with repeat embolization. The likelihood of recurrent bleeding is determined by the nature of the underlying lung disease.

For further information on this topic, please see Teaching File Case 22.

Selected Readings

Cremaschi P, Nascimbene C, Vitulo P, et al. Therapeutic embolization of bronchial artery: a successful treatment of 209 cases of relapse hemoptysis. Angiology 1993; 44:295–299.

Fellows KE, Khaw KT, Schuster S, Shwachman H. Bronchial artery embolization in cystic fibrosis; technique and long-term results. J Pediatr 1979; 95(6):959–963.

Girard P, Baldeyrou P, Lemoine G, Grunewald D. Left main-stem bronchial stenosis complicating bronchial artery embolization. Chest 1990; 97:1246–1248.

Ivanick MJ, Thorwarth W, Donohue J, Mandell V, Delany D, Jaques PF. Infarction of the left main-stem bronchus: a complication of bronchial artery embolization. AJR 1983; 141:535–537.

Jardin M, Remy J. Control of hemoptysis: systemic angiography and anastomoses of the internal mammary artery. Radiology 1988; 168:377–383.

Katoh O, Kishikawa T, Yamada H, Matsumoto S, Kudo S. Recurrent bleeding after arterial embolization in patients with hemoptysis. Chest 1990; 97:541–546.

Kaufman SL, Kan JS, Mitchell SE, Flaherty JT, White RI. Embolization of systemic to pulmonary artery collaterals in the management of hemoptysis in pulmonary atresia. Am J Cardiol 1986; 58:1130–1132.

Keller, FS, Rosch J, Loflin TG, Nath PH, McElvein RB. Nonbronchial systemic collateral arteries: significance in percutaneous embolotherapy for hemoptysis. Radiology 1987; 164:687–692.

Lois JF, Gomes AS, Smith DC, Laks H. Systemic-to-pulmonary collateral vessels and shunts: treatment with embolization. Radiology 1988; 169:671–676.

Mauro MA, Jaques PF, Morris S. Bronchial artery embolization for the control of hemoptysis. Semin Intervent Radiol 1992; 9:45–51.

Rabkin JE, Astafjev VI, Gothman LN, Grigorjev YG. Transcatheter embolization in the management of pulmonary hemorrhage. Radiology 1987; 163:361–365.

Remy J, Arnaud A, Fardou H, Giraud R, Voisin C. Treatment of hemoptysis by embolization of bronchial arteries. Radiology 1977; 122:33–37.

Sweezey NB, Fellows KE. Bronchial artery embolization for severe hemoptysis in cystic fibrosis. Chest 1990; 97:1322–1326.

Tadavarthy SM, Klugman J, Castaneda-Zuniga WR, Nath PH, Amplatz K. Systemic-to-pulmonary collaterals in pathologic states: a review. Radiology 1982; 144:55–59.

Uflacker R, Kaemmerer A, Neves C, Picon PD. Management of massive hemoptysis by bronchial artery embolization. Radiology 1983; 146:627–634.

Uflacker R, Kaemmerer A, Picon PD, et al. Bronchial artery embolization in the management of hemoptysis: technical aspects and long-term results. Radiology 1985; 157:637–644.

Vujic I, Pyle R, Parker E, Mithoefer J. Control of massive hemoptysis by embolization of intercostal arteries. Radiology 1980; 137:617–620.

Wedzicha JA, Pearson MC. Management of massive haemoptysis. Respir Med 1990; 84:9–12.

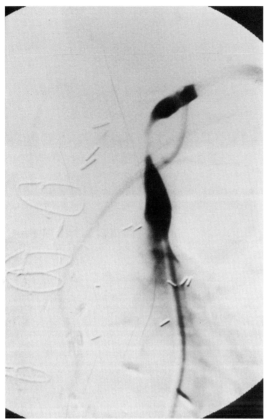

Figure 1. Focal proximal left subclavian artery stenosis. The vertebral artery is not opacified due to retrograde flow ("subclavian steal").

TUTORIAL 7
SUPRA-AORTIC PERCUTANEOUS TRANSLUMINAL ANGIOPLASTY AND STENTS
Donald E. Schwarten, M.D.

Introduction
Despite the success of angioplasty in patients with lesions in the coronary, renal, and peripheral vascular territories, there has been considerable reluctance to employ angioplasty of atherosclerotic lesions in the portions of the brachiocephalic arteries whose target organ is the brain because of the risk of cerebral embolization of debris from the angioplasty site and the perception that this will result in clinically significant neurologic events. However, before peripheral and coronary angioplasty became widely used and accepted, similar concerns about embolic complications were expressed and ultimately proven to be minor or clinically insignificant.

In the past few years percutaneous angioplasty techniques have been used successfully in the craniocerebral vessels. A number of reports, including some substantial case series, have been published indicating excellent anatomic and clinical results with cerebrovascular percutaneous transluminal angioplasty (PTA). Most of these studies have selected patients who had angiographic anatomy that would minimize the risk of cerebral embolization. For example, carotid bifurcation PTA would only be performed in patients who have no angiographic evidence of ulceration within or adjacent to the stenosis, or in patients who have a subclavian steal phenomenon with retrograde vertebral flow, thus essentially eliminating the risk of posterior fossa embolization **(Fig. 1)**.

CEA Versus Medical Therapy

Event Defining Failure	Patients Treated Medically (N=331)	Patients Treated by CEA (N=328)	Relative-Risk Reduction
Any stroke	64 (27.6%)	34 (12.6%)	54%
Any ipsilateral stroke	61 (26.0%)	26 (9.0%)	65%
Any major stroke or death	38 (18.1%)	19 (8.0%)	56%

Figure 2. Impact of surgical carotid endarterectomy (CEA) versus medical therapy alone on the incidence of stroke and death at 2 years following a symptomatic neurologic event. Population consisted of 659 patients with angiographically documented 70%–99% stenosis (NASCET data).

Carotid bifurcation angioplasty is being reported with increasing frequency, most notably in the cardiology literature. Numerous reports of carotid bifurcation stenting have been published, but no prospective trials exist to document the safety or efficacy of these procedures. The North American Symptomatic Carotid Endarterectomy Trial (NASCET) and other trials have made it abundantly clear that carotid endarterectomy is the treatment of choice for patients with symptomatic high-grade carotid bifurcation disease **(Fig. 2)**. Results from the Asymptomatic Carotid Atherosclerosis Study (ACAS) suggest that a similar conclusion is warranted for patients with asymptomatic moderate- to high-grade lesions, although the data are not as compelling, particularly for female patients. Because the issue of carotid bifurcation angioplasty is awash in controversy, this tutorial will focus on the endovascular treatment of other supra-aortic vessels. Carotid bifurcation angioplasty does deserve discussion, however, because there is a place for this procedure in selected patients.

Preprocedure Diagnostic Studies

In addition to a complete history and physical examination, potential cerebrovascular angioplasty candidates should undergo **(Fig. 3)**, at the minimum: 1) cerebrovascular duplex ultrasonography; 2) cross-sectional imaging of the brain; and 3) complete four-vessel arteriography including arch aortography, bilateral common carotid arteriography to delineate the cervical and intracranial anatomy, and vertebral arteriography. The vertebral artery study may be performed digitally during a subclavian artery injection except when the angioplasty is to be performed for posterior fossa symptoms; in that case, the entire course of both vertebral arteries should be examined.

Supra-Aortic PTA: Preprocedural Evaluation

1. Cerebrovascular duplex ultrasound

2. Cerebral CT or MR imaging

3. Complete diagnostic arteriography

Figure 3.

```
┌─────────────────────────────────────────┐
│           Supra-Aortic PTA:               │
│         Pharmacologic Agents              │
├─────────────────────────────────────────┤
│                                           │
│   • Anticoagulation                       │
│   — Aspirin (pre- and post-PTA)           │
│   — Heparin (during PTA)                  │
│                                           │
│   • Antispasmodic                         │
│   — Transdermal nitroglycerin (pre-PTA)   │
│   — Intraarterial nitroglycerin (during PTA) │
│                                           │
│   • Antiarrhythmic                        │
│   —Atropine (for internal carotid PTA)    │
│                                           │
└─────────────────────────────────────────┘
```

Figure 4.

Pharmacologic Adjuncts in Supra-Aortic PTA and Stenting

As with PTA in the peripheral vasculature, antiplatelet therapy remains the mainstay in the supra-aortic vessels (Fig. 4). A single daily dose of 325 mg of aspirin is standard for all patients undergoing extracranial angioplasty and/or stenting. Because of the large caliber of the extracranial supra-aortic vessels and their high flow rates, it is unnecessary to employ routine postprocedural anticoagulation with heparin. Moreover, postprocedural anticoagulation with agents such as ticlopidine or warfarin is seldom warranted.

Significant vasospasm in the intrathoracic segments of the supra-aortic vessels is seldom encountered. On the other hand, the vertebral arteries and the internal carotid arteries are highly susceptible to guide wire and catheter-induced vasospasm, which can be managed with 100 mcg intraarterial boluses of nitroglycerin. We seldom use calcium channel antagonists for prophylaxis of vasospasm. The latter is better achieved with use of transdermal nitroglycerin.

When endovascular procedures are performed at or near the carotid bifurcation, patients should be premedicated with intravenous atropine to protect against severe and potentially fatal bradyarrhythmias induced by stimulation of the carotid body.

Anticoagulation is more important during angioplasty and stenting of the supra-aortic vessels than in other peripheral arteries. Patients should be heparinized to therapeutic levels for the procedure. The anticoagulation should not be reversed with intravenous protamine after the procedure, and it is a good practice to retain sheath position within the approach artery for approximately 30 minutes after the procedure before relinquishing arterial access. As with PTA of other vascular territories, anticoagulation therapy may be extended for 24 hours or more at the discretion of the interventional radiologist based on the presence or absence of a vascular dissection or other notable findings.

Complications associated with lower extremity angioplasty include an acutely ischemic lower extremity that may be managed by the interventionalist but frequently requires surgical intervention. Complications associated with supra-aortic angioplasty **(Fig. 5)** may result in cerebral ischemia which will usually require aggressive management by the interventionalist. It would be the rare case indeed in which even the most skilled vascular surgeon could prevent a stroke in a patient with a complication resulting from carotid angioplasty and/or stenting. It is even less likely that procedural complications of vertebrobasilar interventions could be successfully managed by a surgical approach.

The skills that are necessary to perform peripheral angioplasty successfully fall far short of the skills that must be mastered in order to safely perform angioplasty and stenting in supra-aortic vessels that provide the blood supply to the brain. As yet, there are no credentialing criteria established for percutaneous management of extracranial athero-occlusive disease. At the very least, interventionalists who aspire to perform angioplasty and stenting in these territories must have fundamental knowledge and skills in neuroanatomy and neurophysiology. An awareness of the need and the methods to achieve therapeutic hypertension and hypervolemia is essential, as is a thorough understanding of all methods for neuronal preservation. Interventionalists must also have the training and skill to quickly negotiate microcatheters into intracranial vessels for attempted emergent thrombolysis of iatrogenically-occluded vessels **(Fig. 6)**.

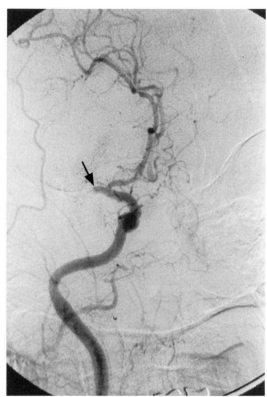

Figure 5. Iatrogenic occlusion of the right middle cerebral artery (arrow).

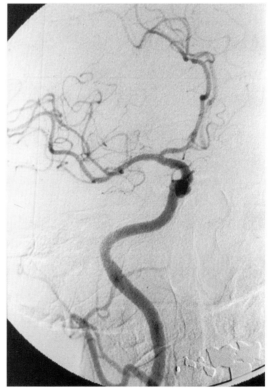

Figure 6. The artery is restored to patency after local thrombolysis through a microcatheter.

```
+------------------------------------------+
|      Subclavian Angioplasty:             |
|            Indications                   |
+------------------------------------------+
|                                          |
|  • Upper extremity claudication          |
|                                          |
|  • Atheroembolic digital ischemia        |
|                                          |
|  • Subclavian steal phenomenon causing   |
|    cerebral or post-CABG myocardial      |
|    ischemia                              |
|                                          |
+------------------------------------------+
```

Figure 7.

Catheter and Guide Wire Technology for Supra-Aortic PTA

In the major supra-aortic vessels, the innominate, common carotid, and subclavian arteries, 0.035-inch guide wire/angioplasty systems that are employed in the peripheral vasculature are appropriate. Some vertebral arteries are large enough to permit the use of 0.018-inch based "infrapopliteal" angioplasty systems. However, whenever possible, ie, in vertebral arteries smaller than 4.5 mm in diameter, it is best to use a guiding catheter and an 0.014-inch-based angioplasty system.

Angioplasty of the carotid bifurcation can be accomplished in most cases with the 0.035-inch-based systems. Clearly, use of these systems with or without stents at the carotid bifurcation has received neither Food and Drug Administration (FDA) nor Health Care Financing Administration approval. The FDA considers a stent in the carotid artery to be a significant risk device that requires an investigational device exemption.

Subclavian Artery Angioplasty

Clinical indications for subclavian artery angioplasty **(Fig. 7)** include atheroembolic digital ischemia, upper extremity claudication, and most commonly, subclavian steal phenomenon. The steal phenomenon may be the classic vertebral artery steal with posterior fossa symptoms. Alternatively, in patients who have undergone left internal mammary artery (LIMA) to coronary artery bypass grafting, the left anterior descending (LAD) coronary artery may flow retrograde through the LIMA to supply the post-stenosis subclavian artery. These patients may present with angina pectoris with or without posterior fossa symptoms. In patients with retrograde flow in the vertebral artery, the posterior fossa is protected because the steal persists briefly after a successful angioplasty. In patients who do not exhibit retrograde vertebral artery flow during pre-angioplasty arteriography, every effort should be made to induce retrograde flow by creating reactive hyperemia in the upper extremity. This can be done mechanically with prolonged suprasystolic inflation of a blood pressure cuff and angioplasty during subsequent cuff deflation, or with intraarterial papaverine or nitroglycerin administration.

Angioplasty of subclavian artery stenoses is usually accomplished from the transfemoral route with the use of standard guide wire exchange techniques. In the simplest scenario, a head-hunter catheter is used to engage the orifice of a stenotic left subclavian artery. The catheter is then exchanged over an exchange-length guide wire for the angioplasty balloon catheter and the procedure is completed **(Figs. 8, 9)**. When the vertebral artery origin is normal there is probably little need to be concerned if the angioplasty balloon crosses the vertebral artery orifice. However, when the vertebral artery orifice is pathologic or in close proximity to the subclavian artery stenosis, as in **Figures 10** and **11**, the vertebral artery should be protected regardless of the status of the contralateral vertebral artery. This may be accomplished by placing a second catheter and a safety guide wire into the vertebral artery through a transaxillary approach or by placing a safety wire into the artery through an ipsilateral or contralateral transfemoral approach. If the vertebral artery is compromised during subclavian angioplasty, it can be balloon dilated using the safety wire for access.

The left subclavian artery is seven times more likely to have atherosclerotic involvement than the right. However, in the patient with a right subclavian artery origin stenosis, the right common carotid artery may be compromised by the angioplasty procedure. A safety wire should be placed in the right common carotid artery to permit immediate angioplasty if its origin is compromised by the subclavian procedure. In this instance it is best to approach the common carotid artery from the transfemoral route. The right subclavian artery can be approached from either the transfemoral or the right axillary route.

Subclavian artery occlusions deserve special mention because it is frequently impossible to traverse a subclavian occlusion from the transfemoral approach. Treatment of subclavian occlusions should be planned so that simultaneous transfemoral and transaxillary approaches can potentially be used. If the occlusion cannot be crossed, transaxillary access is gained from the transfemoral approach. If an attempt to traverse the occlusion from this approach is successful, the transfemoral catheter is replaced with a snare and the guide wire from the transaxillary approach is snared and retrieved into the transfemoral sheath. An appropriate sized stent is then deployed in the recanalized segment of the subclavian artery, as shown in **Figures 12** and **13**. This seemingly cumbersome technique is used because of the reported high recurrence rate for balloon angioplasty of subclavian artery occlusions, and because of the desire to maintain the smallest possible puncture in the axillary artery.

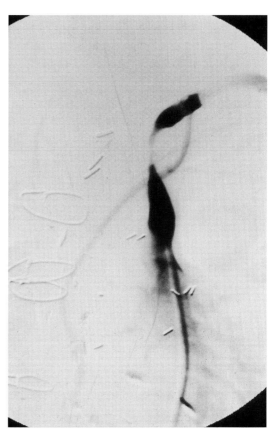

Figure 8. Uncomplicated left subclavian artery stenosis with no vertebral artery filling.

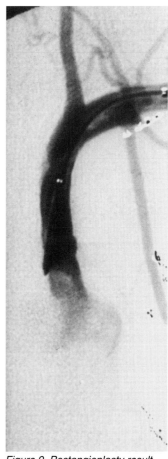

Figure 9. Postangioplasty result.

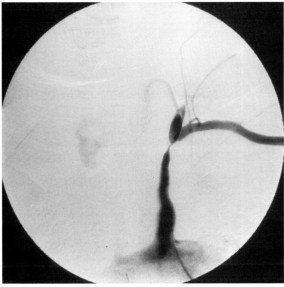

Figure 10. Left subclavian arteriogram demonstrates the vertebral artery to be bridged by a subclavian artery stenosis.

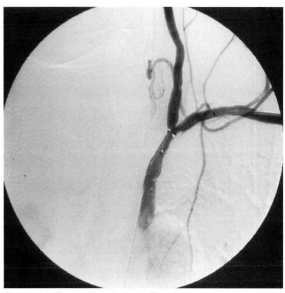

Figure 11. The postangioplasty film shows catheters in both vessels.

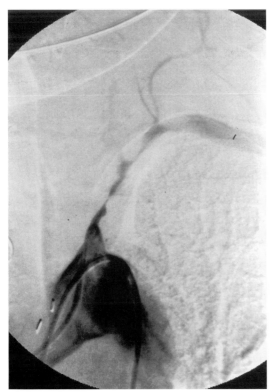

Figure 12. Partial recanalization of a left subclavian artery occlusion. The catheter would not cross the site from the transfemoral approach. A transaxillary catheter was used to snare and guide the transfemoral catheter across the lesion.

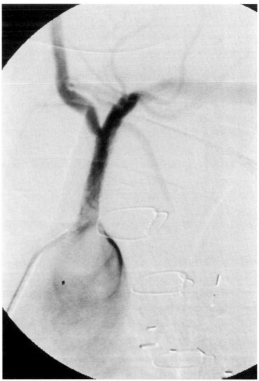

Figure 13. Arteriogram after stent deployment shows restoration of vessel patency. The safety wire is in place.

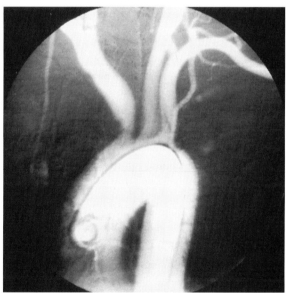

Figure 14. Arch aortogram reveals a proximal innominate artery stenosis suitable for angioplasty without requiring protection of the innominate bifurcation.

Figure 15. Postangioplasty residual stenosis. The patient had equal arm blood pressures immediately after the procedure and at 2-year follow-up.

Innominate Artery Angioplasty

The clinical indications for innominate artery angioplasty also include upper extremity claudication, atheroembolic digital ischemia, and neurologic symptoms. Retrograde flow in the cerebral branches of the innominate artery in the presence of a proximal innominate artery stenosis makes for an angioplasty procedure that is as straightforward as its subclavian counterpart. The presence of antegrade flow in the right common carotid artery adds the risk of right hemispheric embolization. Several techniques to avoid neurologic consequences have been described and include compression of the right common carotid artery during the angioplasty procedure, the use of a second balloon placed into the right common carotid artery for cerebral protection, and finally, surgical exposure of the cervical segment of the right carotid artery to permit "washout" of embolic debris.

A review of the literature suggests that these adjuncts are unnecessary. The risk of a clinically significant neurologic deficit developing from an innominate artery angioplasty in the presence of antegrade flow in the right carotid artery appears to be less than 1%. When the innominate artery lesion is at or near the innominate bifurcation, a second safety system should be in place with the lead guide wire for the angioplasty catheter in either the subclavian or the right common carotid artery.

It is not necessary and may not be desirable to use a balloon segment equal to the diameter of the innominate artery. Slight underdilatation is the goal as shown in **Figures 14** and **15**. This technique not only has a low restenosis rate, but late follow-up arteriograms usually reveal no residual stenosis.

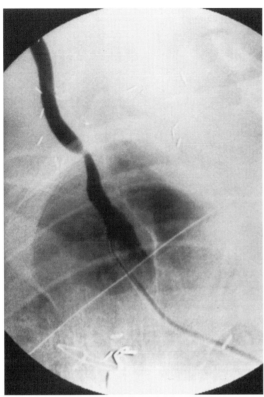

Figure 16. Right common carotid artery and intimal hyperplasia.

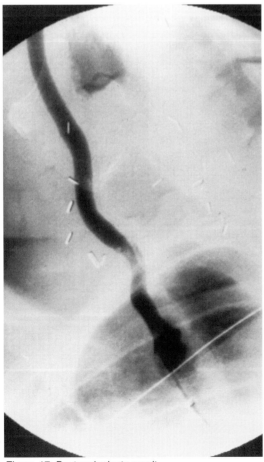

Figure 17. Postangioplasty result.

Carotid Artery Angioplasty

Angioplasty of the proximal segments of the common carotid arteries **(Figs. 16, 17)** can and should be treated differently from angioplasty of the carotid bifurcation. At this time the endovascular management of atherosclerotic carotid bifurcation lesions is considered investigational and should be limited in scope. In a review of over 2,000 extracranial angioplasty procedures, it appears that the risk of carotid bifurcation angioplasty is low, possibly as low as the risk of endarterectomy. It appears that the risk of restenosis is less than 10%, but as yet, there are no data on the long-term results of carotid angioplasty with or without stenting that would permit its comparison with carotid endarterectomy as an effective deterrent to future neurologic or ophthalmic events.

The clinical indications for carotid artery angioplasty can be summarized succinctly. For common carotid artery angioplasty, patients should have a greater than 75% common carotid artery stenosis with ipsilateral hemispheric symptoms. For carotid bifurcation angioplasty, the patient should also have an "unacceptable operative risk." Carotid bifurcation angioplasty should only be performed as an investigational procedure under an approved protocol. At our institution, we have somewhat arbitrarily decided that if the neurosurgeon or vascular surgeon consulted to perform carotid endarterectomy feels that the patient has more than a 5% risk for major morbidity or mortality, angioplasty of the carotid bifurcation/internal carotid artery lesion should be considered.

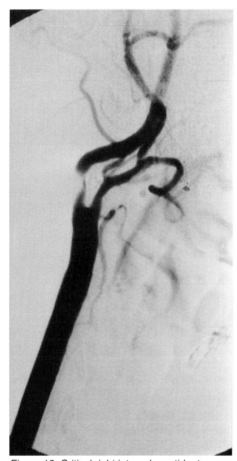

Figure 18. Critical right internal carotid artery stenosis.

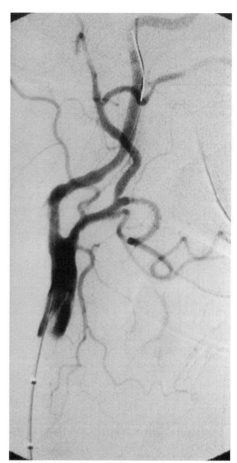

Figure 19. Postangioplasty arteriogram shows the safety wire at the base of the skull.

The techniques of common carotid and internal carotid artery angioplasty **(Figs. 18, 19)** are similar. Vessel sizing in brachiocephalic angioplasty in general is based on the measurement of the nearest normal caliber segment of vessel permitting up to 20% oversizing of the angioplasty balloon. Correct magnification assessment is more important in the brachiocephalic territory than in other regions for obvious reasons. For carotid bifurcation and internal carotid artery stenoses, the degree of internal carotid artery stenosis has been determined based on the methodology employed by NASCET; the narrowest point of the stenosis is measured and compared to the post-bulbar internal carotid artery cervical segment where it first returns to a normal diameter.

Common carotid artery angioplasty is accomplished by the initial selection of the common carotid artery with the diagnostic catheter most suited to the anatomy. Then, as with subclavian and innominate artery angioplasty, an exchange is made over an exchange-length guide wire for the angioplasty catheter. Every attempt is made to maintain the position of the guide wire below the carotid bifurcation during these maneuvers.

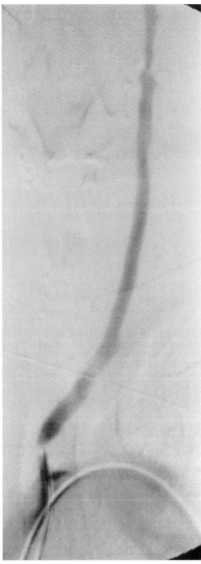

Figure 20. A Simmons catheter has been selected to access and image this proximal left common carotid artery stenosis.

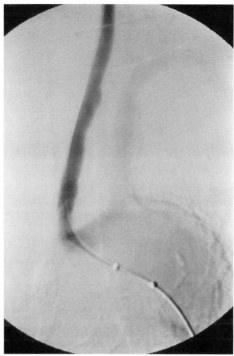

Figure 21. Postangioplasty study obtained with an 0.018-inch guide wire in place.

The origin of the left common carotid artery is frequently resistant to dilatation, but with persistence (not increasing balloon size), an acceptable anatomic result can be achieved in more than 85% of cases **(Figs. 20, 21)**. If a patient has tandem lesions, it may not be possible to ascertain whether the common carotid artery lesion or the carotid bifurcation lesion is responsible for the symptoms. In this circumstance, it may be appropriate to perform the common carotid angioplasty in conjunction with a carotid endarterectomy so that any angioplasty-related debris can be dealt with at the endarterectomy site.

Carotid bifurcation angioplasty, in most series, is accomplished without the use of a second "cerebral protection" balloon. In the series of innominate and carotid artery angioplasty procedures reported by Theron et al, 9% of patients who underwent angioplasty without the benefit of a second protecting balloon suffered a significant neurologic deficit. Among those patients who had the benefit of the second balloon, the incidence of fixed neurologic deficits dropped to near zero. However, this has not been the experience of other authors who have not used a second protecting balloon. Transcranial Doppler has clearly shown that emboli do occur during carotid angioplasty procedures. Transcranial Doppler has also shown that emboli occur during carotid endarterectomy procedures. With all of this information in mind, we and others have elected not to employ a second protecting balloon during carotid artery angioplasty.

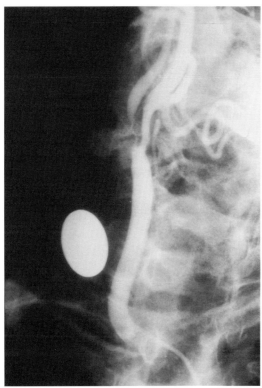

Figure 22. Right common carotid arteriogram before angioplasty. The opaque marker is of known diameter and has been placed in the plane of the carotid bifurcation.

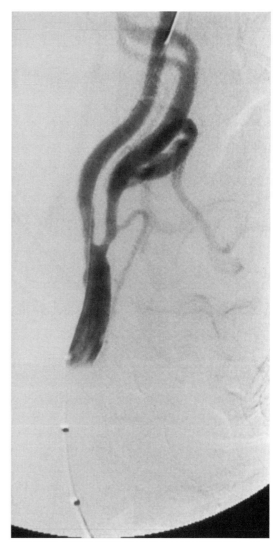

Figure 23. Postangioplasty arteriogram obtained over an 0.018-inch guide wire.

During the procedure, it is important to minimize movement of the exchange guide wire in the internal carotid artery to reduce the risk of vasospasm and/or guide wire-induced dissection. Balloon inflation time should be limited to the amount of time necessary to achieve normal balloon configuration. Following deflation of the balloon, a guide wire exchange is made and an 0.018-inch guide wire is advanced into the distal cervical internal carotid artery. The angioplasty catheter is retracted into the common carotid artery, and arteriography of the angioplasty site and intracranial vasculature is accomplished prior to removal of the safety wire **(Figs. 22–24)**. Even with prolonged balloon inflation (longer than 1 minute), it is uncommon for patients to exhibit neurologic symptoms. Nevertheless, qualified individuals should perform a neurologic assessment of the patient every 3–5 minutes during the procedure.

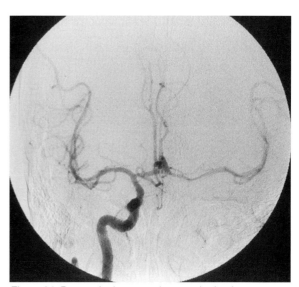

Figure 24. Postangioplasty arteriogram obtained to assess intracranial anatomy. The left internal carotid artery is occluded.

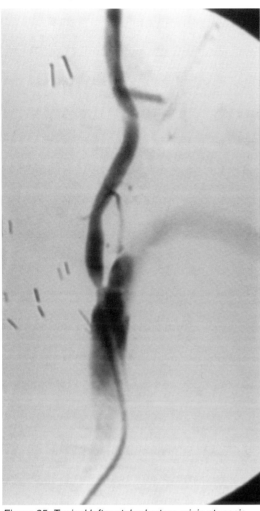

Figure 25. Typical left vertebral artery origin stenosis with adjacent subclavian artery plaque.

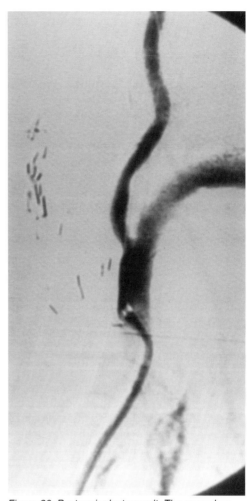

Figure 26. Postangioplasty result. The procedure was performed through a vertebral-configured guiding catheter.

Vertebral Artery Angioplasty

Ninety-five percent of vertebral artery pathology is located at the origin of the vertebral artery, a site easily accessible and treatable by angioplasty **(Figs. 25, 26)**. The risk of developing a fixed neurologic deficit following extracranial vertebral artery angioplasty is reported to be less than 1%, with more than three quarters of patients exhibiting clinical benefit 1 year after the procedure. However, the 85% technical success rate for vertebral artery angioplasty is lower than the technical success rate for angioplasty of any other stenotic brachiocephalic arteries. It seems that plaque on the superior wall of the subclavian artery may engulf the origin of the vertebral artery and, at least, contribute to vertebral artery stenosis. Therefore, vertebral origin angioplasty may be somewhat similar to angioplasty of renal artery ostial lesions.

The clinical indications for vertebral artery angioplasty **(Fig. 27)** include vertebrobasilar insufficiency, global symptoms in the presence of unreconstructable carotid artery disease, and hemispheric symptoms in the presence of unreconstructable ipsilateral carotid artery disease with a patent posterior communicating artery providing the sole straight line inflow to the hemisphere.

Classic teaching is that both vertebral arteries must be significantly diseased or one of the vertebral arteries must be hypoplastic before posterior fossa symptoms can be attributed to reduced posterior fossa flow. This anatomy must be documented prior to vertebral artery angioplasty.

From the angiographer's point of view, the left vertebral artery is the easiest to treat, as shown in **Figures 25** and **26**. Therefore, as long as the left vertebral artery is patent and provides an adequate conduit to the posterior fossa, we approach the left vertebral artery first. This may be done from the transbrachial, transaxillary, or transfemoral approach. The latter is favored, as is the use of a guiding catheter. The guiding catheter permits maintenance of guide wire position throughout the procedure; it also permits the interventionalist to administer pharmacologic agents, and in general it provides some versatility. Clearly, the disadvantage is the increased diameter at the access site. There are a number of precurved guiding catheters designed for vertebral artery access that will engage the subclavian artery easily and can be placed at the orifice of the vertebral artery with equal ease.

An appropriately shaped guide wire is placed past the stenosis well into the mid to distal cervical segment of the vertebral artery. An angioplasty catheter with an appropriately sized balloon is placed over the wire into the stenosis and the procedure is completed. The balloon inflation times tend to be longer than those required to achieve a successful anatomic result at the carotid bifurcation, but symptoms are no more common when they do occur. However, symptoms may be profound and require skilled pharmacologic management. As with other territories, the angioplasty site and the intracranial upstream vasculature are examined before guide wire position is relinquished **(Fig. 28)**.

Vertebral Angioplasty: Indications

• Vertebrobasilar insufficiency

• Global symptoms in the presence of inoperable carotid artery disease

• Hemispheric symptoms in the presence of inoperable ipsilateral carotid artery disease with a patent ipsilateral posterior communicating artery

Figure 27.

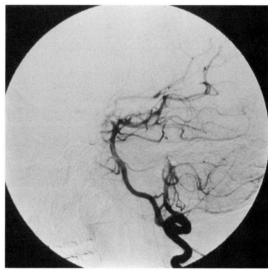

Figure 28. Postangioplasty intracranial anatomy.

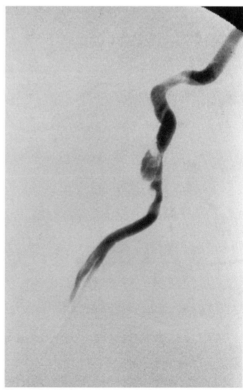

Figure 29. Right internal carotid artery dissection/ false aneurysm.

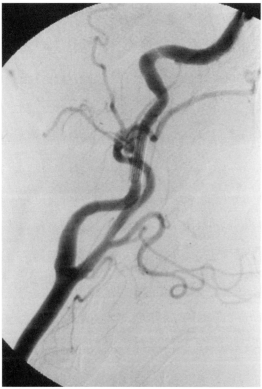

Figure 30. Two years after stent placement.

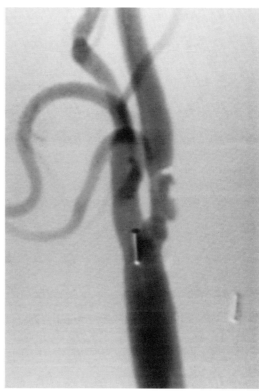

Figure 31. Ulcerated internal carotid artery stenosis.

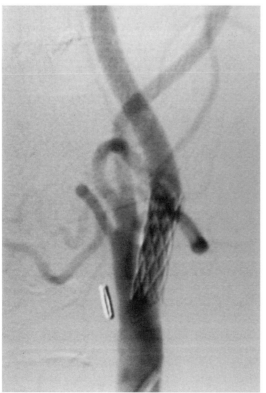

Figure 32. Arteriogram obtained after placement of a Palmaz stent (Johnson & Johnson Interventional Systems, Warren, NJ).

The Role of Stents in the Brachiocephalic Arteries

Except for treatment of subclavian artery occlusions, we have only used stents as "bail-out" devices for spontaneous or angioplasty-induced dissections with threatened abrupt occlusion **(Figs. 29, 30)**. Trials are currently underway to assess the role of stents at the carotid bifurcation **(Figs. 31, 32)** but it will be several years at least before these results are available. In addition to the organized efforts to evaluate carotid bifurcation stenting, an unknown number of sporadic procedures are being performed. The FDA is justifiably concerned about these events and has issued statements indicating that it considers the stent in the carotid territory a significant risk device which requires an investigational device exemption (IDE). Information regarding an IDE package is being developed by the Society of Cardiovascular and Interventional Radiology. Advances in stent design may yield a stent that is ideal for ostial vertebral artery pathology and is an improved stent for the carotid bifurcation.

Conclusion

The percutaneous treatment of atherosclerotic disease of the supra-aortic arteries has a role in clinical practice. Angioplasty, with or without stenting, may reasonably be considered as the first option in the management of intrathoracic disease, particularly for the subclavian artery in the presence of a steal phenomenon.

Our experience with vertebral artery angioplasty has been excellent. Despite a slightly lower technical success rate (86%) than that typically seen in subclavian and carotid artery angioplasty procedures, the long-term results (75% asymptomatic at 1 year) have made vertebral artery PTA our treatment of choice for patients with vertebrobasilar insufficiency who have appropriate anatomy.

Carotid bifurcation angioplasty, with or without stenting, remains controversial, and the results of ongoing and forthcoming trials are eagerly awaited.

Finally, it must be emphasized that competency in peripheral and/or coronary interventions does not imply competency in cerebrovascular angioplasty. As noted previously, additional training should, and perhaps, will be required before the interventionalist can undertake percutaneous cerebrovascular interventions for occlusive disease.

For further information on this topic, please see Teaching File Cases 13, 14, 17, and 18.

Selected Readings

Baker RN, Ramseyer JC, Schwartz WS. Prognosis in patients with transient cerebal ischemic attacks. Neurology 1968; 18:1157–1165.

Executive committee for the asymptomatic carotid atherosclerosis study. Endarterectomy for asymptomatic carotid artery stenosis. JAMA 1995; 273:1421–1428.

Ferguson RDG, Ferguson JG, Lee LT. Extracranial carotid and vertebral artery stenosis: the future of angioplasty in cerebrovascular disease. Batjer HH, ed. Cerebrovascular disease. Philadelphia: Lippincott-Raven, 1996.

Ferguson RDG, Lee LI, Connors JJ, Ferguson JG. Angioplasty in the extracranial and intracranial vasculature. Semin Intervent Radiol 1994; 11:64–82.

Kachel R. Results of balloon angioplasty in the carotid arteries. J Endovasc Surg 1996; 3:22–30.

North American symptomatic carotid endarterectomy trial collaborators. Beneficial effect of carotid endarterectomy in symptomatic patients with high-grade stenosis. New Engl J Med 1991; 325:445–453.

Theron J, Melancon D, Ethier R. "Pre" subclavian steal syndromes and their treatment by angioplasty: hemodynamic classification of subclavian artery stenoses. Neuroradiology 1985; 27:265–270.

Tsai FY, Matovich VB, Hieshima G, et al. Practical aspects of percutaneous transluminal angioplasty of the carotid artery. Acta Radiol Suppl 1986; 369:127–130.

Vitek JJ. Subclavian artery angioplasty and the origin of the vertebral artery. Radiology 1989; 170:407–409.

End Note

Figures 12 and 13 courtesy of Robert Ferguson, M.D., Baptist Memorial Hospital, Memphis, TN.

Causes of Stroke

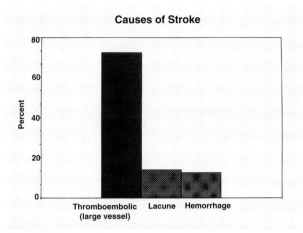

Figure 1.

Mechanisms of Focal Ischemia

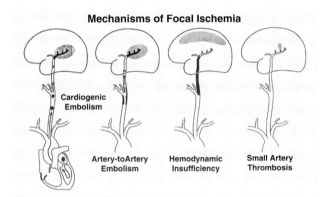

Cardiogenic Embolism

Artery-to-Artery Embolism

Hemodynamic Insufficiency

Small Artery Thrombosis

Figure 2.

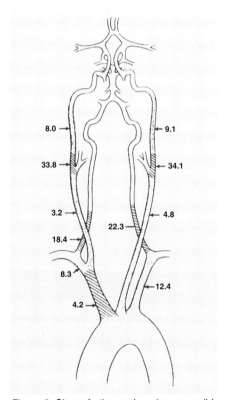

Figure 3. Sites of atherosclerosis responsible for emboli or thrombotic occlusion. Numbers indicate percentages.

TUTORIAL 8
INTRAARTERIAL THROMBOLYSIS FOR ACUTE CEREBRAL INFARCTION
Robert W. Hurst, M.D.

Introduction
The subjects addressed in this tutorial include:
1. Pathophysiology of ischemic cerebral infarction and hemorrhagic transformation
2. The rationale for intraarterial thrombolysis in acute cerebral ischemia
3. Patient selection criteria for intraarterial thrombolysis in acute cerebral ischemia
4. Technique and examples of intraarterial thrombolysis in acute cerebral ischemia
5. Results of acute intraarterial thrombolysis for cerebral ischemia.

Stroke
"Stroke" is the sudden onset of a nonconvulsive neurological deficit of cerebrovascular etiology. Permanent ischemic injury is termed "infarction." The vast majority of strokes (60%–75%) result from ischemia due to thromboembolic occlusion of large intracranial vessels. Thrombotic occlusion of small perforating brain vessels (<200 microns in diameter) is less common an etiology of ischemic stroke (10%–20%) and is termed "lacunar" infarction. Intracranial hemorrhage may also present in a fashion clinically identical to cerebral ischemia **(Fig. 1)**. The different mechanisms underlying stroke require different therapies.

Mechanisms of Ischemia
Large vessel occlusion resulting in cerebral ischemia is usually caused by thromboemboli arising in the extracranial vessels of the neck or by cardiogenic emboli **(Fig. 2)**. Thrombotic occlusion of small vessels (lacunar infarct) and hemodynamic insufficiency are less common mechanisms for cerebral ischemia. Focal atherosclerosis involving extracranial vessels supplying the brain is responsible for the majority of artery-to-artery emboli as well as for thrombotic occlusion of the internal carotid artery **(Fig. 3)**. The bifurcation of the common carotid artery is the most common site of extracranial atherosclerotic involvement of vessels to the brain.

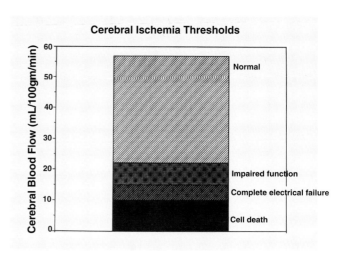

Figure 4. Cerebral blood flow and ischemia.

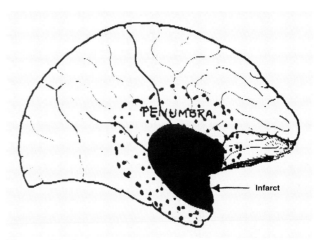

Figure 5. The ischemic penumbra surrounds the infarcted zone.

Thresholds of Ischemia

Vessel occlusion results in central nervous system injury, the severity of which is dependent on the duration and magnitude of the ischemia. As cerebral blood flow declines from normal values (approximately 50 mL/100 gm/minute), failure of neuronal function, initially reversible, occurs **(Fig. 4)**. The tissue may remain viable, however, unless blood flow decreases to approximately 10 mL/100 gm/minute, when irreversible cell death or infarction occurs. Regions of the brain that are receiving insufficient blood flow for normal function but enough blood flow to maintain cell viability may be salvaged by prompt reperfusion. The ischemic area capable of functional recovery with reperfusion has been termed the "ischemic penumbra."

Ischemic Penumbra

The ischemic penumbra is usually adjacent to the more profoundly ischemic and irreversibly damaged area of infarction **(Fig. 5)**. Both the degree and duration of the ischemia are important in determining the extent of neuronal damage **(Fig. 6)**. Even severe ischemia is reversible within a short time, while infarction will develop in areas of less severe ischemia if the time of the ischemia is prolonged. Therefore, the size of the infarction and of the ischemic penumbra depend on the severity and duration of the ischemia. With increased duration of ischemia, more brain tissue becomes irreversibly damaged and moves from the salvageable ischemic penumbra into irreversible infarction.

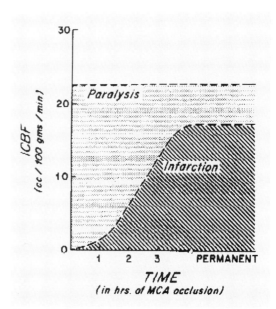

Figure 6. The relationship of intracranial blood flow (ICBF) and the duration of middle cerebral artery (MCA) occlusion.

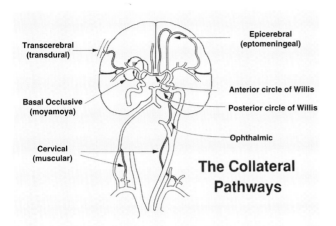

Figure 7. Collateral pathways that aid brain perfusion.

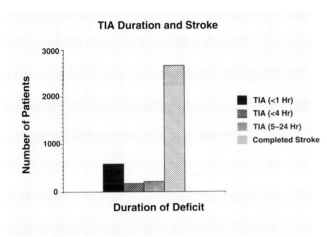

Figure 8. The duration of ischemia and resultant transient ischemic attack and stroke.

Contraindications to Thrombolytic Therapy

Absolute
Intracranial hemorrhage
Active internal bleeding
Recent major trauma (including some surgical procedures)

Relative
CT evidence of acute infarction
Recent surgical procedures
Ulcer disease/recent GI bleeding
Pregnancy and postpartum
Diabetic retinopathy
Uncontrolled severe hypertension
Uncorrectable coagulation defect

Figure 9.

Collaterals and Fibrinolysis

Several mechanisms decrease the severity and duration of cerebral ischemia and thereby limit the development of infarction. A number of collateral pathways can aid brain perfusion when vessel occlusion occurs **(Fig. 7)**. In addition, thrombus or embolus occluding cerebral vessels may be lysed by the fibrinolytic system. The long-term natural history of embolic occlusion of intracranial vessels is usually lysis of the embolus with reopening of the occluded vessel. In some cases of thromboembolic ischemia, these mechanisms successfully limit the ischemia and prevent infarction. The speed and completeness of protection from these mechanisms are unpredictable, however, and often do not permit reperfusion in time to prevent cerebral infarction.

Transient Ischemic Attacks

The presence of collateral pathways and the tendency for occluding thromboemboli to be lysed accounts for the spontaneous reversibility of some episodes of cerebral ischemia. Approximately 28% of ischemic neurological deficits will resolve spontaneously within 24 hours and are defined as "transient ischemic attacks" or TIAs. Most TIAs, however, approximately 60%, last less than 1 hour, and 80% of TIAs last less than 4 hours. If a patient has a neurological deficit persisting more than 4 hours after the onset, his chance of going on to completed infarction is over 90% **(Fig. 8)**. The longer a neurological deficit lasts, the less likely it is to resolve spontaneously.

Rationale for Thrombolysis in Cerebral Ischemia

The rationale for thrombolysis of cerebral vessels, as for thrombolysis in the peripheral and coronary circulations, is based on the assumption that the reopening of an occluded vessel can restore function to areas of surviving tissue (the ischemic penumbra). Shortening the duration of ischemia minimizes the amount of infarction and maximizes potential neurological recovery. Consequently, intraarterial thrombolysis for acute stroke must be performed as soon as possible after the onset of neurological deficit, usually within 6–8 hours. Rapid but complete history and physical examination should include the determination of conditions predisposing to stroke and contraindications to thrombolytic therapy with urokinase **(Fig. 9)**.

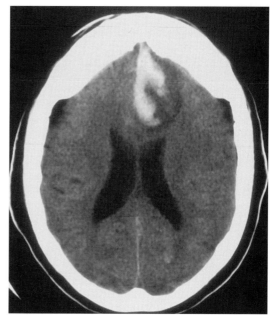

Figure 10. Noncontrast CT scan demonstrates hemorrhagic transformation of a frontal lobe stroke.

Hemorrhagic Transformation

Upon reperfusion, areas of recent infarction are exposed to the force of arterial blood pressure. Extravasation of red blood cells from the damaged vascular bed into the adjacent infarcted area may occur. Extravasation of small amounts of red blood cells into the infarcted area, a phenomenon known as "hemorrhagic transformation," predominately affects gray matter and is seen in up to 40% of untreated embolic infarcts on follow-up computed tomography (CT) scanning **(Fig. 10)**. Spontaneous hemorrhagic transformation is usually clinically insignificant and develops more than 24 hours after the onset of ischemia. The severity of hemorrhagic transformation, however, depends on the volume of brain tissue infarcted and may be minimized by reperfusion before irreversible infarction develops.

Parenchymal Hemorrhage

Less frequently, more bleeding into an area of infarction may result in frank parenchymal hemorrhage associated with mass effect and clinical neurological deterioration **(Fig. 11)**. Hemorrhagic transformation or parenchymal hemorrhage may follow either spontaneous or iatrogenic reopening of occluded cerebral vessels. Because the incidence of hemorrhagic complications increases with the amount and severity of ischemic damage, earlier reperfusion may minimize the chance for hemorrhagic complications. Nevertheless, patients should be monitored closely during thrombolysis for hemorrhagic complications so that a CT scan and neurosurgical consultation can be obtained if necessary.

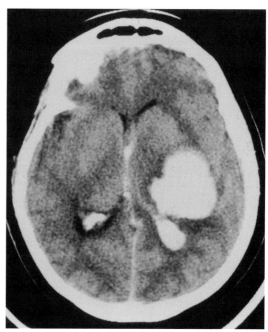

Figure 11. Noncontrast CT scan demonstrates intraparenchymal hemorrhage and mass effect.

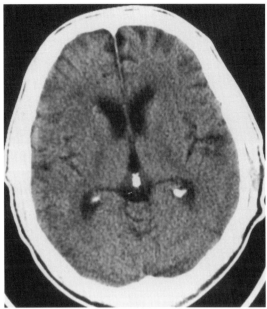

Figure 12. Normal noncontrast CT scan obtained within 6 hours of the onset of ischemic symptoms.

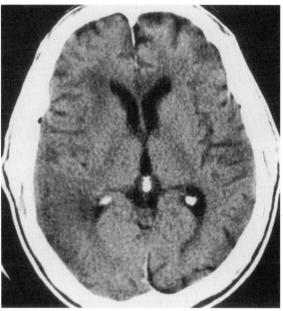

Figure 13. Same patient as in Figure 12. CT scan obtained 24 hours after the onset of ischemia demonstrates loss of gray-white matter discrimination, low attenuation, and mass effect upon the right lateral ventricle.

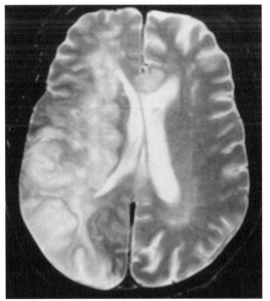

Figure 14. Same patient as in Figure 12. T2-weighted magnetic resonance image obtained 48 hours later demonstrates marked gyral swelling and mass effect.

Imaging Evaluation

Thrombolysis is not believed to be of value in lacunar infarction and is obviously contraindicated in intracranial hemorrhage. Determining the mechanism of stroke in each patient is therefore essential before thrombolysis is performed. An unenhanced CT scan is usually normal within 6 hours of onset of the ischemia (Fig. 12). By 12 to 24 hours, developing infarcts demonstrate mass effect and become hypodense on CT scanning (Fig. 13). Swelling of the infarcted brain tissue reaches its maximum in 48 to 72 hours, when mass effect from large infarcts may cause midline shift, herniation, and death (Fig. 14). An established infarct on the admission CT scan suggests an increased risk of hemorrhage with vessel reopening and is a contraindication to thrombolysis.

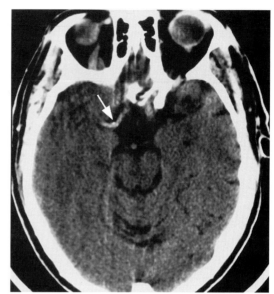

Figure 15. Noncontrast CT scan demonstrates increased density within the right middle cerebral artery, suggesting acute large vessel occlusion (arrow).

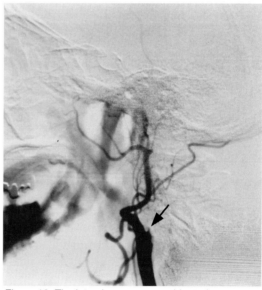

Figure 16. The lateral common carotid arteriogram demonstrates occlusion of the internal carotid artery at its origin (arrow). Only the external carotid artery branches are visible.

Thrombolytic Therapy

Occasionally, hyperdense embolus may be visible within the intracranial vessels, suggesting large vessel occlusion **(Fig. 15)**. While useful, this sign is uncommon and most patients with acute cerebral ischemia have no abnormalities on CT scanning. After excluding contraindications to thrombolysis, arteriography of the symptomatic vascular distribution is performed. A normal arteriogram suggests small vessel infarction and thrombolysis is not indicated. Most patients studied within 6 hours from the onset of ischemic deficit will have a large vessel occlusion causing the deficit. If a large vessel occlusion is identified, heparin is administered.

Technique—Case 1

Thromboembolic occlusion may involve either the extracranial or intracranial vessels supplying the brain. This patient with the new onset of left hemiplegia had complete acute occlusion of the right internal carotid artery **(Fig. 16)**. The diagnostic catheter (6 F or 7 F) is perfused with heparinized saline using a pressure flush system. A microcatheter is advanced through the diagnostic catheter to the level of the occlusion, and urokinase is infused directly into the occluding clot.

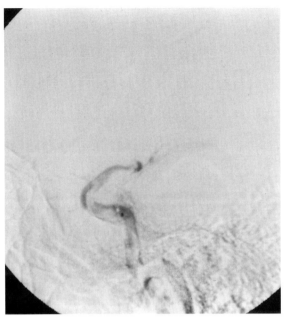

Figure 17. Image of the intracerebral portions of the internal carotid artery demonstrates progressive restoration of flow during thrombolysis.

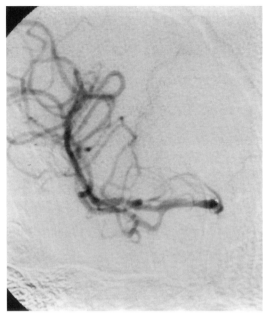

Figure 18. Image of the intracerebral portions of the internal carotid artery demonstrates progressive restoration of flow during thrombolysis.

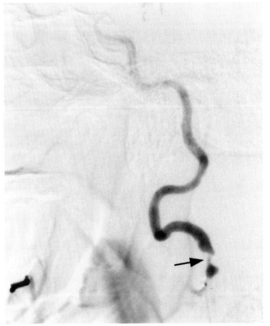

Figure 19. After successful thrombolysis, an underlying severe proximal internal carotid artery stenosis is revealed (arrow).

Later views show progressive reopening of the cavernous internal carotid artery (ICA) and mid carotid artery (MCA) **(Figs. 17, 18)** with lysis of clot. Injection of the reopened right ICA shows high-grade stenosis responsible for thrombus formation and occlusion **(Fig. 19)**.

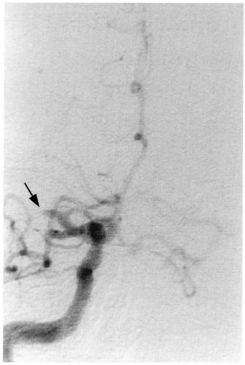

Figure 20. Right middle cerebral artery arteriogram demonstrates proximal occlusion (arrow).

Technique—Case 2

This patient developed left hemiparesis following embolic occlusion of the proximal right MCA during cerebral arteriography **(Fig. 20)**. The microcatheter tip is embedded within or placed proximal to the obstructing clot **(Figs. 21, 22)**. Initial boluses of 25,000–50,000 units of urokinase are followed by 5,000–10,000 units/minute by hand injection until clot lysis occurs with distal filling **(Fig. 23)**, or until a total dose of approximately 1,000,000 units has been given. After thrombolysis, normal filling of all branches was seen and there was complete neurological recovery **(Fig. 24)**.

Technique—Case 3

Right hemiparesis and loss of speech resulted from cardioembolic occlusion of the left MCA **(Fig. 25)**. The tip of the microcatheter was placed at the level of the occlusion **(Figs. 26, 27)**. Mechanical disruption of the clot by the guide wire in conjunction with urokinase infusion may aid clot lysis, and can be performed until clot lysis occurs with filling of distal branches **(Fig. 28)**. After thrombolysis, there was normal filling of MCA branches **(Fig. 29)**. In cases where there is a risk of recurrent emboli (especially cardiac emboli), patients may be maintained on heparin. After thrombolysis, monitoring in the intensive care unit, follow-up CT scanning, and laboratory evaluation of coagulation parameters including prothrombin time, partial thromboplastin time, platelet count, and fibrinogen level are necessary.

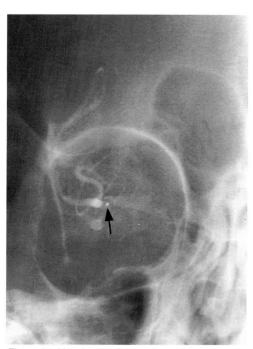

Figure 21. Unsubtracted view of a middle cerebral arteriogram obtained through a microcatheter placed proximal to the occlusion. The radiopaque leading tip of the catheter is faintly visible (arrow).

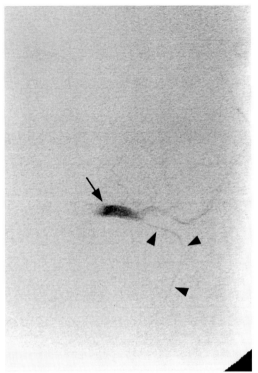

Figure 22. Digital subtraction image of an occluded MCA (arrow). The catheter is faintly visible (arrowheads).

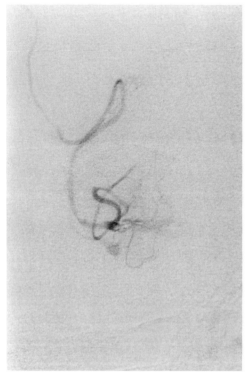

Figure 23. After partial lysis, increased flow into the MCA branches is visible.

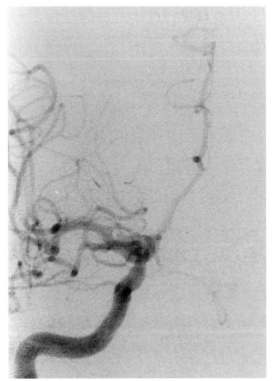

Figure 24. At completion of thrombolysis, normal flow has been restored to all MCA branches.

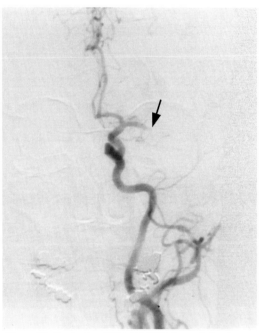

Figure 25. Occlusion of the left MCA (arrow) due to an embolus from the heart.

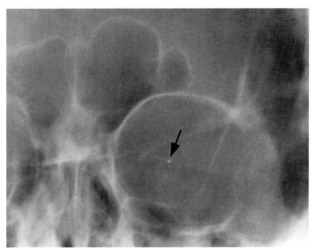

Figure 26. Unsubtracted view of the microcatheter tip at the level of the occlusion (arrow).

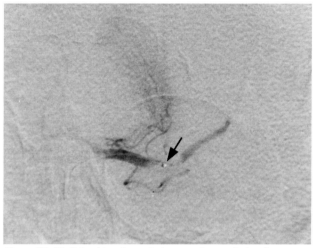

Figure 27. Digital subtraction arteriogram demonstrates the catheter tip within the occluded segment.

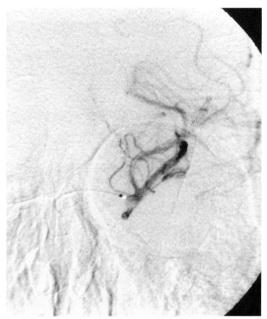

Figure 28. Digital subtraction arteriogram obtained during partial lysis of the embolus reveals increased flow to the distal MCA branches.

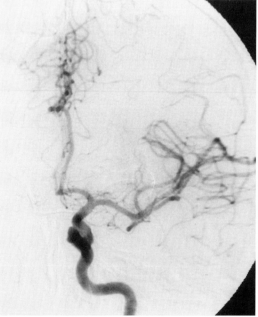

Figure 29. The completion arteriogram reveals normal flow to the left MCA.

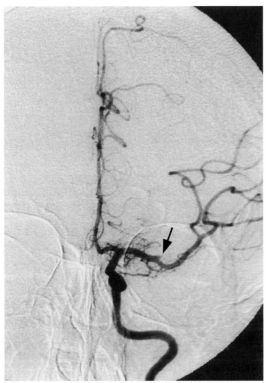

Figure 30. This occlusion of a peripheral MCA branch (arrow) resulted in a significant neurologic deficit.

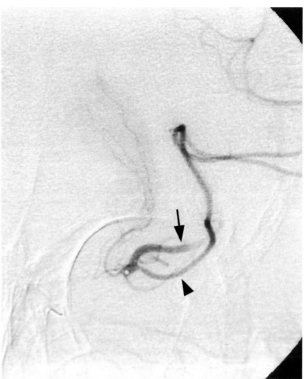

Figure 31. Digital subtraction arteriography performed at the level of the occlusion (arrow) demonstrates preserved flow to the inferior trunk (arrowhead) and lenticulostriate arteries.

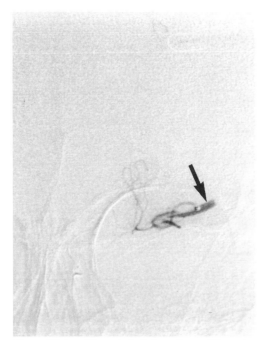

Figure 32. Local thrombolysis is performed through a catheter placed within the occlusion (arrow).

Technique—Case 4

Significant deficits may also result from peripheral cerebral vessel occlusion **(Fig. 30)**. Catheter placement proximal to the occluded branch **(Fig. 31)** shows good filling of the open inferior trunk and reflux into the lenticulostriate arteries. Selective placement into the occluded trunk shows clot **(Fig. 32)**.

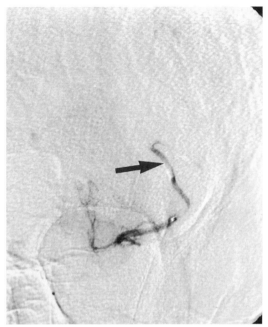

Figure 33. Progressive lysis of the embolus (arrow).

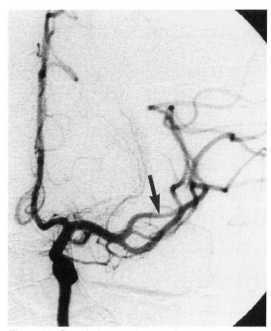

Figure 34. Completion arteriogram demonstrates vessel patency.

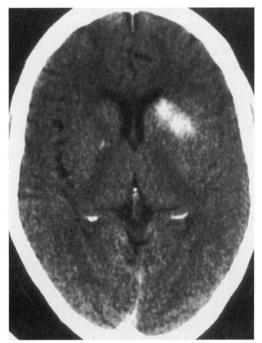

Figure 35. CT scan obtained immediately after thrombolysis reveals focal high density due to contrast material injections during thrombolysis.

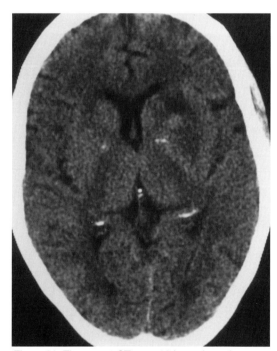

Figure 36. The repeat CT scan 12 hours later demonstrates no residual high density, distinguishing the transient finding from hemorrhagic transformation.

Progressive lysis of the embolus occurs with filling of distal branches **(Fig. 33)**. After thrombolysis, there is complete reopening **(Fig. 34)**. In some cases, CT scanning performed immediately after thrombolysis shows high density without mass effect from selective local injection of contrast material **(Fig. 35)**. Contrast resolves on a CT scan obtained 12 hours later, allowing differentiation from hemorrhagic transformation **(Fig. 36)**.

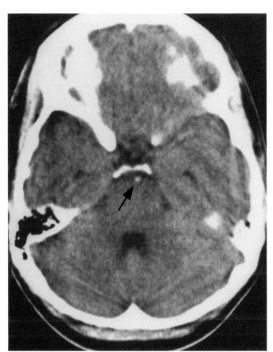

Figure 37. Noncontrast CT scan demonstrates high density in the basilar artery (arrow), indicating acute occlusion.

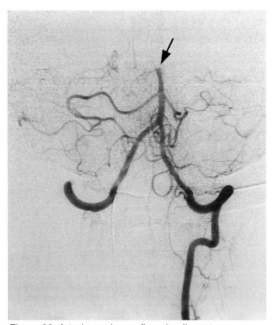

Figure 38. Arteriography confirms basilar artery occlusion (arrow).

Thrombolysis in the Vertebrobasilar Circulation—Case 5

Evidence suggests that thrombolysis in the vertebrobasilar circulation may be performed safely after longer periods of deficits (up to 24 hours) if no evidence of infarction is present on CT scanning. An unenhanced CT scan may demonstrate high-density clot occluding the basilar artery which is confirmed on arteriography **(Figs. 37, 38)**. A microcatheter was embedded in the basilar artery clot **(Figs. 39, 40)**; this was followed by progressive reopening of the distal basilar artery and branches **(Fig. 41)**. Injection of the left vertebral artery after thrombolysis confirmed reopening, and there was significant recovery of neurological deficits **(Fig. 42)**.

Results

At present, a number of clinical trials are evaluating the ultimate role of intracranial thrombolysis for acute cerebral ischemia. Available reports suggest that recanalization may be accomplished in 50%–75% of cases with an incidence of hemorrhage or hemorrhagic transformation (mostly asymptomatic) of 3.5%–10%. Clinical improvement may be expected in up to 75% of patients with recanalization of anterior circulation occlusions. Acute recanalization of vertebrobasilar occlusions in one study was associated with a 70% survival rate, compared to a 13% survival rate for patients treated with conventional therapy.

Selected Readings

Bozzao L, Fantozzi L, Bastianello S, et al. Ischemic supratentorial stroke: angiographic findings in patients examined in the very early phase. J Neurol 1989; 236:340–342.

del Zoppo GJ, Ferbert A, Otis S, et al. Local intra-arterial fibrinolytic therapy in acute carotid territory stroke: a pilot study. Stroke 1988; 19:307–313.

Friday G, Lai SM, Alter M, et al. Stroke in the Lehigh Valley: racial/ethnic differences. Neurology 1989; 39:1165–1168.

Hacke W, Zeumer H, Ferbert A, Bruckmann H, del Zoppo GJ. Intra-arterial thrombolytic therapy improves outcome in patients with acute vertebrobasilar occlusive disease. Stroke 1988; 19:1216–1222.

Hornig CR, Dorndorf W, Agnoli AL. Hemorrhagic cerebral infarction: a prospective study. Stroke 1986; 17:179–185.

Koudstaal P, van Gijn J, Frenken C, et al. TIA, RIND, minor stroke: a continuum, or different subgroups. J Neurol Neurosurg Psychiatry 1992; 55:95–97.

Levy DE. How transient are transient ischemic attacks? Neurology 1988; 38:674–677.

Matsumoto K, Satoh K. Topical intraarterial urokinase infusion for acute stroke. In: Hacke W, del Zoppo G, Hirschberg M, eds. Thrombolytic therapy in acute ischemic stroke. Berlin: Springer-Verlag, 1991; 207–212.

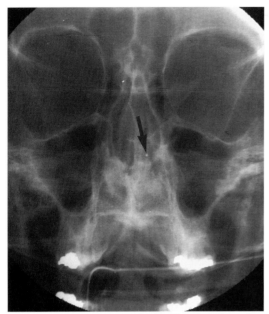

Figure 39. Microcatheter embedded in a thrombosed vessel (arrow).

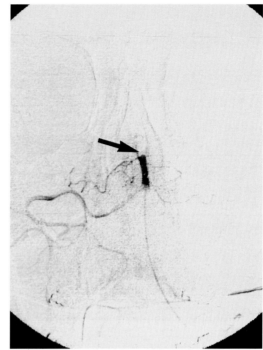

Figure 40. Digital subtraction arteriography performed through the microcatheter confirms its position within the thrombus (arrow).

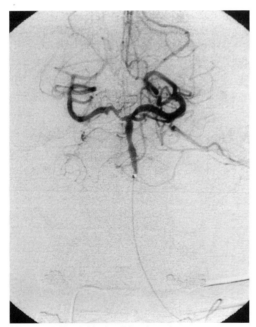

Figure 41. Partial lysis of the thrombus.

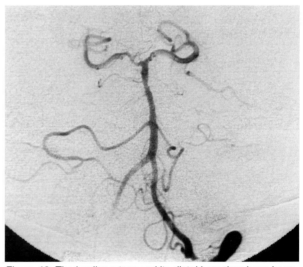

Figure 42. The basilar artery and its distal branches have been restored to patency.

Mohr JP, Caplan LR, Melski J, et al. The Harvard cooperative stroke registry: a prospective registry. Neurology 1978; 28:754–762.

Mori E, Tabuchi M, Yoshida T, Yamadori A. Intracarotid urokinase with thromboembolic occlusion of the middle cerebral artery. Stroke 1988; 19:802–812.

Theron J, Courtheoux P, Casasco A, et al. Local intraarterial fibrinolysis in the carotid territory. Am J Neuroradiology 1989; 10:753–756.

End Notes
Figures 2 and 7 from Awad I, ed. Cerebrovascular occlusive disease and brain ischemia. Park Ridge, IL: American Association of Neurological Surgeons, 1992; 284, 285. Used with permission.

Figure 3 from Hass WK, Fields WS, North RR, Kircheff II, Chase NE, Bauer RB. Joint study of extracranial arterial occlusion. II. Arteriography, techniques, sites, and complications. JAMA 1968; 203:963. Used with permission.

Figure 4 from Symon L. The relationship between CBF, evoked potentials, and the clinical features in cerebral ischemia. Acta Neurol Scand 1980; 78:179. Used with permission.

Figure 6 from Jones TH, Morawetz RB, Crowell RM. Threshold of focal ischemia in awake monkeys. J Neurosurg 1981; 54:781. Used with permission.

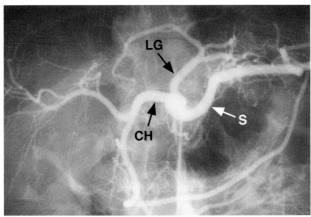

Figure 1. The celiac artery is most frequently the origin of the left gastric (LG), splenic (S), and common hepatic (CH) arteries.

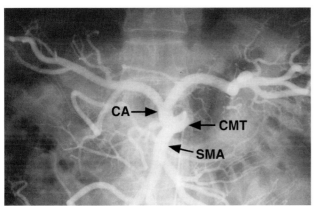

Figure 2. The celiacomesenteric trunk (CMT) is a common origin of the celiac artery (CA) and the superior mesenteric artery (SMA).

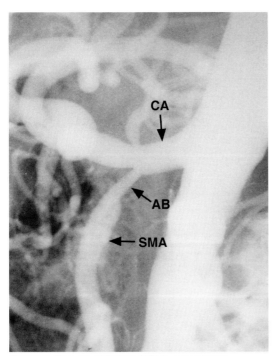

Figure 3. The arc of Buhler (AB) is a persistent embryonic ventral anastomosis between the celiac artery (CA) and the SMA, seen as a bridging vessel connecting the two origins.

TUTORIAL 9
DIAGNOSTIC VISCERAL NORMAL AND VARIANT ANATOMY— CELIAC, SUPERIOR MESENTERIC, AND INFERIOR MESENTERIC ARTERIES
Joseph Bonn, M.D.

Introduction
The subjects addressed in this tutorial include:
1. Normal and variant celiac artery anatomy
2. Normal and variant superior mesenteric artery (SMA) anatomy
3. Normal and variant inferior mesenteric artery (IMA) anatomy.

N.B.: In each example, "normal" is defined as the most common anatomical arrangement, while "variant" defines those arrangements present in the minority of cases.

Normal Celiac Artery
The celiac artery, axis, or trunk originates from the abdominal aorta just caudal to the diaphragmatic crura, typically at the level of the inferior margin of the left pedicle of the T12 vertebra. After a short caudal segment, it turns ventral and is most commonly the origin of three vessels: the left gastric artery, the splenic artery, and the common hepatic artery **(Fig. 1)**. In 55%–75% of the population, these three arteries originate independently, with the left gastric artery usually arising as the first branch.

Variant Celiac Artery
In approximately 25% of cases, the three branches originate not independently but as a true trifurcation. In the remaining small percentage, variants consist mostly of branches replaced elsewhere, such as the left gastric artery (2%) or the common hepatic artery (3%), or of vessels joined together, such as the celiacomesenteric trunk **(Fig. 2)**, a common origin of the celiac artery and the SMA. This is not to be confused with the arc of Buhler, a persistent embryonic ventral anastomosis between the celiac artery and the SMA, seen as a bridging vessel connectingthe two origins **(Fig. 3)**.

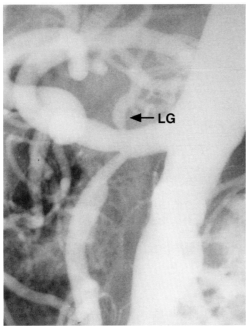

Figure 4. The left gastric artery (LG) is the first and smallest branch of the celiac artery, and supplies the lesser curvature and cardia of the stomach.

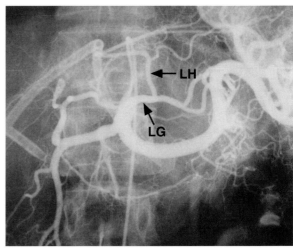

Figure 5. A variant lateral segmental branch of the left hepatic artery (LH) arises from the left gastric artery (LG).

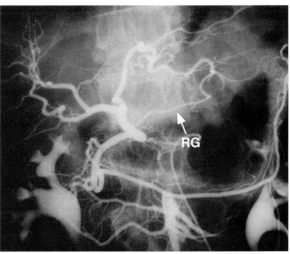

Figure 6. The normal right gastric artery (RG) traverses the lesser curve of the stomach before anastomosing with the left gastric artery.

Normal Left Gastric Artery

The left gastric artery is the first and smallest branch of the celiac artery, traveling in a cephalad direction **(Fig. 4)** to supply the lesser curvature and cardia of the stomach, where it usually divides into anterior and posterior branches, the latter often anastomosing with the right gastric artery. Distal left gastric branches also serve the distal esophagus.

Variant Left Gastric Artery

Variations include the site of origin of the left gastric artery and the uncommon branches that may arise from the left gastric artery. Examples of the former are the left gastric artery originating directly from the abdominal aorta in 3% of cases, from a lienogastric trunk (splenic and left gastric arteries arising together from the aorta) in 4% of cases, and a hepatogastric trunk (common hepatic and left gastric arteries arising together from the aorta) in 2% of cases. Examples of the branches that uncommonly arise from the left gastric artery include left hepatic branches, either completely or partially in 23% of cases **(Fig. 5)**, and inferior phrenic arteries in 3%–4% of cases.

Normal Right Gastric Artery

The right gastric artery has two common origins: the proper hepatic artery in 40% of cases and a left or middle hepatic artery in 40% of cases. It travels along the lesser curve of the stomach to supply the pylorus and posterior body, then anastomoses with the posterior branches of the left gastric artery **(Fig. 6)**.

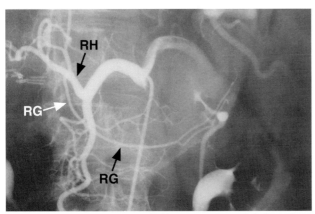

Figure 7. A right gastric artery (RG) has a variant origin from the right hepatic artery (RH).

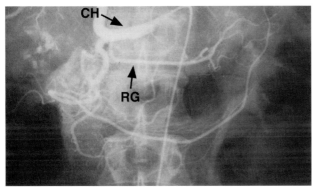

Figure 8. A right gastric artery (RG) has a variant origin from the common hepatic artery (CH).

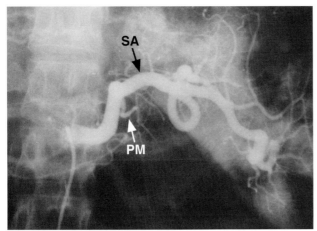

Figure 9. The pancreatica magna artery (PM) originates at the mid portion of the splenic artery (SA).

Variant Right Gastric Artery

The right gastric artery varies in its origin, arising from the right hepatic artery in 10% of cases **(Fig. 7)**, the gastroduodenal artery in 8%, and the common hepatic artery in 2% **(Fig. 8)**.

Normal Splenic Artery

The splenic artery originates from the celiac artery in 99% of cases, traveling superior and anterior to the splenic vein before dividing into parenchymal branches in the splenic hilum. The main splenic artery commonly gives rise to the dorsal pancreatic artery, the pancreatica magna artery **(Fig. 9)** (from the mid-splenic, and the largest pancreatic branch), several short gastric arteries to the gastric cardia and fundus, a superior polar splenic artery, and the left gastroepiploic artery, which runs along the lesser curvature of the stomach to anastomose with the right gastroepiploic artery. The inferior polar splenic artery usually arises from the left gastroepiploic artery.

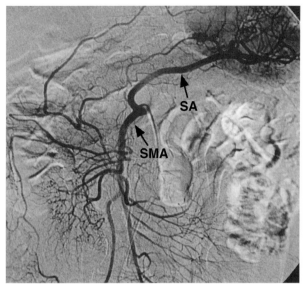

Figure 10. The lienomesenteric trunk is a variant origin of the splenic artery (SA) from the SMA.

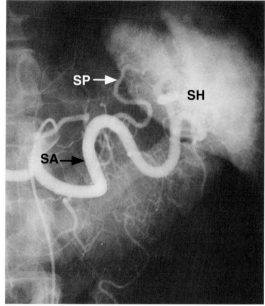

Figure 11. The superior polar branch (SP) of the splenic artery (SA) may originate separately from the splenic hilum (SH).

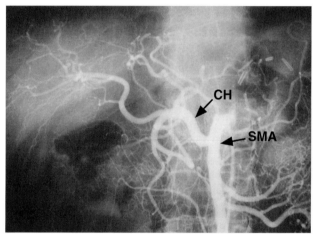

Figure 12. A common hepatic artery (CH) has a variant origin from the SMA.

Variant Splenic Artery

In less than 1% of cases, the splenic artery arises from the superior mesenteric artery, otherwise known as a lienomesenteric trunk **(Fig. 10)**. Even more rarely, the superior polar splenic artery arises from the proximal splenic artery rather than distally by the hilum **(Fig. 11)**.

Normal Common Hepatic Artery

The common hepatic artery usually arises from the celiac artery, traveling anteriorly and to the right, where it reaches the superior duodenum, gives off the gastroduodenal artery, and becomes the proper hepatic artery. In 55% of cases, all hepatic arteries arise from the common hepatic artery.

Variant Common Hepatic Artery

Uncommon origins of the common hepatic artery include from the superior mesenteric artery in 2.5% of cases **(Fig. 12)**, the aorta in 2%, and very rarely from the left gastric artery.

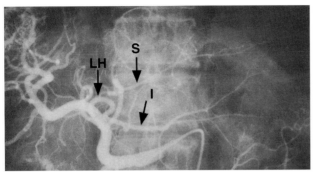

Figure 13. A lateral segmental branch of the left hepatic artery (LH) divides into superior (S) and inferior (I) subsegmental arteries.

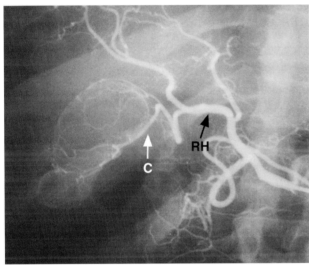

Figure 14. The most frequent gallbladder supply is a single cystic artery (C) originating from the right hepatic artery (RH).

Normal Proper Hepatic Artery

The proper hepatic artery normally originates from the common hepatic artery after the origin of the gastroduodenal artery. It travels as part of the portal triad anterior to the portal vein and to the left of the common bile duct. After reaching the porta hepatis it divides into the intrahepatic segmental arteries, including the right ventrocranial, right dorsocaudal, left medial (sometimes called the middle hepatic), and the left lateral (sometimes called the left hepatic), which divides into characteristic parallel superior and inferior branches **(Fig. 13)**. In 40% of cases the right gastric artery arises from the proper hepatic artery.

The cystic artery, supplying the gallbladder, varies considerably; however, the most common presentation, seen in 45% of cases, is a single artery originating from the right hepatic artery **(Fig. 14)**.

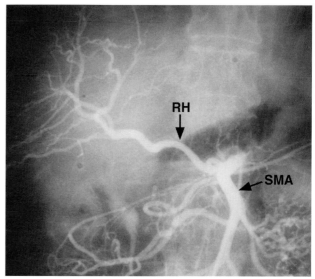

Figure 15. The right hepatic artery (RH) is completely replaced to the SMA.

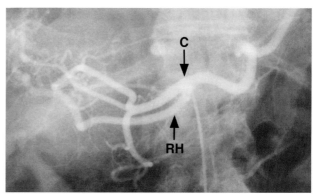

Figure 16. A proximal origin of the right hepatic artery (RH) directly from the celiac artery (C).

Variant Proper Hepatic Artery

The right hepatic artery can be completely replaced to the SMA in 12%–14% of cases **(Fig. 15)**, or originate from the SMA as an accessory in 6%–8%. In less than 2% of cases, it can originate directly from the aorta, or from the celiac artery as an early common hepatic artery bifurcation **(Fig. 16)**. The left hepatic artery can be entirely replaced to the left gastric artery in 11%–12% of cases, or an accessory left hepatic artery can arise from the left gastric artery in a similar percentage **(Fig. 17)**. Rarely, in 1%–2% of cases, the combined left hepatic/left gastric trunk can arise directly from the aorta. Variations in a single cystic artery (80%) include origins from a right hepatic artery replaced to the SMA (12%), from the proximal (2%) or distal (10%) common hepatic artery, proper hepatic or gastroduodenal arteries each (2%), or the left hepatic artery (5%). There are two cystic arteries in 19% of cases and three cystic arteries in 1% of cases.

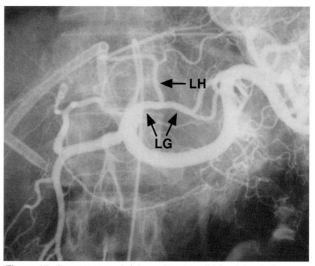

Figure 17. An accessory left hepatic artery (LH) arising independently from the left gastric artery (LG).

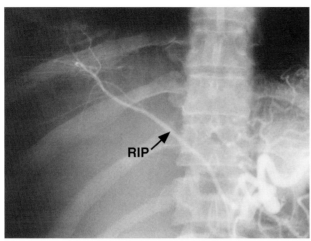

Figure 18. A right inferior phrenic artery (RIP) originating directly from the aorta.

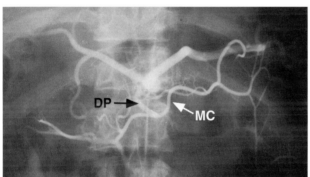

Figure 19. The dorsal pancreatic artery (DP) can provide a variant supply to the middle colic artery (MC).

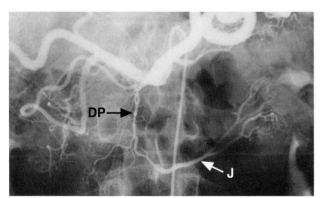

Figure 20. The dorsal pancreatic artery (DP) can provide a variant supply to the jejunum (J).

Normal Inferior Phrenic Arteries

The inferior phrenic arteries originate from the celiac artery, as the first branch, in 55% of cases, with the second most common origin being from the aorta **(Fig. 18)**.

Variant Inferior Phrenic Arteries

In 3%–4% of cases, the inferior phrenic arteries originate from the left gastric artery.

Normal Pancreatic Arteries

The dorsal pancreatic artery originates most commonly from the splenic artery (40%) from which it travels to the dorsal surface of the pancreas, contributing a branch to the uncinate process, and in 75% of cases giving rise to the transverse pancreatic artery supplying the tail of the pancreas. The pancreatica magna usually arises from the splenic artery and supplies the distal body and the tail of the pancreas.

Variant Pancreatic Arteries

Variant origins of the dorsal pancreatic artery include the celiac artery (22%), the common hepatic artery (20%), and the superior mesenteric artery or the aorta (14% each). In 4% of cases, the dorsal pancreatic artery gives rise to the middle colic artery **(Fig. 19)**, or jejunal branches **(Fig. 20)**.

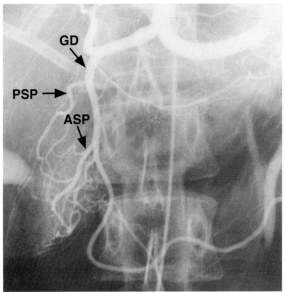

Figure 21. Major branches of the gastroduodenal artery (GD) that contribute to the pancreaticoduodenal arcade, including the posterior superior (PSP) and the anterior superior (ASP) pancreaticoduodenal arteries.

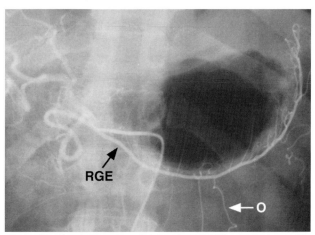

Figure 22. The right gastroepiploic artery (RGE) contributes to the abundant supply to the stomach and the omentum (O).

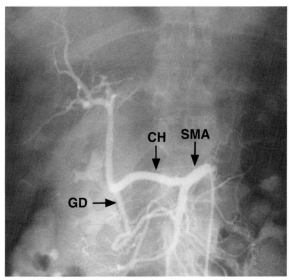

Figure 23. A variant gastroduodenal artery (GD) originates from a replaced common hepatic artery (CH) to the SMA.

Normal Gastroduodenal Artery

The gastroduodenal artery originates in 75% of cases from the common hepatic artery, beginning posterior to the duodenum and giving off four major branches: the right gastroepiploic artery, the posterior superior pancreaticoduodenal (PSP) artery, the anterior superior pancreaticoduodenal (ASP) artery **(Fig. 21)**, and the supraduodenal artery. The PSP artery travels to the posterior surface of the head of the pancreas where it anastomoses with the posterior inferior pancreaticoduodenal artery. The ASP artery travels to the anterior surface of the head of the pancreas where it anastomoses with the anterior inferior pancreaticoduodenal artery. The supraduodenal artery supplies the pylorus and the first portion of the duodenum. The right gastroepiploic artery supplies the greater curvature of the stomach, the pylorus, the first portion of the duodenum, and the omentum **(Fig. 22)**. The arc of Barkow is an epiploic arc in the omentum which parallels the gastroepiploic vessels to serve as a collateral network.

Variant Gastroduodenal Artery

The second most common origin of the gastroduodenal artery is as part of a replaced or accessory hepatic artery from the SMA or aorta (11%) **(Fig. 23)**. Other variants include origins from the right (6%) or left (4%) hepatic, or superior mesenteric arteries (4%) directly.

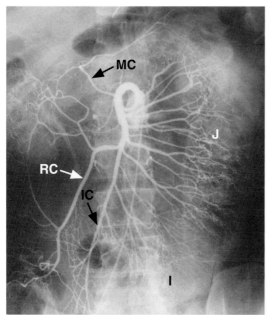

Figure 24. The superior mesenteric artery divides into inferior pancreaticoduodenal, jejunal (J), and ileal (I) arteries, supplying the duodenum, pancreas, and small intestine. The ileocolic (IC), right colic (RC), and middle colic (MC) arteries serve the distal ileum and the ascending and transverse colon.

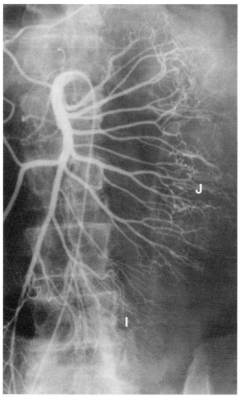

Figure 26. Jejunal (J) and ileal (I) arteries divide into arterial arcades that become the vasa recta of the small intestine.

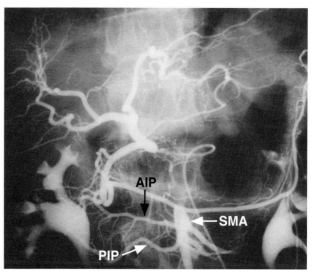

Figure 25. In this variant, there are separate origins from the SMA for the anterior (AIP) and posterior (PIP) inferior pancreaticoduodenal arteries.

Normal Superior Mesenteric Artery

The superior mesenteric artery arises from the abdominal aorta at approximately the L1 vertebral level, about 1 cm distal to the origin of the celiac artery. It passes anteriorly from the aorta, traveling posterior to the pancreas and splenic vein, supplying the distal duodenum, the head and body of the pancreas, and the jejunum, ileum, and the large intestine to the splenic flexure **(Fig. 24)**.

The first major branch of the SMA is a single inferior pancreaticoduodenal artery in 60% of cases, which then divides into the anterior and posterior branches, which anastomose with their superior pancreaticoduodenal counterparts.

Variant Superior Mesenteric Artery

Variations in the SMA pertain to the individual branching arteries, the replaced hepatic arteries which were described earlier, and the small intestine and large intestine arteries which will be covered below. One variant worth describing here is that in 40% of cases the anterior and posterior branches of the inferior pancreaticoduodenal artery have separate origins off the SMA **(Fig. 25)**.

Normal Jejunal and Ileal Arteries

The normal small bowel has between ten and twenty jejunal and ileal branches, arising from the left margin of the SMA and coursing toward the right lower quadrant. Distally, the separate branches join as the arterial arcades which then give rise to the vasa recta of the bowel **(Fig. 26)**.

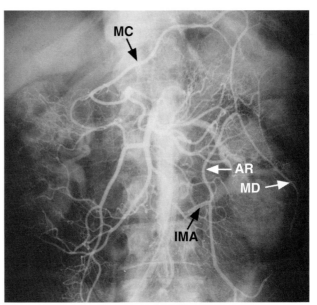

Figure 27. The middle colic artery (MC) divides into an anastomosis with the right colic artery (RC) and the supply for the transverse colon.

Variant Jejunal and Ileal Arteries

Rarely, the dorsal pancreatic or gastroduodenal arteries can supply branches to the jejunum **(Fig. 20)**.

Normal Middle Colic Artery

The middle colic artery typically arises as the second branch of the SMA after the inferior pancreaticoduodenal artery, beginning anterior and to the right, and turning right before dividing into right and left branches which follow the mesenteric border of the transverse colon **(Fig. 27)**. The right branch anastomoses with the ascending branch of the right colic artery at the hepatic flexure. The left branch anastomoses with the left colic branch at the splenic flexure, where the marginal artery of Drummond along the mesenteric border, and the arc of Riolan within the mesentery, form an anastomosing network between the SMA and the IMA **(Fig 28)**.

Variant Middle Colic Artery

In 10% of cases the middle colic artery arises from the dorsal pancreatic artery or celiac arteries **(Fig. 29)**. Other more rare middle colic artery variations include a common right colic/middle colic trunk, a middle colic artery arising from the SMA alongside a replaced right hepatic artery, an accessory middle colic artery serving the left colic artery directly, and absence of the middle colic artery.

Normal Right Colic/Ileocolic Arteries

The right colic artery originates from the SMA distal to the middle colic artery, and supplies the upper ascending colon and the proximal transverse colon. Its descending branch anastomoses with the ileocolic artery, and the ascending branch anastomoses with the descending branch of the middle colic artery. The ileocolic artery supplies the cecum, the appendix, a descending branch that anastomoses with ileal branches, and an ascending branch that anastomoses with the descending branch of the right colic artery **(Fig. 30)**.

Figure 28. Two important anastomotic branches between the SMA and the IMA are the marginal artery of Drummond (MD), and the arc of Riolan (AR).

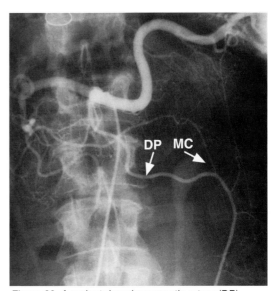

Figure 29. A variant dorsal pancreatic artery (DP) supplies the middle colic artery (MC).

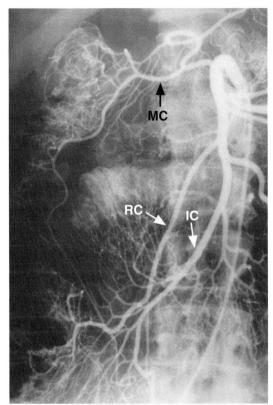

Figure 30. The right colic artery (RC) divides into ascending and descending branches to anastomose with the ileocolic (IC) and middle colic (MC) arteries, respectively.

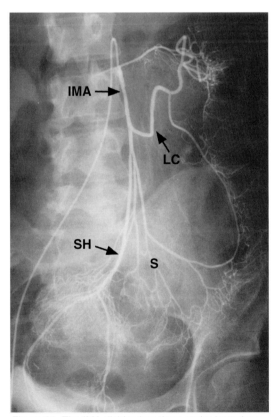

Figure 31. The IMA divides into three major branches: the left colic (LC), the sigmoid (S), and the superior hemorrhoidal (SH) arteries.

Variant Right Colic/Ileocolic Arteries

Rarely, the right colic artery may be absent or may originate in common with the ileocolic artery or the middle colic artery.

Normal Inferior Mesenteric Artery

The inferior mesenteric artery originates from the anterior abdominal aorta at the L3 vertebra, traveling caudally and to the left where it divides into the left colic artery, the sigmoid artery, and the superior hemorrhoidal arteries **(Fig. 31)**. The IMA supplies the distal transverse colon, the splenic flexure, the descending colon, the sigmoid colon, and the upper rectum.

Variant Inferior Mesenteric Artery

In about 5% of cases, the distal sigmoid artery branches do not anastomose with the superior hemorrhoidal artery.

For further information on this topic, please see Teaching File Cases 28 and 49.

Selected Readings

Abrams HL, ed. Abrams angiography: vascular and interventional radiology. 3rd edition. Boston: Little, Brown and Company, 1983.

Johnsrude IS, Jackson DC. A practical approach to angiography. 2nd edition. Boston: Little Brown and Company, 1987.

Kadir S. Atlas of normal and variant angiographic anatomy. Philadelphia: W.B. Saunders Company, 1991.

Netter FH. Atlas of human anatomy. Summit, NJ: Ciba-Geigy Corporation, 1989.

Reuter SR, Redman HC, Cho KJ. Gastrointestinal angiography. 3rd edition. Philadelphia: W.B. Saunders Company, 1986.

End Notes

Figure 10 courtesy of Donald Logan, M.D., and Michael Amygdalos, M.D.

TUTORIAL 10
MESENTERIC ISCHEMIA
Adam B. Winick, M.D., and
Anthony C. Venbrux, M.D.

Introduction
The subjects addressed in this tutorial include:
1. The definition of mesenteric ischemia
2. The etiology of mesenteric ischemia
3. Therapy by radiologic, medical, and surgical means
4. Complications of therapy.

Mesenteric ischemia can be a devastating condition associated with high morbidity and mortality. The patient with this disorder must be rapidly diagnosed and treated to maintain bowel viability.

Mesenteric ischemia results from decreased blood flow to all or part of the small bowel and colon. Ischemia may be acute or chronic. Clinically, patients can have complex and variable signs and symptoms. The most frequent clinical finding in a patient with mesenteric ischemia is a syndrome of abdominal pain disproportionate to the physical examination, nausea, vomiting, and diarrhea. The wide variety of symptoms is thought to be related to the diverse etiologies of ischemia, the duration of the ischemia, the pathophysiologic response of the bowel, the region of the gastrointestinal tract affected, the extent of the ischemia, and the patient's underlying medical condition. Most importantly, the physician(s) caring for the patient must have a high clinical index of suspicion in order to make the correct diagnosis and to institute prompt therapy so that early intervention by radiologic, medical, or surgical means may correct insufficient flow of blood to the bowel.

Mesenteric ischemia can be caused by an acute event, or it can develop insidiously, with or without an acute clinical exacerbation. Classification into acute or chronic forms has been based on the onset and type of clinical symptomatology. The acute form can be classified according to whether the ischemia arises from occlusive or nonocclusive causes. In both instances, the viability of the bowel is at risk. In a review of the incidence of mesenteric ischemia from Montefiore Medical Center, New York, **(Fig. 1)**, acute mesenteric ischemia was second to colonic ischemia in incidence; however, it is the most life-threatening of the ischemic disorders involving the intestine. A spectrum of pathologic findings can be associated with mesenteric ischemia, ranging from completely reversible alterations of bowel function to transmural hemorrhagic necrosis of the wall of the bowel. The end result of the ischemic episode and the extent of injury to the bowel is dependent on a number of factors, as listed in **Figure 2**.

Incidence of Different Etiologies of Mesenteric Ischemia	
Type of Ischemia	*Incidence*
Acute mesenteric ischemia	30%
Superior mesenteric artery embolus	(50%)
Nonocclusive mesenteric ischemia	(25%)
Superior mesenteric artery thrombosis	(10%)
Mesenteric venous thrombosis	(5%)
Miscellaneous (vasculitis, etc.)	(5%)
Colonic ischemia	60%
Focal segmental ischemia	5%
Chronic mesenteric ischemia	5%

Figure 1.

Factors in Determining the Extent of Intestinal Injury Due to Ischemia
1. The state of the systemic circulation.
2. The degree of functional or anatomic compromise.
3. The number and caliber of the vessels affected.
4. The response of the vascular bed to diminished perfusion.
5. The nature and capacity of the collateral circulation to supply the needs of the dependent segment of bowel.
6. The duration of the insult.
7. The metabolic needs of the dependent segment as dictated by its function and bacterial population.

Figure 2.

Types and Risk Factors for Mesenteric Infarction	
Type	*Risk Factors*
Superior mesenteric artery (SMA) embolus	Myocardial infarction (MI), arrhythmias, ventricular aneurysm, endocarditis, atheroma
SMA thrombosis	Atheroma, congestive heart failure, hypotension, oral contraceptives
Nonocclusive infarction	MI, shock, sepsis, hypotension, digoxin or propranolol overdose, unknown
SMV thrombosis	Primary mesenteric occlusion, sepsis, oral contraceptives, thrombocytosis, disseminated intravascular coagulation, postsplenectomy

Figure 3.

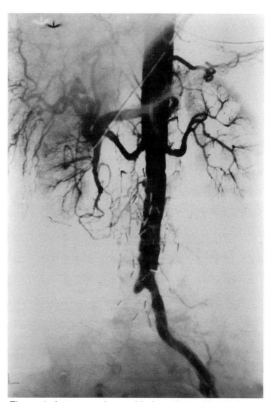

Figure 4. Aortogram in an elderly patient with atrial fibrillation, chronic right iliac occlusion, and recent onset of abdominal pain. Contrast material fills the celiac axis, and there is no collateral flow to any of the other mesenteric vessels.

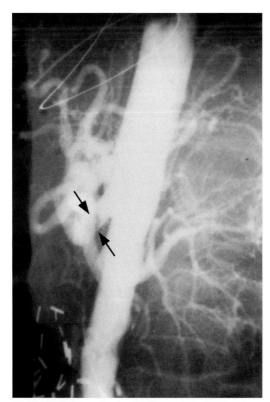

Figure 5. Same patient as in Figure 4. Lateral aortogram demonstrates patency of the celiac axis. An embolus fills the proximal SMA (arrows).

Clinical Findings of Mesenteric Ischemia

Acute mesenteric ischemia is a life-threatening vascular emergency that has a mortality rate of 60%–100%. If diagnosis and treatment are delayed, the ischemic insult to the bowel can progress to fatal infarction. The small bowel can withstand up to 6 hours of ischemia before changes start to become irreversible. Infarction occurs within 8–10 hours after complete arterial occlusion. The diagnosis of ischemia should be entertained in any patient more than 50 years of age who has abdominal pain and any of the risk factors listed in **Figure 3**. The abdominal pain is usually acute in onset and out of proportion to the minimal findings on abdominal examination. Unexplained gastrointestinal bleeding or abdominal distention may be the only early clinical findings. Leukocytosis may be seen in 75% of patients, and metabolic acidosis may be found in 50%. Classic peritoneal findings and shock are found after the ischemia has progressed to infarction.

Classification of Mesenteric Ischemia

Acute mesenteric ischemia can be classified into one of the following three types: 1) embolic occlusion of the superior mesenteric artery (SMA) **(Figs. 4–8)**; 2) thrombotic occlusion of a major visceral branch; or 3) nonocclusive ischemia, which is usually due to cardiac dysfunction causing a low-flow state within the mesenteric vasculature **(Figs. 9, 10)**.

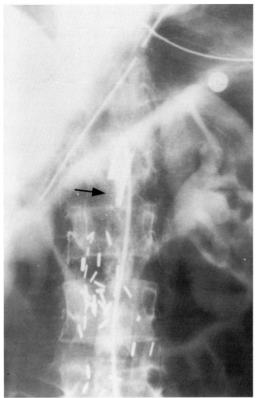

Figure 6. Same patient as in Figure 4. Selective catheterization of the SMA demonstrates the occlusive embolus (arrow). Surgical embolectomy and resection of infarcted bowel were performed.

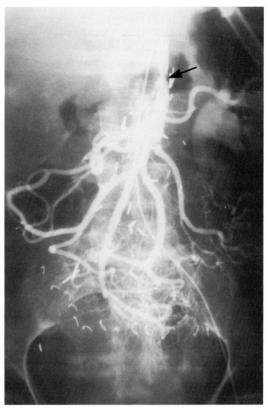

Figure 7. Same patient as in Figure 4. The postoperative superior mesenteric arteriogram demonstrates narrowing at the site of surgical embolectomy (arrow). Note the limited number of peripheral branches and numerous surgical clips due to resection of infarcted bowel.

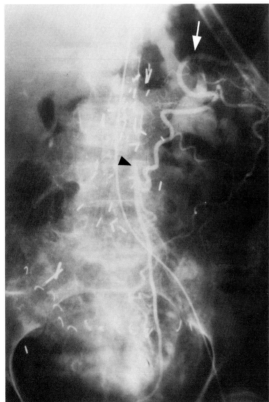

Figure 8. Same patient as in Figure 4. Delayed image shows collateral circulation reconstituting the inferior mesenteric artery (arrowhead) through the arc of Riolan (arrow). Blood flows from the SMA to the middle colic artery, and then the left colic artery to provide flow to the sigmoid colon.

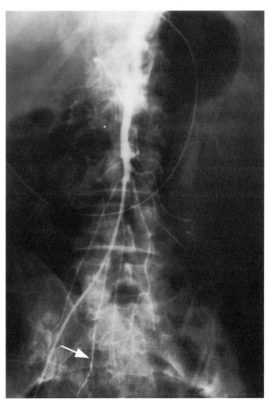

Figure 9. Selective catheterization of the SMA in an elderly patient with septic shock demonstrates marked pruning of SMA branches. Discrete focal areas of narrowing are best seen in the peripheral ileal branches (arrow).

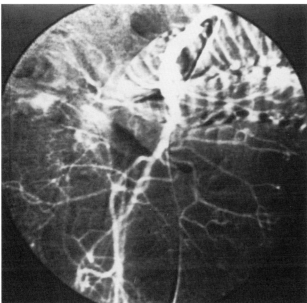

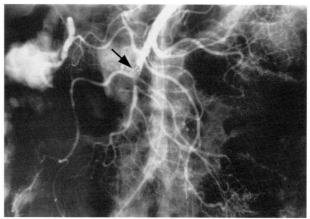

Figure 11. Partially occlusive embolus (arrow) in the SMA in a patient with atrial fibrillation.

Figure 10. Same patient as in Figure 9. Repeat superior mesenteric arteriogram after infusion of a vasodilator. Opacification of the branches is improved due to the pharmacologic vasodilation. Volume resuscitation and antibiotics are also critical in the treatment of this patient with nonocclusive mesenteric ischemia.

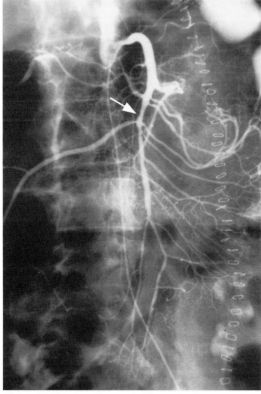

Figure 12. Same patient as in Figure 11. Repeat arteriogram after surgical embolectomy shows mild narrowing at the site of prior embolus (arrow). Despite the removal of the embolus, areas of discrete arterial narrowing and fusiform dilation suggest ongoing nonocclusive ischemic changes.

Embolic Occlusion of the SMA

Embolic occlusion of the SMA is the classic example of acute occlusive mesenteric ischemia. The sudden and severe onset of symptoms occurs when the relatively normal SMA vessel becomes occluded by the embolus and there is insufficient collateral circulation to divert blood to the distal mesenteric vessels. The embolus will usually lodge within the main vessel at sites of normal narrowing, just distal to the origin of major vessel branching; however, in 10%–15% of cases, the embolus will lodge peripherally in branches of the SMA. The embolus may occlude the vessel only partially, and vasospasm may occur proximal and distal to the embolus, accelerating the ischemia and impairing collateral blood flow. Twenty percent of patients with an SMA embolus will develop synchronous emboli in other arteries. On arteriography, the embolus appears as a sharp, rounded filling defect within the SMA, causing complete or partial occlusion (Figs. 11, 12).

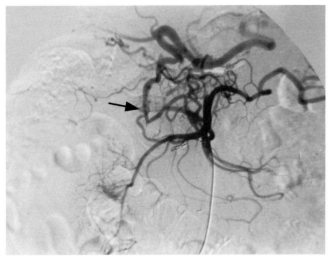

Figure 13. Selective catheterization of the SMA demonstrates pancreaticoduodenal arcade collaterals (arrow) which reconstitute celiac arterial branches.

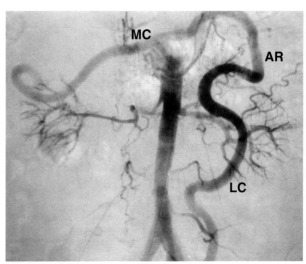

Figure 14. Abdominal aortogram demonstrates collateral circulation between the IMA and SMA. A prominent arc of Riolan (AR) provides the vascular "bridge" between the middle colic branch (MC) of the SMA and the left colic branch (LC) of the IMA.

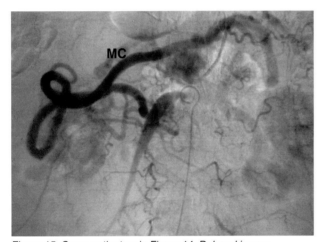

Figure 15. Same patient as in Figure 14. Delayed image demonstrates retrograde flow through the middle colic artery (MC) into the SMA.

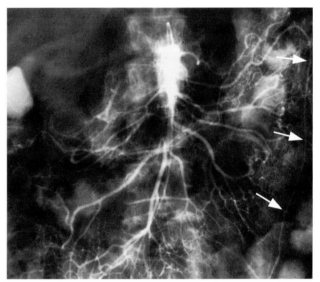

Figure 16. Superior mesenteric arteriogram demonstrates the marginal artery of Drummond (arrows) along the mesenteric border of the bowel, an important collateral pathway between the SMA and left colon.

Thrombotic Occlusion of Visceral Vessels

Thrombotic occlusion of the main visceral vessels is generally gradual; it may not cause abrupt symptoms of mesenteric ischemia because of the rich collateral networks that connect the celiac, SMA, and inferior mesenteric artery (IMA) circulations. The major collateral pathways between the various mesenteric circulations are as follows: the pancreaticoduodenal arcades connect the celiac and SMA circulations (**Fig. 13**), and the marginal artery of Drummond and the arc of Riolan connect the SMA (middle colic artery) and the IMA (left colic artery) (**Figs. 14–16**).

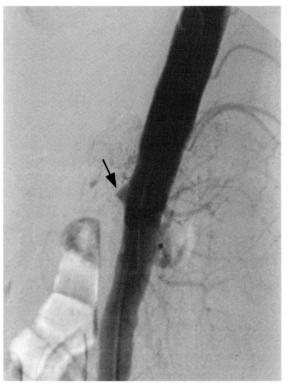

Figure 17. Lateral abdominal aortogram shows total occlusion of the SMA.

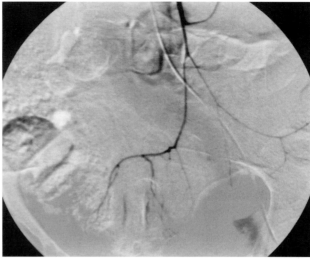

Figure 18. Inferior mesenteric arteriogram in a 60-year-old woman demonstrates extensive narrowing of peripheral IMA branches. The intramural vessels and the arcade vasculature are not visualized. A local papaverine infusion was begun after a test injection revealed improvement in vessel caliber.

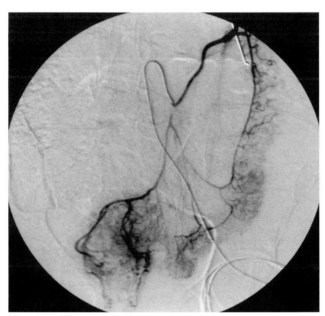

Figure 19. Follow-up arteriogram after a 12-hour papaverine infusion demonstrates marked improvement in the mesenteric vasculature with visualization of the intramural vessels and mucosal blush. Bowel resection was averted.

Most of the thrombotic occlusions that result in mesenteric ischemia are associated with underlying atherosclerotic disease, with chronic occlusion of the celiac artery, and a thrombotic occlusion of a high-grade narrowing of the proximal segment of the SMA. Because the acute event is superimposed on a chronic process, approximately 20%–50% of patients will describe a history of prior abdominal pain and weight loss. On arteriography, an abrupt vessel cut-off is usually seen within the first 2 cm of the SMA trunk **(Fig. 17)**. Occasionally, the thrombus will occlude the vessel only partially, causing decreased blood flow to the bowel.

Nonocclusive Mesenteric Ischemia
Nonocclusive mesenteric ischemia is caused by splanchnic artery vasoconstriction in response to multiple systemic factors. Clinical conditions associated with nonocclusive mesenteric ischemia include heart failure, arrhythmias, hypovolemia from dehydration or bleeding, hypotension from shock or sepsis, rapid administration of digitalis, or a reaction to vasopressor therapy. Vasoconstriction may persist even after the underlying condition has been corrected.

Arteriographic findings in patients with nonocclusive mesenteric ischemia can include vasoconstriction in patients thought to have mesenteric ischemia, who are not in shock, not on vasopressors, and do not have pancreatitis; a "pruned" appearance of the mesenteric vasculature; localized spasm; narrowing of the origins of two or more branches of the SMA; alternating areas of dilatation and constriction; narrowed arcades; and loss of intramural vessels within segments of the intestine **(Figs. 18, 19)**.

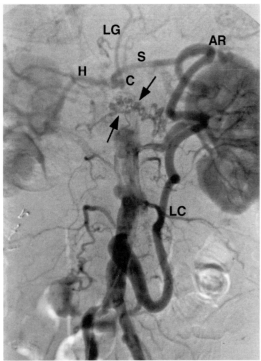

Figure 20. Aortogram of a 66-year-old man with lower extremity claudication. Incidental findings include a markedly enlarged IMA with retrograde flow in the left colic artery (LC) and a prominent arc of Riolan (AR). Multiple tiny collaterals (arrows) course toward the celiac artery and the SMA. Reconstitution of flow in the celiac (C), splenic (S), common hepatic (H), and left gastric (LG) arteries is seen.

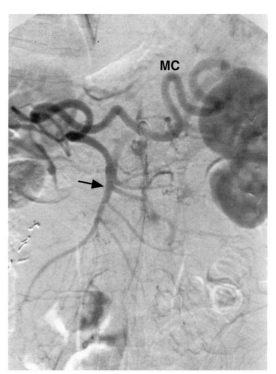

Figure 21. Same patient as in Figure 20. Later image reveals retrograde flow through the middle colic artery (MC) filling the SMA (arrow) and its branches.

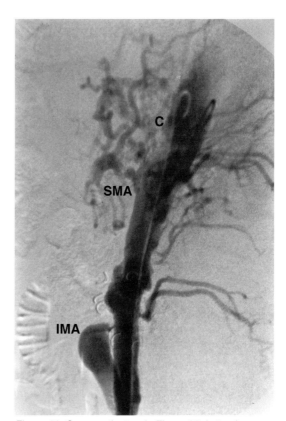

Figure 22. Same patient as in Figure 20. Lateral aortogram documents critical stenoses of the celiac (C), SMA (SMA), and IMA (IMA) ostia. There is marked post-stenotic dilatation of the IMA.

Chronic Mesenteric Ischemia

Chronic ischemia occurs in patients with significant atherosclerotic disease. Some investigators believe that two out of the three main mesenteric vessels must be occluded before symptoms appear. In a series of patients with chronic ischemia, 98%–99% of patients had occluded celiac and SMA vessels, and 50% had significant stenosis of the IMA. Because of the chronicity, a collateral vessel network is present which often prevents progression to infarction **(Figs. 20–22)**. The viability of the bowel is usually not compromised, but blood flow is inadequate to support the functional demands of the bowel. The clinical symptoms have commonly been chronic in nature. The pain is generally postprandial (intestinal angina), occurring 15–30 minutes after a meal and continuing for 1–4 hours. As the disease continues, smaller amounts of food precipitate more severe and persistent abdominal pain. Significant weight loss can occur, as well as food avoidance due to a fear of eating.

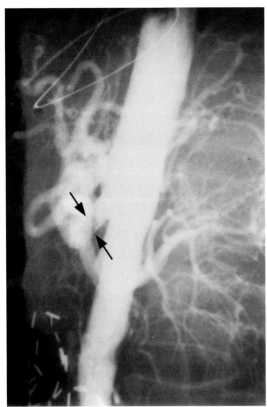

Figure 23. Lateral aortogram of the patient shown in Figure 4. The celiac axis is visualized; a filling defect occludes the proximal SMA (arrow).

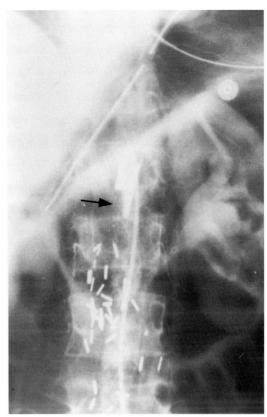

Figure 24. Selective catheterization of the SMA demonstrates the occlusive embolus (arrow) within the proximal SMA. Surgical bowel resection and embolectomy were performed.

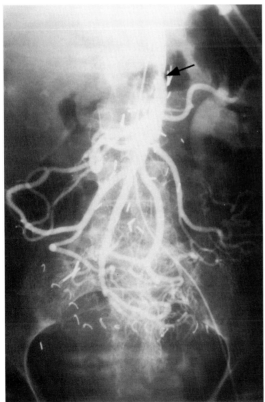

Figure 25. Same patient as in Figure 24. Postoperative superior mesenteric arteriogram demonstrates narrowing at the site of surgical embolectomy (arrow). Note the limited number of peripheral branches and numerous surgical clips due to resection of infarcted bowel.

Treatment of Mesenteric Ischemia

In patients who have an embolic cause of the ischemia with no collateral network to provide blood flow to the bowel, and in whom there is clinical suspicion of infarction, the treatment is emergency surgical embolectomy to restore flow **(Figs. 23–25)**. The surgeon can use the preoperative arteriogram to pinpoint the exact location of the embolus. From case reports in the radiologic literature, patients with partial or near total occlusion of the SMA without clinical evidence of infarction may also be candidates for thrombolytic therapy if a channel through the thrombus for antegrade flow can be rapidly restored. If peritoneal signs or symptoms of infarction are found during the infusion, emergency laparotomy is warranted.

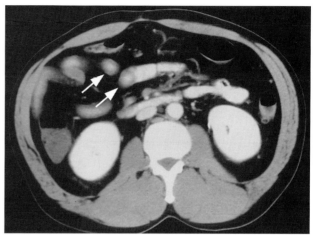

Figure 26. CT image from a 58-year-old man with acute abdominal pain demonstrates thickened bowel loops within the right mid abdomen (arrows) suggesting mesenteric ischemia.

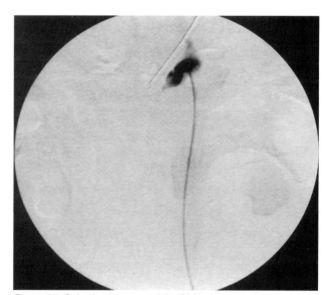

Figure 27. Selective injection of the SMA shows total occlusion due to thrombus.

In patients with thrombosis of a chronically diseased mesenteric vessel, thrombolytic therapy may be indicated if there are no signs or symptoms of bowel infarction **(Figs. 26–29)**. Once the clot has been lysed and flow restored, the decision must be made whether to treat the underlying atherosclerotic lesion with angioplasty or with surgical repair of the vessel. There have been a number of small series and case reports in the radiologic literature of mesenteric vessel angioplasty, with results of 86%–100% technical success with follow-up of 6–28 months **(Figs. 30, 31)**. Complication rates have been low. Recurrence of the stenosis has occurred within 4–48 months of the angioplasty in 10%–50% of patients. Repeat angioplasty of the recurrent stenosis appears to improve patency significantly. If the lesion is not amenable to angioplasty, surgical repair of the vessel can be attempted with endarterectomy or bypass grafting **(Fig. 32)**.

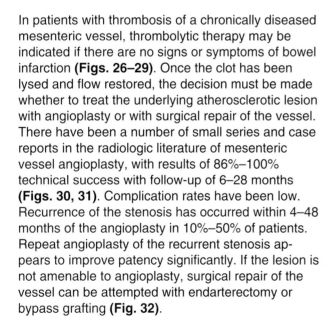

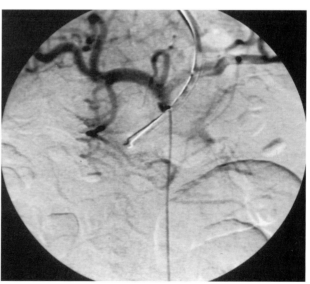

Figure 28. Selective injection of the celiac axis reveals no collateral flow to the SMA.

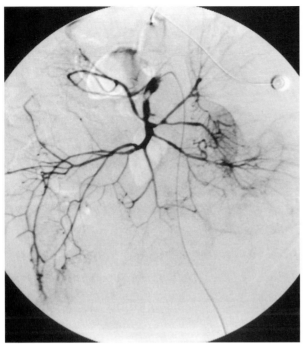

Figure 29. Superior mesenteric arteriogram after a 13-hour infusion of urokinase into the proximal SMA reveals near complete lysis of the clot and restoration of intestinal perfusion. At laparotomy only 80 cm of small bowel required resection.

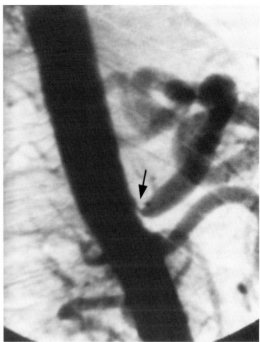

Figure 30. Critical stenosis of the celiac axis (arrow) shown on the lateral aortogram. In this asymptomatic patient an angioplasty was performed in order to allow selective hepatic arterial chemotherapy infusion.

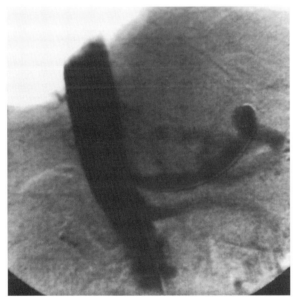

Figure 31. The aortogram after celiac angioplasty performed from a left brachial approach documents improved flow into the celiac axis. Such interventional techniques may be used to treat patients with mesenteric ischemia.

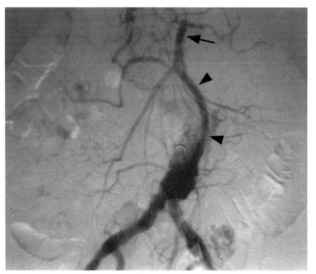

Figure 32. Pelvic arteriogram in a patient surgically treated for chronic mesenteric ischemia. A tubular prosthetic graft (arrowheads) courses from the aorta just above its bifurcation to the SMA (arrow).

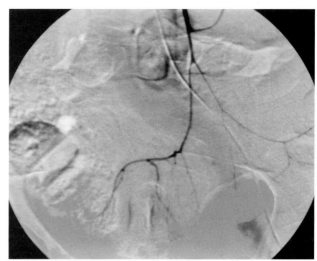

Figure 33. The effect of vasodilator therapy for treatment of nonocclusive ischemia. The initial IMA study demonstrates extensive narrowing and pruning of peripheral IMA branches.

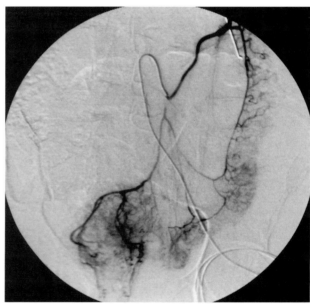

Figure 34. A repeat IMA study after a 12-hour infusion of papaverine into the IMA reveals marked improvement in the mesenteric flow. The patient did not require bowel resection.

In nonocclusive mesenteric ischemia, papaverine can be instilled into the main mesenteric vessel in an attempt to relieve the vasoconstriction. Papaverine can also be infused in patients with embolic or thrombotic occlusion of the vessels to improve flow by relieving any vasospasm that might be present (Figs. 33, 34). The concentration can be adjusted based on the patient's fluid requirements. Clinical circumstances dictate the duration of the infusion. The infusion should be switched to saline 30 minutes prior to a follow-up arteriogram. While the patient is on papaverine, close intensive care monitoring is needed.

Summary

In the past, only surgical treatment of mesenteric ischemia was available. However, with better testing procedures, monitoring, heightened awareness of the clinical presentation, and advancements in angiographic and interventional techniques, an interdisciplinary approach to therapy has arisen. At Montefiore Medical Center in New York City, a diagnosis and treatment algorithm has been developed using an aggressive multimodality approach to acute mesenteric ischemia (Figs. 35, 36). Using this algorithm, 50% or more of patients with acute mesenteric ischemia survive, and 70%–90% of patients lose less than 1 meter of intestine.

For further information on this topic, please see Teaching File Cases 29 and 30.

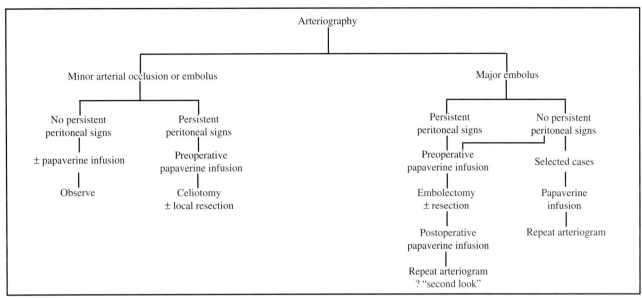

Figure 35. Algorithm for aggressive multimodality approach to acute mesenteric ischemia from Montefiore Medical Center.

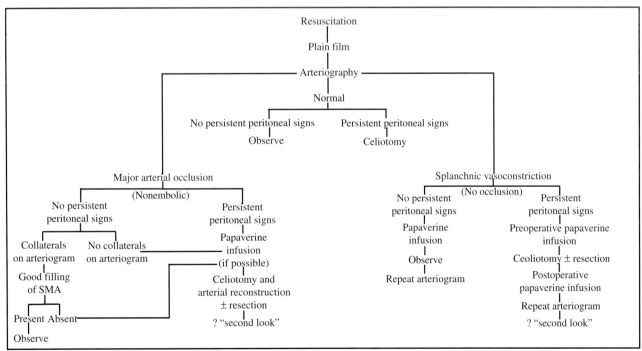

Figure 36. Algorithm for aggressive multimodality approach to acute mesenteric ischemia from Montefiore Medical Center.

Selected Readings

Bakal CW, Sprayregen S, Wolf EL. Radiology in intestinal ischemia: angiographic diagnosis and management. Surg Clin North Am 1992; 72:125–141.

Boyer L, Delorme JM, Alexandre M, et al. Local fibrinolysis for superior mesenteric artery thromboembolism. Cardiovasc Intervent Radiol 1994; 17:214–216.

Brandt LJ, Boley SJ. Nonocclusive mesenteric ischemia. Annu Rev Med 1991; 42:107–117.

Corder AP, Taylor I. Acute mesenteric ischaemia. Postgrad Med J 1993; 69:1–3.

Crotch-Harvey MA, Gould DA, Green AT. Case report: percutaneous transluminal angioplasty of the inferior mesenteric artery in the treatment of chronic mesenteric ischaemia. Clin Radiol 1992; 46:408–409.

Cunningham CG, Reilly LM, Rapp JH, Schneider PA, Stoney RJ. Chronic visceral ischemia: three decades of progress. Ann Surg 1991; 214:276–287.

Cunningham CG, Reilly LM, Stoney R. Chronic visceral ischemia. Surg Clin North Am 1992; 72:231–244.

Gharagozloo F, Bulkley GB, Zuidema GD, O'mara CS, Alderson PO. The use of intraperitoneal xenon for early diagnosis of acute mesenteric ischemia. Surgery 1984; 95:404–411.

Golden DA, Ring EJ, McLean GK, Freiman DB. Percutaneous transluminal angioplasty in the treatment of abdominal angina. AJR 1982; 139:247–249.

Heys SD, Brittenden J, Crofts TJ. Acute mesenteric ischaemia: the continuing difficulty in early diagnosis. Postgrad Med J 1993; 69:48–51.

Jones PF. Emergency abdominal surgery. Oxford: Blackwell Scientific Publications, 1987; 481–487.

Kaleya RN, Sammartano RJ, Boley SJ. Aggressive approach to acute mesenteric ischemia. Surg Clin North Am 1992; 72:157–182.

Kornblith PL, Boley SJ, Whitehouse BS. Anatomy of the splanchnic circulation. Surg Clin North Am 1992; 72:1–30.

Moore WM Jr, Hollier LH. Mesenteric artery occlusive disease. Cardiol Clin 1991; 9:535–541.

Odurny A, Sniderman KW, Colapinto RF. Intestinal angina: percutaneous transluminal angioplasty of the celiac and superior mesenteric arteries. Radiology 1988; 167:59–62.

Roberts L, Wertman DA, Mills SR, Moore AV, Heaston DK. Transluminal angioplasty of the superior mesenteric artery: an alternative to surgical revascularization. AJR 1983; 141:1039–1042.

Schoenbaum SW, Pena C, Koenigsberg P, Katzen BT. Superior mesenteric artery embolism: treatment with intraarterial urokinase. J Vasc Interv Radiol 1992, 3:485–490.

Stoney RJ, Cunningham CG. Acute mesenteric ischemia. Surgery 1993; 114:489–90.

Tytle TL, Prati RC. Percutaneous recanalization in chronic occlusion of the superior mesenteric artery. J Vasc Interv Radiol 1995; 6:133–136.

End Note

Figures 26–29 courtesy of E. Druy, M.D., George Washington University Medical Center, Washington, D.C.

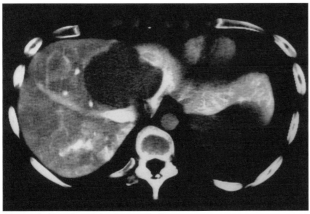

Figure 1. Focal nodular hyperplasia.

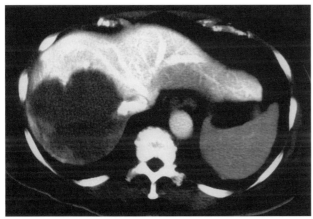

Figure 2. Cavernous hemangioma.

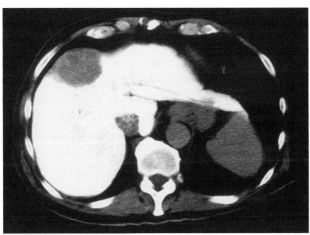

Figure 3. Hepatocellular carcinoma.

TUTORIAL 11
COMPUTED TOMOGRAPHY–
ARTERIAL PORTOGRAPHY

Emily K. Folz, M.D.,
Richard D. Redvanly, M.D.,
Vincent G. McDermott, M.D., and
Rendon C. Nelson, M.D.

Introduction

The subjects addressed in this tutorial include:
1. Rationale and indications for computed tomography-arterial portography
2. Arteriography and computed tomography techniques
3. Interpretation of the images
4. Diagnostic and technical pitfalls.

Rationale for Computed Tomography-Arterial Portography

Normal hepatic parenchyma has a dual blood supply, with the majority of its blood derived from the portal vein ($\approx$75%), and a minority from the hepatic artery ($\approx$25%). Conversely, hepatic tumors, whether benign or malignant, primary or metastatic, derive the majority if not all of their blood supply from the hepatic artery. Computed tomography-arterial portography (CTAP) capitalizes on this difference in dominant perfusion to maximize lesion conspicuity. In general, hepatic tumors, whether primary or metastatic, are of low attenuation compared to normal hepatic parenchyma on CTAP **(Figs. 1–3)**.

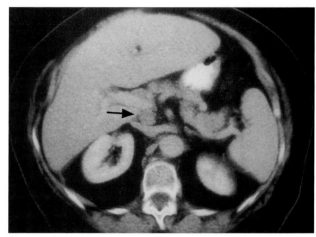

Figure 4. Porta hepatis node on dynamic CT scan (arrow).

Indications for CTAP

Metastatic Colorectal Carcinoma

CTAP is used in the preoperative evaluation of patients with isolated hepatic metastases from colorectal cancer who are being considered for partial hepatic resection. Extrahepatic metastases, including tumors of the hepatic lymph nodes **(Fig. 4)**, should already have been excluded. Criteria for resectability include the presence of 4 or fewer hepatic metastases, the ability to achieve tumor-free margins, and the ability to preserve enough liver to sustain adequate hepatic function following resection of the hepatic metastases **(Fig. 5)**. Approximately 160,000 new cases of colorectal cancer are diagnosed each year. Of these, about 8,000 patients meet the criteria for partial hepatic resection. These patients have improved long-term survival rates after successful resection of their hepatic metastases (20%–40% 5-year survival) compared to similar patients who do not undergo resection (<5% 5-year survival).

Hepatocellular Carcinoma

CTAP has been used in the preoperative evaluation of patients with hepatocellular carcinoma (HCC) to assess the potential for tumor-free surgical margins. However, 70% of hepatocellular carcinomas develop in cirrhotic livers and CTAP may be of limited value in this group of patients because portosystemic shunting can cause major portions of liver parenchyma to be poorly enhanced, thereby diminishing diagnostic efficacy **(Fig. 6)**. Patients with cirrhosis also frequently have multifocal HCC. The sensitivity of CTAP for detecting the dominant neoplastic mass in these patients ranges from 81% to 94%. However, the sensitivity for detecting small satellite lesions or intrahepatic metastases is probably less than 60%. Furthermore, because of limited liver function and regenerative capacity, many of these patients cannot survive a major parenchymal resection.

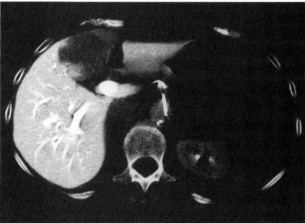

Figure 5. Colorectal cancer resection candidate with an isolated hepatic metastasis.

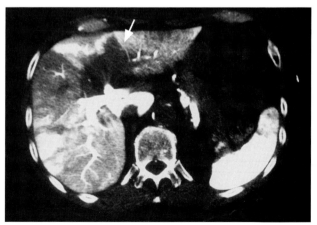

Figure 6. Hepatocellular carcinoma (arrow) within a heterogeneously enhancing cirrhotic liver.

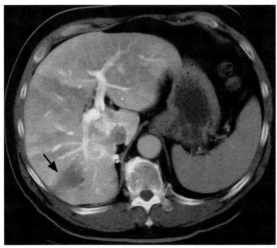

Figure 7. SMA injection with streaming artifact (arrow).

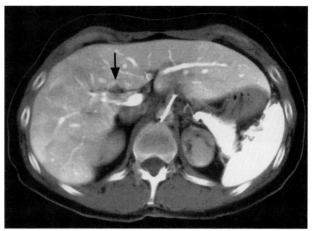

Figure 8. SA injection with streaming artifact (arrow).

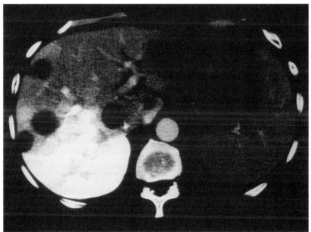

Figure 9. SMA injection with artifactual hyperenhancement of the right lobe.

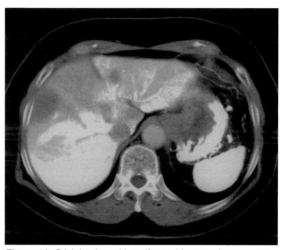

Figure 10. SA injection with artifactual hyperenhancement of the right lobe.

Arteriographic Technique

Superior Mesenteric Versus Splenic Artery Injection
CTAP technique has not been standardized. Contrast material may be injected through a catheter secured in the superior mesenteric artery (SMA) or in the splenic artery (SA). A recent comparative study of SMA and SA injections suggests that SA injections result in fewer artifacts related to differential flow of contrast material within the portal vein as well as fewer nontumorous perfusion abnormalities. However, these artifacts are seen with both SMA and SA injections **(Figs. 7–10)**. Another recent study found no difference in the number or types of artifacts seen when comparing CTAP exams performed with SMA versus SA injections. Use of a catheter with both end- and side-holes may reduce artifacts caused by streaming. Further investigation will be necessary to define optimal catheter position. This will remain an issue since catheter placement in the SA tends to be more technically challenging than placement in the SMA.

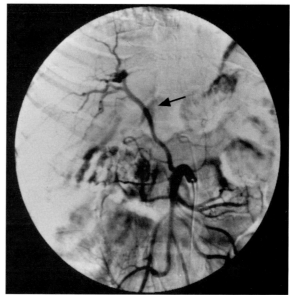

Figure 11. DSA of a replaced right hepatic artery (arrow).

Detection of Anatomic Variants

The Seldinger technique is used to gain access to the common femoral artery. Using a 5-F catheter, (typically a Simmons-type catheter), digital subtraction arteriograms (DSA) of the celiac artery and SMA are obtained to assess for the presence of anatomical variants. One fourth of patients examined will have some hepatic arterial supply originating from the SMA. Approximately 14% of patients have a replaced right hepatic artery **(Fig. 11)**, 6% of patients have an accessory right hepatic artery, and 2.5% of patients have a common hepatic artery arising from the SMA. If the SMA is chosen for catheter placement, the tip must be positioned distal to the origin of these anomalous hepatic arteries to prevent contrast material from reaching the liver through both hepatic arterial and portal venous pathways **(Fig. 12)**. Similarly, if contrast material is injected via the splenic artery, the catheter tip must be positioned distal to the origin of any hepatic artery branch arising from the splenic or left gastric arteries.

CT Technique

Injection of Contrast Material

Once the 5-F catheter has been secured either in the superior mesenteric artery or the splenic artery, 150–200 mL of 60% iodinated contrast material is administered through the catheter at a rate of 1.5–3.0 mL per second using a mechanical power injector. Dynamic CT scanning is begun 10–20 seconds after the start of the contrast material injection. A longer scan delay of approximately 30 seconds is preferred when spiral CT technique is used, because the acquisition time is shorter. Seven- to 10-mm-thick contiguous axial sections of the entire liver are obtained **(Fig. 13)**.

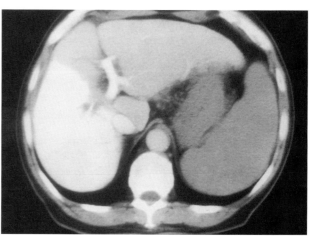

Figure 12. CTAP of inadvertent injection into the replaced right hepatic artery off the SMA.

CTAP Technique	
Contrast Material	150–200 mL 60% iodinated contrast material
Injection Rate	2 mL/sec (range 1.5–3.0 mL/sec)
Scan Delay	10–20 seconds for nonspiral CT 30 seconds for spiral CT
Section Thickness	7–10 mm

Figure 13.

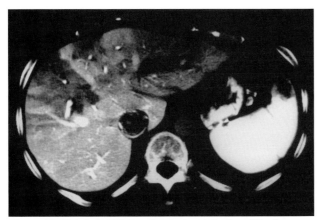

Figure 14. "Striated" CTAP makes lesion detection difficult.

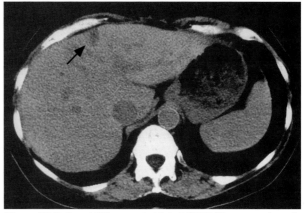

Figure 15. Delayed CT scan of striated CTAP. The parenchymal inhomogeneity has resolved and the lesion is now clearly visible (arrow).

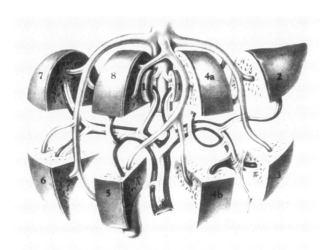

Figure 16. Liver segment diagram.

Anatomic Subsegment	Nomenclature		
	Couinaud	Bismuth	Goldsmith & Woodburne
Caudate lobe	I	I	Caudate lobe
Left lateral superior subsegment	II	II	Left lateral segment
Left lateral inferior subsegment	III	III	Left lateral segment
Left medial superior subsegment	IV	IVa	Left medial segment
Left medial inferior subsegment	IV	IVb	Left medial segment
Right anterior inferior subsegment	V	V	Right anterior segment
Right anterior superior subsegment	VIII	VIII	Right anterior segment
Right posterior inferior subsegment	VI	VI	Right posterior segment
Right posterior superior subsegment	VII	VII	Right posterior segment

Figure 17. Segmental nomenclature chart.

Delayed CT

Hepatocytes excrete 1%–2% of the contrast material administered during CTAP. On CT images obtained 4–6 hours after the CTAP, normal liver will be hyperattenuating compared to tumors which do not contain functioning hepatocytes. Exceptions include regenerative nodules, hepatic adenomas, focal nodular hyperplasia, and well-differentiated HCC, which may contain functioning hepatocytes resulting in a variable amount of enhancement on delayed CT. Delayed CT technique consists of 7–10-mm-thick contiguous axial sections of the entire liver similar to those obtained for CTAP except no additional contrast material is administered. Delayed CT scanning is primarily useful for proving or disproving equivocal lesions and for differentiating nontumorous perfusion abnormalities from neoplastic deposits. It is also useful when heterogeneous parenchymal enhancement during CTAP makes lesion detection difficult **(Figs. 14, 15)**.

Image Interpretation

Segmental Anatomy of the Liver

The Goldsmith and Woodburne nomenclature divides the liver into three lobes—right, left, and caudate. The plane extending from the middle hepatic vein to the gallbladder fossa divides the right and left lobes. The right lobe is further divided into anterior and posterior segments along the vertical plane of the right hepatic vein. The left lobe is further divided into medial and lateral segments along the vertical plane of the left hepatic vein. In the Bismuth and Couinaud nomenclatures, the anterior and posterior segments of the right hepatic lobe and the medial and lateral segments of the left hepatic lobe are further divided into subsegments along the plane of the right and left portal veins. Thus, each of these segments is divided into inferior and superior subsegments **(Fig. 16)**. The Bismuth nomenclature describes a total of nine sectors—eight subsegments plus the caudate lobe **(Fig. 17)**.

Image Interpretation

Localizing Lesions

It is important to describe the precise location of a lesion using a system such as the Bismuth system because modern surgical techniques permit resection of specific subsegments of the liver, thereby preserving as much normal liver as possible. Resection of a fraction of a subsegment is typically avoided since it is likely to result in excessive bleeding, bile leaks, and devascularized parenchyma. It is equally important to describe the proximity of a lesion to major blood vessels. If a lesion is immediately adjacent to a large vessel, achieving a tumor-free margin may not be possible if only the subsegment containing the lesion is resected **(Fig. 18)**.

Lesion Detection

As previously discussed, both primary and metastatic hepatic tumors are predominantly supplied by the hepatic artery, while normal liver parenchyma is predominantly supplied by the portal vein. Because of this, the appearance of both primary and metastatic tumors on CTAP will be of low attenuation and normal liver will be of high attenuation. Regenerative nodules are an exception because they are predominantly supplied by the portal vein **(Fig. 19)**. The sensitivity for detecting lesions with use of CTAP has been estimated at 85%–93%, which is superior to that of noncontrast multisequence magnetic resonance, dynamic contrast-enhanced CT, and transabdominal ultrasound imaging. Although CTAP is quite sensitive, its specificity is relatively low and is not reliable for differentiating between benign and malignant lesions. The false positive rate for detecting malignant disease is estimated to be 15%.

Lesion Interpretation

Tumor Versus Perfusion Defect

Hypoattenuating areas on CTAP may be due to benign or malignant lesions, or to perfusion defects. Perfusion defects are seen in areas that receive blood from sources other than the hepatic artery or the portal vein. For example, cystic veins and gastric veins may drain into the liver. Areas receiving blood from these aberrant veins may be seen as hypoattenuating areas on CTAP because the blood containing contrast material in the portal venules is diluted by the noncontrasted blood from the aberrant veins. Perfusion defects may also be seen in areas of the liver which are preferentially supplied by the hepatic artery rather than the portal vein. Delayed CT may differentiate true lesions from pseudolesions because true lesions remain hypoattenuating but perfusion defects become isoattenuating to normal liver on delayed CT **(Fig. 20)**.

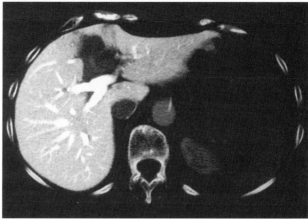

Figure 18. Metastasis immediately adjacent to the right portal vein.

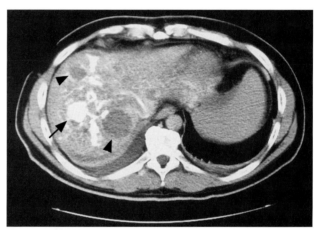

Figure 19. CTAP of a regenerative nodule (arrow) and HCC (arrowheads).

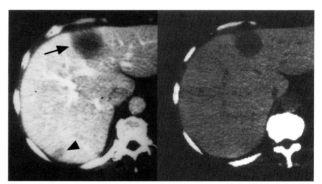

Figure 20. Metastasis (arrow) and perfusion defect (arrowhead). Delayed CT scan of metastasis and perfusion defect.

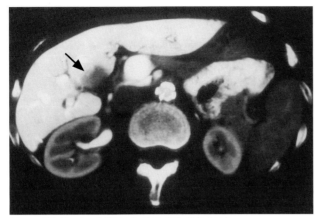

Figure 21. Segment IV perfusion defect (arrow).

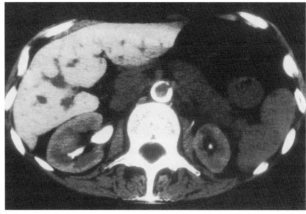

Figure 22. Same patient as in Figure 21. Delayed CT scan shows resolution of the perfusion defect.

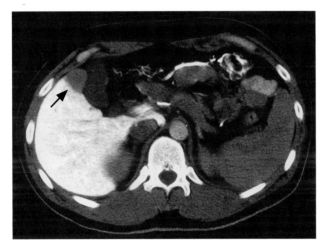

Figure 23. Perfusion defect near the gallbladder (arrow).

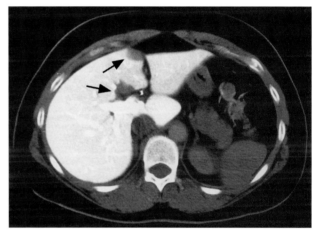

Figure 24. Two segment IV perfusion defects.

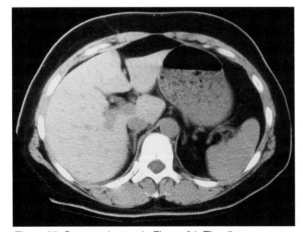

Figure 25. Same patient as in Figure 24. The disappearance of the lesions on the delayed scan suggests benignity.

Features Which Suggest A Benign Lesion
Many perfusion abnormalities can be differentiated from malignant lesions because they occur at typical locations. Approximately 8%–14% of patients who undergo CTAP have flat or wedge-shaped low-attenuation lesions in the medial segment of the left hepatic lobe, just anterior to the porta hepatis **(Figs. 21, 22)**, an area supplied by aberrant gastric veins. Similarly, perfusion defects are common about the gallbladder, probably due to aberrant drainage from cystic veins **(Fig. 23)**. Another common location for nontumorous hypoattenuating defects is anteromedial to the fissure which divides the medial and lateral segments of the left hepatic lobe **(Figs. 24, 25)**. Some of these defects may be caused by focal fatty infiltration, while others are probably due to aberrant drainage from sources such as capsular or internal mammary veins.

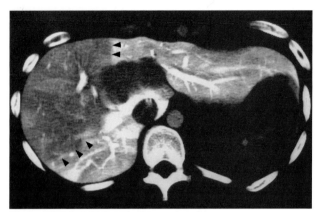

Figure 26. "Straight line sign" (arrowheads).

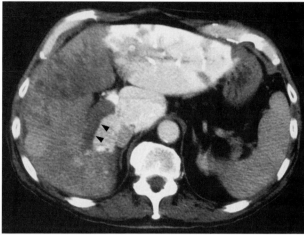

Figure 27. CTAP of right portal vein obstruction (arrowheads) shows lack of enhancement of right hepatic lobe.

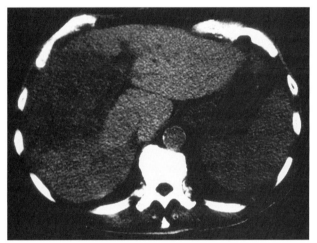

Figure 28. Same patient as in Figure 27. Delayed CT scan shows hypoattenuation and atrophy of the right lobe from chronic portal vein obstruction.

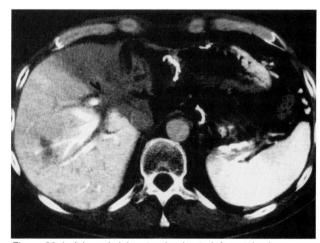

Figure 29. Left hepatic lobe atrophy due to left portal vein obstruction.

Features Which Suggest Malignancy

The "straight line sign" describes a low-attenuation lesion that has straight margins. These straight lines tend to extend from the central portion of the liver to the capsule and are typically caused by a centrally-located tumor which obstructs a branch of the portal vein **(Fig. 26)**. Portal venous invasion is typical with hepatocellular carcinoma, but it can also occur with metastases. Even peripherally-located tumors may obstruct a distal branch of the portal vein and cause a wedge-shaped subcapsular defect. On delayed CT scanning, the nontumorous area may become isoattenuating to normal parenchyma while the centrally-located tumor usually remains hypoattenuating and therefore more discernible. However, with long-standing portal venous obstruction and progressive hepatocyte damage, the wedge-shaped defect may undergo atrophy and may continue to be of low attenuation on delayed CT scanning **(Figs. 27–31)**.

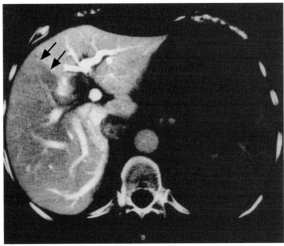
Figure 30. CTAP with straight line (arrows) and no apparent cause.

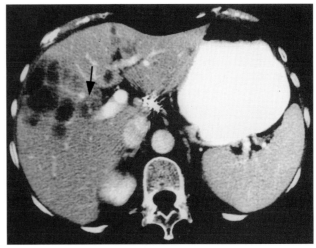
Figure 31. Dynamic CT scan 1 month later shows the lesion (arrow) now clearly compressing the portal vein.

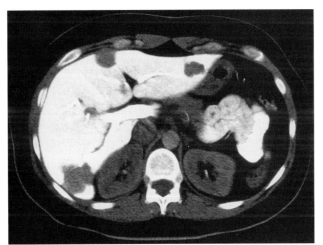
Figure 32. Subcapsular perfusion defects on CTAP.

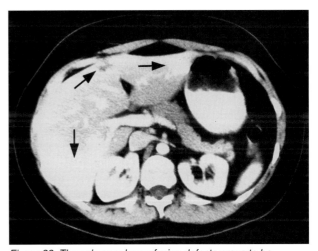
Figure 33. The subcapsular perfusion defects prove to be hemangiomas on the dynamic CT scan (arrows).

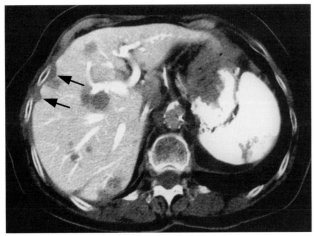
Figure 34. Subcapsular tumor deposits (arrows).

Subcapsular Abnormalities

CTAP frequently demonstrates small subcapsular hypoattenuating lesions. Many of these are perfusion defects which are linear or wedge-shaped and can be distinguished from the rounded contour of tumor deposits. However, perfusion defects can appear round and mass-like and may be difficult to differentiate from neoplastic lesions without the use of delayed CT scanning. Some of these subcapsular lesions are hemangiomas or cysts which, unless they are very small, can be characterized with use of magnetic resonance imaging by their very high signal intensity on heavily T2-weighted images. Alternatively, dynamic CT scanning may be used to show the typical peripheral nodular enhancement characteristic of a hemangioma **(Figs. 32, 33)**. However, subcapsular tumor implants may also occur and those lesions which cannot be adequately characterized preoperatively must be thoroughly investigated with use of intraoperative palpation or ultrasound **(Fig. 34)**.

Causes of Suboptimal Liver-to-Lesion Contrast	
Problem	*Solution*
Excessive contrast material used during arteriogram	Limit contrast material volume used during DSA to 50 mL or less
Catheter malposition	Obtain CT images of catheter tip prior to initiating contrast material injection to ensure proper positioning in the SMA or SA
Suboptimal scan delay	Use scan delay of 10–20 seconds for nonspiral technique, and 30 seconds for spiral technique

Figure 35.

Causes of Suboptimal Liver-to-Lesion Contrast
Excessive Contrast Material
Contrast material administered during arteriography seeps into the interstices of both primary and metastatic lesions, raising their attenuation values and narrowing the difference between the lesions and the enhancing normal parenchyma. Therefore, use of excessive contrast material during arteriography can diminish lesion conspicuity. Ideally, the volume of contrast material administered during the arteriogram should be limited to 20–30 mL but a more realistic value is probably 50 mL (≈20 g of iodine) or less. Normal saline instead of contrast material should be used to insure the catheter is secure for transport of the patient. In some centers, the only contrast material used prior to CTAP is that required to position the catheter. The patient is transferred to the CT scanner with the catheter *in situ*, then returns to the angiography suite for the DSA after the CTAP. This is more cumbersome but may improve lesion detection **(Fig. 35)**.

Catheter Malposition
A second cause of suboptimal liver-to-lesion contrast is catheter malposition. For example, if the catheter is positioned in the SMA proximal to a replaced right hepatic artery, contrast material will be delivered to the right hepatic lobe through both the portal venous and hepatic arterial systems, thereby obscuring lesions. Alternatively, the catheter can become dislodged while the patient is being transported from the vascular interventional suite to the CT scanner **(Fig. 36)**. Therefore, it is prudent to obtain a few CT images at the level of the catheter tip to ensure that proper placement has been maintained during the transfer **(Fig. 37)**.

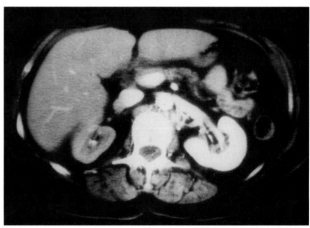

Figure 36. Catheter malposition in the left renal artery.

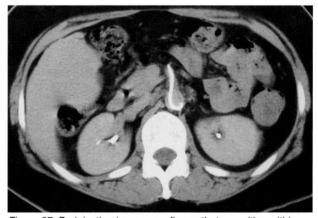

Figure 37. Preinjection images confirm catheter position within the SMA.

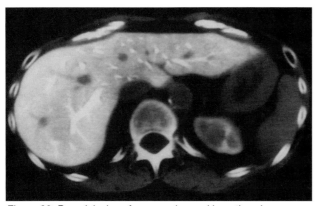
Figure 38. Pseudolesions from unenhanced hepatic veins.

Suboptimal Scan Delay
Problems can arise with nonspiral dynamic CT scanning if the delay between the initiation of contrast material injection and the initiation of imaging is suboptimal. If the scan delay is too short, areas of the liver may be scanned before there is adequate contrast enhancement **(Fig. 38)**. If the scan delay is too long, areas of the liver may be scanned during the equilibrium phase. A scan delay of 10–20 seconds and a caudocranial scanning direction is usually optimal for nonspiral technique. With spiral CT, it makes no difference whether scanning begins at the dome or the inferior edge of the liver since the entire liver can typically be scanned during 1 or 2 breathholds and scanning is easily completed prior to the equilibrium phase. The major technical issue with spiral CT is to choose a scan delay which is not too short. The optimal scan delay is typically 30 seconds for spiral CT scanners.

For further information on this topic, please see Teaching File Case 48.

Selected Readings

Abrams HL, ed. Abrams angiography: vascular and interventional radiology. 3rd edition. Boston: Little, Brown and Company, 1983.

Freeny PC, Nghiem HV, Winter TC. Helical CT during arterial portography: optimization of contrast enhancement and scanning parameters. Radiology 1995; 194:83–90.

Little AF, Baron RL, Peterson MS, et al. Optimizing CT portography: a prospective comparison of injection into the splenic versus superior mesenteric artery. Radiology 1994; 193:651–655.

Matsui O, Takahashi S, Kadoya M, et al. Pseudolesion in segment IV of the liver at CT during arterial portography: correlation with aberrant gastric venous drainage. Radiology 1994; 193:31–35.

Nelson RC. Techniques for computed tomography of the liver. Radiol Clin North Am 1991; 29:1199–1212.

Nelson RC, Chezmar JL, Sugarbaker PH, Murray DR, Bernardino ME. Preoperative localization of focal liver lesions to specific liver segments: utility of CT during arterial portography. Radiology 1990; 176:89–94.

Nelson RC, Thompson GH, Chezmar JL, Harned II RK, Fernandez MD. CT during arterial portography: diagnostic pitfalls. Radiographics 1992; 12:705–720.

Paulson EK, Baker ME, Hilleren DJ, et al. CT arterial portography: causes of technical failure and variable liver enhancement. AJR 1992; 159:745–749.

Peterson MS, Baron RL, Dodd III GD, et al. Hepatic parenchymal perfusion defects detected by CTAP: imaging-pathologic correlation. Radiology 1992; 185:149–155.

Soyer P. Segmental anatomy of the liver: utility of a nomenclature accepted worldwide. AJR 1993; 161:572–573.

Soyer P, Bluemke DA, Hruban RH, Sitzmann JV, Fishman EK. Primary malignant neoplasms of the liver: detection with helical CT during arterial portography. Radiology 1994; 192:389–392.

Soyer P, Levesque M, Caudron C, Elias D, Zeitoun G, Roche A. MRI of liver metastases from colorectal cancer vs. CT during arterial portography. J Comput Assist Tomogr 1993; 17:67–74.

Sugarbaker PH. Surgical decision making for large bowel cancer metastatic to the liver. Radiology 1990; 174:621–626.

Vogel SB, Drane WE, Ros PR, Kerns SR, Bland KI. Prediction of surgical resectability in patients with hepatic colorectal metastases. Ann Surg 1994; 219:508–516.

End Notes

Figures 12, 21, and 22 from Nelson RC, Thompson GH, Chezmar JL, Harned II RK, Fernandez MD. CT during arterial portography: diagnostic pitfalls. Radiographics 1992; 12:708, 713. Used with permission.

Figure 16 from Nelson RC, Chezmar JL, Sugarbaker PH, Murray DR, Bernardino ME. Preoperative localization of focal liver lesions to specific liver segments: utility of CT during arterial portography. Radiology 1990; 176:90. Used with permission.

Angiographic Manifestations of Visceral Tumors

Invasion of Arteries and Veins
- Encasement and Occlusions
- Displacement of Vessels
- Neovascularity
- Increased Accumulation of Contrast Material
- Arteriovenous Shunting

Figure 1.

TUTORIAL 12
DIAGNOSTIC ANGIOGRAPHY OF VISCERAL TUMORS
Richard R. Saxon, M.D., and
Steven R. Maxfield, M.D.

Introduction
The subjects addressed in this tutorial include:
1. Angiographic manifestations of visceral tumors
2. Alimentary tract tumors
3. Pancreatic tumors
4. Hepatic tumors
5. Renal tumors.

Angiographic Manifestations of Visceral Tumors
With the advent of computed tomography (CT) scanning, magnetic resonance (MR) imaging, ultrasound imaging, and percutaneous biopsy, the role of angiography in the diagnostic evaluation of most visceral tumors has diminished. However, visceral arteriography is still extremely useful for the detection, diagnosis, and staging of visceral tumors when cross-sectional imaging modalities prove inconclusive. Understanding the manifestations of visceral tumors seen during arteriography performed for other indications is also essential (eg, renal cell carcinoma seen prior to a renal percutaneous transluminal angioplasty). Although generalizations are hard to make, five findings **(Fig. 1)** are the main arteriographic manifestations exhibited by most visceral tumors.

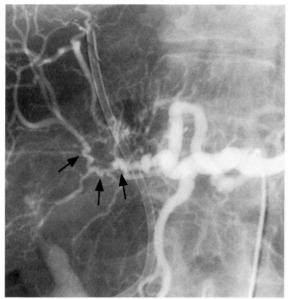

Figure 2. Serrated, saw-toothed appearance of malignant arterial encasement in the right hepatic artery (arrows). An endoscopic stent has been placed for treatment of biliary obstruction.

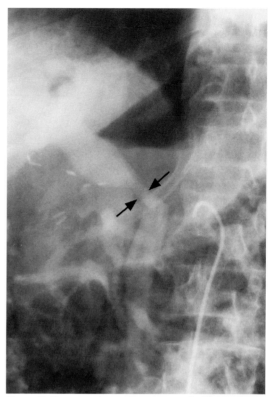

Figure 3. Compression and encasement of the main portal vein near the mesenteroportal junction (arrows).

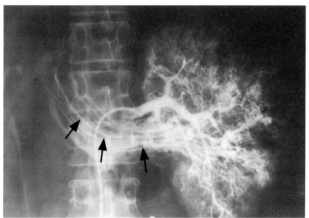

Figure 4. Renal cell carcinoma extending into the renal vein. The "thread and streak" sign is pathognomonic of malignant vascular supply to an intraluminal tumor (arrows).

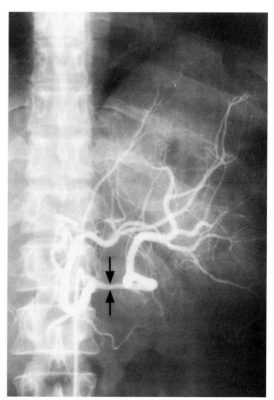

Figure 5. Pancreatic carcinoma. The smooth narrowing of the splenic artery (arrows) is nonspecific and can arise from benign or malignant disease.

Invasion of Arteries and Veins

Encasement and Occlusions

Vascular invasion or "encasement" is a reliable sign of malignancy that occurs with most adenocarcinomas of the pancreas, stomach, bowel, liver, and colon. Arterial encasement can appear serrated (saw-toothed) **(Fig. 2)** or serpiginous. With extensive invasion, arterial or venous occlusions occur. Venous changes include compression and encasement **(Fig. 3)**. A "thread and streak" sign (arterial supply to an intraluminal tumor) is pathognomonic of malignant invasion **(Fig. 4)**. Smooth narrowing of vessels is a less specific finding **(Fig. 5)** and can be seen in benign or malignant neoplasia, atherosclerosis, or inflammation.

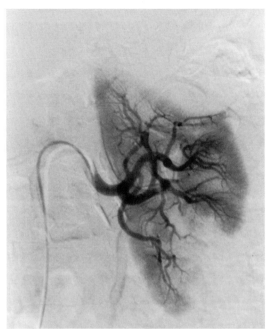

Figure 6. Simple renal cysts. Nonspecific displacement of the upper and lower pole vessels is present.

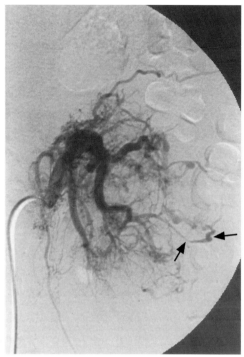

Figure 7. Neovascularity in a patient with renal cell carcinoma. Serpiginous, angulated vessels of varying diameter are present (arrows).

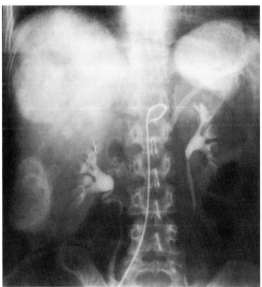

Figure 8. The venous phase of a celiac arteriogram demonstrates the tumor blush of multiple islet cell metastases to the liver.

Displacement of Vessels

Although vascular displacement clearly outlines masses, it may be caused by cysts, abscesses, or neoplasms. Therefore, displacement is a nonspecific finding **(Fig. 6)**. Sometimes displacement is the most striking finding on the arteriogram and serves to direct attention to other less apparent but more specific findings, such as neovascularity or vascular encasement.

Neovascularity

Many nonscirrhous malignant and sometimes benign tumors develop their own blood supply. These vessels, often called "tumor vessels," lack a normal muscular wall and therefore do not vasoconstrict in response to epinephrine. Tumor vessels are short and serpiginous with abrupt angulations and variable diameter **(Fig. 7)**. Neovascularity is often diagnostic of a neoplasm and usually appears as "increased vascularity" relative to surrounding tissue. Tumor vessels can occasionally be mimicked by the abnormal channels that develop near inflammation, hemorrhage, and granulation tissue.

Increased Accumulation of Contrast Material

Increased accumulation of contrast material within the substance of the tumor during the parenchymal phase of the arteriogram is called "tumor blush" **(Fig. 8)**. Although poorly understood, this process may be caused by accumulation of contrast material within the interstitium of the tumor. Tumor blush is usually seen in the more vascular tumors as opposed to the scirrhous/infiltrating neoplasms. Tumor blush is a nonspecific finding that can also be seen with inflammatory diseases.

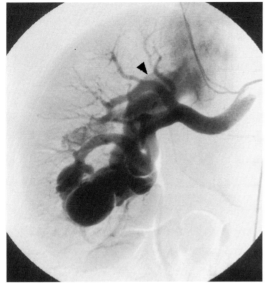

Figure 9. Arteriovenous shunting due to a renal arteriovenous malformation. Early filling of the renal vein (arrowhead) is present.

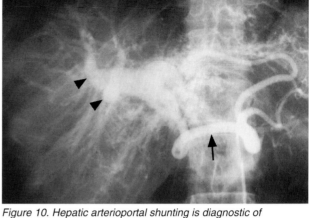

Figure 10. Hepatic arterioportal shunting is diagnostic of hepatoma. Portal vein filling (arrowheads) is visible during the arterial phase (arrow) of the study.

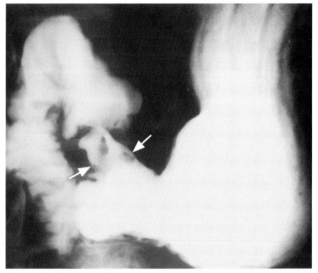

Figure 11. Antral gastric adenocarcinoma (arrows).

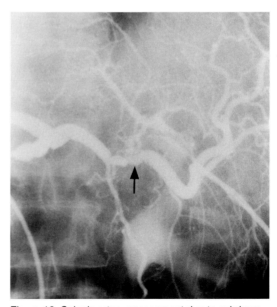

Figure 12. Splenic artery encasement due to scirrhous gastric carcinoma (arrow).

Arteriovenous Shunting

Visceral veins are not normally seen during the arterial phase of an arteriogram. Early, dense venous opacification can be seen in "vascular" tumors, inflammatory diseases, and arteriovenous malformations **(Fig. 9)**. Arteriovenous shunting seen in association with displacement of vessels and/or tumor vascularity can be very specific for malignancy. For example, portal vein opacification during the arterial phase of hepatic arteriography seen in association with a liver mass **(Fig. 10)** is essentially diagnostic of a hepatoma.

Alimentary Tract Neoplasms—Adenocarcinoma

Adenocarcinoma is the most frequently occurring tumor of the alimentary tract. Tumors in the alimentary tract with similar histology tend to have similar angiographic appearances. Gastric adenocarcinomas **(Figs. 11, 12)** are scirrhous; thus, the angiographic feature is predominantly vascular encasement **(Fig. 13)**. On the other hand, colon carcinomas usually exhibit marked tumor vascularity **(Fig. 14)**, a prominent tumor blush **(Fig. 15)**, as well as vascular encasement **(Fig. 16)**. Encasement of mesenteric vessels by adenocarcinoma of the small bowel or colon and of the gastroepiploic vessels by gastric carcinoma indicates malignant invasion.

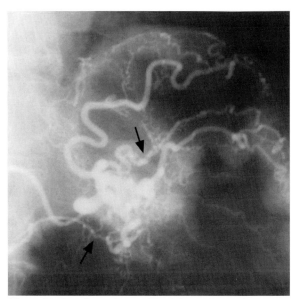

Figure 13. Gastric carcinoma. The left gastric arteriogram demonstrates arterial encasement of lesser curvature vessels (arrows).

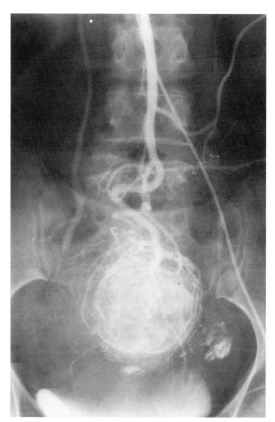

Figure 14. Tumor vascularity of sigmoid carcinoma.

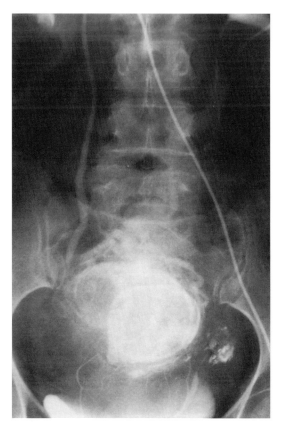

Figure 15. Same patient as in Figure 14. Prominent tumor blush is seen on the parenchymal phase arteriogram.

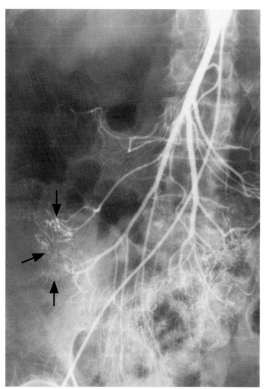

Figure 16. Vascular encasement by a cecal carcinoma (arrows).

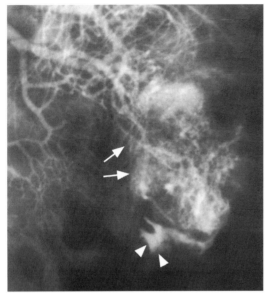

Figure 17. Magnified view of a jejunal leiomyoma. Tumor blush (arrows) and extravasation of contrast material (arrowheads) was seen during an acute episode of gastrointestinal bleeding.

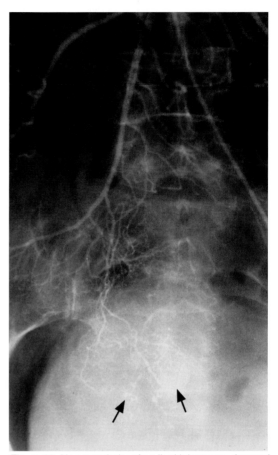

Figure 18. Neovascularity of an ileal leiomyoma (arrows).

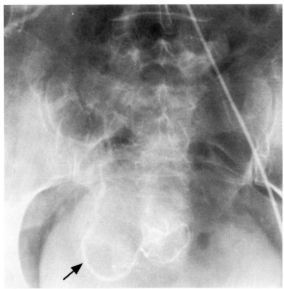

Figure 19. Same patient as in Figure 18. Prominent draining vein (arrow).

Alimentary Tract—Myomatous Neoplasms

Leiomyomas and leiomyosarcomas are tumors of smooth muscle that can arise anywhere in the alimentary tract. Patients with myomatous tumors often experience chronic, recurrent gastrointestinal bleeding and occasional massive acute hemorrhage **(Fig. 17)**. When these tumors occur in the small bowel, the source of bleeding may be cryptic, and diagnostic arteriography can be quite helpful. These tumors tend to be hypervascular with a dense tumor blush, occasional pooling of contrast material, and dense venous drainage **(Figs. 18, 19)**. Distinguishing benign from malignant tumors is often very difficult. Leiomyosarcomas are generally large and irregular **(Fig. 20)**. Vascular encasement is a sign of malignancy.

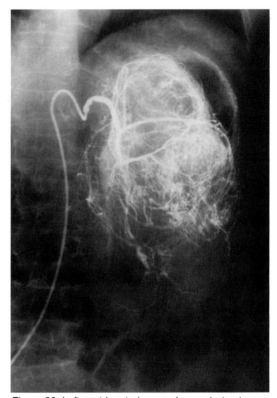

Figure 20. Left gastric arteriogram demonstrates tumor vessels within a large gastric leiomyosarcoma.

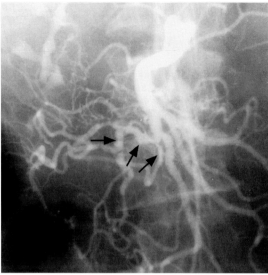

Figure 21. Superior mesenteric arteriogram demonstrates arterial irregularity due to a carcinoid tumor (arrows).

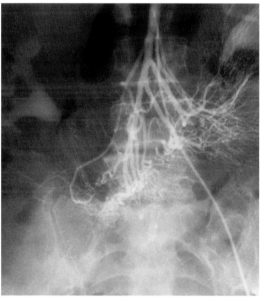

Figure 22. Arterial retraction and straightening due to mesenteric shortening by carcinoid tumor.

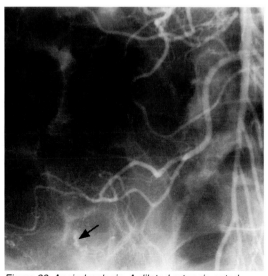

Figure 23. Angiodysplasia. A dilated artery is noted (arrow).

Alimentary Tract—Carcinoid
Carcinoid tumors tend to arise in the ileum. When the tumors ulcerate, they can cause gastrointestinal bleeding that prompts a request for diagnostic angiography. Angiographic features are related to the desmoplastic nature of the tumor and include arterial narrowing "arteritis" **(Fig. 21)** distant from the site of the tumor, vascular displacement *toward* the tumor, and, occasionally, neovascularity **(Fig. 22)**. Malignant carcinoid tumors are usually larger and near the terminal ileum. Due to mesenteric shortening and thickening, vessels may become kinked and retracted toward a central point, producing a "stellate" or "sunburst" appearance.

Alimentary Tract—Angiodysplasia
Known by a number of names including telangiectasias, angiomas, vascular ectasias, and arteriovenous malformations, these lesions are not true neoplasms but rather clusters of ectatic submucosal vascular spaces. They are a common angiographic finding in chronic recurrent gastrointestinal hemorrhage and can be multiple (as in hereditary hemorrhagic telangiectasia). Angiographic features vary with size. Small lesions may demonstrate only a slightly dilated artery and early draining vein **(Fig. 23)**. Larger lesions demonstrate a vascular nidus with a dense blush that drains early into a large vein.

195

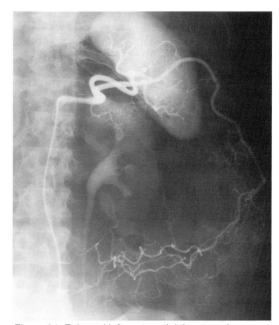

Figure 24. Enlarged left gastroepiploic artery due to omental metastases from ovarian carcinoma.

Alimentary Tract—Metastases

Some metastases to the alimentary tract occur by direct extension from an adjacent organ. Choriocarcinoma and melanoma commonly metastasize to the alimentary tract via the hematogenous route. Metastases have a variable appearance that depends on the site of origin. For example, choriocarcinoma metastases are hypervascular whereas ovarian carcinoma metastases are hypovascular and cause vascular distortion **(Fig. 24)**.

Pancreatic Neoplasms

The indications for pancreatic arteriography have greatly diminished since the advent of percutaneous biopsy, cross-sectional imaging, and endoscopic retrograde cholangiopancreatography. However, subselective arteriography with catheterization and injection of branches such as the splenic, hepatic, gastroduodenal, dorsal pancreatic **(Fig. 25)**, and pancreaticoduodenal arteries can be up to 90% accurate in detecting pancreatic neoplasms **(Fig. 26)**. Arteriography is useful in evaluating small carcinomas where a cure is possible and an assessment of resectability and arterial roadmapping is desired. It is also useful when a tumor is suspected but other imaging modalities have been inconclusive.

Figure 25. Normal dorsal pancreatic arteriogram.

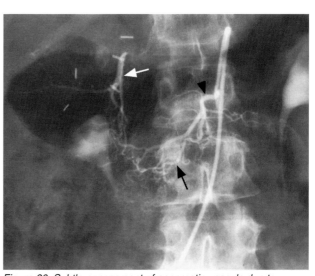

Figure 26. Subtle encasement of pancreatic vessels due to pancreatic carcinoma (black arrow). Gastroduodenal artery (white arrow); dorsal pancreatic artery (arrowhead).

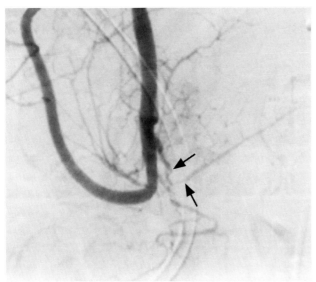

Figure 27. Pancreatic carcinoma. Magnified gastroduodenal arteriogram demonstrates encasement of the superior pancreaticoduodenal artery (arrows).

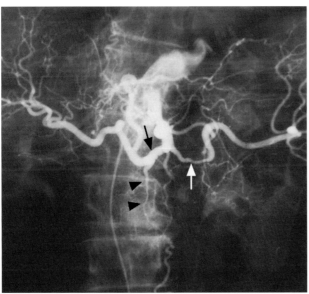

Figure 28. Extensive arterial encasement due to pancreatic carcinoma. The splenic (white arrow), gastroduodenal (arrowheads), and common hepatic (black arrow) arteries are involved.

Pancreas—Adenocarcinoma

Pancreatic carcinoma is a scirrhous, infiltrating, poorly vascularized tumor. The primary angiographic abnormality is invasion of arteries and veins **(Fig. 27)**. Major vessel encasement (eg, superior mesenteric artery, superior mesenteric vein, celiac artery) implies that the tumor is not resectable for cure **(Fig. 28)**. In a series of ninety patients with periampullary tumors, Dooley et al found that 77% of tumors were resectable when encasement was absent, 35% when vessel encasement was present, and none were resectable when vascular occlusion was present. Serpiginous and saw-toothed vascular encasement are accurate predictors of pancreatic carcinoma. Smooth narrowing of the vessels is a less specific finding that requires other evidence to confirm malignancy.

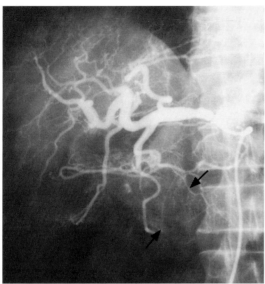

Figure 29. Neovascularity due to pancreatic carcinoma (arrows).

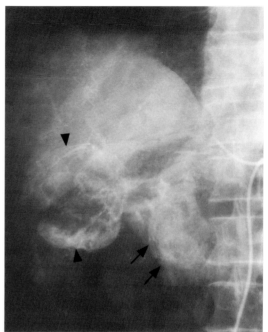

Figure 30. Same patient as in Figure 29. The venous phase hepatic arteriogram demonstrates the tumor blush of the pancreatic cancer (arrows) and a large liver metastasis (arrowheads).

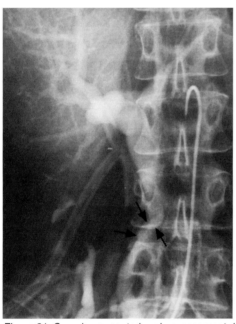

Figure 31. Superior mesenteric vein encasement due to carcinoma within the pancreatic head (arrows).

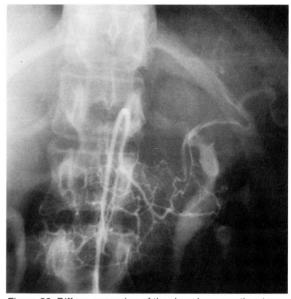

Figure 32. Diffuse narrowing of the dorsal pancreatic artery due to chronic pancreatitis.

Neovascularity is seen in approximately 60% of patients with pancreatic adenocarcinoma **(Figs. 29, 30)**. Venous invasion, distortion, or occlusion can also occur. For example, the superior mesenteric vein is involved in 85%–99% of pancreatic head carcinomas **(Fig. 31)**. The differential diagnosis includes pancreatitis, which often involves large areas of the pancreas and may appear hypervascular with alternating dilatation and narrowing of normal sized vessels **(Fig. 32)**. Neoplasms tend to cause more focal and irregular vascular changes. Atherosclerosis can mimic encasement but usually causes more smooth, eccentric or circumferential narrowing in arteries; the veins appear normal.

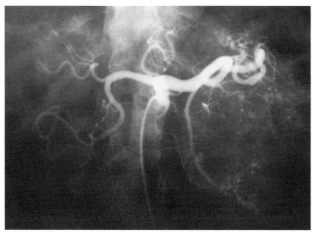

Figure 33. Early arterial phase of celiac arteriography demonstrates a large pancreatic cystadenoma.

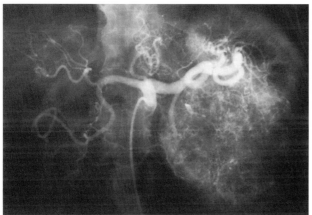

Figure 34. Same patient as in Figure 33, late arterial phase.

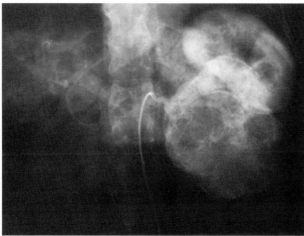

Figure 35. Same patient as in Figure 33, venous phase.

Pancreas—Cystic Tumors

Cystadenomas and cystadenocarcinomas are rare tumors that lack early symptomatology and are therefore large at presentation. They are often well encapsulated with cystic spaces. Arteriography demonstrates hypervascularity with a dilated arterial supply and fine tumor vessels leading to increased accumulation of contrast material **(Figs. 33–35)**. Vessels may be displaced by the tumor. It is not possible to distinguish benign from malignant disease unless there is invasion of large arteries. Hepatic arterial injections should be performed to look for hypervascular hepatic metastases.

199

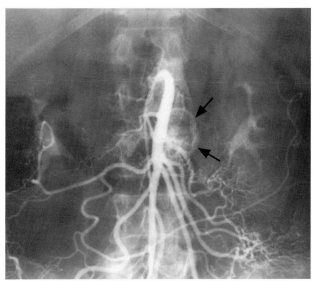

Figure 36. Hypervascular well-circumscribed blush typical of an islet cell tumor (arrow).

Pancreas—Endocrine Neoplasms

Pancreatic islet cell tumors can be divided into functional and nonfunctional types. Functional tumors can secrete insulin, gastrin, glucagon, vasoactive intestinal polypeptide (VIP), and other hormones. The clinical presentation depends on the type of hormone secreted by the tumor. The diagnosis is confirmed by biochemical assay. Insulinomas are the most common functional pancreatic endocrine tumor (60%) and cause symptoms of fasting hypoglycemia. They are usually benign but multiple lesions occur in one third of cases. Alpha-1 islet cell tumors are fairly common, often malignant, and secrete gastrin, causing Zollinger-Ellison syndrome. Other islet cell tumors are rare.

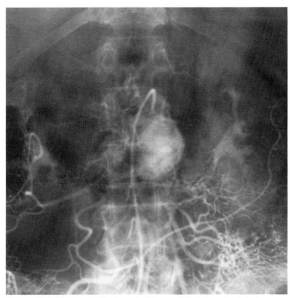

Figure 37. Same patient as in Figure 36, late arterial phase. Dense opacification of the tumor is maintained.

Pancreas—Functional Islet Cell Tumors

Because most functional islet cell tumors are small and similar in tissue consistency to the normal pancreas, they are difficult to detect by cross-sectional imaging techniques. Arteriography is frequently helpful. Most islet cell tumors have a typical angiographic appearance regardless of cell type. The lesions tend to be well-circumscribed and hypervascular; they opacify early in the arterial phase, blush densely, and stay opacified into the venous phase **(Figs. 36, 37)**. Subselective arteriography with high-quality technique, adequate bowel preparation, and multiple different views are all essential to detecting small, subtle adenomas.

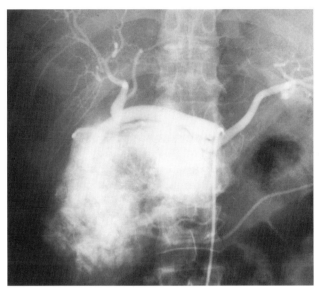

Figure 38. This large malignant islet cell neoplasm escaped early detection because the tumor was hormonally nonfunctional.

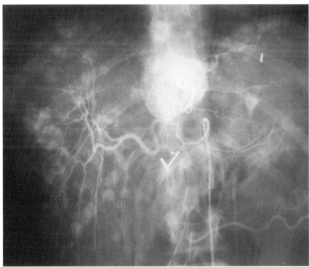

Figure 39. Highly visible hypervascular hepatic metastases from islet cell cancer.

Pancreas—Nonfunctioning Islet Cell Tumors

Differentiation between benign and malignant islet cell tumors can be quite difficult. Nonfunctioning tumors are more commonly malignant and often become very large before they are detected **(Fig. 38)**. Size is one criterion that is useful in differentiating benign from malignant islet cell tumors: if a lesion is larger than 5 cm, it is most likely malignant. If a malignancy is suspected, hepatic arteriography should be performed. Because liver metastases are usually quite hypervascular, very small lesions can be detected **(Fig. 39)**.

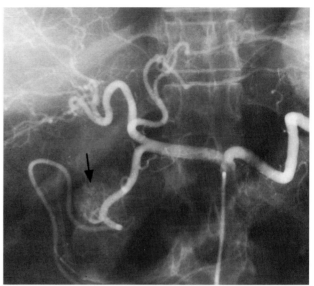

Figure 40. Hypervascular gastrinoma within the duodenal wall (arrow).

Islet Cell Tumor—Diagnostic Accuracy

Arteriographic detection of small functional islet cell tumors varies with the type of adenoma. Localization of insulinomas with high-quality arteriography is successful in up to 90% of cases, because these tumors are usually discrete and hypervascular. Arteriographic localization of gastrinomas is significantly less accurate (as low as 15%). Gastrinomas can be hypovascular, are often multiple, can exist in the form of generalized alpha-1 hyperplasia (not detectable by arteriography), and can occur in the duodenal wall (10%–15%), a location easily missed by arteriography **(Figs. 40, 41)**. Causes of false-positive diagnosis include accessory spleens and the pancreatic tail seen en face.

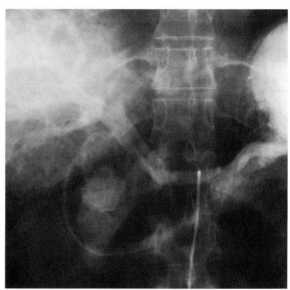

Figure 41. Same patient as in Figure 40. Venous phase of a celiac arteriogram.

Venous Sampling for Islet Cell Tumors

When selective arteriography fails to localize an islet cell tumor, percutaneous transhepatic portal vein catheterization with hormone assays can be extremely accurate. A sensitivity of 94% has been reported for localization of insulinomas when CT scanning and arteriography were negative or equivocal. Detailed anatomical mapping of the sites that are sampled is mandatory to accurately localize the tumor to the head, body, or tail of the pancreas **(Fig. 42)**. Another elegant and accurate technique has been described that combines subselective intraarterial hormone injections with timed hepatic venous sampling for detection of cryptic islet cell tumors, most often gastrinomas.

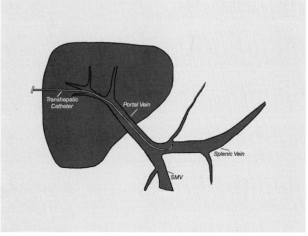

Figure 42. Venous sampling for detection of islet cell tumors.

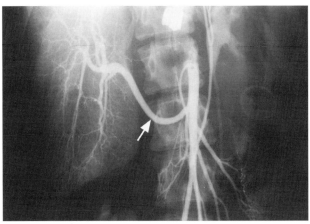

Figure 43. Replaced right hepatic artery originating from the superior mesenteric artery. Knowledge of variant hepatic arterial anatomy is crucial for complete arteriographic evaluation of the liver.

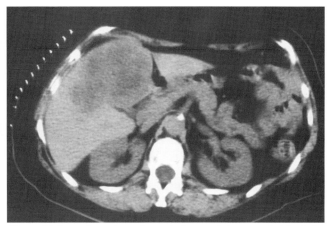

Figure 44. Large hypodense tumor in the medial segment of the left lobe of the liver.

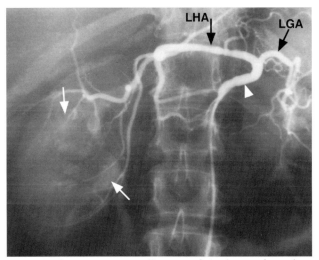

Figure 45. Same patient as in Figure 44. Selective arteriography of the left gastric–left hepatic common arterial trunk (arrowhead). Branches from this left hepatic artery feed the hepatoma (arrows). LHA="replaced" left hepatic artery; LGA=left gastric artery.

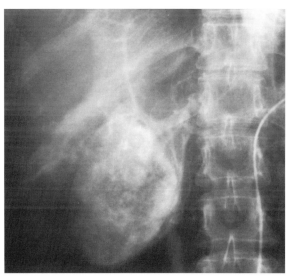

Figure 46. Same patient as in Figure 44, parenchymal phase.

Hepatic Neoplasms

Hepatic arteriography is performed both for diagnostic purposes and prior to an intervention. Benign and malignant liver tumors have angiographic features which can be quite specific. Therapy for primary and metastatic liver tumors includes surgery, chemotherapy, chemoembolization, and percutaneous ablation. It is important to be aware of the variants of arterial anatomy in order to obtain adequate diagnostic arteriograms (Fig. 43). In only 60% of patients can the entire liver be evaluated by injection of the common hepatic artery alone. Injection of the left gastric (Figs. 44–46), replaced right hepatic, accessory right hepatic, and other variant arteries may be required.

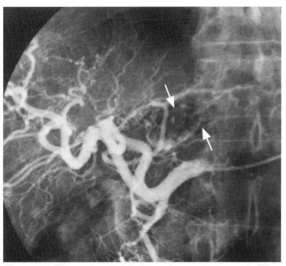

Figure 47. The early arterial phase demonstrates early filling of the dilated vascular lakes ("cotton wool" spots) of cavernous hemangioma (arrows).

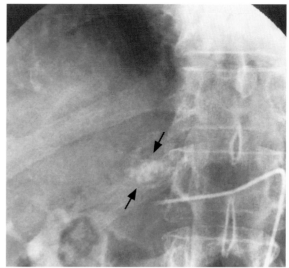

Figure 48. Same patient as in Figure 47. The delayed image demonstrates the characteristic persistent pooling of contrast material within the vascular spaces of the hemangioma.

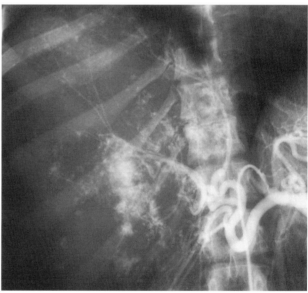

Figure 49. Large right lobe hemangioma. There is no evidence of hypervascularity or vascular invasion. The hepatic arteries are not increased in size.

Hepatic Cavernous Hemangioma

Cavernous hemangiomas, usually seen in middle-aged women, are the most common benign hepatic tumors. They can be single or multiple. Their angiographic appearance is very characteristic. The feeding arteries are normal in caliber regardless of the size of the tumor. Small, dilated amorphous vascular spaces begin to fill in the mid arterial phase and remain opacified well into the venous phase ("cotton wool" appearance) **(Figs. 47, 48)**. Hemangiomas show no evidence of vascular infiltration or neovascularity but can displace vessels **(Fig. 49)**. Although they are almost always asymptomatic, very large lesions can bleed or become painful, requiring treatment by either embolization or resection.

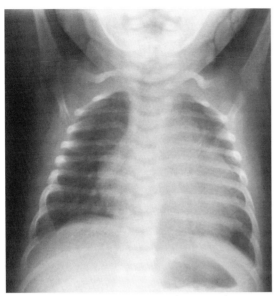

Figure 50. Chest radiograph of an infant with a hemangioendothelioma. The arteriovenous shunting through the tumor has caused cardiomegaly and pulmonary edema.

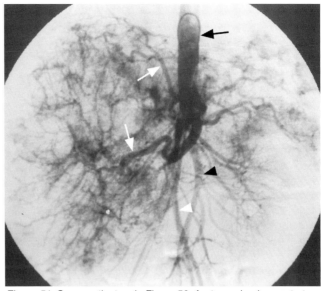

Figure 51. Same patient as in Figure 50. Aortography demonstrates marked enlargement of the supraceliac aorta (black arrow) and hepatic arteries (white arrows) to supply the massive liver tumor. The superior mesenteric (black arrowhead) and iliac arteries (white arrowhead) approach normal caliber.

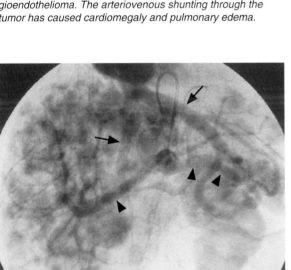

Figure 52. Same patient as in Figure 50, venous phase. The extensive liver involvement is shown. Prominent portal veins (arrowheads) and draining hepatic veins (arrows) are seen.

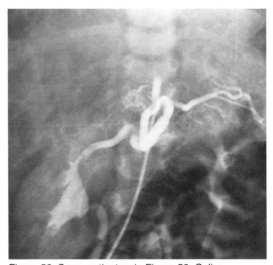

Figure 53. Same patient as in Figure 50. Celiac arteriogram after hepatic artery embolization.

Hepatic Hemangioendothelioma

Hemangioendotheliomas are in general benign neoplasms of infants. Patients have signs and symptoms of congestive heart failure (Fig. 50). As the lesions involute spontaneously over the first year of life, symptoms often resolve. One third of patients also have extrahepatic lesions. They are extremely vascular lesions (Fig. 51) with large amorphous spaces similar to cavernous hemangiomas. However, these lesions differ in that the feeding arteries are markedly dilated, contrast material does not persist in the vascular spaces, and arteriovenous shunting to the hepatic veins is a prominent feature (Fig. 52). In infants with severe congestive heart failure, arterial embolization can be life-saving (Fig. 53).

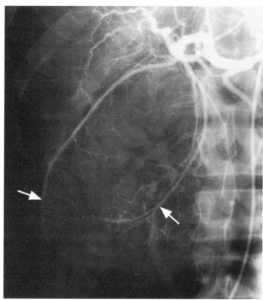

Figure 54. Abnormal vessels enter the hepatic adenoma from its periphery (arrows).

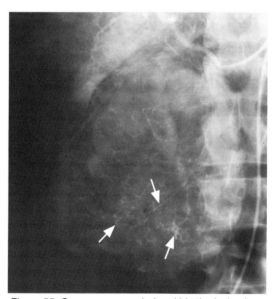

Figure 55. Coarse neovascularity within the lesion is noted later in the filming sequence (arrows).

Hepatic Adenoma

Hepatic adenomas are associated with oral contraceptive use in young women and type 1 glycogen storage disorder. They frequently rupture and hemorrhage and are therefore resected even when the patient is asymptomatic. Arteriography demonstrates a homogeneous hypervascular mass fed by enlarged arteries that enter from the periphery of the lesion and penetrate to a central area of coarse neovascularity **(Figs. 54, 55)**. These lesions do not demonstrate pooling of contrast material, arteriovenous shunting, or portal vein invasion. The center of the mass may be relatively lucent when there is hemorrhage within the tumor.

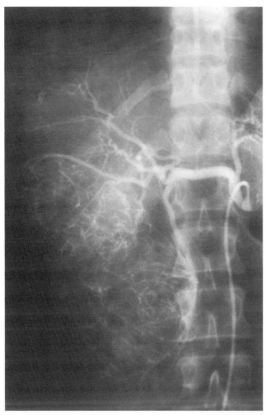

Figure 56. Focal nodular hyperplasia. A more reticular pattern of vessels is present near the center of the tumor.

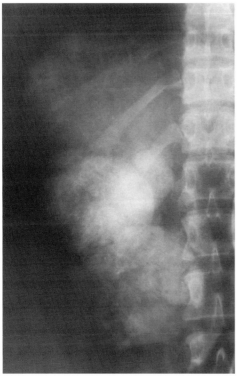

Figure 57. Same patient as in Figure 56, venous phase. Faint central lucencies may occasionally be visible, corresponding to the central scar.

Hepatic Focal Nodular Hyperplasia

Focal nodular hyperplasia (FNH) is a benign lesion that occurs in men and women of all ages. Tumors tend to occur near the capsule and can be multiple. At arteriography, the arteries divide into small penetrating branches with a reticular pattern in the center of the tumor **(Fig. 56)**. No arterial dilatation or neovascularity is seen, but lesions can possess a lucent ring or "pseudocapsule." The parenchymal phase shows fine homogeneous granularity, often with a linear lucency from a central scar **(Fig. 57)**. Distinguishing FNH from adenomas can be difficult and nuclear medicine imaging with technetium-99-labeled sulfur colloid is essentially diagnostic of FNH if the lesion is isointense or hyperaccumulating.

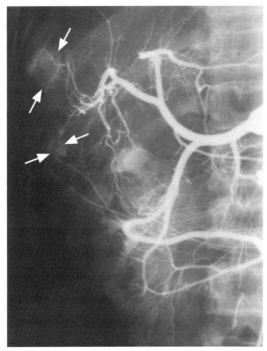

Figure 58. Multifocal hepatoma (arrows).

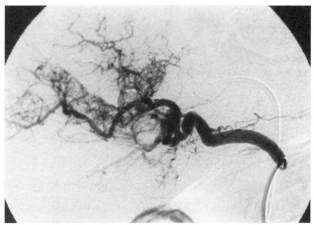

Figure 59. Hepatic neovascularity from hepatocellular carcinoma.

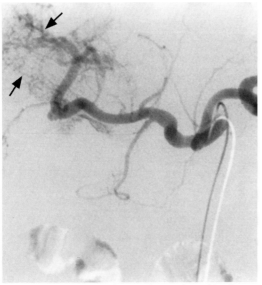

Figure 60. A celiac arteriogram in a patient with a hepatoma demonstrates the "thread and streak" sign of arterial supply to an intraluminal tumor (arrows). See also Figure 4.

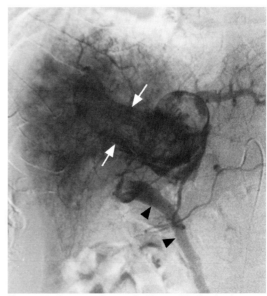

Figure 61. Same patient as in Figure 60. On the later image, the right portal vein is markedly enlarged and filled with tumor thrombus (arrows). Portal hypertension has led to recanalization of the umbilical vein (arrowheads).

Hepatoma

Hepatomas tend to occur in patients with cirrhosis and in patients with chronic active hepatitis B. They can be single, multiple **(Fig. 58)**, or diffuse. Angiographic features include enlargement of the hepatic artery and neovascularity **(Fig. 59)**. Approximately 30% demonstrate arterial to portal vein shunting (nearly pathognomonic). Portal vein invasion is characteristic of hepatoma and is very rare with metastases or other neoplasms **(Figs. 60, 61)**. Hepatic or portal vein invasion with a "thread and streak" sign can occur. Rarely, other lesions such as regenerative nodules and hypervascular metastases (choriocarcinoma and renal cell carcinoma) can mimic hepatomas.

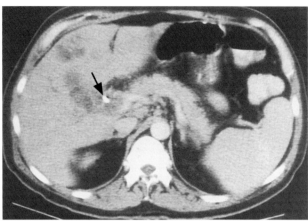

Figure 62. Common bile duct stent placement (arrow) for palliation of biliary obstruction. Repeated periductal biopsies failed to demonstrate tumor.

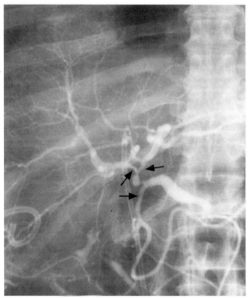

Figure 63. Same patient as in Figure 62. Hepatic arteriogram demonstrates conclusive findings of arterial encasement (arrows). The endoscopic biliary stent is visible.

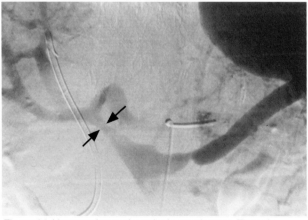

Figure 64. Venous phase of a splenic arteriogram. There is encasement of the main portal vein at the liver hilum (arrows).

Cholangiocarcinoma

Cholangiocarcinomas are scirrhous infiltrating tumors. They typically do not show neovascularity or dilated sinusoids (unlike hepatomas). Cross-sectional imaging **(Fig. 62)**, cholangiography, and biopsy can all be inconclusive, particularly when sclerosing cholangitis is also present. Arteriography is positive in 60%–70% of cases and is important in staging, preoperative planning, and diagnosis. Arterial invasion is the main arteriographic finding **(Fig. 63)**. When large, these tumors may show increased vascularity and a tumor blush. Lesions are generally unresectable when major arteries or veins, such as the main portal vein or proper hepatic artery, are encased or occluded **(Fig. 64)**.

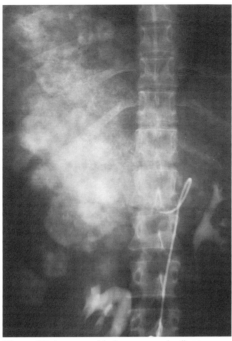

Figure 65. Innumerable hypervascular liver metastases.

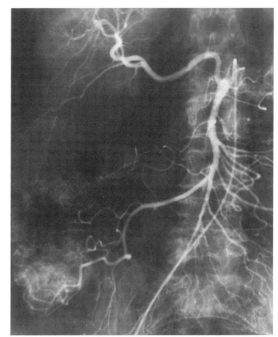

Figure 66. The superior mesenteric arteriogram demonstrates a cecal carcinoma. A replaced right hepatic artery is present.

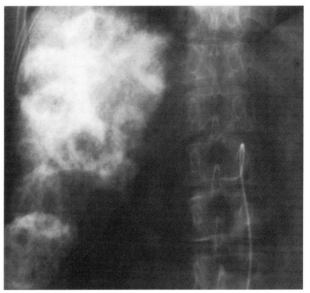

Figure 67. Same patient as in Figure 66. Capillary phase image from a select infusion arteriogram of the right hepatic artery. Multiple hypovascular liver metastases are evident.

Hepatic Metastases

Metastases are the most common malignant hepatic tumor. Metastases show variable vascularity depending on the organ of origin. They are most often multiple, but can be single. Hypervascular metastases are most easily identified against the homogeneous parenchymal phase of the liver. Some show pooling of contrast material and a tumor blush. Lesions as small as 0.5–1.0 cm can be detected with high-quality arteriography. Hypervascular metastases include choriocarcinoma, renal cell carcinoma, endocrine tumors, carcinoid, and leiomyosarcoma **(Fig. 65)**.

"Hypovascular" liver metastases create filling defects in the capillary phase of the injection and are therefore much harder to identify **(Fig. 66)**. These tumors can typically be diagnosed more easily with CT or MR imaging. Infusion hepatic arteriograms with long, slow injections can be quite helpful (40–60 mL over 10–15 seconds with filming out to 30 seconds). Infusion arteriography makes hypovascular metastases stand out relative to the normal liver **(Fig. 67)**. The normal parenchyma appears less dense because the contrast material becomes diluted in the hepatic sinusoids by portal vein inflow. Hypovascular metastases arise from most forms of adenocarcinoma of the bowel and pancreas.

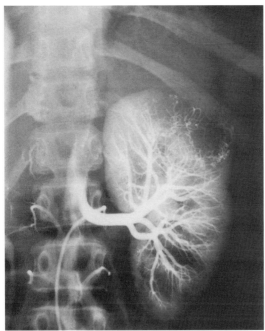

Figure 68. Renin-secreting juxtaglomerular upper pole mass. This was detected during screening arteriography in a patient with severe hypertension.

Renal Neoplasms

Although diagnostic arteriography is rarely needed for renal tumors, it is commonly performed for a number of other indications (aortography, renal donors, hypertension) and may coincidentally reveal a tumor **(Fig. 68)**. Because of this, understanding the manifestations of the various renal tumors is essential. Diagnostic renal arteriography is also helpful in equivocal cases of carcinoma and when elucidation of vascular anatomy is needed prior to a partial nephrectomy (such as in patients with recurrent renal cell carcinoma after a contralateral nephrectomy). High-quality renal arteriograms and venograms/cavograms are very accurate for detecting and staging renal cell carcinoma.

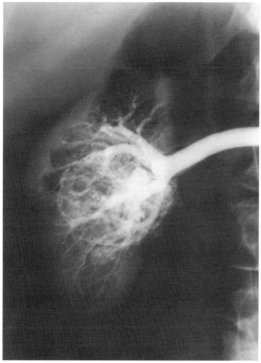

Figure 69. Renal cell carcinoma, arterial phase.

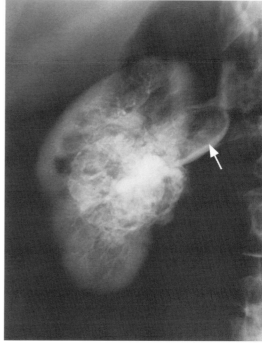

Figure 70. A later image demonstrates a filling defect within the right renal vein (arrow).

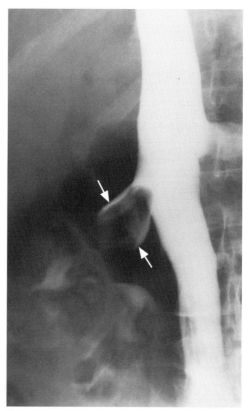

Figure 71. Inferior vena cavogram confirms the presence of tumor thrombus within the right renal vein (arrows).

Renal Cell Carcinoma

Hypernephromas are derived from tubular epithelium. They account for 85% of renal malignancies in the non-pediatric population. Most of these tumors are hypervascular at arteriography and readily diagnosed with 94%–100% sensitivity. Since bilateral malignancy is present in approximately 10% of patients, the contralateral kidney should always be evaluated. Angiographic features include neovascularity with irregular arteries (92%), vessel displacement (91%), tumor blush/stain, and venous invasion **(Figs. 69–71)**. Differential diagnosis includes lymphoma, benign vascular tumors (particularly angiomyolipomas) and occasionally abscesses or xanthogranulomatous pyelonephritis.

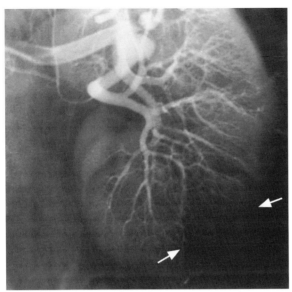

Figure 72. The arterial phase demonstrates a cystic-appearing lesion in the lower pole (arrows).

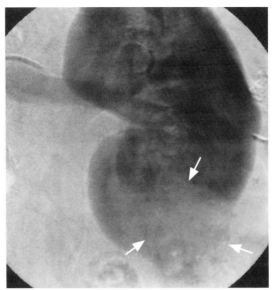

Figure 73. The parenchymal phase confirms the presence of a hypovascular lesion with ill-defined margins.

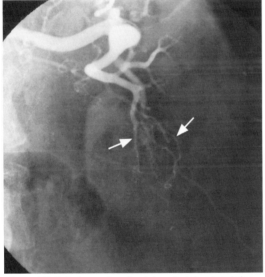

Figure 74. Arteriography after intraarterial epinephrine injection clearly demonstrates the tumor vascularity. These vessels, unlike the normal parenchymal vasculature, do not vasoconstrict in response to epinephrine.

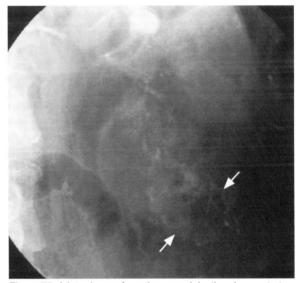

Figure 75. A later image from the same injection demonstrates neovascularity.

Renal Pharmacoangiography and Embolization

Epinephrine injected immediately prior to arteriography can help localize subtle renal neoplasms. Vasoconstriction of normal vessels emphasizes the blood flow to the tumor via abnormal vessels that lack a responsive muscular wall and do not vasoconstrict **(Figs. 72–75)**. Occasionally, renal venograms are also helpful to look for invasion, an essential component of staging the tumor. Hepatic arteriograms for detection of metastasis can be helpful in selected cases. The value of preoperative embolization for renal neoplasms is still debated. Preoperative embolization of large vascular lesions clearly decreases intraoperative bleeding.

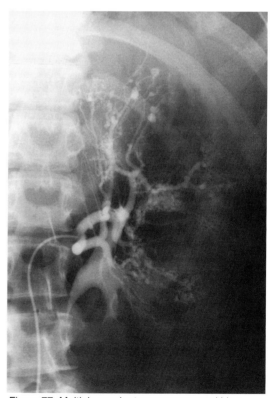

Figure 76. "Spoke-wheel" appearance of arteries and a central lucent scar are characteristic of a renal oncocytoma.

Renal Neoplasms—Adenomas

Oncocytomas are the most common benign renal tumor and are usually asymptomatic. Preoperative distinction from renal cell carcinoma is often difficult or impossible. Angiographic features that are very characteristic of this tumor include a "spoke-wheel" appearance with centrally radiating arteries and a lucent scar in the center of the mass **(Fig. 76)**. Larger adenomas may have malignant features. Because angiographic features overlap significantly with renal cell carcinomas, these tumors are rarely definitively diagnosed prior to nephrectomy.

Renal Neoplasms—Angiomyolipomas

Angiomyolipomas tend to occur in females and are associated with tuberous sclerosis. Often incidentally detected on imaging studies, they can be definitively diagnosed when fat density is detected on CT scanning. Angiomyolipomas can present with hemorrhagic complications, and embolization may be indicated. Angiographic features include a hypervascular mass with large, tortuous feeding arteries arranged circumferentially, multiple small arterial aneurysms, a "sunburst" or "whorled" appearance in the parenchymal and venous phases, as well as venous lakes **(Fig. 77)**. Arterial-venous shunting is not typical. Angiographic differentiation from hypernephroma is usually not definitive.

Figure 77. Multiple renal artery aneurysms within a large angiomyolipoma.

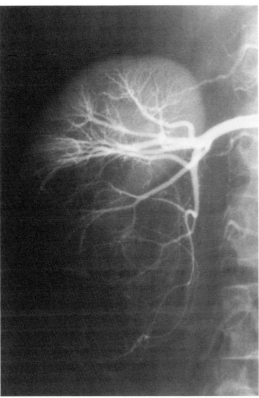

Figure 78. Breast cancer metastatic to the lower pole of the right kidney.

Renal Neoplasms—Other Tumors

Less common renal tumors include fibromas, leiomyomas, intrarenal transitional cell neoplasms, and neurogenic tumors (neurofibromas and schwannomas). These tumors may have markedly increased vascularity suggesting a malignancy. Metastases to the kidney are twice as common as primary renal tumors; however, they are rarely found ante mortem. Angiographic features are typically similar to that of the primary tumor from which the metastasis arose **(Fig. 78)**.

For further information on this topic, please see Teaching File Cases 40–45, 48, 51, 54, 55, 59, and 60.

Selected Readings

Abrams HL. Renal tumor versus renal cyst. In: Abrams HL, ed. Abrams angiography: vascular and interventional radiology. 3rd edition. Boston: Little, Brown and Company, 1983; 1123–1174.

Aspestrand F, Kolmannskog F. CT compared to angiography for staging of tumors of the pancreatic head. Acta Radiol 1992; 33:556–560.

Aspestrand F, Kolmannskog F, Jacobsen M. CT, MR imaging and angiography in pancreatic APUDomas. Acta Radiol 1993; 34:468–473.

Chait A. Current status of renal angiography. Urol Clin North Am 1985; 12(4):687–698.

Dooley WC, Cameron JL, Pitt HA, Lillemoe KD, Yue NC, Venbrux AC. Is preoperative angiography useful in patients with periampullary tumors? Ann Surg 1990; 211(6):649–655.

Doppman JL, Miller DL, Chang R, et al. Gastrinomas: localization by means of selective intraarterial injection of secretin. Radiology 1990; 174:25–29.

Freeny PC. Radiologic diagnosis and staging of pancreatic ductal adenocarcinoma. Radiol Clin North Am 1989; 27(1):121–128.

Levine E. Renal cell carcinoma: radiological diagnosis and staging. Semin Roentgenol 1987; 22:248–259.

Miller DL. Endocrine angiography and venous sampling. Radiol Clin North Am 1993; 31(5):1051–1067.

Pasieka JL, McLeod MK, Thompson NW, Burney RE. Surgical approach to insulinomas: assessing the need for preoperative localization. Arch Surg 1992; 127:442–447.

Reuter SR, Redman HC, Cho KJ. Tumors. In: Reuter SR, Redman HC, Cho KJ. Gastrointestinal angiography. 3rd edition. Philadelphia: W.B. Saunders Company, 1986; 128–247.

Rossi P, Allison DJ, Bezzi M, et al. Endocrine tumors of the pancreas. Radiol Clin North Am 1989; 27(1):129–161.

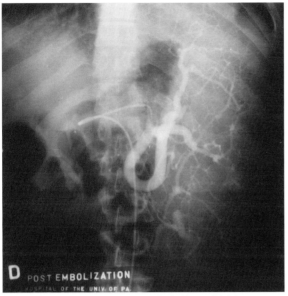

Figure 1. Splenic embolization with Gelfoam (Upjohn, Kalamazoo, MI) and coils for treatment of hypersplenism.

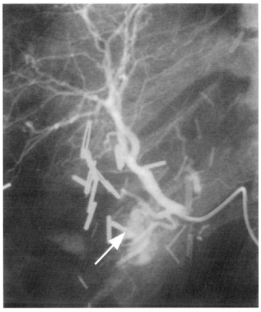

Figure 2. Uncontrollable hemorrhage and hypotension following segmental hepatic resection for tumor. Extravasation is present (arrow).

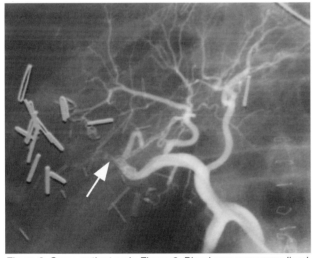

Figure 3. Same patient as in Figure 2. Blood pressure normalized after hepatic artery embolization (arrow).

TUTORIAL 13
EMBOLIZATION— GENERAL PRINCIPLES AND TECHNIQUES
Constantin Cope, M.D.

Introduction
Embolization is an appropriate treatment for hemorrhage, vascular malformations, arteriovenous fistulas, and malignant and functioning tumors, as well as for hypersplenism **(Fig. 1)** and renovascular hypertension. It can also be used to divert blood flow. Embolization can obviate surgery, render surgery less hazardous, or complement difficult surgical procedures **(Figs. 2, 3)**.

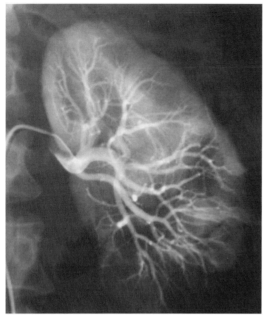

Figure 4. Renal AV fistula; the lesion was not seen on the main renal arteriogram.

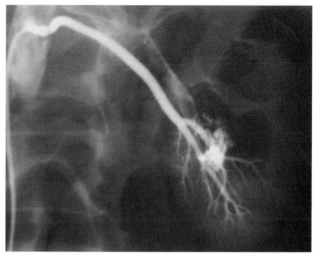

Figure 5. Selective arteriography of the lower pole artery. The fistula is fed by an accessory renal artery.

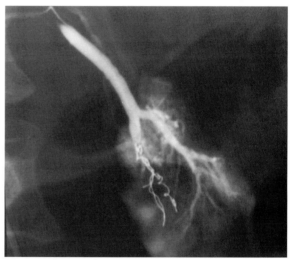

Figure 6. Superselective embolization of the fistula with minimal renal tissue loss.

Efficacy

The efficacy of embolic therapy for arresting localized bleeding, thrombosing aneurysms and arteriovenous (AV) malformations, or devitalizing tumors depends greatly on the operator's ability to assess and control the vascular inflow from various sources while compromising as little normal tissue as possible **(Figs. 4–6)**.

Patient Preparation for Embolization

The patient should be rendered as physiologically stable as possible with fluid, blood products, vaso-pressors, antibiotics, etc **(Fig. 7)**. Adequate fluid intake is especially important to offset the renal toxicity caused by the large volume of contrast material which may need to be administered for diagnosis and procedural and postprocedural arteriographic documentation. It must be appreciated that selective embolization may not be effective for arresting bleeding if severe coagulopathy cannot be at least partially corrected.

Periprocedural Precautions

The patient should be carefully and continuously monitored **(Fig. 8)**. The procedure should be discontinued immediately if there is symptomatic evidence of errant emboli to nerves, brain, spinal cord, or limbs. Sedation and pain medications should be administered in the smallest doses that are sufficient to provide patient comfort and cooperation. Deep narcosis should be avoided.

Patient Preparation
1. Baseline liver function tests, blood count, creatinine 2. Normalize coagulation 3. Stabilize blood pressure, oxygenation 4. Antibiotic coverage? 5. Intravenous fluids

Figure 7.

Patient Monitoring
1. Blood pressure, electrocardiography 2. Oxygen saturation 3. Errant emboli (assess limb color, temperature, pulses, pain, numbness)

Figure 8.

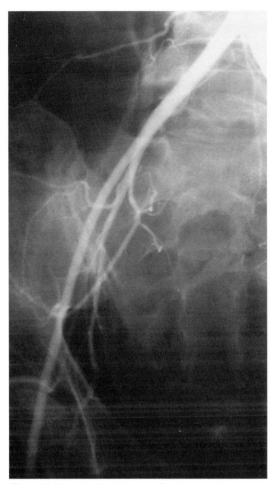

Figure 9. Hypotension 6 hours after hysterectomy; normal pelvic arteriogram.

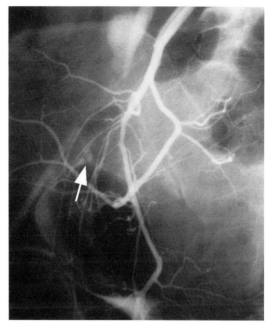

Figure 10. A bleeding point becomes visible upon selective hypogastric arteriography (arrow).

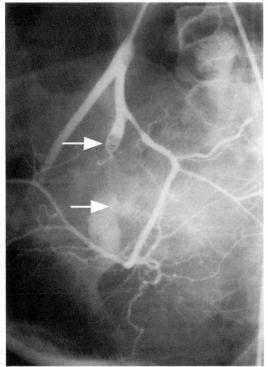

Figure 11. Bleeding was arrested by distal and proximal coil embolization of the anterior hypogastric artery (arrows).

Life-Threatening Hemorrhage

There should be minimal delay in bringing patients with active hemorrhage to the interventional suite, *especially* if they are hemodynamically unstable. Resuscitative measures can be carried out just as efficiently in a well-equipped angiography section as in an intensive care unit **(Figs. 9–11)**.

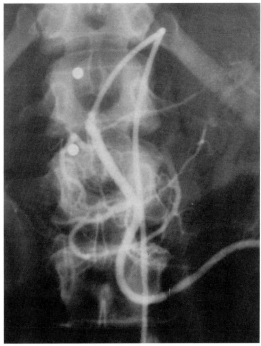

Figure 12. Vigorous duodenal bleeding seen by endoscopy; the gastroduodenal artery (GDA) is normal. No extravasation is seen.

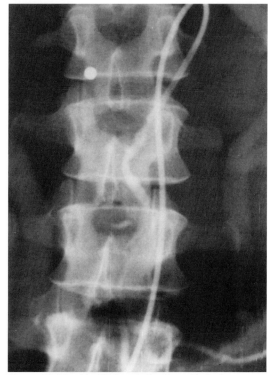

Figure 13. Empiric GDA embolization with Gelfoam was performed after endoscopically visualized bleeding; blood pressure normalized immediately.

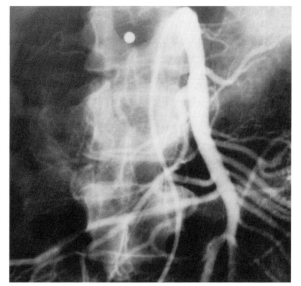

Figure 14. Same patient as in Figure 13. Superior mesenteric arteriogram shows no retrograde filling of the GDA through the pancreaticoduodenal arcade.

Clinical Localization of Bleeding Lesion

When the arteriogram shows no bleeding point, the following clinical examination(s) can provide a clue as to the most appropriate vessel(s) to embolize: hemoptysis: bronchoscopy, chest radiography, chest CT. Upper GI bleed: nasogastric tube aspiration, upper endoscopy, radionuclide scans **(Figs. 12–14)**. Lower GI bleed: lower endoscopy, radionuclide scans. Hematuria: CT scan. Abdominal trauma: CT scan. Bleeding from percutaneous catheters: temporary removal of a nephrostomy or biliary drain over a safety wire **(Figs. 15–20)**.

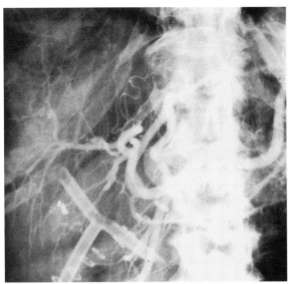

Figure 15. Severe intermittent hemobilia through T-tube following cholecystectomy; the celiac arteriogram is normal.

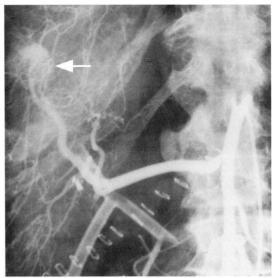

Figure 16. Same patient as in Figure 15. Intrahepatic bleeding (arrow) fed by an accessory hepatic artery arising from the SMA. A locked loop drain pulled out during surgery was thought to be the cause of bleeding.

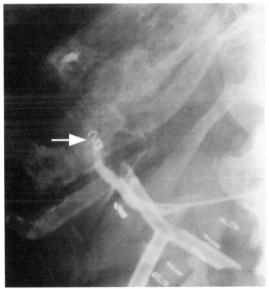

Figure 17. Same patient as in Figure 15. Accessory right hepatic artery was embolized with coils and Gelfoam (arrow).

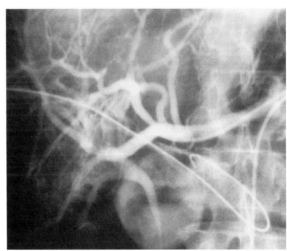

Figure 18. History of severe bleeding during biliary drain exchange. Bleeding was not seen on this celiac arteriogram even after withdrawing the drain over the wire.

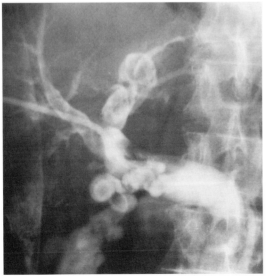

Figure 19. Same patient as in Figure 18. Cholangiogram after drain reinsertion shows that blood clots have filled the biliary tree in the interim.

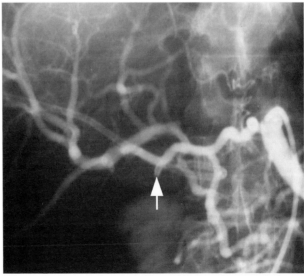

Figure 20. Same patient as in Figure 18. Superior mesenteric arteriogram shows transection of the pancreaticoduodenal branch (arrow) by the drain.

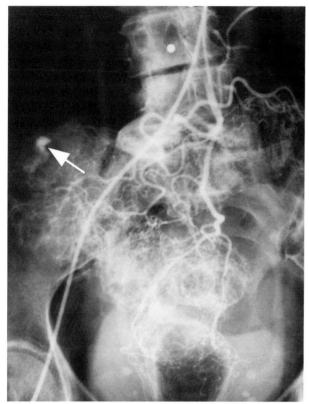

Figure 21. Diverticular bleeding of the sigmoid colon (arrow).

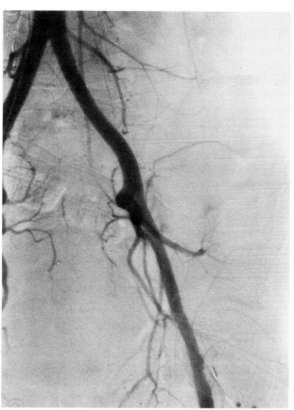

Figure 22. Motorcycle injury; the initial pelvic arteriogram was normal.

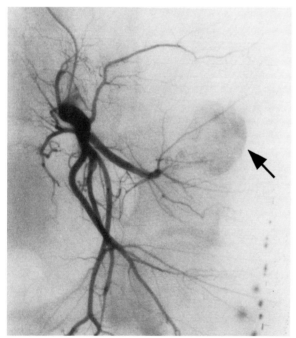

Figure 23. A selective internal iliac arteriogram demonstrates a large gluteal artery pseudoaneurysm (arrow).

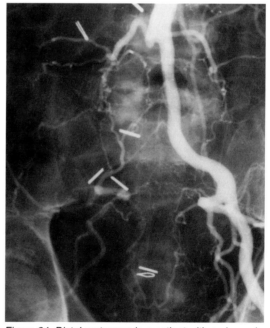

Figure 24. Distal aortogram in a patient with prolonged rectal bleeding despite ligation of the right iliac artery. No lesion is seen.

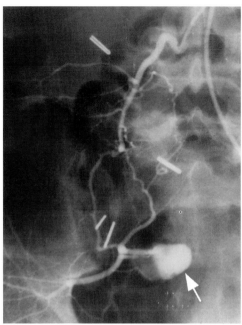

Figure 25. Selective catheterization of the 5th lumbar artery demonstrates a pseudoaneurysm (arrow) from an internal iliac artery branch.

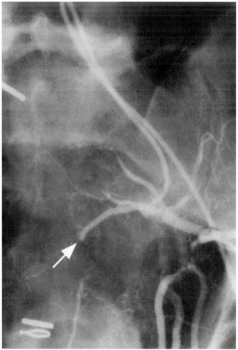

Figure 27. A feeding left hypogastric artery branch is also embolized with Gelfoam (arrow).

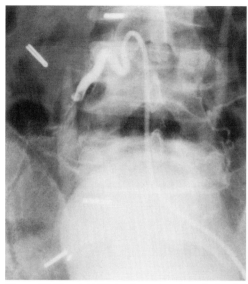

Figure 26. The right 5th lumbar artery is embolized.

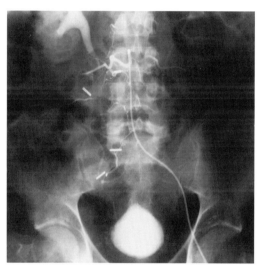

Figure 28 .The pseudoaneurysm was not opacified from the 3rd or 4th lumbar (shown here) or inferior mesenteric arteries.

Vascular Hemorrhage

Possible bleeding points can appear as extravasation of contrast material **(Fig. 21)**, tumor or inflammatory blush, aneurysms or pseudoaneurysms, varicosities, vascular malformations, and localized arterial spasm.

Arteriographic Localization of a Bleeding Lesion

Although a bleeding point may not be identified until subselective or superselective arteriography is performed **(Figs. 22, 23)**, it is most important to first map out the area of interest by mid stream aortography and/or main trunk opacification for the following reasons:

1. To dispel any confusion caused by guide wire-induced vascular spasm.
2. To allow identification of all possible feeding vessels **(Figs. 24–28)**.
3. To localize the presence of potential multiple bleeding points or metastases.

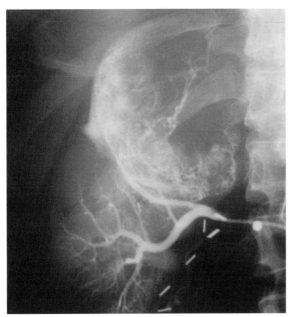

Figure 29. Inoperable large renal carcinoma with lung metastases.

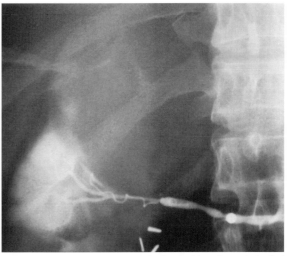

Figure 30. Main renal artery embolized with coils and alcohol. Coil embolization may be disadvantageous in this setting because the resulting proximal vessel occlusion may permit distal tissue perfusion through existing and newly recruited collateral vessels.

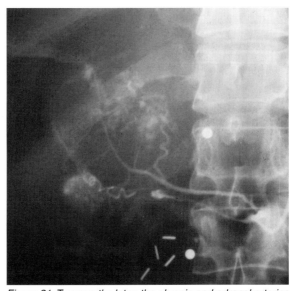

Figure 31. Two months later, the phrenic and adrenal arteries were major tumor feeders and were embolized.

Unusual Arterial Feeders

It is important to study unusual potential sources of blood supply in patients who have had previous embolization **(Figs. 29–31)** or surgical arterial ligation. For example, in patients undergoing repeated hepatic chemoembolization, the lumbar, phrenic, and internal mammary arteries **(Figs. 32, 33)** may provide substantial feeders to the liver.

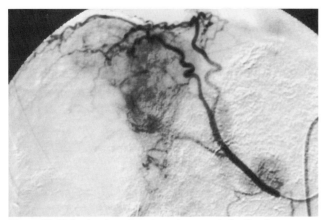

Figure 32. Following hepatic artery chemoembolization for hepatoma, residual tumor is supplied by the phrenic artery.

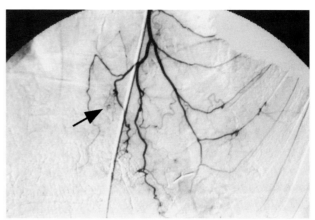

Figure 33. The hepatoma is also fed by the right internal mammary artery (arrow).

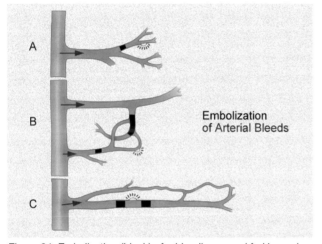

Figure 34. Embolization (black) of a bleeding vessel fed by end artery (A), dual arteries (B), and feeding collaterals (C).

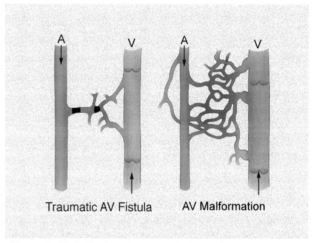

Figure 35. Embolization of a traumatic fistula. Vascular malformation should be sclerosed.

Local Anatomic Considerations for Embolization

The efficacy of embolization of a lesion depends greatly on the ability of the operator to control all its vascular feeders, eg:

1. The kidney has end arteries **(Fig. 34A)**;
2. The pancreas, duodenum, and liver have dual blood supplies **(Fig. 34B)**;
3. Collateral blood supply distal to the bleeding point must be controlled when most major arteries are being occluded to prevent backbleeding **(Fig. 34C)**.
4. Traumatic arteriovenous fistulas can usually be successfully embolized **(Fig. 35)**. Vascular malformations are best sclerosed with alcohol by percutaneous or catheter techniques. In short, except for lesions supplied by end arteries, most need to be managed with embolization of one or more proximal and/or distal feeders in addition to the main supply artery.

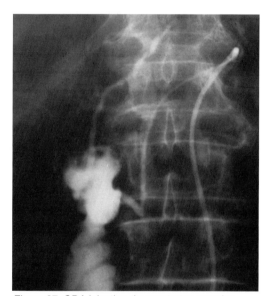

Figure 36. Aneurysm embolization techniques (A,B,C); preliminary embolization of feeding vessel (D); compression of fresh pseudoaneurysm with ultrasound transducer (E).

Aneurysms

Aneurysms and pseudoaneurysms must be excluded from their efferent, afferent, and feeding vessels **(Fig. 36)**. Narrow-neck aneurysms can be embolized safely **(Fig. 36)** with coils and/or thrombin used directly. Wide-neck aneurysms need to have their mouths covered with a tight-mesh stent before coil embolization. Fresh, accessible traumatic pseudoaneurysms can often be occluded with use of compression under ultrasound monitoring **(Fig. 36)**.

Embolic Agents

Particulate

Agents for embolization can be classified into those used for short-term occlusion for decreasing or temporarily arresting blood flow, and those employed for permanent occlusion. Temporary embolic agents are often preferred as the first line of therapy because they generally lead to less tissue damage and allow future repeat embolization through recanalized vessels **(Figs. 37, 38)**. The release of particles dispersed in contrast material must always be performed by slow controlled injection under careful fluoroscopic control to prevent reflux. Embolization is contraindicated immediately following ineffective vasopressin infusion because it may lead to organ infarction.

Figure 37. GDA injection demonstrates massive extravasation into the duodenum.

Blood Clots

Autologous blood clot formed by stasis or with the addition of thrombin or e-aminocaproic acid can be injected through a standard size selective catheter with a 1 mL syringe. This method is most useful in patients with fairly normal clotting factors who are oozing from superficial ulcers, minor vascular trauma, or post-needle biopsy bleeds. Clot emboli are especially useful for arresting minor bleeding sites of the kidney due to trauma. Because of the high fibrinolytic potential of this organ, the bleeding point will remain occluded while the neighboring embolized vessels will recanalize early enough to minimize renal infarction.

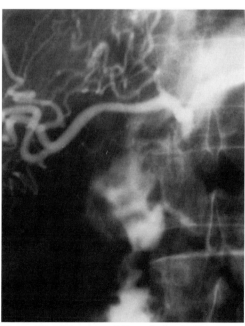

Figure 38. GDA successfully embolized with Gelfoam.

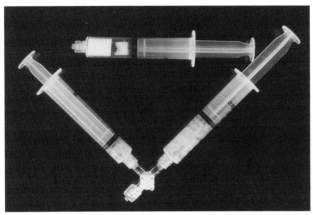

Figure 39. Gelfoam slurry formed from small slabs by back and forth injection through a 3-way stopcock.

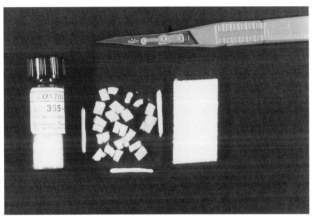

Figure 40. Gelfoam cubes and torpedoes (right); polyvinyl alcohol bottle (left).

Gelfoam

Gelfoam is surgical absorbable sponge commercially available in slabs or in powder form (40–60 microns). It can provide vascular occlusion lasting from a few days to a few weeks. The powder form can lead to serious complications, such as infarction of bowel, nerves, etc, when accidental reflux embolization occurs. Gelfoam **(Fig. 39)** is most commonly used as a slurry, or in 1 x 1-mm cubes **(Fig. 40)**. Larger 1–2 cm-long "torpedoes" are used in preference to smaller particles when there is a potential for accidental embolization of small branches to sensitive organs such as the spinal cord. Gelfoam particles can be sandwiched between two Gianturco coils (Cook, Bloomington, IN) for the more permanent vascular occlusion of larger vessels.

Permanent Particulate Agents

Silicone, steel, acrylic, and ceramic microspheres of various diameters have been used to embolize vascular malformations and certain tumors. These agents have been largely replaced by polyvinyl alcohol (PVA) particles **(Fig. 40)**, which are available in sterile form in a wide variety of sub-millimeter sizes. PVA emboli incite sufficient vascular thrombosis and fibrosis of the vessel wall to prevent recanalization. They are often used in combination with metal coil emboli. In order to prevent PVA particles from clogging microcatheters, they must be kept uniformly suspended in contrast material. This can be accomplished by repeatedly injecting the contents of one syringe into another through a three-way stopcock just before injection.

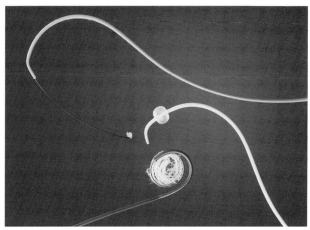

Figure 41. Occlusion balloon; deployment of fiber-wrapped coils.

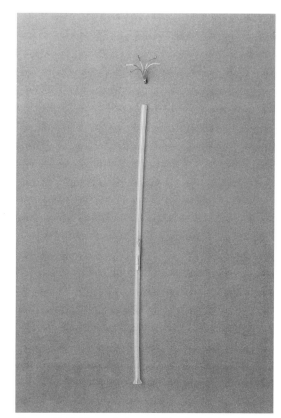

Figure 42. Spider embolus outside of retaining sleeve.

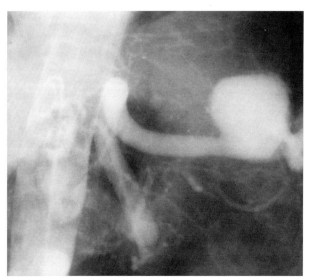

Figure 43. Congenital splenic artery aneurysm.

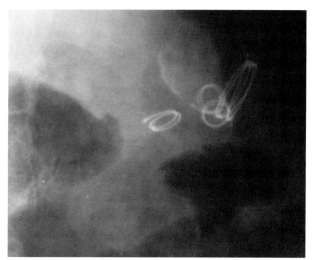

Figure 44. Splenic aneurysm occluded with large coils.

Occlusive Agents for Larger Vessels
Occlusive agents for larger vessels include ends of bristle brushes, silk tufts, catheter segments, metal spring coils, and detachable and nondetachable balloons **(Fig. 41)**. Stainless steel spider emboli can serve as nonocclusive baffles to prevent migration of coils or balloons in large high-flow arteries **(Fig. 42)**.

Gianturco Coils
Stainless steel Gianturco coils, which are threaded with Dacron filaments to induce clotting, are available in 3–20-mm diameters and in various lengths **(Figs. 43, 44)**. To prevent possible migration, the diameter of the expanded coil should be slightly larger than the diameter of the segment of vessel to be embolized. The coil length must be chosen so that, when the coil is deployed in the vessel, it will not protrude back into the main feeding vessel.

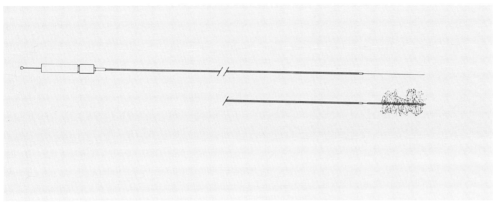

Figure 45. The coil is straightened when loaded on the coil positioner wire.

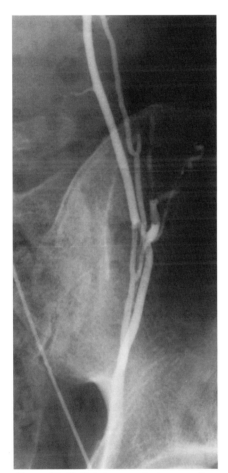

Figure 46. Multiple incompetent spermatic veins.

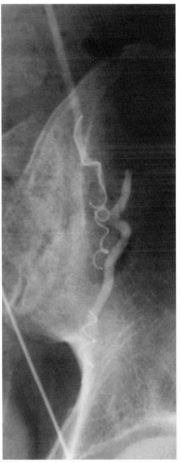

Figure 47. The spermatic veins are easily embolized with a coil positioner.

Large-vessel occlusion is performed by engaging several coils end-to-end in progressively diminishing diameters. Distal small vessel particulate embolization is often used in combination with coils to prevent backflow through collateral vessels. Coils may also be used to protect non-target vessels from particulate embolization. Coil positioners (Cook) are helpful devices for more accurate advancement, placement, and release of coils **(Figs. 45–47)**.

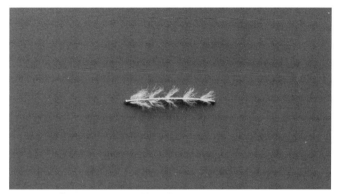

Figure 48. Straight microcoil (Cook).

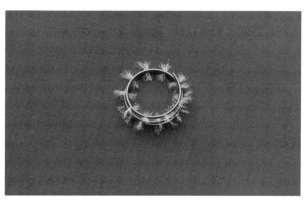

Figure 49. Circular microcoil (Cook).

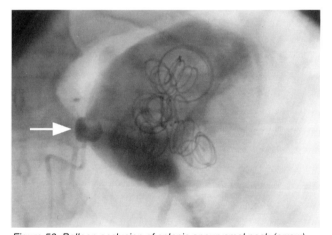

Figure 50. Balloon occlusion of splenic aneurysmal neck (arrow) to allow safe injection of thrombin.

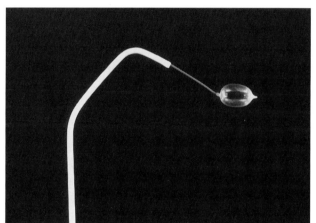

Figure 51. Detachable balloon.

Microcoils
Microcoils, made of platinum alloy and coated with Dacron threads, are designed to be threaded through superselective catheters as small as 2.2-F or less. Microcoils are available in a wide variety of lengths, diameters, and configurations from straight **(Fig. 48)** to a floral or ring design which can expand to as wide as a 6-mm diameter **(Fig. 49)**.

Balloons
Small-diameter fixed occlusion balloon catheters can be used to slow rapid arterial flow in arteriovenous malformations and to prevent untoward reflux during liquid or particulate embolization **(Fig. 50)**. Detachable balloon catheters are very effective for managing high-flow vascular lesions, aneurysms, and major arterial lacerations. They can be flow-directed, positioned and repositioned very accurately, and exchanged for a larger balloon size if necessary. They are still considered investigational devices in the United States **(Fig. 51)**.

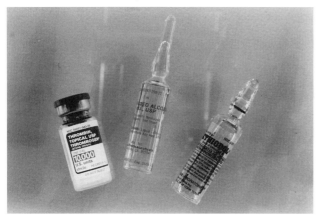

Figure 52. Thrombin, absolute alcohol, and Ethiodol (Savage Laboratories, Melville, NY) for liquid embolization.

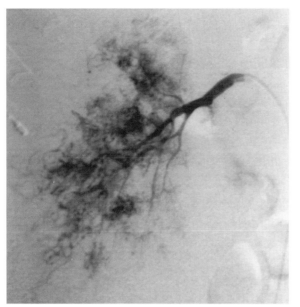

Figure 53. Renal carcinoma embolized with an alcohol/Ethiodol 3:1 mixture.

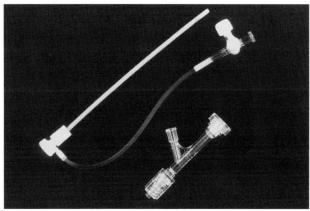

Figure 54. Introducing sheath (top); Tuohy-Borst adapter (bottom).

Embolic Agents—Liquid

Liquid embolic agents **(Fig. 52)** include coagulants (thrombin, collagen material, and fibrin adhesives), sclerosing agents (hypertonic glucose and contrast material, hot contrast material, pure ethanol, Ethibloc [Ethnor Laboratories/Ethicon, Neuilly, France], sodium tetradecyl sulfate, and glues [N-butyl-2-cyanoacrylate]). Sclerosing agents not only induce vascular thrombosis by intimal denudation but also exert a beneficial cytotoxic effect on the target organ. They are administered either percutaneously or intravascularly. Alcohol can be opacified with metrizamide powder or iodinated oil **(Fig. 53)**. Since many of these agents are cytotoxic, reflux to adjacent tissue must be minimized with use of slow injections, very selective peripheral infusion, proximal balloon occlusion, or by wedging the catheter.

Catheter Delivery Systems

Introduction Sheaths

Catheter-introducing sheaths, by reducing trauma to the entry vessel and decreasing frictional forces for selective catheter maneuvers, should be used for any complex vascular interventions. The sheath diaphragm should remain leak-proof even in the presence of micro guide wires and repeated catheter exchanges. Tuohy-Borst adapters, an integral part of coaxial catheterization systems, are used for irrigation to prevent blood reflux around microcatheters and guide wires as well as to opacify the vascular territory to be embolized **(Fig. 54)**.

Diagnostic Catheters

Standard 5- to 6-F diagnostic catheters with hockey stick, cobra, and sidewinder tip configurations are commonly used for embolization of second and third order arterial branches **(Fig. 55)**. The recent introduction of slippery hydromer coatings for these catheters as well as for Nitinol guide wires has greatly improved the ease with which complex subselective catheterization can be performed without resorting to the more expensive microcatheter kits.

Superselective Catheters and Guide Wires

With the introduction of 2- to 3-F microcatheters and platinum-tipped micro guide wires **(Figs. 56, 57)** with diameters from 0.010–0.018 inch and graduated flexibility, it is now possible to reach and embolize almost any branch vessel down to as small as 1–2 mm in diameter with relative ease and safety. Superselective catheters are introduced through standard selective guiding catheters **(Fig. 58)** and advanced to follow the coaxial torqueable curved-tipped micro guide wire to the target vessels for embolization. Injectable guide wires (eg, the 0.038-inch Cragg wire, [Medi-Tech, Boston Scientific Corporation, Watertown, MA]) although not quite as flexible, may allow injection of larger embolic particles than some superselective catheters.

Immediate Complications of Embolization Procedures

Catheter-Related Complications

Since embolization requires that the catheter tip be as close as possible to the bleeding point or tumor, the operator must be experienced in performing selective and superselective catheterization. Vascular complications, which include dissection, perforation, and severe spasm with thrombosis, can be largely avoided with use of the coaxial catheter technique, micro guide wires, and frequent opacification of the vascular route to be taken **(Fig. 59)**. Superselective catheters can be easily perforated during injections if excessive pressure is used or when they are kinked or partially occluded by clot or particulate emboli. Micro guide wire tips are easily distorted, kinked, or even broken if they are advanced too forcefully.

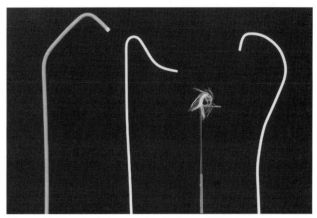
Figure 55. Standard shapes of selective catheters.

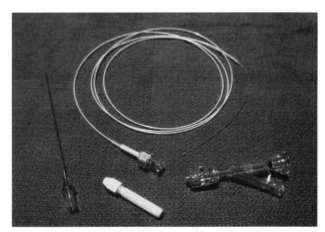
Figure 56. Superselective catheter set (Target Therapeutics, Fremont, CA).

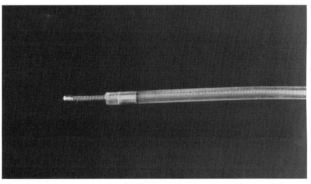
Figure 57. Superselective 0.016-inch guide wire within a platinum-tipped 3-F microcatheter (Target).

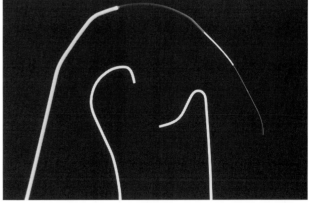
Figure 58. Typical guiding catheters for superselective catheterization.

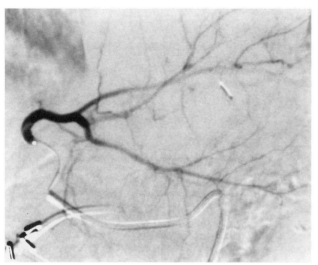

Figure 59. Superselective catheterization of the left hepatic artery using a coaxial system.

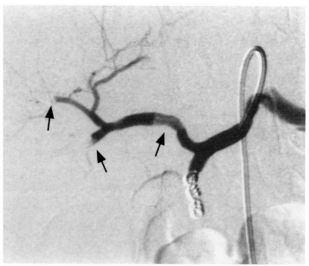

Figure 60. Duodenal bleeder treated with coil and Gelfoam embolization. There is accidental Gelfoam reflux into the hepatic artery (arrows).

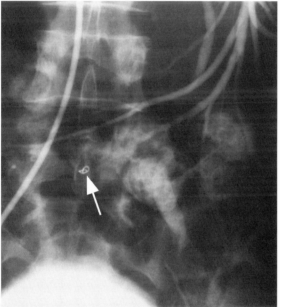

Figure 61. Accidental coil embolization of a superior mesenteric artery branch (arrow) with no complications.

Complications Related to Particulate Embolization
Complications of particulate embolization are related to premature release or reflux of embolic particles to non-target vessels **(Fig. 60)**. This can result in excessive tissue damage and dysfunction or injury to nerve tissue, with sensory or motor loss.

Complications Related to Coil Embolization
Improper sizing of the coil to the vessel diameter can lead to proximal or distal coil migration **(Fig. 61)**. The use of too long or too wide a coil can lead to retrograde displacement of the introducing catheter, with resulting protrusion of the proximal end of the coil into the main vascular trunk. Since these misplaced coils are unstable or become a source of emboli, they should be extracted with a snare. Misjudgment of vessel diameter when there is spasm (eg, spermatic vein) can lead to the use of undersized coils which may subsequently migrate. Coil-induced vascular thrombosis is occasionally subject to recanalization.

Sclerosant-Related Complications
Since sclerosants denature proteins and can reach down to the capillary level, tissue infarction and necrosis due to accidental reflux into non-target vessels can be devastating when such organs as bowel, gallbladder, adrenal glands, spinal cord, and major nerve trunks are affected.

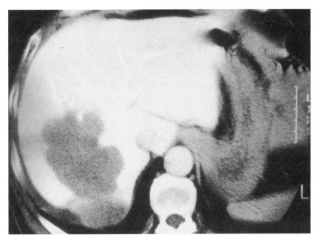

Figure 62. Colon metastases to the liver.

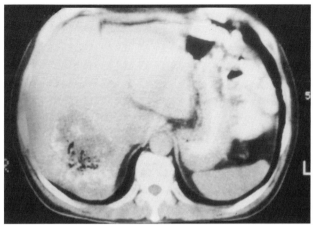

Figure 63. After chemoembolization, there is asymptomatic gas formation within the tumor.

Delayed Complications of Embolization

Postembolization Syndrome

Postembolization syndrome follows embolization of the liver, kidney, spleen, and, in more severe form, after hepatic chemoembolization. It includes pain, fever, nausea and vomiting, and adynamic ileus, and can last 3–5 days. Gas formation can occur in the ischemic area and usually resolves without treatment **(Figs. 62, 63)**. Dehydration and hyperkalemia may develop in severe cases. A true abscess manifested by high spiking fever and chills and septicemia is uncommon except in splenic embolization. It is managed by antibiotics, drainage, and, if necessary, splenectomy. Chemoembolization of the liver can lead to a more severe degree of postembolization syndrome and greater toxicity to the gallbladder, stomach, and duodenum when these are unintentionally embolized.

Nephrotoxicity

Because some embolization procedures are preceded by long, detailed diagnostic arteriographic studies to localize the bleeding point and/or by complex catheterization procedures, some patients with pre-existing renal risk factors may develop some degree of renal failure even if they are well-hydrated, due to the large volume of contrast material which may have to be administered to successfully complete the procedure. Patients undergoing hepatic chemoembolization may be in a higher risk category because of the potential nephrotoxicity of cisplatin and the products of necrotic tissue breakdown.

For further information on this topic, please see Teaching File Cases 16, 49, 52, 53, 56, 63, 66, and 69.

Selected Readings

deSouza NM, Reidy JF, Koffman CG. Arteriovenous fistulas complicating biopsy of renal allografts: treatment of bleeding with superselective embolization. AJR 1991; 156:507–510.

Dion JE. Principles and methodology. In: Vinuela F, ed. Interventional neuroradiology: endovascular therapy of the central nervous system. New York: Raven Press, 1992.

Encarnacion CE, Kadir S, Beam CA, Payne CS. Gastrointestinal bleeding: treatment with gastrointestinal arterial embolization. Radiology 1992; 183:505–508.

Palmaz JC, Walter JF, Cho KJ. Therapeutic embolization of small-bowel arteries. Radiology 1984; 152:377–382.

Pentecost MJ, Teitelbaum GP, eds. Embolotherapy. Semin Intervent Radiol 1992; 9:1–71.

Pollak JS, Egglin TK, Rosenblatt MM, Dickey KW, White RI. Clinical results of transvenous systemic embolotherapy with a neuroradiologic detachable balloon. Radiology 1994; 191:477–482

Quinn SF, Frau DM, Saff GN, et al. Neurologic complications of pelvic intraarterial chemoembolization performed with collagen material and cisplatin. Radiology 1988; 167:55–57.

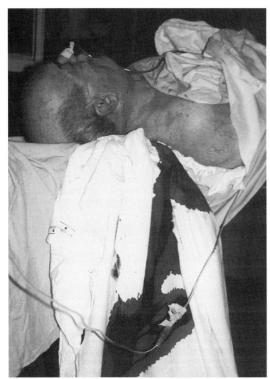

Figure 1. A patient comes to the emergency department vomiting blood. Immediate clinical evaluation and hemodynamic stabilization follow.

TUTORIAL 14
UPPER GASTROINTESTINAL BLEEDING—DIAGNOSTIC EVALUATION AND MANAGEMENT
Anthony C. Venbrux, M.D.

Introduction
This tutorial is a review of percutaneous transcatheter management of patients with upper gastrointestinal hemorrhage. The subjects addressed include:
1. Indications
2. Methods of treatment
3. Embolic materials
4. Complications
5. Contraindications
6. Specific technical points.

Patient Preparation
Gastrointestinal bleeding is a potentially life-threatening condition necessitating immediate medical attention. A distressed patient may come to the emergency department complaining of having vomited blood **(Fig. 1)** or "coffee ground material," or of having passed a "black" or "tarry" stool.

The goals of the physician are to evaluate, stabilize, and treat the patient with gastrointestinal bleeding. Evaluation includes a careful physical examination and a history not only of the acute episode but of any underlying medical condition (ie, a history of liver disease, excessive alcohol intake, recent ingestion of medications such as aspirin, etc). As part of the diagnostic work-up, laboratory data should include the patient's hemoglobin, hematocrit, platelet count, and coagulation profile.

Additional blood should be drawn and sent for typing and cross-matching, as well as an analysis of the patient's electrolytes and renal and liver functions. If the patient is hemodynamically unstable, intravenous fluids and blood products should be given immediately. Once they are stable, patients are generally admitted to the intensive care unit for hemodynamic monitoring and further work-up. If a patient cannot be stabilized, emergency surgical or interventional therapy is required. The location and severity of gastrointestinal bleeding determine therapy.

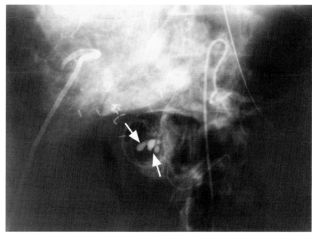

Figure 2. The late image from a celiac arteriogram demonstrates extravasation (arrows) in this patient with actively bleeding duodenal ulcers.

The need for upper gastrointestinal endoscopy is generally based on the patient's history. Upper gastrointestinal endoscopy may demonstrate esophageal ulceration with bleeding, a Mallory-Weiss tear (a laceration at the gastroesophageal junction), esophageal varices, gastric ulcers, gastritis, or duodenal ulcers.

If the patient is not a surgical candidate because of underlying medical conditions such as severe chronic obstructive pulmonary disease or severe cardiac disease, the radiologist is frequently asked to perform arteriography and transcatheter embolotherapy. The precise site of bleeding can be determined by arteriography. A site of contrast material extravasation on the delayed images obtained during arteriography (Fig. 2) determines the next course of action.

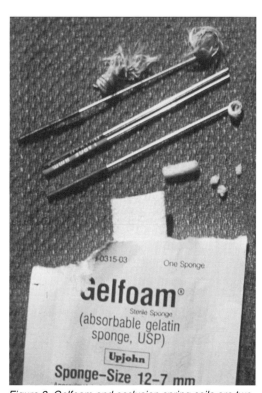

Figure 3. Gelfoam and occlusion spring coils are two embolic agents frequently used to stop bleeding in a patient with an upper gastrointestinal hemorrhage.

Superselective catheters/guide wires facilitate precise deployment of embolic agents such as Gelfoam (Upjohn, Kalamazoo, MI) and/or occlusion spring coils (Cook, Bloomington, IN) (Fig. 3) to stop bleeding in the upper gastrointestinal tract. The rich collateral circulation in the upper gastrointestinal tract renders embolization a safe therapeutic option. However, in those patients whose collaterals have been disrupted by gastric surgery, embolization must be approached with caution because organ infarction is a major potential complication. An upper gastrointestinal bleeding site is generally not treated with a vasoconstrictor such as vasopressin. This may prove risky in patients with coronary artery disease, hypertension, or other medical conditions. Transcatheter embolotherapy is generally definitive, with a relatively low incidence of rebleeding.

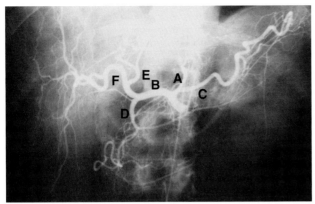

Figure 4. Normal anatomy of the celiac artery. A=left gastric artery; B=common hepatic artery; C=splenic artery; D=gastroduodenal artery; E=left hepatic artery; F=right hepatic artery.

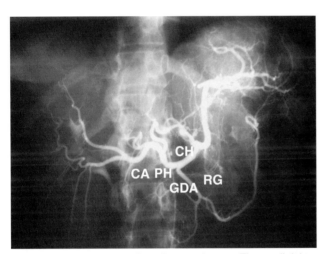

Figure 6. RAO projection of a celiac arteriogram. The small right gastric artery (RG) courses along the lesser curvature of the stomach. The common hepatic (CH), proper hepatic (PH), and gastroduodenal arteries (GDA) are identified. In this particular patient, the cystic artery (CA) arises from the left hepatic artery (ie, a variation in anatomy).

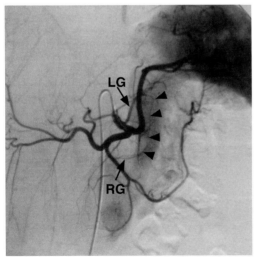

Figure 7. Celiac arteriogram shows the anastomoses (arrowheads) of the right (RG) and left gastric (LG) arteries along the lesser curvature of the stomach.

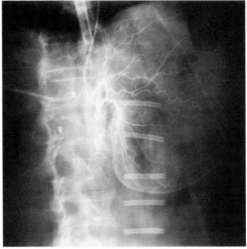

Figure 5. Right anterior oblique (RAO) projection of a left gastric arteriogram obtained in a postoperative patient with an upper gastrointestinal bleed using an axillary artery approach. The stomach is distended with blood. Bleeding was demonstrated during gastroduodenal arteriography. The left gastric artery supplies the region of the gastroesophageal junction, the gastric fundus, and a portion of the body of the stomach.

Vascular Anatomy of the Upper Gastrointestinal Tract

Fluoroscopically, the celiac axis arises from the ventral surface of the aorta at the level between the lower half of the T12 vertebral body and the level of the T12–L1 disc space.

The celiac axis "classically" has three major branches **(Fig. 4)**:
1. the left gastric artery (4A)
2. the common hepatic artery (4B)
3. the splenic artery (4C).

There are several common important variants in arterial anatomy. Knowledge of these is essential so that serious complications can be avoided during embolization procedures. Normal and variant visceral arterial anatomy are reviewed in Tutorial 9 entitled "Normal and Variant Visceral Arterial Anatomy."

Gastric Blood Supply—Left and Right Gastric Arteries

The gastroesophageal junction is supplied primarily by small vessels arising from the left gastric artery. The fundus and a portion of the body of the stomach are also supplied by the left gastric arterial branches **(Fig. 5)**. Terminal branches of the left gastric artery anastomose with the right gastric artery, forming an arcade along the lesser curvature of the stomach **(Figs. 6, 7)**. The right gastric artery generally arises at the bifurcation of the proper hepatic artery and the gastroduodenal artery. Variant anatomy may also be found at this location, and the right gastric artery may arise from the common hepatic artery, etc. The right gastric artery may be very small and overlooked during routine celiac arteriography.

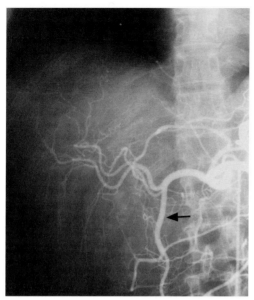

Figure 8. The gastroduodenal artery (arrow) supplies a portion of the stomach, the duodenum, and the pancreas.

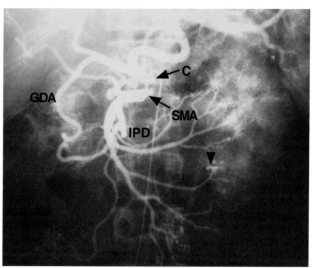

Figure 9. Superior mesenteric arteriogram in a woman with a celiac origin stenosis and polyarteritis nodosa. Microaneurysms (arrowhead) are seen in jejunal and ileal branches of the SMA. The inferior pancreaticoduodenal artery (IPD) arises from the proximal SMA and fills the celiac artery (C) through the pancreaticoduodenal branches of the gastroduodenal artery (GDA).

A rich anastomotic arcade exists between the right and left gastric arteries along the lesser curvature of the stomach. This provides an important collateral pathway in the event of occlusion of the left gastric artery, common hepatic artery, etc. This in part also explains why transcatheter embolotherapy in patients with upper gastrointestinal tract bleeding is possible: the rich anastomotic arcade reduces the risk of organ ischemia or infarction.

Gastric Blood Supply—Gastroduodenal Artery
The gastroduodenal artery **(Fig. 8)** supplies a portion of the stomach, the duodenum, and the pancreas. A rich anastomotic arcade is found between the pancreaticoduodenal blood supply arising from the gastroduodenal artery and the superior mesenteric artery via the inferior pancreaticoduodenal artery. The inferior pancreaticoduodenal artery arises from the proximal superior mesenteric artery (SMA) **(Fig. 9)** and forms an anastomosis with the pancreaticoduodenal arteries arising from the gastroduodenal artery. The terminal branch of the gastroduodenal artery is the right gastroepiploic artery **(Fig. 10)**.

Similar to the right gastric/left gastric arterial arcade, the right gastroepiploic artery has a rich anastomotic network (arcade) with the left gastroepiploic artery along the greater curvature of the stomach. The left gastroepiploic artery is the terminal branch of the splenic artery.

In summary, there are important arcades along the lesser curvature (ie, right gastric/left gastric arteries) and greater curvature (ie, right gastroepiploic/left gastroepiploic arteries) of the stomach and there is the anastomotic arcade between the celiac axis and the superior mesenteric artery (ie, via the pancreaticoduodenal branches).

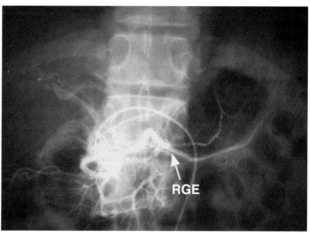

Figure 10. Selective catheterization of the gastroduodenal artery. The terminal branch of the GDA is the right gastroepiploic artery (RGE). The RGE courses along the greater curvature of the stomach and forms an anastomotic arcade with the left gastroepiploic artery, the latter being a terminal branch of the splenic artery (not shown).

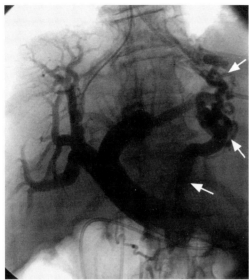

Figure 11. Transjugular portal venogram performed during a TIPS procedure. Note hepatofugal filling of the coronary vein and varices (arrows).

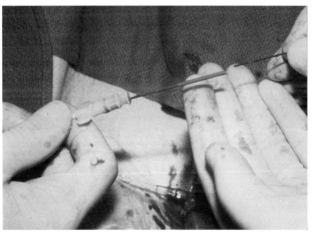

Figure 12. A Gianturco spring coil (Cook) is advanced through the catheter using a guide wire.

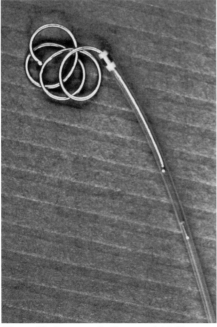

Figure 13. A superselective coaxial 3-F microcatheter. Microcoils can be advanced through the catheter lumen.

Esophageal Variceal Hemorrhage

Hemorrhage from esophageal varices results from advanced liver disease and accounts for approximately 15,000 annual hospital admissions in the United States. Treatment of esophageal variceal hemorrhage consists of endoscopic sclerotherapy/banding, aggressive medical therapy including use of balloon tamponade catheters, surgical decompression via portosystemic shunts (eg, portacaval, mesocaval, and distal splenorenal [Warren] shunts), and transjugular intrahepatic portosystemic shunting (TIPS) **(Fig. 11)**. Intravenous systemic vasopressin may be valuable in controlling esophageal variceal bleeding. Somatostatin and somatostatin-like analogues in combination with other modes of medical therapy have also been shown to be effective.

Please refer to the SCVIR syllabus Volume 2: "Portal Hypertension: Options for Diagnosis and Treatment" for an in-depth discussion of the management of variceal hemorrhage.

Indications for Transcatheter Embolotherapy in the Gastrointestinal Tract

In general, transcatheter embolotherapy **(Fig. 12)** is indicated in a patient who is not a surgical candidate, in a patient who may be a surgical candidate but requires stabilization prior to surgery, or as a definitive means of therapy. Transcatheter arterial embolotherapy may be used in patients with upper gastrointestinal bleeding from ulcer disease, gastritis, trauma, or a Mallory-Weiss tear.

Present clinical and past surgical and medical histories are important. To re-emphasize, if a patient has had a prior Billroth surgical procedure for ulcer disease, the normal arterial arcades (collateral blood supply) of the upper gastrointestinal tract may be disrupted. Collateral vessels are frequently ligated during surgery. Transcatheter embolotherapy in such patients must be performed as superselectively as possible and with great caution **(Fig. 13)** as there is a greater risk of gastrointestinal tract infarction. In the event of bowel infarction, surgical intervention will be necessary.

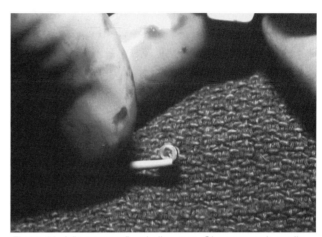

Figure 14. A "permanent" embolic agent, Gianturco spring coils, are advanced through a catheter using a guide wire (not shown).

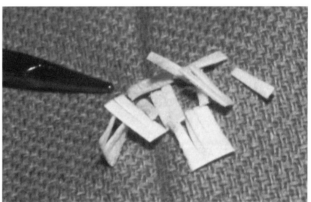

Figure 15. A "temporary" embolic agent, Gelfoam pledgets (also known as "torpedoes"—small strips of Gelfoam), may be injected through the catheter. Smaller particles or a "slurry" may be also be used (not shown).

Embolic Materials

Several types of embolic materials have been developed. These include:

1. Gianturco spring coils (Cook)—stainless steel coils with embedded synthetic fibers—permanent **(Fig. 14)**;

2. Gelfoam—protein foam which is cut into small cubes or "torpedoes" or made into a "slurry"—temporary; 2–4 weeks **(Fig. 15)**;

3. Clot—temporary, usually lasting only hours;

4. Ivalon (Unipoint, High Point, NC) (particulate polyvinyl alcohol) **(Fig. 16)**—permanent;

5. Polymerizing tissue "glues" (eg, N-butyl cyanoacrylate). This is not presently approved by the Food and Drug Administration for use but reports in the literature document its effectiveness.

6. Detachable balloons—permanent. Detachable balloons require placement of a guiding catheter. The balloons may be "floated" to the site of bleeding and used to "bridge" the bleeding site. Currently, there are no commercially available detachable balloons in the United States. Detachable silicone balloons were commercially available as recently as 3 years ago but production has ceased. Safety and efficacy trials evaluating other detachable balloons are currently underway.

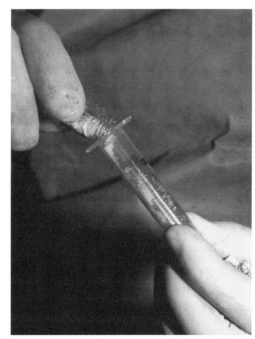

Figure 16. A "permanent" embolic agent, polyvinyl alcohol particles (Ivalon). Graded particle sizes are commercially available. These can be poured into a syringe and emulsified with contrast material or saline.

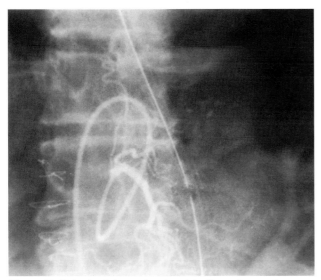

Figure 17. Selective left gastric artery injection using a cobra catheter and Waltman's loop technique. The patient has a Mallory-Weiss tear and distal esophageal ulceration. Intraarterial vasopressin was infused for control of bleeding.

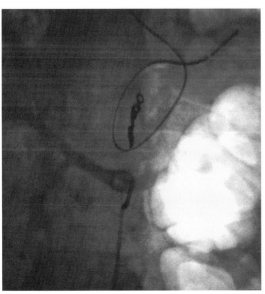

Figure 18. Celiac axis arteriogram after successful coil embolization of the left gastric artery in a patient with a Mallory-Weiss tear.

Transcatheter Embolotherapy in the Upper Gastrointestinal Tract—Technique

The goal of embolotherapy is to use large particles to occlude vessels at bleeding sites. A curved catheter is introduced into the celiac artery through a femoral approach. The catheter is directed into a specific vessel (eg, the gastroduodenal artery). With the catheter tip precisely placed in the vessel to be embolized, occlusion of the vessel in the upper gastrointestinal tract is generally accomplished with use of Gianturco coils or Gelfoam. Gianturco coils are permanent embolic agents; Gelfoam is temporary. Gelfoam is occlusive for several weeks, and vessels embolized with Gelfoam are subject to recanalization. In some cases, however, Gelfoam may cause local inflammatory changes sufficient to result in permanent vessel occlusion. Particulate ("solid") polyvinyl alcohol (ie, Ivalon), is another permanent embolic material which may be used, although extreme caution should be exercised. Gelfoam powder or extremely small (ie, "dust-like") Ivalon should not be used because of the risk of tissue-level infarction. Because of the risk of tissue necrosis, alcohol should *not* be used to embolize vessels in the gastrointestinal tract.

Occasionally a pharmacologic vasoconstrictor such as vasopressin **(Fig. 17)** may be infused directly through the arterial catheter. This method may be useful in patients who have had collaterals disrupted by previous gastrointestinal surgery.

Patients with the following bleeding sites may be treated with transcatheter embolotherapy of the indicated vascular distribution.
1. Bleeding peptic ulcer—embolization of the gastroduodenal artery
2. Gastritis—embolization of the left gastric artery, or direct intraarterial infusion of vasopressin into the left gastric artery
3. Trauma—embolization of the vessel at the site of injury
4. Mallory-Weiss tear—embolization of the left gastric artery **(Fig. 18)**.

Esophageal and gastric varices are not treated with transcatheter embolotherapy techniques. Frank bleeding from varices during arteriography is virtually never visible unless massive bleeding is present. Endoscopic sclerotherapy or banding is used for initial control of esophageal variceal hemorrhage. Endoscopic therapy is not used in cases of gastric or intestinal varices.

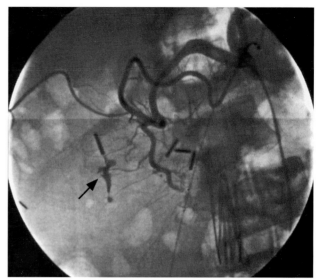

Figure 19. Gastroduodenal arteriogram in a patient with peptic ulcer disease. Extravasation of contrast material is identified in the duodenum (arrow).

Perhaps the easiest and most rapid transcatheter technique for occluding blood flow is the use of Gelfoam or Gianturco coils. It is important to "bridge" a bleeding site so that collateral flow does not cause rebleeding. For example, if the patient has peptic ulcer disease and a bleeding duodenal ulcer **(Fig. 19)** and the gastroduodenal artery is embolized proximally, the bleeding may stop for a period of time only to recur several hours later. This may be due to reconstitution of flow through the gastroduodenal artery via the left and right gastroepiploic arteries along the greater curvature of the stomach.

In this example, blood flows through the splenic artery, through the left gastroepiploic artery, retrograde through the right gastroepiploic artery, and then into the gastroduodenal artery.

Another pathway for reconstitution of gastroduodenal artery blood flow is via the inferior pancreaticoduodenal artery blood (from the superior mesenteric artery) with flow through the pancreaticoduodenal arteries to the gastroduodenal artery and to the site of hemorrhage. Several other collateral pathways may also contribute. It is therefore important to begin embolization distal to the bleeding site (if technically possible), and to occlude across the bleeding site. This reduces the chance of collateral blood flow to the bleeding site causing recurrent hemorrhage **(Fig. 19)**.

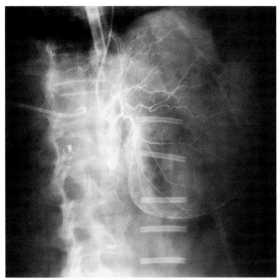

Figure 20. RAO projection of a left gastric arteriogram.

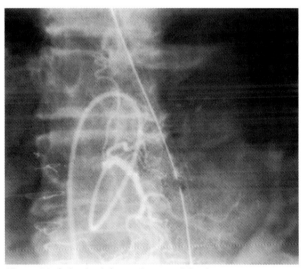

Figure 21. Selective left gastric artery injection.

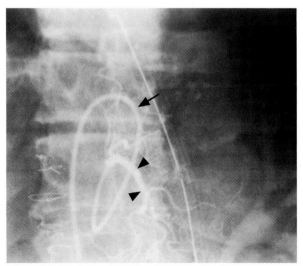

Figure 22. A cobra catheter has been used to form a "Waltman's loop." Note the loop in the abdominal aorta (arrow). The left gastric artery has been selectively catheterized (arrowheads).

Technical Hints—Left Gastric Artery

Selective catheterization of the left gastric artery **(Figs. 20, 21)** may be the most technically challenging procedure for the interventional radiologist. Because the left gastric artery typically arises from the proximal celiac artery and points cephalad, engaging the orifice with a catheter may be difficult. In general, three techniques are used.

1. A Simmons-type catheter may be pulled caudally and partially deformed. If the anatomy is favorable, the orifice of the left gastric artery may be selectively catheterized.

2. A Rösch left gastric catheter (Cook) may be used. Like the Simmons-type catheter, it must be formed into its hook-shaped configuration. The tip engages the celiac access. The "upturned tip" is then used to engage the orifice of the left gastric artery as the catheter is pulled down slightly.

3. The cobra catheter is formed into a "Waltman's loop" **(Fig. 22)**. For this, a cobra catheter is advanced over a floppy-tipped guide wire into the celiac access. The tip is directed toward the splenic or common hepatic artery. By withdrawing the guide wire and continuing to advance the shaft of the cobra catheter, a loop is formed in the aorta with the tip still in the celiac vascular distribution. By advancing and withdrawing the cobra catheter, the loop in the aorta tightens or enlarges, dragging the cephalad-pointing tip into the left gastric artery orifice. Again, if the anatomy is favorable, this may allow secure catheterization of the left gastric artery for transcatheter embolotherapy or infusion of vasoconstricting drugs.

Technical Hints—Right Gastric Artery

The right gastric artery may also be difficult to catheterize selectively. The right gastric artery is frequently small and its anatomic origin is variable. A cobra catheter may be used to engage the common hepatic artery and the origin of the right gastric artery; however, a coaxial microcatheter system may be required to selectively catheterize this vessel beyond its origin.

Technical Hints—Gastroduodenal Artery

Most often, a cobra catheter is of the appropriate configuration to selectively catheterize the gastroduodenal artery. The catheter is advanced over a floppy-tipped guide wire into the common hepatic artery. Its downward-pointing tip usually engages the gastroduodenal artery quite readily. When the artery is small or distal catheterization is desired, a coaxial microcatheter system may be used.

Diagnostic Angiography in Cases of Occult Bleeding

If the cause of upper gastrointestinal bleeding is obscure, arteriography may identify a structural abnormality and should be performed as part of the comprehensive evaluation when other diagnostic tests (eg, endoscopy) are negative. For example, intermittently bleeding intraluminal, mural, or mesenteric masses, or arteriovenous malformations may be missed on endoscopy yet readily identified with arteriography. In general, nuclear medicine studies (eg, tagged red blood cells or technetium-99 sulfur colloid studies) may not be useful in patients with suspected upper gastrointestinal hemorrhage.

Complications of Embolotherapy

Complications of transcatheter embolotherapy in the upper gastrointestinal tract are infrequent but may include gastrointestinal infarction or ischemia. The risk of tissue necrosis is increased in patients who have had prior upper gastrointestinal tract surgeries (eg, Billroth or Siguira procedures). The risk/benefit ratio must be considered, and dialogue with referring physicians is essential for the selection of appropriate therapy and management of potential complications. Non-target organ embolization and infarction is the major complication of transcatheter embolotherapy in the upper gastrointestinal tract.

Complications of Vasopressin Infusion

Complications of intraarterial vasopressin infusions include:
1. Cardiovascular complications (arrhythmias, myocardial infarction, hypertension)
2. Metabolic complications (cerebral edema, electrolyte disturbances)
3. Catheter-related complications (sepsis from chronic indwelling catheters, puncture site hematoma, femoral arteriovenous fistulas, etc) **(Fig. 23)**
4. Bowel infarction and ischemia
5. Peripheral vascular complications due to the systemic vasoconstrictive effects of vasopressin (eg, digit ischemia).

Contraindications to Transcatheter Therapy in the Upper Gastrointestinal Tract

Contraindications are relative. The risk of allergy to the contrast material must be considered in any patient with a more generalized allergic history (eg, hives). In a patient with a strong allergic history to contrast material (ie, anaphylaxis) and life-threatening upper gastrointestinal hemorrhage, the arteriographic studies can be performed with an anesthesiologist or anesthetist present.

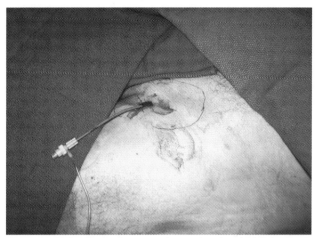

Figure 23. Indwelling catheters and vascular sheaths left in place during lengthy vasopressin therapy may lead to complications such as hematomas, sepsis, pseudoaneurysm formation, vessel thrombosis, or distal embolization.

In patients with coagulopathies, attempts must be made to correct clotting parameters prior to or during arteriography. This intervention alone may aid in controlling upper gastrointestinal hemorrhage. However, even if the coagulopathy cannot be controlled, arteriography should still be performed. An arterial vascular sheath used during the procedure may be left in place afterwards to reduce the risk of hematoma and provide arterial access for blood pressure transduction by the intensive care unit staff. Once the patient has been stabilized with transcatheter embolotherapy, the coagulopathy can then be aggressively treated with medical therapy (eg, vitamin K) and blood products.

Pitfalls and Hints

During an episode of gastrointestinal bleeding, contrast material may occasionally "track" down the mucosa in between the folds, creating a "pseudo-vein sign." If a linear or gently curved "abnormal vessel" is noted during arteriography that has the appearance of a vein (or follows the course of mucosal folds), be suspicious for a site of bleeding. Extravasated contrast material may track along the dependent region of a hollow viscus.

It is useful to place an arteriographic sheath in the common femoral artery. The sheath can be flushed with heparinized saline and kept in place while the patient is in the intensive care unit. The sheath permits the removal of catheters that have become clogged with embolic material, without sacrificing arterial access. In the event of recurrent bleeding, percutaneous access is already present.

During a typical 1–3-day vasopressin infusion, it is useful to cover the percutaneous puncture site with a sterile, adhesive, clear dressing. The clear dressing allows the nurses and physicians to evaluate the region for possible groin hematoma while preserving the sterility of the catheter and puncture site.

Conclusion

The nonsurgical approach to the treatment of patients with upper gastrointestinal bleeding requires knowledge of basic angiographic techniques. Monitoring of patients in an intensive care unit is mandatory. Transcatheter embolotherapy or infusion of vasopressin may be life-saving in patients who are not surgical candidates, or may be a definitive means of therapy. A multidisciplinary team effort is essential in managing such patients. The radiologist is an essential part of this team.

For further information on this topic, please see Teaching File Cases 31–34, 56, and 57.

Selected Readings

Athanasoulis CA. Interventional radiology. Philadelphia: W.B. Saunders Company, 1982; 55–156.

Dempsey DT, Burke DR, Reilly RS, McLean GK, Rosato EF. Angiography in poor-risk patients with massive nonvariceal upper gastrointestinal bleeding. Am J Surg 1990; 159:282–6.

LaBerge JM, Ring EJ, Gordon RL, et al. Creation of transjugular intrahepatic portosystemic shunt (TIPS) with the Wallstent endoprosthesis: results in 100 patients. Radiology 1993; 187:413–420.

Lang EV, Picus D, Marx MV, Hicks ME, Friedland GW. Massive upper gastrointestinal hemorrhage with normal findings on arteriography: value of prophylactic embolization of the left gastric artery. AJR 1992; 158:547–549.

Mauro MA, Jaques P. Transcatheter management of pseudoaneurysms complicating pancreatitis. J Vasc Interv Radiol 1991; 2:527–532.

Reuter SR, Redman HC, Cho KJ. Gastrointestinal angiography. 3rd edition. Philadelphia: W.B. Saunders Company, 1986; 282–338.

Reilly HF, al-Kawas FH. Dieulafoy's lesion. Diagnosis and management. Dig Dis Sci 1991; 36:1702–1707.

Rollins ES, Picus D, Hicks ME, Darcy MD, Bower BL, Kleinhoffer MA. Angiography is useful in detecting the source of chronic gastrointestinal bleeding of obscure origin. AJR 1991; 156:385–388.

Rosen RJ, Sanchez G. Angiographic diagnosis and management of gastrointestinal hemorrhage: current concepts. Radiol Clin North Am 1994; 32:951–67.

Sebrechts C, Bookstein JJ. Embolization in the management of lower gastrointestinal hemorrhage. Semin Intervent Radiol 1988; 5:39–48.

Toyoda H, Nakano S, Takeda I, et al. Transcatheter arterial embolization for massive bleeding from duodenal ulcers not controlled by endoscopic hemostasis. Endoscopy 1995; 27:304–307.

End Notes

The authors wish to acknowledge the assistance and expertise of Debbie Offenbacker and Kay Marseglia in the preparation of this manuscript.

Figure 3 courtesy of Sally E. Mitchell, M.D.

Figure 9 courtesy of Ms. Peg Cooper, C.V.R.T.

Figure 19 courtesy of Gunnar B. Lund, M.D.

Appendix 1
Gastrointestinal Bleeding: Protocol for Vasopressin Infusion

A variety of protocols exist for superior mesenteric arterial infusion. In general, most regimens are based upon dose titration to a level at which bleeding is arrested yet ischemic complications are avoided. Most physicians advocate a slow tapering of the infusion once the desired effect has been achieved. A sample protocol for vasopressin infusion is as follows:

1. Selective arteriogram shows extravasation.
2. Mixture of vasopressin solution is prepared: 100 U/vasopressin is mixed with 500 mL of normal saline or 5% dextrose, giving a concentration of 0.2 U/mL. Alternatively, 200 U/vasopressin may be mixed in 500 mL of solution for a concentration of 0.4 U/mL.
3. Infusion is delivered with a constant arterial infusion pump at the rate of 30–60 mL/hr, depending on the dose rate to be delivered.
4. Infusion of vasopressin is initiated at 0.2 U/min for 20 minutes.
5. After 20 minutes of infusion, a repeat arteriogram is performed. The films are assessed for the presence of extravasation and for evidence of excessive constriction of mesenteric arterial branches. If constriction is excessive, the dose rate is reduced by half and the arteriogram is repeated 20 minutes later. If there is no extravasation, the catheter is secured in the groin, and the patient is transferred to the ICU for continued infusion. If extravasation is still present after 20 minutes of infusion, the infusion dose rate is doubled to 0.4 U/min, and a repeat arteriogram is performed 20 minutes later.
6. If bleeding is not controlled after infusion of 0.4 U/min, a further increase in the dose rate will generally not be beneficial and may be dangerous, and alternative methods for controlling bleeding should be considered.
7. Once the initial infusion dose rate has been established and control of bleeding confirmed, a usual infusion regimen is as follows:

> Vasopressin at 0.2 U/min for 24 hours.
> Vasopressin at 0.1 U/min for 24 hours.

Infusion is discontinued if there is no clinical evidence of further bleeding. If the initial infusion dose rate is 0.4 U/min, the regimen is as follows:

> Vasopressin at 0.4 U/min for 6–8 hours.
> Vasopressin at 0.3 U/min for 16 hours.
> Vasopressin at 0.2 U/min for 16 hours.
> Vasopressin at 0.1 U/min for 16 hours.

Infusion is discontinued if there is no clinical evidence of further bleeding. After vasopressin has been tapered, saline should be infused for approximately 6–8 hours through the indwelling catheter. In this way, the catheter is already in place and vasopressin may be restarted if bleeding recurs. At this point an alternate therapy should be considered (eg surgery, superselective catheterization and embolization, or a repeat course of vasopressin therapy).

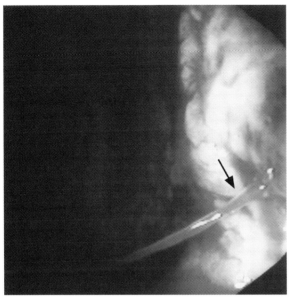

Figure 1. Colonoscopy with lower GI bleeding (arrow).

TUTORIAL 15
LOWER GASTROINTESTINAL BLEEDING—DIAGNOSTIC EVALUATION AND MANAGEMENT
Daniel Picus, M.D.

Introduction
The subjects addressed in this tutorial include:
1. Diagnosis of lower gastrointestinal bleeding
2. Etiologies of lower gastrointestinal bleeding
3. Transcatheter management of lower gastrointestinal bleeding.

Lower Gastrointestinal Bleeding— Presentation
Rectal bleeding is a sign of both upper and lower gastrointestinal (GI) bleeding. The treatment of these two entities differs considerably, however, and it is therefore very important to differentiate between them. Bright red blood per rectum usually indicates a lower GI source, but occasionally a brisk upper GI bleed can manifest itself in this fashion. Hematemesis almost always indicates an upper GI source. When the source of bleeding is unclear from the history, the patient should undergo upper endoscopy to rule out the common causes of upper GI bleeding such as ulcers, gastritis, or varices. If the upper endoscopy is negative, lower GI bleeding is confirmed. Endoscopy is often less useful in patients with lower GI bleeding because a colon filled with blood can make endoscopic visualization difficult. **Figure 1** shows a colonoscopic view of brisk colonic bleeding from diverticulosis.

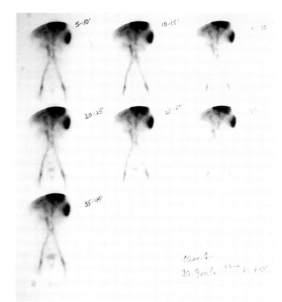

Figure 2. Radionuclide scan. Initial images fail to reveal a bleeding site.

Lower GI Bleeding—Stabilization

For patients with acute bleeding, the most important first step is resuscitation. Patients who are hemodynamically unstable must be transferred to an intensive care unit (ICU) and large-bore intravenous access obtained. A nasogastric tube is helpful both to differentiate upper from lower GI bleeding and to empty the stomach of blood in order to minimize the risk of aspiration. Although stabilization is a critical first step, it is important not to wait for the patient to stop bleeding before beginning the search for a source. Lower GI bleeding is often intermittent and once it stops, it can be very difficult to determine the cause until it starts again (frequently in the middle of the night). Modern angiographic facilities must be equipped to care for patients with acute bleeding. This includes appropriately trained nursing personnel and monitoring equipment such as noninvasive blood pressure monitors, electrocardiography, and pulse oximetry.

Diagnosis—Radionuclide Scanning

Radionuclide scanning with technetium-labeled red blood cells is widely used for the diagnosis of GI bleeding. Its primary advantage is that by scanning over extended periods of time it can detect intermittent bleeding. Arteriography, on the other hand, must be performed during active bleeding in order to yield a diagnosis. Unfortunately, radionuclide scanning is often unable to localize the bleeding to a specific anatomic region. Extravasated blood is frequently moved rapidly forward and backward from the bleeding site by bowel peristalsis. Additionally, scintigraphy lacks the precise anatomic detail provided by arteriography. **Figures 2** and **3** show a positive radionuclide scan demonstrating bleeding in the distal small bowel. Note that no bleeding is seen on the initial scans **(Fig. 2)**. Arteriography performed at that time would have been negative. The diagnosis was determined only by scanning for 2 hours.

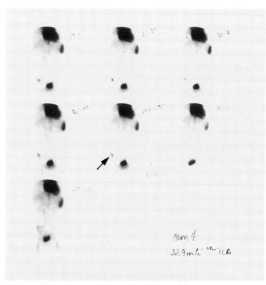

Figure 3. Radionuclide scan. Delayed images obtained at 2 hours show accumulation of the radioisotope in the right lower quadrant (arrow).

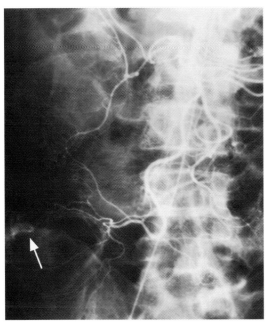

Figure 4. The early phase of a superior mesenteric arteriogram performed for lower GI bleeding shows extravasation (arrow).

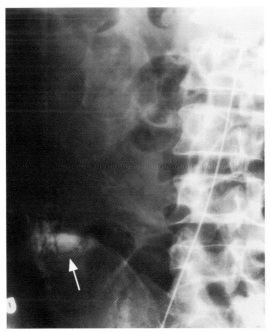

Figure 5. Same patient as in Figure 4. A later phase of the superior mesenteric artery injection shows persistent accumulation of contrast material (arrow) at the bleeding site.

Diagnosis—Arteriography

Arteriography for lower GI bleeding must be performed while the patient is actively hemorrhaging. A complete arteriographic examination requires injection of both the superior and inferior mesenteric arteries. If no bleeding is seen from either of these territories, the celiac artery should be evaluated for aberrant anatomy (eg, celiac artery giving rise to the middle colic artery), as well as to exclude bleeding from the upper GI tract. Active extravasation of contrast material into the bowel lumen defines the site of bleeding. The extravasation should persist throughout the entire injection and may change in size and shape on serial films as it flows into the bowel lumen **(Figs. 4, 5)**. Other associated findings may include the vascular tuft and prominent draining veins of angiodysplasia, hypervascularity associated with inflammation, or tumor vascularity seen with various malignant and benign conditions (see below).

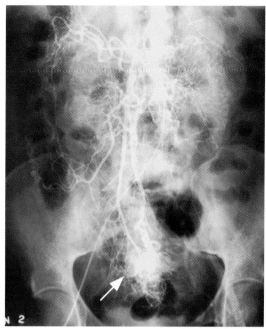

Figure 6. Early phase injection shows a small bowel leiomyoma with hypervascular blush (arrow).

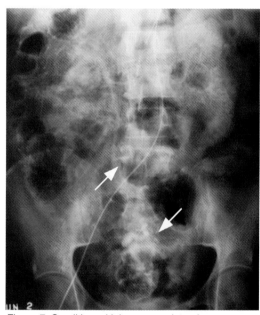

Figure 7. Small bowel leiomyoma—late phase. There are early draining veins (arrows).

Arteriography is also useful in determining the source of bleeding in patients with chronic GI bleeding. Both Sheedy et al and Rollins et al have shown that the etiology of chronic lower GI bleeding can be established by arteriography in greater than 30% of patients after other diagnostic measures have been exhausted. Most of the patients in these series were not actively bleeding at the time of arteriography and were diagnosed by structural abnormalities on the arteriogram. Examples of such abnormalities include angiodysplasia, small bowel tumors, and other inflammatory conditions. **Figures 6** and **7** show the typical hypervascular blush of an ileal leiomyoma with a large draining vein. This patient had an extensive negative work-up for chronic lower GI bleeding. Obviously, arteriography in the setting of chronic GI bleeding is an elective procedure but one that should not be overlooked.

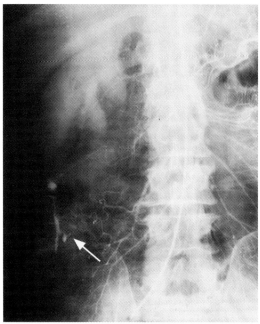

Figure 8. Provocative superior mesenteric arteriogram shows extravasation in the right lower quadrant (arrow).

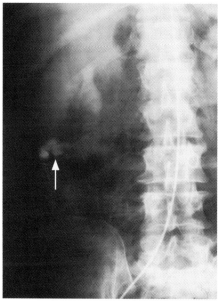

Figure 9. Same patient as in Figure 8. The late image demonstrates persistent accumulation of extravasated contrast material (arrow).

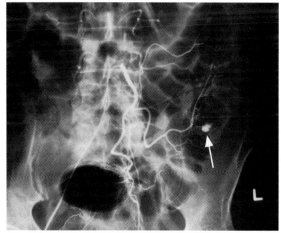

Figure 10. Inferior mesenteric arteriogram shows extravasation in the left lower quadrant (arrow).

Arteriography—Provocative Maneuvers

A variety of pharmacologic agents have been tried in an effort to increase the yield of arteriography in GI bleeding. Heparin may be useful to keep a patient bleeding between an initial diagnostic study (eg, radionuclide scan) and a definitive localization of the bleeding with arteriography. A more aggressive approach is to try to start a patient bleeding with thrombolytic therapy. This should be done only if the patient has had a complete work-up including upper and lower endoscopy. A formal diagnostic arteriogram should also be obtained to ascertain that catheterization of the vessel is possible, and to look for structural lesions. The thrombolytic agent is given in the nuclear medicine department with the patient under the gamma camera. Obviously, the arteriography and surgical teams should be standing by. **Figures 8** and **9** show active bleeding in the ascending colon.

Etiologies of Lower GI Bleeding

Diverticulosis

In elderly patients, diverticulosis is the most common cause of lower GI bleeding. While the majority of diverticular disease is located in the descending and sigmoid colons, bleeding diverticuli are more common in the ascending colon. The reason for this is unknown. Some authors postulate that it is related to the wider necks of right-sided colonic diverticuli, which expose more of the submucosal artery to injury. In 80%–90% of patients, the bleeding stops spontaneously, but it can recur in up to 25% of individuals. The classic arteriographic finding is extravasated contrast material filling the diverticulum **(Fig. 10)**. Intraarterial vasopressin is considered the treatment of choice for diverticular bleeding.

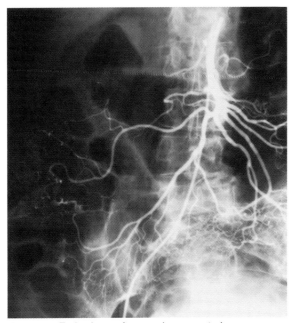

Figure 11. Early phase of a superior mesenteric arteriogram shows right colon angiodysplasia.

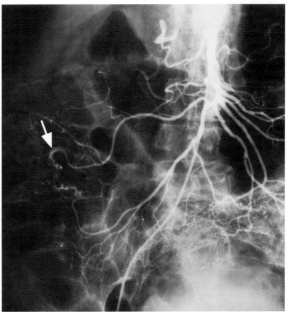

Figure 12. Right colon angiodysplasia—middle phase. An early draining vein is visualized (arrow).

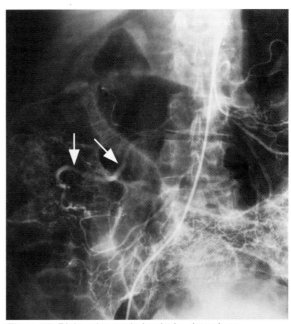

Figure 13. Right colon angiodysplasia—late phase. The early draining vein is well seen (arrows).

Angiodysplasia

Angiodysplasia is also a lesion seen in elderly patients and is probably an acquired rather than congenital lesion. The cause of angiodysplasia is unknown, but it may be due to repeated obstruction of the submucosal veins from increases in intraluminal bowel pressure. The lesion of angiodysplasia is most commonly found in the cecum or ascending colon, but it may occur in the descending colon, sigmoid colon, or small bowel. Twenty-five percent of patients have multiple lesions. Patients typically present with chronic intermittent lower GI bleeding. The classic arteriographic findings are a vascular tuft of small arteries associated with early opacification of a prominent draining vein **(Figs. 11–13)**. Actual extravasation of contrast material is rarely seen. Definitive therapy for angiodysplasia is surgical resection. However, stabilization with intraarterial vasopressin may be useful. Pathological confirmation is difficult because the lesion is only seen with meticulous specimen preparation.

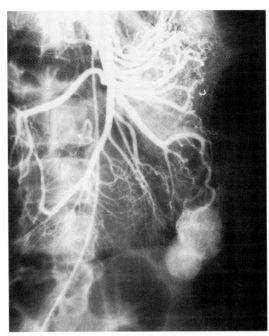

Figure 14. The early phase injection of a superior mesenteric arteriogram shows a jejunal leiomyoma with well-circumscribed hypervascular blush (arrow).

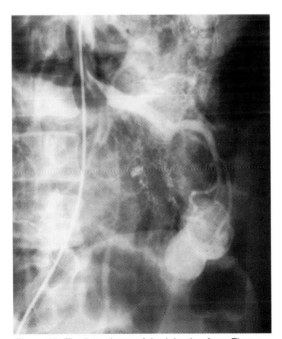

Figure 15. The late phase of the injection from Figure 14 shows persistent blush and an early draining vein.

Tumors

Tumors are an unusual cause of lower GI bleeding. By far, the most common bowel tumor is adenocarcinoma of the colon, which rarely causes clinically significant bleeding and is usually diagnosed easily with barium and endoscopic studies. Small bowel tumors are more difficult to identify and can lead to chronic lower GI bleeding. Leiomyoma and leiomyosarcoma of the small bowel have a classic angiographic appearance consisting of an extremely hypervascular, well-circumscribed mass **(Figs. 14, 15)**. Carcinoid tumors are more difficult to identify but can be diagnosed by the associated desmoplastic reaction which results in retraction and occlusion of multiple mesenteric arteries and veins. Lymphoma and metastases are very difficult to detect arteriographically unless a hypervascular mass is seen.

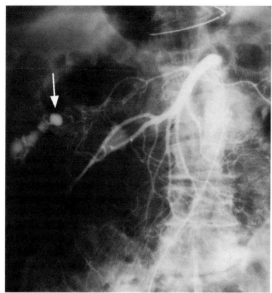

Figure 16. The early phase of a superior mesenteric artery (SMA) injection shows postpolypectomy bleeding with extravasation (arrow).

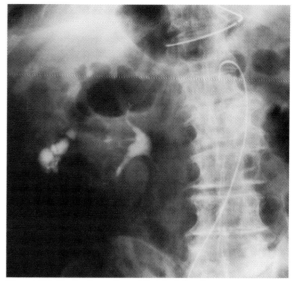

Figure 17. Postpolypectomy bleed—late phase.

Postpolypectomy Bleeding

Major bleeding following a colonic polypectomy is unusual, but can be seen in 0.5%–2% of patients. Hemorrhage may occur immediately, or may be delayed for up to 7–10 days. Most postpolypectomy hemorrhages are self-limited and require no intervention. Delayed hemorrhage can be treated with vasopressin therapy. Arteriographic findings are limited to active extravasation of contrast material into the bowel lumen **(Figs. 16, 17)**.

Other Causes of Lower GI Bleeding

Colonic varices are rarely associated with lower GI bleeding. Usually, this diagnosis is made in association with other findings of portal hypertension, including cirrhosis and varices in the esophagus and stomach. Mesenteric varices can be seen on the venous phase of both the superior mesenteric and inferior mesenteric artery injections. **Figure 18** shows massive duodenal and proximal jejunal varices in a patient with post-traumatic superior mesenteric vein (SMV) occlusion. Actual extravasation from the varices is almost impossible to document. Transjugular intrahepatic portosystemic shunting has been shown to be an effective method for treating lower GI bleeding from colonic varices. Other unusual causes for lower GI bleeding include postoperative anastomotic lesions, small bowel or colonic ulcers, visceral artery aneurysms, inflammatory bowel disease, Meckel's diverticulum, and aortoenteric fistulas.

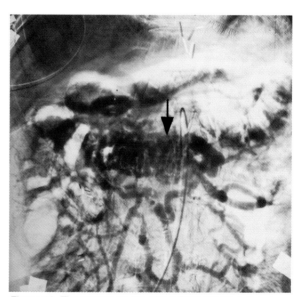

Figure 18. The venous phase of the SMA injection shows SMV occlusion and duodenal varices (arrows).

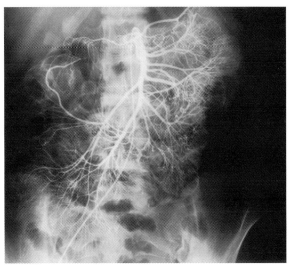

Figure 19. Normal SMA.

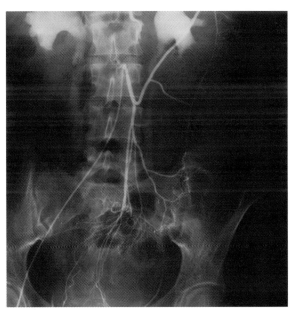

Figure 20. Normal inferior mesenteric artery.

Transcatheter Management of Lower GI Bleeding

Transcatheter techniques, including direct intraarterial infusion of vasoconstrictive agents (eg, vasopressin) and embolotherapy, are both useful in the management of lower GI bleeding. Both techniques require that the patient's hemostatic mechanism be intact to enable the formation of a stable clot over the area of bleeding without causing irreversible ischemic damage. Vasopressin is more widely used for lower GI bleeding (as opposed to embolotherapy) since the collateral arterial supply to the colon and small bowel is limited and the risk of infarction with embolotherapy is higher. Normal vascular anatomy is shown on **Figures 19** and **20**. Embolotherapy is more widely used in patients with upper GI bleeding where multiple arterial collaterals to the stomach and duodenum make infarction less of a risk.

Vasopressin

Vasopressin is a pressor compound secreted by the posterior pituitary gland. It also has significant antidiuretic properties. It causes arterial and capillary vasoconstriction, which results in a decrease in perfusion pressure at the site of bleeding. Transcatheter selective arterial infusion of vasopressin is therapeutic at smaller doses than those needed for traditional intravenous therapy. With this smaller dose, the risk of significant systemic side effects (eg, coronary and peripheral vasoconstriction, arrhythmia, etc) is less. Vasopressin also stimulates contraction of the smooth muscle of the GI tract. Therefore, it is not unusual for patients to experience transient abdominal cramps and a grossly bloody bowel movement shortly after the vasopressin therapy begins. It is important to distinguish these transient symptoms from the more prolonged symptoms of mesenteric ischemia.

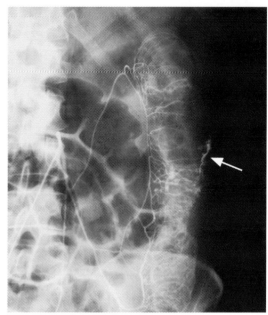

Figure 21. Before vasopressin therapy the inferior mesenteric arteriogram shows extravasation of contrast material (arrow).

Transcatheter Vasopressin Infusion—Technique

Depending on the site of bleeding, the catheter is placed in the main trunk of the superior mesenteric artery (SMA) or inferior mesenteric artery (IMA). Intraarterial vasopressin is then started at a rate of 0.2–0.3 U/minute. Follow-up arteriography is performed 20–30 minutes later and should show cessation of bleeding with significant arterial vasoconstriction and preservation of perfusion to distal arterial branches. **Figures 21** and **22** show the typical arteriographic appearance before and after vasopressin therapy. Note the decrease in peripheral perfusion on **Figure 22**. If vasoconstriction is excessive, the vasopressin dose should be reduced. If active hemorrhage is still seen, the vasopressin dose should be increased up to a maximum of 0.4 U/minute. At rates higher than 0.4 U/minute, systemic effects begin to occur. The patient must be monitored carefully for signs and symptoms of mesenteric ischemia. These should not be confused with the typical transient abdominal cramping seen upon initiation of vasopressin therapy.

Transcatheter Vasopressin Infusion—Management

Patients on intraarterial vasopressin must be monitored in an ICU setting. Generally, the vasopressin dose is slowly tapered over 12–24 hours and then discontinued if there is no further bleeding. During infusion, the patient must be carefully monitored for local and systemic complications. Local complications include puncture site complications and distal embolization. Systemic complications include myocardial, mesenteric, and peripheral ischemia, brady- and tachyarrhythmias, as well as hyponatremia and water retention. If severe, these may require cessation of the vasopressin infusion. Significant underlying coronary or mesenteric arterial disease should be considered a relative contraindication to intraarterial vasopressin therapy. However, these risks must be weighed against the risk of continued GI bleeding requiring possible surgical therapy.

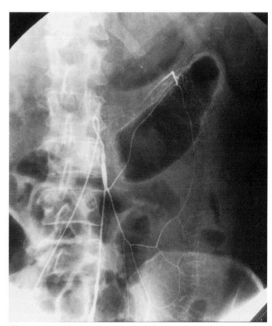

Figure 22. After vasopressin infusion the inferior mesenteric arteriogram shows vasoconstriction due to the vasopressin.

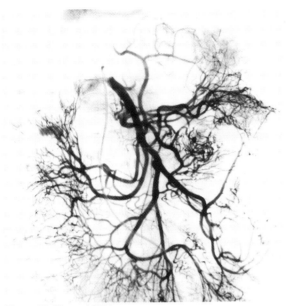

Figure 23. Normal SMA.

Vasopressin Therapy—Results

Vasopressin therapy is effective in up to 90% of patients with bleeding from colonic diverticuli. However, bleeding will recur in 20%–30% of these patients, and surgical resection should be considered (particularly in patients whose bleeding has recurred) once the patient's status is optimized. In patients with angiodysplasia, vasopressin therapy is less likely to be curative but can be very useful in allowing control of the bleeding and stabilization of the patient for elective rather than emergent surgical resection. If the patient's bleeding does not respond to vasopressin therapy and the patient is a poor candidate for surgery, embolization of the bleeding lesion should be considered.

Embolization for Lower GI Bleeding

Embolization for lower GI bleeding must be approached with much greater caution than for embolization of bleeding from the stomach or duodenum where multiple collateral pathways minimize the risk of ischemic injury. The vasa recta of the large and small bowel arise predominantly as a single artery and do not have extensive intercommunications. **Figure 23** shows normal SMA territory anatomy. The lack of extensive arterial collaterals in the small bowel and colon means that embolization for lower GI bleeding carries a significant risk of ischemic injury. The reported risk is 15%–35%. Embolization that is too aggressive can result in either transmural necrosis and bowel infarction or more subtle mucosal ischemia with eventual stricture formation. Bowel ischemia may be kept to a minimum with careful patient selection and attention to technical detail.

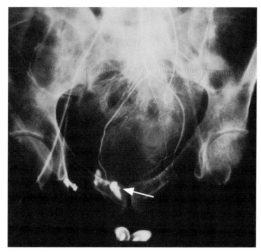

Figure 24. An inferior mesenteric arteriogram for rectal bleeding shows extravasation (arrow).

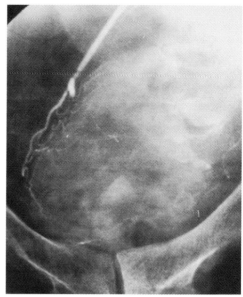

Figure 25. Rectal bleeding study after embolotherapy.

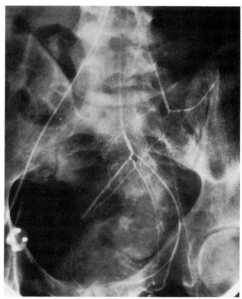

Figure 26. Inferior mesenteric arteriogram after embolotherapy.

Embolization—Patient Selection

The primary indication for embolization in lower GI bleeding is failure of vasopressin therapy in patients who are poor candidates for emergent surgery. Embolization in such debilitated patients can be a life-saving procedure. Embolization is also useful in order to stabilize a patient with massive lower GI bleeding for later elective surgery with a resultant lower morbidity and mortality. Most lesions are amenable to embolotherapy, including diverticulosis, angiodysplasia, tumors, and inflammatory lesions. Lesions in the rectum are particularly well suited to embolotherapy instead of vasopressin infusion. The rich collateral network in this portion of the bowel provided by the internal iliac arteries makes infarction much less likely. **Figures 24–26** show successful embolotherapy in a patient with massive bleeding from a rectal ulcer, using Gelfoam pledgets (Upjohn, Kalamazoo, MI) to occlude the bleeding vessel. **Figures 25** and **26** are postembolization images.

Embolization—Technical Details

The goal of embolization is to decrease the perfusion pressure at the bleeding site to allow formation of a stable clot. This requires that the patient have a functioning hemostatic system. Embolization should be performed at a level distal enough to treat only the involved segment of bowel, but proximal enough to maintain some collateral perfusion. Coaxial catheter systems are extremely useful because they allow such selective catheterization. Generally, agents such as Gelfoam pledgets, larger Ivalon particles (Unipoint, High Point, NC) (>500 microns), or microcoils are most useful. Small particulate matter such as Gelfoam powder or very small Ivalon particles (<300 microns) should not be used in order to avoid the risk of too distal an embolization with subsequent bowel infarction. Antibiotic coverage is recommended during colonic embolization to protect against enteric bacteria which may migrate across the ischemic bowel wall.

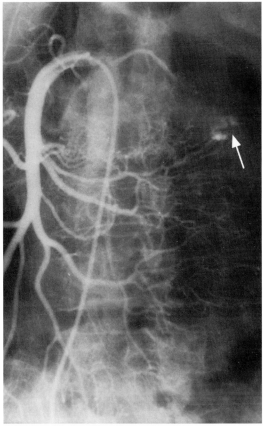

Figure 27. Localization of small bowel bleeding. The superior mesenteric arteriogram shows extravasation (arrow).

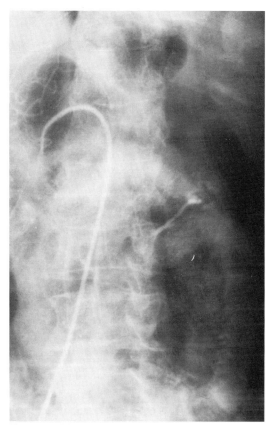

Figure 28. A later phase injection shows continued extravasation.

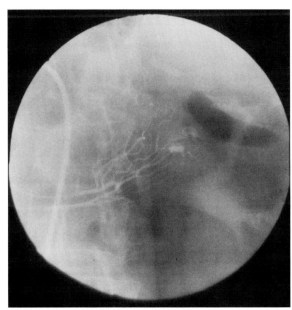

Figure 29. Localization of small bowel bleeding.

Transcatheter Localization for Small Bowel Bleeding

Bleeding lesions in the small bowel are very difficult to localize at surgery. Despite exquisite preoperative arteriographic mapping, once the abdominal cavity is opened the surgeon is confronted with a huge expanse of small bowel loops that have no consistent anatomic relationship to each other. Because of this, a variety of transcatheter techniques have been developed to mark lesions in the small bowel prior to surgical resection. These all involve selective catheterization of the branch artery leading to the bleeding vessel. We prefer to localize the offending segment of small bowel with 1 mL of methylene blue dye injected through the selective catheter. Because the methylene blue dye will diffuse away, the actual injection is done in the operating room once the abdomen has been opened. Other authors have advocated placing microcoils in the feeding artery which are then palpated at laparotomy.

Figures 27 and **28** show a patient with a small bowel arteriovenous malformation causing chronic lower GI bleeding. This lesion would have been very difficult to find at surgery. To aid in localization, a 3-F catheter was placed selectively into the feeding vessel **(Fig. 29)**.

The patient was then taken to the operating room where 1 mL of methylene blue dye was injected into the catheter, staining the target segment of small bowel blue **(Fig. 30)**. The segment of small bowel was successfully resected, resulting in resolution of the patient's bleeding **(Fig. 31)**.

For further information on this topic, please see Teaching File Cases 35–39.

Selected Readings

Conn HO, Ramsby GR, Storer EH, et al. Intraarterial vasopressin in the treatment of upper gastrointestinal hemorrhage: a prospective, controlled clinical trial. Gastroenterology 1975; 68:211–221.

Encarnacion CE, Kadir S, Beam CA, Payne CS. Gastrointestinal bleeding: treatment with gastrointestinal arterial embolization. Radiology 1992; 183:505–508.

Jasinski RW, Smith DC, Chase DR, Field FI. Angiographic preoperative bowel segment localization using methylene blue, isosulfan blue, and fluorescein. Invest Radiol 1987; 22:462–466.

Mills B, Zuckerman G, Sicard G. Discrete colon ulcers as a cause of lower gastrointestinal bleeding and perforation in end-stage renal disease. Surgery 1981; 89:548–552.

Palmaz JC, Walter JF, Cho KJ. Therapeutic embolization of the small bowel arteries. Radiology 1984; 152:377–382.

Rollins ES, Picus D, Hicks ME, Darcy MD, Bower BL, Kleinhoffer MA. Angiography is useful in detecting the source of chronic gastrointestinal bleeding of obscure origin. AJR 1991; 156:385–388.

Rösch J, Keller FS, Wawrukiewicz AS, Krippaehne WW, Dotter CT. Pharmacoangiography in the diagnosis of recurrent massive lower gastrointestinal bleeding. Radiology 1982; 145:615–619.

Rösch J, Kozak BE, Keller FS. Interventional diagnostic angiography in acute lower gastrointestinal bleeding. Semin Intervent Radiol 1988; 5:10–17.

Rosenkrantz H, Bookstein JJ, Rosen RJ, Goff WB, Healy JF. Postembolic colonic infarction. Radiology 1982; 142:47–51.

Veidenheimer MC, Schoetz DJ. Vascular disorders: lower gastrointestinal hemorrhage. Semin Colon Rectal Surg 1994; 5.

Zuckerman DA, Bocchini TP, Birnbaum EH. Massive hemorrhage in the lower gastrointestinal tract in adults: diagnostic imaging and intervention. AJR 1993; 161:703–711.

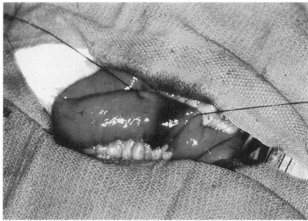

Figure 30. Localization of small bowel bleeding.

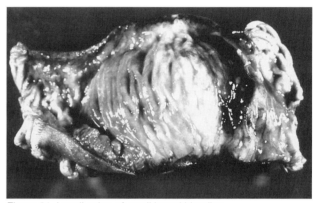

Figure 31. Localization of small bowel bleeding.

Epidemiology
• Colorectal cancer —155,000 cases/60,000 deaths annually (U.S.) • Hepatoma — 1,250,000 deaths worldwide/10,000–14,000 U.S. • Ocular melanoma — 2,000 cases, death in 2–6 months from liver mets • Neuroendocrine — 1,200 cases/year, long survival

Figure 1.

TUTORIAL 16 CHEMOEMBOLIZATION OF HEPATIC MALIGNANCIES

Michael C. Soulen, M.D.

Introduction

The subjects addressed in this tutorial include:

1. Theory, anatomy, and physiology of chemoembolization
2. Patient selection and preoperative evaluation
3. Procedural and periprocedural management
4. Results and complications.

The Problem of Hepatic Malignancies

Hepatoma is the most common fatal malignancy in the world. Colon cancer is the second leading cause of cancer death in the United States, and about half of these deaths are due to liver metastases. Other cancers which commonly develop fatal hepatic metastases despite resection of the primary tumor include ocular melanoma, neuroendocrine tumors, and gastrointestinal sarcomas **(Fig. 1)**. Systemic chemotherapy and radiation therapy have negligible impact on all these diseases. The only hope for cure is surgery, but most hepatic tumors are unresectable at presentation.

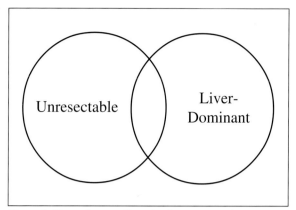

Figure 2. Venn diagram: liver-dominant tumors that are unresectable are candidates for regional therapy.

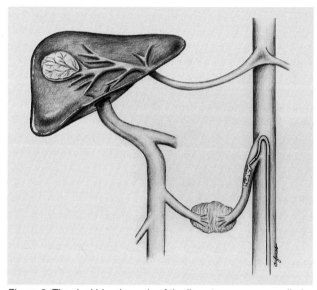

Figure 3. The dual blood supply of the liver: tumors are supplied by the hepatic artery, while the liver parenchyma is predominantly fed by the portal vein.

Regional Therapies

Various novel therapies have been developed to treat these unresectable malignancies that are nonetheless liver-dominant **(Fig. 2)**, meaning that the tumor is confined to the liver or that the dominant mass in the liver is what will lead to the major morbidity and death of the patient. These approaches include infusion of drugs into the hepatic artery or portal vein, embolization, chemo-embolization, infusion or injection of radioactive substances, and percutaneous tumor ablation with physical or chemical agents. These techniques share a local or regional approach.

Regional Hepatic Therapy—
Anatomy and Physiology

Anatomic studies from the 1950s showed that the liver has a dual blood supply, receiving three quarters of its blood from the portal vein, while tumors in the liver obtain nearly all their blood supply from the hepatic artery **(Fig. 3)**. Subsequent physiologic studies confirmed this concept. Fluorodeoxyuridine uptake in colorectal metastases is fifteen times higher with intraarterial infusion than with intraportal infusion. This disparity in blood supply between the tumor and normal liver, combined with the ease of catheterizing the hepatic artery, led to the development of catheter-based techniques for regional hepatic therapy such as embolization and intraarterial chemoinfusion.

Randomized Trials of Intravenous vs Intraarterial Infusion for Colon Cancer

| | *Response* | | |
	IA	IV	Survival Benefit
Kemeney, 1987	50%	20%	crossover
Chang, 1987	62	17	N.S.
Hohn, 1989	42	10	crossover
Martin, 1990	48	21	N.S.
Rougier, 1992	43	09	N.S.

Figure 4.

Randomized Trials of Intravenous vs Intraarterial Infusion for Colon Cancer

| | *Complications* | |
	GI	Biliary
Kemeney, 1987	25%	19%·
Chang, 1987	21	33
Hohn, 1989	00	52
Martin, 1990	13	26
Rougier, 1992	25	37

Figure 5.

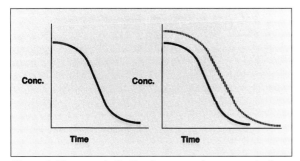

Figure 6. Chemoembolization increases drug concentration and dwell time. The response is proportional to the area under the curve.

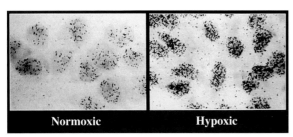

Figure 7. Doxorubicin uptake in human hepatoma cells.

Hepatic Artery Infusion Chemotherapy—Disadvantages

Early experiences with hepatic artery infusion for colorectal metastases reported a 60% response rate. A quarter century elapsed before five separate randomized trials were completed, showing no significant long-term survival benefit over systemic therapy **(Fig. 4)**. The higher early response rate with intraarterial infusion was offset by gastrointestinal and biliary toxicity in 25%–50% of patients **(Fig. 5)** and surgical or pump-related complications in 15%. Overall, 80% of patients receiving intraarterial infusion had to interrupt therapy because of complications, and 30% had to discontinue permanently.

Chemoembolization—Theoretical Advantages

Chemoembolization combines hepatic artery embolization with simultaneous infusion of concentrated chemotherapeutic drugs. Theoretical advantages are fourfold. Embolization increases both the concentration and the dwell time of the drug in the tumor. Tumor response is proportional to the area under the concentration-time curve **(Fig. 6)**. Chemoembolization increases this area by orders of magnitude. Ischemia paralyses the cell membrane pumps that actively eject the drug from the tumor cells. This is one of the mechanisms of drug resistance. Hypoxia increases intracellular drug uptake **(Fig. 7)**. Finally, retention of up to 85% of the drug in the liver minimizes systemic toxicity.

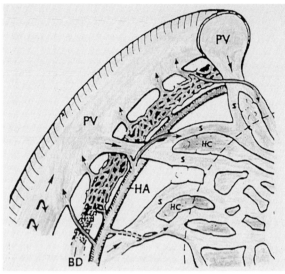

Figure 8. Arterioportal connections.

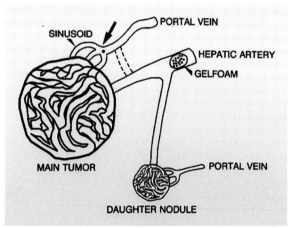

Figure 9. Liver tumor embolization: particle only.

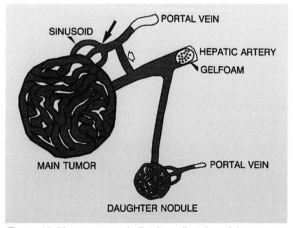

Figure 10. Liver tumor embolization: oil and particle.

Choice of Therapeutic Agents

No compelling evidence exists to support one drug or drug combination, nor one particular embolic particle. Combining particles with iodized oil causes superior tumor necrosis, and in some series improved survival, compared to either agent alone. This may be because hepatic arterial blood passes through presinusoidal arterioportal shunts into the terminal portal venules before entering tumors **(Fig. 8)**. Particle embolization alone leaves the shunts open and permits continued portal blood flow to the tumor **(Fig. 9)**. Use of oil clogs the shunts, and the particles then prevent washout of liquid agents by blocking continued arterial inflow **(Fig. 10)**.

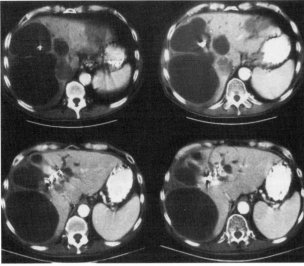

Figure 11. CT scan 6 months after chemoembolization of metastatic colon cancer in a patient with stented biliary strictures from prior intraarterial chemotherapy. A giant biloma replaces most of the right lobe.

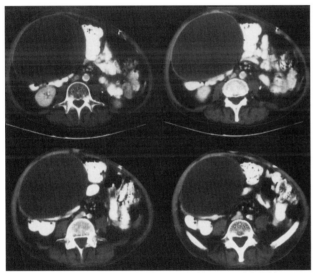

Figure 12. Same patient as in Figure 11. More caudal CT image demonstrates the intraabdominal extent of the giant biloma.

Preoperative Evaluation

- Abdominal computed tomography, magnetic resonance imaging
- Chest radiography
- Laboratory studies
— Complete blood count
— Coagulation studies
— Creatinine
— Liver function tests
- Tumor markers

Figure 13.

Patient Selection—Contraindications
Chemoembolization is palliative therapy. It is important to avoid complications that worsen rather than sustain quality of life. Patients who cannot tolerate hepatic artery embolization should be excluded. This includes anyone with encephalopathy or jaundice. Patients with the constellation of 50% liver replacement by tumor, aspartate transaminase >100, lactate dehydrogenase >425, and bilirubin >2 are at unacceptable risk of hepatic failure. Any degree of biliary obstruction, even with a normal serum bilirubin, can lead to biliary necrosis. **Figures 11** and **12** show massive biloma formation in a patient despite successful stenting of biliary strictures. Portal vein obstruction by tumor is acceptable as long as hepatopetal flow is present.

Preprocedure Assessment
Before chemoembolization is performed, imaging studies must be reviewed to determine the location and extent of tumor within the liver and to exclude significant extrahepatic disease. Preprocedure laboratory studies should include a complete blood count, a creatinine level, liver function tests, coagulation studies, and tumor markers **(Fig. 13)**. Patients should be carefully counseled regarding the palliative role of therapy, given the significant discomforts, risks, and cost of the procedure.

Patient Preparation
• Informed consent • Overnight fast • Intravenous normal saline 200–300 mL/hr • Foley catheter • Premedications: Ancef, Flagyl, Zofran   Decadron, Benadryl

Figure 14. Sample regimen.

Patient Preparation

At our institution, patients fast overnight, then are hydrated with normal saline. A Foley catheter is placed to monitor urine output. Prophylactic antibiotics, antiemetics, sedatives, and narcotics are administered **(Fig. 14)**.

Pre-embolization Arteriography

Careful visceral arteriography is performed to assess portal flow and hepatic arterial anatomy, and to identify gastroenteric branches. Variant supply to the liver must be noted, so that all tumor-feeding branches can be treated. Catheters must be placed well beyond the origins of the gastroduodenal artery, right gastric artery, and supraduodenal branches to avoid non-target embolization to the gut. **Figure 15** shows a large left hepatic artery originating from a left gastric/left hepatic common trunk. The right gastric artery arises from the medial segment left hepatic artery. The right hepatic artery and each left hepatic artery will have to be chemoembolized separately to avoid non-target embolization.

The Cystic Artery

Figure 16 shows the same patient as in **Figure 15**, with the catheter tip in the right hepatic artery. This illustrates the importance of obtaining a final arteriogram prior to injecting chemotherapeutic agents: a large cystic artery is now identified which was not seen on the celiac run. It is safe to chemoembolize proximal to the origin of the cystic artery, because surgical cholecystitis is rare; however, embolizing the gallbladder may substantially increase the pain of the procedure. In this case, terminal branches of the cystic artery communicated with the right gastric artery, so the catheter tip was advanced distally before chemoembolization was performed.

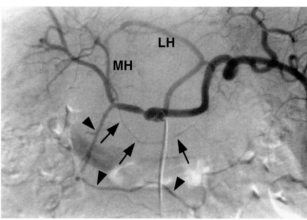

Figure 15. Celiac axis arteriogram demonstrates a large left hepatic artery (LH) that originates from a left gastric/left hepatic common arterial trunk. The right gastric artery (arrows) arises from the medial segment left hepatic artery (MH). The gastroduodenal artery (arrowheads) lies caudal to the right gastric artery.

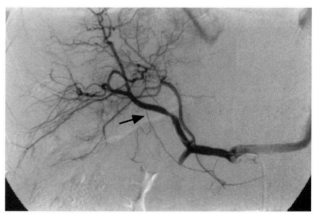

Figure 16. Same patient as in Figure 15. The common hepatic arteriogram shows the unusual cystic artery (arrow).

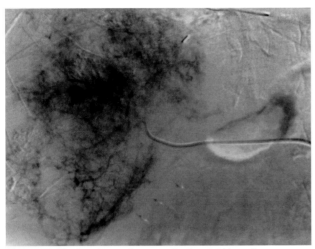

Figure 17. The late image from a selective right hepatic arteriogram prior to chemoembolization demonstrates the abnormal vasculature of a hepatoma.

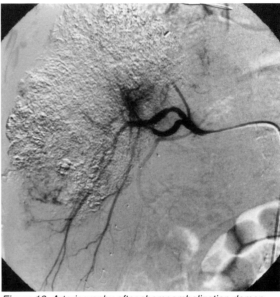

Figure 18. Arteriography after chemoembolization demonstrates intended subtotal stasis within the hepatic arteries. The granular artifact within the liver parenchyma results from the iodized oil.

PREMEDS FOR CHEMOEMBOLIZATION	CHEMOTHERAPY ORDERS
Ondansetron 24 mg IV	Mitomycin 10 mg
Dexamethasone 10 mg IV	Adriamycin 50 mg
Cefazolin 1 gm IV	Cisplatinum 100 mg
Metronidazole 500 mg IV	Sterile Contrast Solution 8.5 mL
Diphenhydramine 50 mg IV	Sterile Water for Injection 1.5 mL

ADMIT TO INTERVENTIONAL RADIOLOGY

DX: Liver metastases, s/p chemoembolization

CONDITION: [   ] ALLERGIES: [   ]

VS: q 15' x 4, q 30' x 4, q 1 hr x 4, then q shift/

ACT: Bedrest with _____ leg straight x 6 hr, then ad lib

Check _____ groin for pulse and hematoma with each VS

Foley to gravity

I and O

DIET: Clears, advance to regular as tolerated

IVF: NSS @ 150 cc/hr x 3 liters, then D 5 1/2 NSS @ 80 cc/hr

MEDS: Cefazolin 500 mg IV q 8 hr

    Metronidazole 500 mg IV q 12 hr

    Morphine Sulfate 10 mg IM q 4 hr prn severe pain

    Tylenol #3 2 tabs po q 4 hr prn moderate pain

    Tylenol 650 mg po or pr q 4 hr prn fever

    Prochlorperazine 25 mg pr q 8 hr prn nausea

    Ondansetron 8 mg IV q 8 hr and Dexamethasone 8 mg IV q 8 hr x 2 days,

      starting at 7 a.m.

Figure 19. Sample hospital admission orders.

Procedural Endpoints

Lobar chemoembolization is much better tolerated than treatment of the whole liver at once, and complications are less likely to be fatal. Once the catheter is placed into the left or right hepatic artery and safe catheter position is confirmed arteriographically **(Fig. 17)**, the chemoembolic mixture is injected until the magical "90% stasis" is achieved. The goal is a "pruned tree" or "tree-in-winter" appearance, with preservation of flow in the main hepatic arterial trunks **(Fig. 18)**. This prevents thrombosis of the hepatic artery, permitting repeated therapy from this route, and minimizes extrahepatic collateral formation.

Postprocedure Care

Eighty to ninety percent of patients will suffer postembolization syndrome, characterized by pain, nausea, vomiting, and fever. The severity of these symptoms varies dramatically. Vigorous intravenous hydration and prophylaxis with narcotics, antiemetics, and antipyretics permits discharge of half of patients within 24 hours, and most within 48 hours. Sample admitting orders for chemoembolization are shown in **Figure 19**; details vary among institutions. At our institution, patients are discharged on a 5-day course of oral antibiotics (ciprofloxacin or Augmentin), with oral narcotics and antiemetics to be taken as needed.

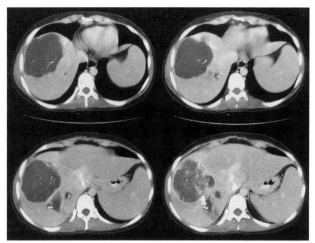

Figure 20. Hepatic necrosis peripheral to a large right lobe hepatoma is seen.

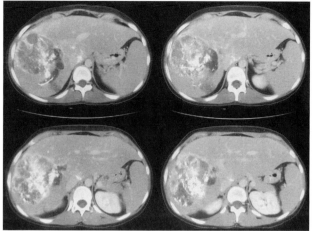

Figure 21. Oil uptake in a right lobe hepatoma. Local portal vein occlusion caused hepatic necrosis peripheral to the tumor (Figure 20).

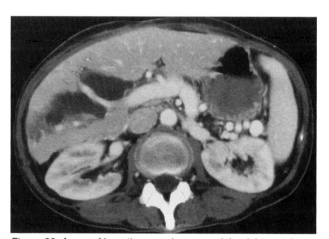

Figure 22. Areas of hepatic necrosis surround the right portal vein.

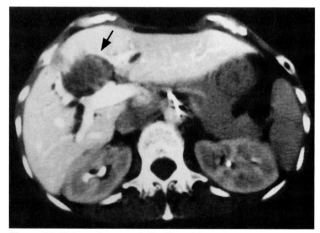

Figure 23. Before chemoembolization. A tumor mass compresses the left portal vein (arrow).

Complications

Major complications include hepatic and biliary necrosis, abscess, cholecystitis, and embolization to the gut, totaling 3%–4% of all cases. Rarer complications include renal and hematologic toxicity (<1%). **Figures 20** and **21** show infarction of the liver peripheral to a large hepatoma, due to local occlusion of portal venous flow. **Figure 22** shows hepatobiliary necrosis isolating the main right portal vein. **Figures 23** and **24** show atrophy of the left lobe after chemoembolization of an intrahepatic tumor compressing the left portal vein. **Figure 25** shows gastric ulcers after 1 mL of chemoembolic mixture flowed down the right gastric artery. Larger doses cause transmural necrosis.

Results—Hepatoma

The response rate for hepatoma is 60%–85%. Survival averages about 70% at 1 year, 50% at 2 years, and 40% at 3 years, similar to the survival data for resection. Significant prognostic factors include tumor volume, tumor stage, oil uptake and retention, and severity of underlying cirrhosis. **Figures 26** and **27** show a hepatoma occupying the posterior segment of the right lobe, which completely opacified with oil and shrunk by 65% after chemoembolization.

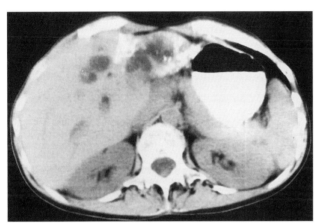

Figure 24. One month after chemoembolization. The left lobe of the liver has undergone significant atrophy.

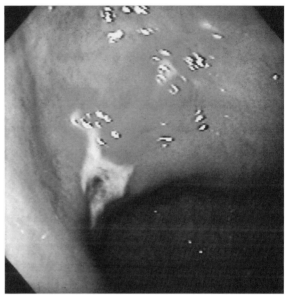

Figure 25. Gastric endoscopy reveals ulcerations due to errant embolization of the right gastric artery.

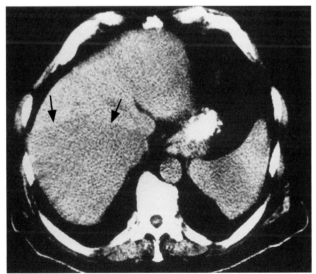

Figure 26. Hepatoma occupying the posterior segment of the right lobe (arrows).

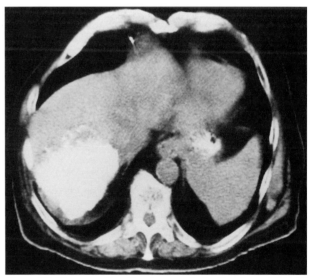

Figure 27. Three months after chemoembolization dense Ethiodol (Savage Laboratories, Melville, NY) uptake is noted within the tumor, which has shrunk by 65%.

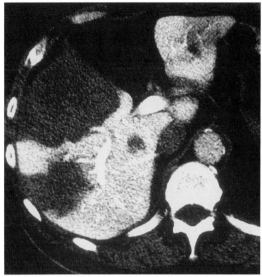

Figure 28. Computed tomography (CT) scan before chemoembolization of metastatic colon cancer.

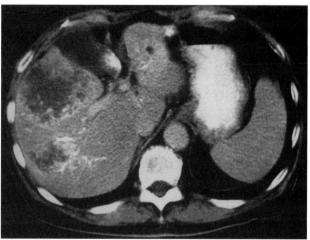

Figure 29. CT scan 1 month after chemoembolization of metastatic colon cancer.

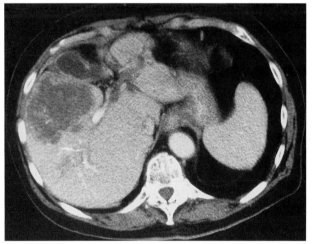

Figure 30. Six months after chemoembolization.

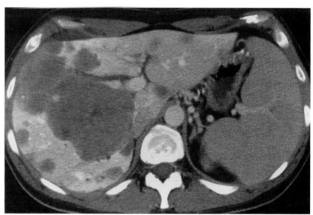

Figure 31. Metastatic colon cancer before chemoembolization.

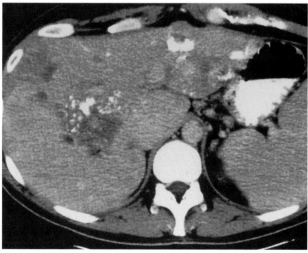

Figure 32. Metastatic colon cancer after chemoembolization.

Results—Colon Cancer

Early response rates of metastatic colon cancer to chemoembolization are 75%–85%. Most lesions remain morphologically stable despite a significant drop in carcinoembryonic antigen levels but develop central necrosis **(Figs. 28, 29)**. Oil uptake and retention is less than with hepatoma, and has a peripheral pattern. Tumor shrinkage can lag behind the biological response by months **(Fig. 30)**. Occasionally lesions regress dramatically **(Figs. 31, 32)**, and can have gaseous necrosis. One-year survival at three different United States centers was about two-thirds. No randomized trials have been reported yet, so survival benefit is unknown.

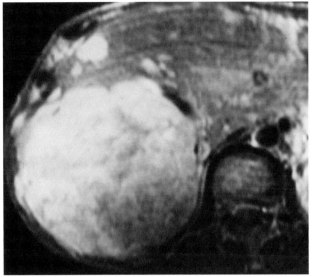

Figure 33. Magnetic resonance (MR) image of a carcinoid tumor before chemoembolization.

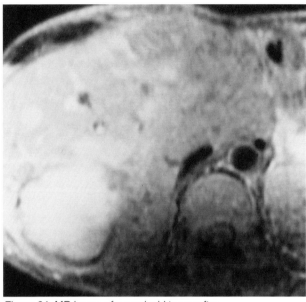

Figure 34. MR image of a carcinoid tumor after chemoembolization.

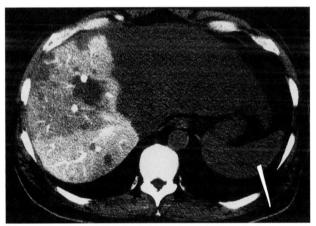

Figure 35. CT scan of metastatic ocular melanoma before chemoembolization.

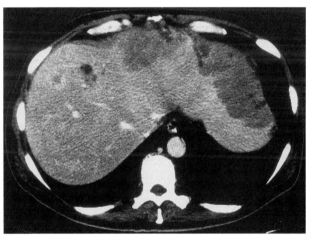

Figure 36. Same patient as in Figure 35 after chemoembolization.

Results—Neuroendocrine Tumors and Ocular Melanoma

Neuroendocrine tumors such as carcinoid and islet cell tumors respond well to particle embolization (93%). Chemoembolization may improve the duration of response based on the few early reports. **Figures 33** and **34** show dramatic regression of carcinoid after chemoembolization in a patient who was not adequately palliated by particle embolization alone. Complications may be increased with chemoembolization of carcinoids. Ocular melanoma has been reported to respond well to chemo-embolization with polyvinyl alcohol particles **(Figs. 35, 36)**, but not to Gelfoam (Upjohn, Kalamazoo, MI) or collagen, which are temporary embolic agents.

271

Results—Other Metastases

A host of other metastatic lesions have been treated with chemoembolization. **Figures 37** and **38** show metastatic breast cancer before and after treatment. There is not sufficient data on any one tumor type to make conclusive statements about response or survival. Overall, response rates run 60%–75% with median survivals of 8–11 months. Treatment of such lesions must done on a case by case, compassionate basis.

The tutorial on advanced chemoembolization will cover pitfalls, problematic cases, management of complications, and other applications.

For further information on this topic, please see Teaching File Cases 45–47.

Selected Readings

Breedis C, Young G. The blood supply of neoplasms in the liver. Am J Pathol 1954; 30:969–985.

Charnsangavej C. Chemoembolization of liver tumors. Semin Intervent Radiol 1993; 10:150–160.

Kan Z, Sato M, Ivancev K, et al. Distribution and effect of iodized poppyseed oil in the liver after hepatic artery embolization: experimental study in several animal species. Radiology 1993; 186:861–866.

Katsumori T, Fujita M, Takahashi T, et al. Effective segmental chemoembolization of advanced hepatocellular carcinoma with tumor thrombus in the portal vein. Cardiovasc Intervent Radiol 1995; 18:217–221.

Groupe d'etude et de traitement du carcinome hepatocellulaire. A comparison of Lipiodol chemoembolization and conservative treatment for unresectable hepatocellular carcinoma. N Engl J Med 1995; 332:1256–1261.

Pentecost MJ, Daniels JR, Teitelbaum GP, Stanley P. Hepatic chemoembolization: safety with portal vein thrombosis. J Vasc Interv Radiol 1993; 4:347–351.

Pentecost MJ, Teitelbaum GP, Katz MD, Daniels JR. Chemoembolization in hepatic malignancy. Semin Intervent Radiol 1992; 9:28–37.

Pentecost MJ. Transcatheter treatment of hepatic metastases. AJR 1993; 160:1171–1175.

Perry LJ, Stuart K, Stokes KR, Clouse ME. Hepatic arterial chemoembolization for metastatic neuroendocrine tumors. Surgery 1994; 116:1111–1117.

Soulen MC. Chemoembolization of hepatic malignancies. Oncology 1994; 8:77–84.

Stuart K, Stokes K, Jenkins R, Trey C, Clouse M. Treatment of hepatocellular carcinoma using doxorubicin/ethiodized oil/gelatin powder chemoembolization. Cancer 1993; 72:3202–3209.

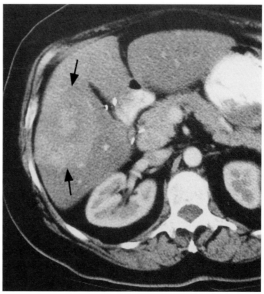

Figure 37. Pretreatment CT scan of a patient with metastatic breast cancer (arrows).

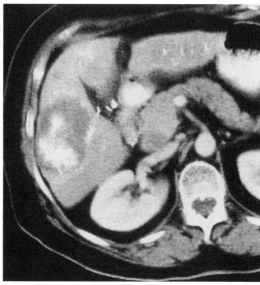

Figure 38. Lesion demarcation and oil uptake is present after chemoembolization.

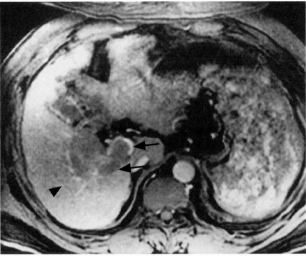

Figure 1. The MR scan demonstrates main and right portal vein invasion by hepatoma (arrows). Flow is present in the more peripheral portal vein branches (arrowhead).

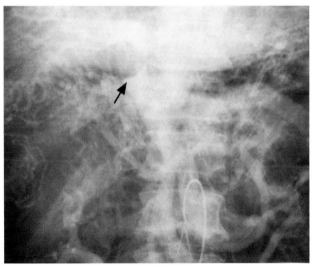

Figure 2. Arterial portography confirms partial portal vein occlusion with adequate flow (arrow).

TUTORIAL 17
ADVANCED CHEMOEMBOLIZATION— ANATOMY, TECHNIQUE, AND COMPLICATIONS

Kevin L. Sullivan, M.D., and
Michael C. Soulen, M.D.

Introduction
The subjects addressed in this tutorial include:
1. Anatomic pitfalls and problems
2. Dose of Ethiodol
3. Selection of percutaneous techniques
4. Assessment of response
5. Recurrence
6. Complications.

Problems
Portal Vein Occlusion
In order for chemoembolization to be performed safely, the portal flow must be adequate to prevent infarction of normal hepatic parenchyma. If the portal vein is occluded, well-developed periportal collateral veins may provide sufficient nutrient hepatic perfusion to permit chemoembolization. In this patient with a right lobe hepatoma, there is invasion of the right and main portal veins on a magnetic resonance (MR) scan, but flow is observed in more peripheral branches **(Fig. 1)**. This was confirmed on arterial portography **(Fig. 2)**, and chemoembolization was performed without complications.

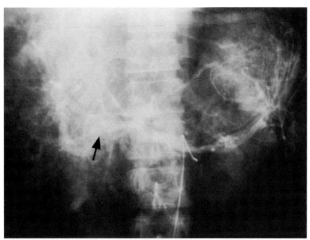

Figure 3. The venous phase of a pretreatment splenic arteriogram shows complete occlusion of the portal vein with numerous periportal collaterals (arrow).

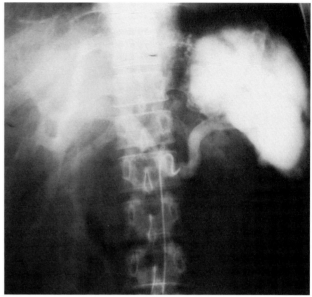

Figure 4. The venous phase of a post-treatment splenic arteriogram shows a normal portal vein.

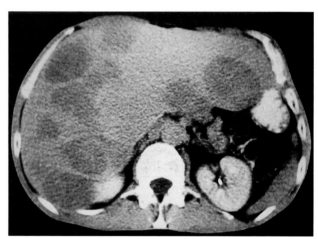

Figure 5. CT scan of a patient with ocular melanoma metastatic to the liver.

Even complete occlusion of the portal vein is not a contraindication to judicious chemoembolization if hepatopetal flow is present **(Fig. 3)**. After twelve segmental chemoembolizations, this patient's hepatoma regressed and the portal vein recanalized completely **(Fig. 4)**.

Variant Hepatic Arterial Anatomy
An understanding of the patient's hepatic arterial anatomy is essential if extrahepatic embolization is to be avoided. In this patient with metastatic melanoma **(Fig. 5)**, a celiac arteriogram **(Fig. 6)** demonstrates that part of the left hepatic artery arises from the same trunk as the left gastric artery. Selective left hepatic arteriography with carbon dioxide gastric distention revealed no gastric branches **(Fig. 7)**. In another patient, arteriography after carbon dioxide gastric distention demonstrate a typical left gastric artery distribution **(Fig. 8)**. Following embolization, continued flow was demonstrated in a left hepatic artery branch **(Fig. 9)**. The chemoembolization catheter was distal to the most proximal branch of the left hepatic artery. Additional chemoembolization was performed. An arteriogram obtained after chemoembolization confirms that all branches supplying the tumor have been embolized.

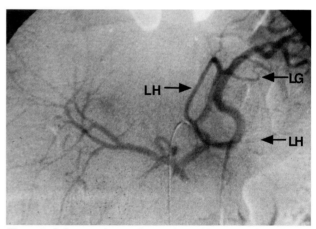

Figure 6. Celiac arteriogram in a patient with metastatic ocular melanoma and variant hepatic arterial anatomy. The left gastric (LG) and left hepatic (LH) arteries arise from a common trunk.

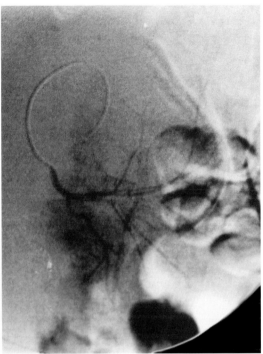

Figure 7. Same patient as in Figure 6. The selective left hepatic arteriogram during carbon dioxide gastric distention demonstrates the left hepatic artery distribution.

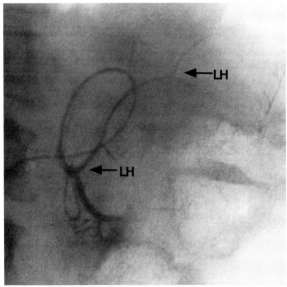

Figure 9. Left gastric-left hepatic trunk injection after chemoembolization.The vessels demonstrated in Figure 7 are occluded, but a branch of the left hepatic artery (LH) proximal to the chemoembolized arteries has antegrade flow. This vessel was subsequently chemoembolized.

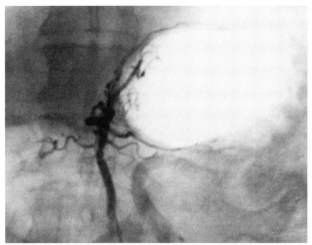

Figure 8. In another patient, a selective left gastric arteriogram during carbon dioxide gastric distention demonstrates the left gastric artery distribution.

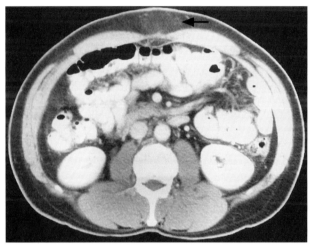

Figure 10. Periumbilical inflammation of fat after chemo-embolization (arrow).

Viscera Other Than the Liver Supplied by the Hepatic Artery

Selective chemoembolization of the right or left hepatic arteries avoids a number of extrahepatic organs. However, the vascular supply to several organs can arise from the right or left hepatic arteries. The right gastric artery generally arises from the left hepatic artery. The cystic artery often arises from the right hepatic artery.

In this case, a periumbilical rash and induration noted after chemoembolization of the left hepatic artery prompted a computed tomography (CT) scan **(Fig. 10)**. The inflammatory changes in the fat were probably due to chemoembolic agents flowing into the falciform artery. Techniques for avoiding such complications include more selective catheter placement when such vessels are observed, or protective proximal "blockade" embolization of these non-target vessels when this can be done safely.

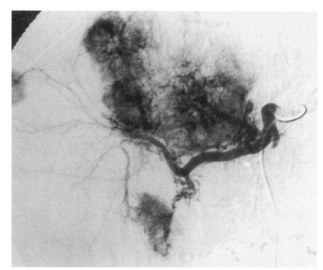

Figure 11. Common hepatic arteriogram shows multiple hypervascular metastases and nonvisualization of the GDA.

Pitfalls

Sumping

Reversal of flow in the gastroduodenal artery (GDA) can occur due to celiac artery stenosis or a sump effect caused by increased flow to large, hypervascular tumors **(Fig. 11)**. In the latter case, embolization of the tumor will result in restoration of antegrade flow in the GDA **(Fig. 12)**. Because the GDA may not be seen on the initial hepatic arteriogram, care must be taken to position the catheter tip well beyond the expected location of the GDA origin (determined from the superior mesenteric artery [SMA] injection). Failure to do so, as in this case, will result in non-target embolization to the stomach, duodenum, or pancreas, as shown in this CT scan **(Fig. 13)**.

Technical Issues

One common problem is excessive embolization. As discussed in the introductory tutorial, it is crucial to preserve some forward flow in the hepatic artery, to permit retreatment at a later time and to prevent formation of numerous extrahepatic collaterals (see below). There is always a milliliter of the chemo-embolic mixture within the catheter lumen. If one does not stop at "90% stasis," the final flush of the catheter will cause complete arterial stasis or reflux into non-target vessels.

Another pitfall to avoid is advancing a 4–5-F hydrophilic catheter too selectively. If the catheter size approaches the vessel diameter, it will artifactually slow flow. When the catheter is removed after embolizing to apparent "near-stasis," rapid flow will be restored to the tumor.

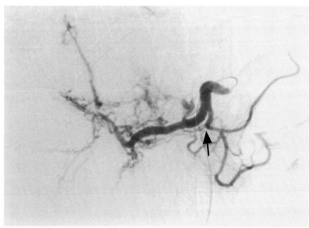

Figure 12. After partial embolization, the GDA now fills antegrade due to elimination of the sump (arrow).

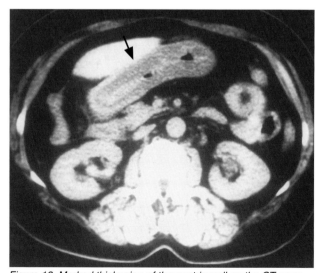

Figure 13. Marked thickening of the gastric wall on the CT scan after non-target embolization of the stomach.

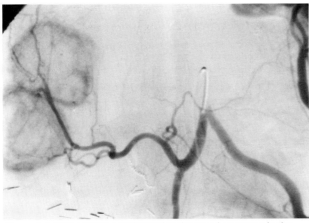

Figure 14. Initial celiac arteriography shows a hepatoma in the right lobe.

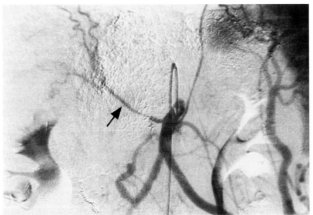

Figure 15. Celiac arteriogram 4 months after treatment demonstrates hepatic artery occlusion. The right inferior phrenic artery now supplies the tumor (arrow).

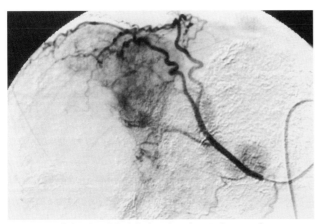

Figure 16. Selective right inferior phrenic arteriogram demonstrates tumor vascularity.

Collaterals

Inferior Phrenic Artery

Tumors can parasitize arteries adjacent to the liver, such as the phrenic, intercostal, lumbar, internal mammary, mesenteric, epiploic, splenic, pancreatic, cystic, and gastroenteric arterial branches. When flow in the hepatic artery is compromised by chemoembolization, collaterals form from these same vessels. **Figure 14** shows a hepatoma prior to chemoembolization. Four months later, the right hepatic artery is occluded. The tumor is fed by the right inferior phrenic artery **(Figs. 15, 16)**. The inferior phrenic artery can usually be chemo-embolized with relative impunity, although symptoms of diaphragmatic pain and irritation are common. Adrenal branches should be avoided.

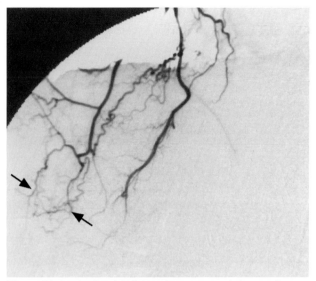

Figure 17. A selective right internal mammary arteriogram 2 months later demonstrates supply to the hepatoma (arrows).

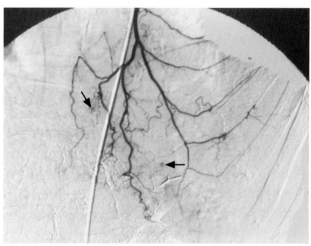

Figure 18. The left internal mammary artery also supplies the hepatoma through its terminal branches (arrows).

Internal Mammary Arteries

Two months later, the same patient now has collateral flow from the right and left internal mammary arteries **(Figs. 17, 18)**. Care must be taken to place a microcatheter distal to anterior intercostal and superior epigastric branches of the terminal internal mammary artery, to avoid chest wall necrosis. When are collaterals large enough to warrant chemoembolization? A good rule of thumb is the "back of the room test." If collaterals to the liver are obvious from the back of the room, they are worth embolizing.

Intercostal Arteries

When tumor recurs in the liver and the hepatic artery is attenuated or occluded, the hunt for collateral supply to the tumor starts with a low thoracic aortogram **(Fig. 19)**. The aortogram will demonstrate all the collateral pathways except for the internal mammary arteries. In this case, multiple intercostal arteries feed recurrent tumor along the margin of the liver. **Figures 20–23** show selective catheterization of intercostal arteries IX–XII. As with internal mammary artery embolization, the catheter must be placed far distally into branches feeding only the liver, to avoid chest wall tissue necrosis. This patient nonetheless developed geographic skin necrosis, which caused significant morbidity despite excellent tumor control.

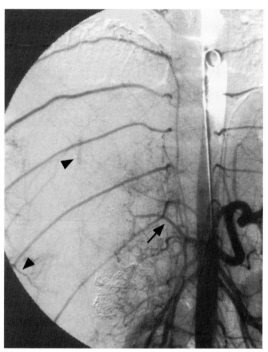

Figure 19. An aortogram shows an attenuated hepatic artery (arrow) and multiple intercostal arteries feeding the liver (arrowheads).

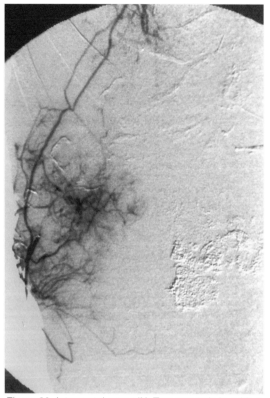

Figure 20. Intercostal artery IX. Tumor supply is evident.

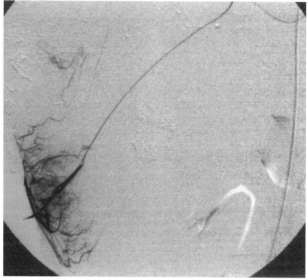

Figure 21. Intercostal artery X.

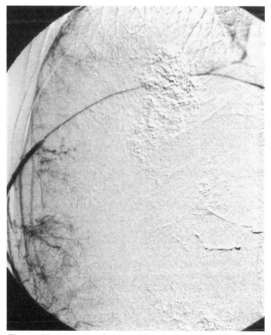

Figure 22. Intercostal artery XI.

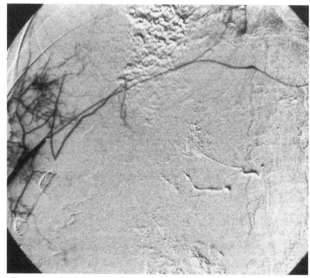

Figure 23. Intercostal artery XII.

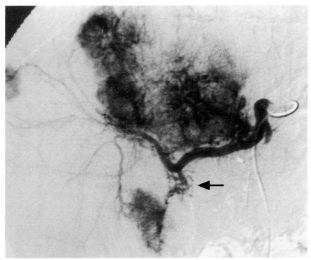

Figure 24. Celiac arteriogram. An enlarged cystic artery supplies a metastasis (arrow).

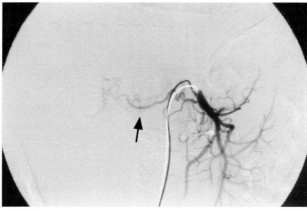

Figure 25. Same patient as in Figure 24. The superior mesenteric arteriogram, early phase, shows communication between the IPDA and the right hepatic artery (arrow) after multiple hepatic artery embolizations.

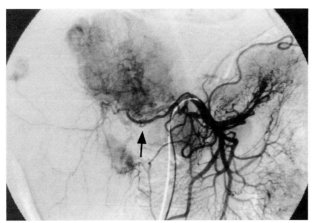

Figure 26. Same patient as in Figure 24. A later image also shows communication between the IPDA and the right hepatic artery (arrow).

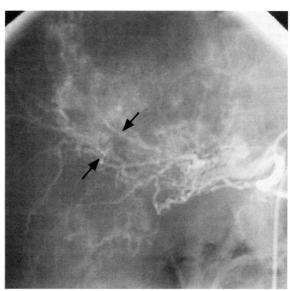

Figure 27. Same patient as in Figure 24. The gastroduodenal artery injection shows numerous small collaterals to the liver (arrows).

Mesenteric and Ligamentous Arteries

A host of collateral arterial pathways exist through the mesenteric and ligamentous attachments between the liver and the stomach, bowel, and gallbladder. **Figure 24** shows a celiac artery injection that reveals an enlarged cystic artery feeding a metastasis adjacent to the gallbladder. An SMA injection **(Figs. 25, 26)** shows collaterals from the inferior pancreaticoduodenal arcade (IPDA) to the right hepatic artery. Selective injection of the GDA **(Fig. 27)** shows a nest of collaterals to the liver. The GDA was embolized with coils. One month later, numerous fine collaterals arise from the stump of the GDA and proper hepatic artery **(Fig. 28)**. A left gastric artery injection at the same time **(Figs. 29, 30)** also shows numerous collaterals feeding the liver.

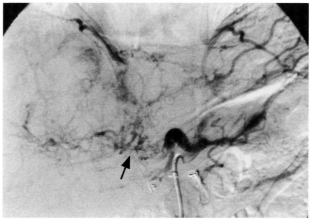

Figure 28. Celiac arteriography 1 month after coil embolization of the GDA. Numerous fine collaterals now arise from the stump of the GDA and the thrombosed proper hepatic artery (arrow).

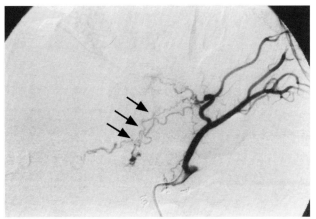

Figure 29. The early image from a selective left gastric artery injection shows numerous collaterals to the left lobe of the liver (arrows).

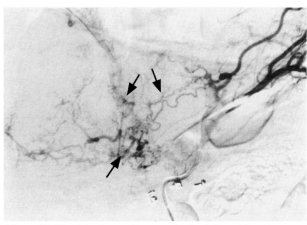

Figure 30. The later image from a selective left gastric artery injection shows numerous collaterals to the left lobe of the liver (arrows).

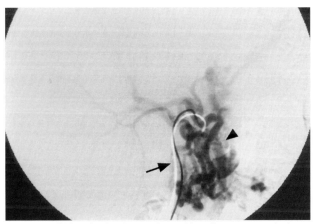

Figure 31. SMA injection in a patient with celiac artery occlusion and diffuse hypervascular hepatic metastases. An enlarged pancreaticoduodenal arcade (arrowhead) fills the hepatic artery (arrow) via retrograde flow up the GDA.

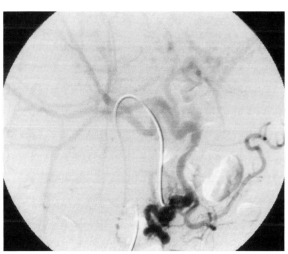

Figure 32. Selective inferior pancreaticoduodenal arcade injection shows the pathway to the liver.

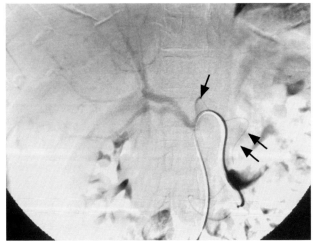

Figure 33. A microcatheter has been advanced into the right hepatic artery (arrows).

Celiac Artery Occlusion
Celiac artery stenosis or occlusion, often due to median arcuate ligament compression, can prevent direct access to the hepatic artery. In such cases, the hepatic artery is usually reconstituted from the SMA via retrograde flow in the pancreaticoduodenal arcade and the GDA **(Fig. 31)**. Often there will be a large enough vessel through this arcade to permit passage of a microcatheter from the SMA into the hepatic artery **(Figs. 32, 33)**.

Ethiodol Dose

Dose for Hypervascular Tumors

Experimental and clinical studies suggest that the addition of Ethiodol (Savage Laboratories, Melville, NY) to chemoembolic mixtures may improve treatment efficacy. The volume of Ethiodol must increase as the volume of hypervascular tumor increases in order to be effective. As a rough estimate, 1 mL of Ethiodol can be administered for each centimeter of largest tumor diameter for hypervascular neoplasms. However, total volumes over 20 mL can lead to pulmonary symptoms due to arteriosystemic venous shunting. Hepatic necrosis can also occur with large volumes of Ethiodol, due to Ethiodol occlusion of portal vein branches. Ethiodol enters the portal vein via normal communications between the arterial and portal systems. A small amount of Ethiodol in portal venules is to be expected, and can be used as a visual endpoint **(Fig. 34)**. More central portal vein branches should not be opacified. This can be monitored with radiographs during chemoembolization when necessary.

Dose for Nonhypervascular Tumors

The native liver tissue has a limited tolerance for oil embolization, especially when oil embolization is combined with particulate embolization. Some experimental data suggest that at doses of 0.2 mL/kg of oil followed by gelatin sponge embolization, areas of necrosis and atrophy develop. At a dose of 0.5 mL/kg, hepatic failure is likely. In patients with large, hypervascular tumors, oil will be taken up preferentially by the tumor, so a higher total dose can be injected. However, metastatic lesions such as those from colon cancer are not usually grossly hypervascular. In such cases, it may be advisable to limit the total dose of Ethiodol to perhaps 7–10 mL (0.1–0.15 mL/kg) to avoid hepatic necrosis.

Complications

Abscess Formation

Following successful chemoembolization, tumor necrosis occurs. This necrotic tissue is at risk for bacterial seeding and abscess formation. This patient had persistent fever and pain following chemoembolization of a hepatoma. A CT scan revealed tissue necrosis with gas **(Fig. 35)**. This pattern can be seen with tissue necrosis alone, but pain and fever that persisted for longer than is typically seen after chemoembolization prompted needle aspiration. Purulent fluid and positive bacterial cultures confirmed the presence of an abscess, which was successfully managed with percutaneous drainage **(Fig. 36)** and antibiotics. This patient did not receive prophylactic antibiotics. Some interventionalists strongly advocate the routine use of prophylactic antibiotics, but the efficacy of antibiotic prophylaxis is uncertain.

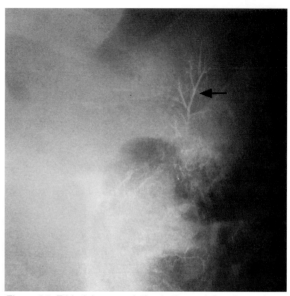

Figure 34. Ethiodol accumulation in the peripheral portal venules after chemoembolization (arrow).

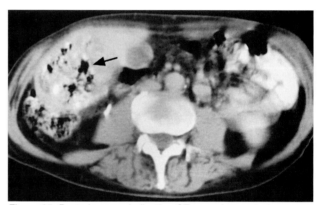

Figure 35. Post-chemoembolization CT scan demonstrates a gas-filled abscess (arrow).

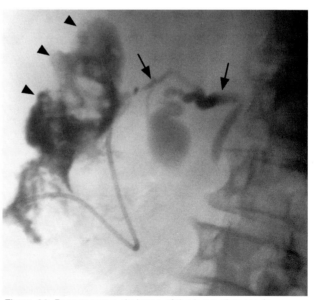

Figure 36. Percutaneous drainage of the large abscess (arrowheads). Communication with the biliary tree is seen (arrows).

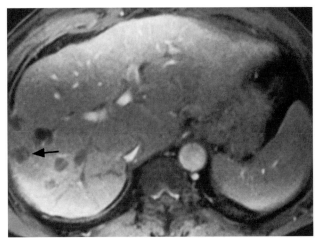

Figure 37. MR scan of bilomas (arrow) and dilated bile ducts after chemoembolization.

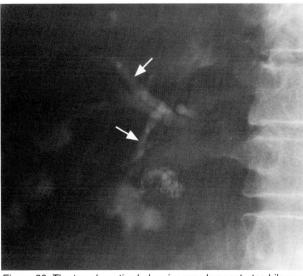

Figure 38. The transhepatic cholangiogram demonstrates bilomas and dilated ducts (arrows).

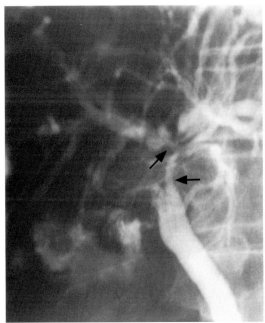

Figure 39. Post-chemoembolization biliary strictures at the hepatic duct confluence (arrows).

Biliary Strictures

This patient with multifocal hepatoma presented with fever and elevated alkaline phosphatase following three right hepatic and one left hepatic chemo-embolizations. There were multiple nonenhancing, fluid-filled structures as well as dilated ducts in the posterior aspect of the right lobe **(Fig. 37)**. These were believed to represent bilomas, probably secondary to a bile duct stricture. Transhepatic cholangiography confirmed this diagnosis **(Fig. 38)**. Strictures were present in the region of the confluence of the common hepatic duct and right and left hepatic ducts **(Fig. 39)**. This condition was managed with a transhepatic biliary drain. Bile ducts derive their blood supply from the hepatic artery and are therefore more prone to injury than the paren-chyma, which is supplied by the hepatic artery and the portal vein.

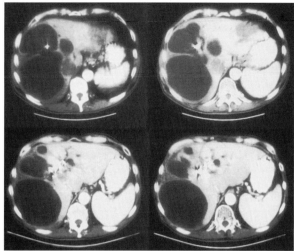

Figure 40. CT scan of the abdomen 6 months after chemoembolization. The patient has biliary stents in place for treatment of strictures which developed after chemotherapy infusions through a surgically placed hepatic artery pump. A large biloma extends from the right lobe into the pelvis.

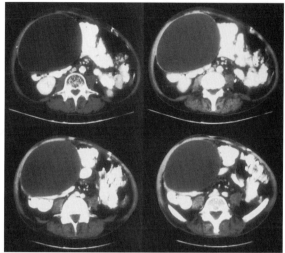

Figure 41. More caudal images demonstrate the extent of the biloma.

Biliary Necrosis

Chemoembolization and arterial chemoinfusion cause destruction of much of the capillary plexus surrounding the bile ducts. Small, clinically unsuspected bilomas are found in 10%–15% of livers on pathological examination. When the bile ducts are necrotic but the surrounding functional liver parenchyma is preserved, bilomas form because the secreted bile has no place to go. This patient developed biliary strictures from intraarterial infusion chemotherapy. A biliary stent was placed, and his serum bilirubin returned to normal. Subsequent chemoembolization caused extensive bile duct necrosis and formation of a huge biloma **(Figs. 40, 41)**. He required external catheter drainage for the rest of his life.

Percutaneous Ablation Technique

Percutaneous injection of alcohol is also an effective method of treating unresectable hepatic neoplasms. It appears to be most effective for hepatomas. The combination of this soft tumor in a hard, cirrhotic liver is ideal, because the alcohol infiltrates yet remains confined within the tumor. Metastases in a normal liver are more difficult to treat. Lesions measuring 3 cm or smaller are ideal, because it is possible to deliver the necessary volume of ethanol in one treatment, with the patient under conscious sedation. Larger lesions must be injected in multiple sessions, or delivered with the patient under general anesthesia for pain control. A single 1.5-cm hepatoma was ablated with percutaneous ethanol under ultrasound guidance in this patient following multiple chemoembolizations **(Figs. 42, 43)**.

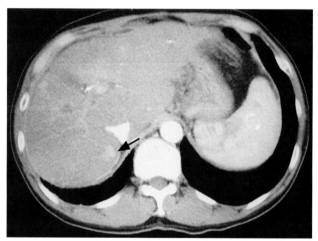

Figure 42. A small hepatoma (arrow) prior to percutaneous ethanol injection.

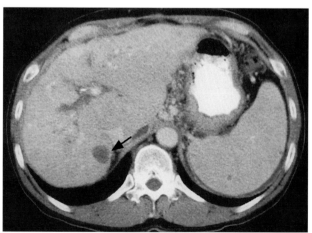

Figure 43. The same hepatoma after percutaneous ethanol ablation (arrow).

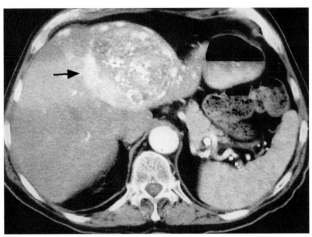

Figure 44. The CT scan 1 month after chemoembolization demonstrates viable, enhancing tumor (arrow) at the lateral margin of the Ethiodol-containing area.

Assessment of Response

After chemoembolization therapy, the presence of viable tumor can be assessed with pre- and post-contrast CT scanning, or with gadolinium-enhanced MR imaging approximately 1 month later. By this time, normal liver tissue will eliminate most of the Ethiodol, whereas tumor will generally still have Ethiodol. Tumor which has retained Ethiodol will be highly radiopaque on the CT scan. Homogeneous uptake of Ethiodol is associated with a higher degree of tumor necrosis. Tumor tissue that shows enhancement with intravenous contrast material should be considered viable, and deserves further therapy.

In this large left lobe hepatoma **(Fig. 44)**, a CT scan obtained 1 month after chemoembolization of the left hepatic artery revealed viable tumor along the right margin of the tumor due to supply from the right hepatic artery. The right hepatic artery was subsequently chemoembolized.

Recurrence

There are two forms of recurrence: regrowth of a treated lesion, and the appearance of new lesion(s). For hepatocellular carcinoma, a new lesion is the more common form of recurrence. For multicentric lesions, repeat chemoembolization is indicated. In this patient with hepatoma, the initial right lobe lesions treated with chemoembolization **(Fig. 45)** remained stable, but multiple new lesions developed, which were treated with chemoembolization **(Fig. 46)**. However, repeat chemoembolizations may cause arteritis. Chemoembolization in such vessels can lead to early stasis, and consequently, the delivery of an inadequate dose of Ethiodol. This patient initially had hepatic arteries of normal caliber **(Fig. 47)**, but after three chemoembolizations on the right, vessel caliber had markedly decreased **(Fig. 48)**. Antegrade flow ceased with less than 1 mL of Ethiodol. Percutaneous alcohol ablation or chemoembolization via collaterals are options in such cases.

Small neoplasms can receive blood supply entirely or partly from the portal vein. With growth, the arterial blood supply predominates. For this reason, small lesions may not be effectively treated by chemoembolization. This also applies to well-differentiated neoplasms, which can derive blood supply from both arterial and portal venous sources. This is probably responsible in part for the pattern of tumor recurrence. Patients must therefore be followed closely with cross-sectional imaging and appropriate tumor markers (eg carcinoembryonic antigen or alpha-fetoprotein). They can be treated again when such small lesions have grown to the point where chemoembolization can be effective.

Neoadjuvant Applications

Some solitary liver tumors are unresectable because of inadequate hepatic reserve or encroachment on critical vascular structures. Chemoembolization may cause sufficient tumor response to permit resection for cure. **Figures 49** and **50** demonstrate such a case in a 31-year-old with fibrolamellar hepatoma. At initial exploration the tumor was found to be unresectable because it was compressing the lateral segment of the left lobe. The tumor diameter decreased from 17 cm to 11 cm after chemoembolization, and resection became possible. Chemoembolization has not been shown to decrease recurrence after resection, however.

For further information on this topic, please see Teaching File Cases 45–47.

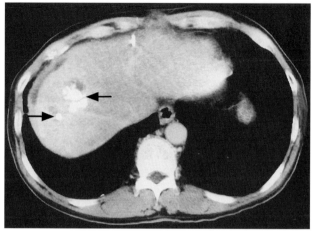

Figure 45. Multifocal hepatoma 1 month after chemoembolization (arrows).

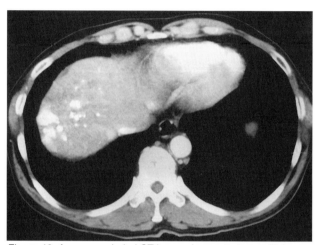

Figure 46. A more cephalad CT image demonstrates multiple new lesions which were treated with chemoembolization.

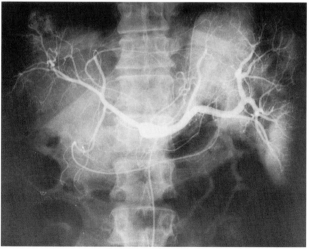

Figure 47. Celiac arteriogram demonstrates the normal caliber of the arteries prior to chemoembolization.

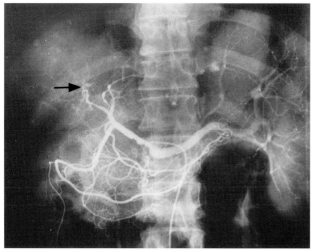

Figure 48. After three treatments, the hepatic arteries are markedly diminished in caliber (arrow).

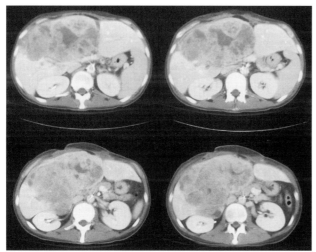

Figure 49. Prechemoembolization CT scan of a fibrolamellar hepatoma that had been deemed unresectable at exploration.

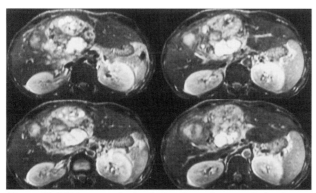

Figure 50. MR images obtained after three chemoembolizations shows partial regression of the tumor, now permitting hepatic trisegmentectomy.

Selected Readings

Bartolozzi C, Lencioni R, Caramella D, et al. Treatment of large HCC: transcatheter arterial chemoembolization combined with percutaneous ethanol injection versus repeated transcatheter arterial chemoembolization. Radiology 1995; 197:812–818.

Choi BI, Kim HC, Han JK, et al. Therapeutic effect of transcatheter oily chemoembolization therapy for encapsulated nodular hepatocellular carcinoma: CT and pathologic findings. Radiology 1992; 182:709–713.

Chung JW, Park JH, Han JK, et al. Hepatic tumors: predisposing factors for complications of transcatheter oily chemoembolization. Radiology 1996; 198:33–40.

Imaeda T, Yamawaki Y, Seki M, et al. Lipiodol retention and massive necrosis after Lipiodol-chemoembolization of hepatocellular carcinoma: correlation between computed tomography and histopathology. Cardiovasc Intervent Radiol 1993; 16:209–213.

Kan Z, Ivancev K, Lunderquist A. Peribiliary plexa—important pathways for shunting of iodized oil and silicon rubber solution from the hepatic artery to the portal vein. An experimental study in rats. Invest Radiol 1994; 29:671–676.

Kan Z, Ivancev K, Lunderquist A, et al. In vivo microscopy of hepatic tumors in animal models: a dynamic investigation of blood supply to hepatic metastases. Radiology 1993; 187:621–626.

Kim JH, Chung JW, Han JK, Park JH, Choi BI, Han MC. Transcatheter arterial embolization of the internal mammary artery in hepatocellular carcinoma. J Vasc Interv Radiol 1995; 6:71–77.

Kishi K, Sonomura T, Satoh M, et al. Acute toxicity of Lipiodol infusion into the hepatic arteries of dogs. Invest Radiol 1994; 10:882–889.

Kobayashi S, Nakanuma Y, Terada T, Matsui O. Postmortem survey of bile duct necrosis and biloma in hepatocellular carcinoma after transcatheter arterial chemo-embolization therapy: relevance to microvascular damage of peribiliary capillary plexus. Am J Gastroenterol 1993; 88:1410–1415.

Livraghi T, Lazzaroni S, Pellicano S, Ravasi S, Torzilli G, Vettori C. Percutaneous ethanol injection of hepatic tumors: single-session therapy with general anesthesia. AJR 1993; 161:1065–1069.

Miller DL. First, do no harm. Radiology 1996; 198:10–12.

Nakoa N, Kamino K, Miura K, et al. Recurrent hepatocellular carcinoma after partial hepatectomy: value of treatment with transcatheter arterial chemoembolization. AJR 1991; 156:1177–1179.

Pentecost MJ, Daniels JR, Teitelbaum GP, Stanley P. Hepatic chemoembolization: safety with portal vein thrombosis. J Vasc Interv Radiol 1993; 4:347–351.

Saitoh S, Ikeda K, Koida I, et al. Small hepatocellular carcinoma: evaluation of portal blood flow with CT during arterial portography performed with balloon occlusion of the hepatic artery. Radiology 1994; 193:67–70.

Sato M, Yamada R, Uchida B, Hedgepeth P, Rösch J. Effects of hepatic artery embolization with Lipiodol and gelatin sponge particles on normal swine liver. Cardiovasc Intervent Radiol 1993; 16:348–354.

Shiina S, Tagawa K, Niwa Y, et al. Percutaneous ethanol injection therapy for hepatocellular carcinoma: results in 146 patients. AJR 1993; 160:1023–1028.

Su YC, Chen LT, Jan CM, et al. Reappraisal of gastroduodenal lesions after transcatheter arterial chemoembolization of liver neoplasms: selective versus superselective method. J Clin Gastroenterol 1994; 18:118–121.

Takayasu K, Wakao F, Moriyama N, et al. Response of early-stage hepatocellular carcinoma and borderline lesions to therapeutic arterial embolization. AJR 1993; 160:301–306.

Ueno K, Miyazono N, Inoue H, Miyake S, Nishida H, Nakajo M. Embolization of the hepatic falciform artery to prevent supraumbilical skin rash during transcatheter arterial chemoembolization for hepatocellular carcinoma. Cardiovasc Intervent Radiol 1995; 18:183–185.

Yeung E, Jackson J, Finn JP, Thomas MG, Benjamin IS, Adam A. Acalculous cholecystitis complicating hepatic intraarterial Lipiodol: case report. Cardiovasc Intervent Radiol 1989; 12:80–82.

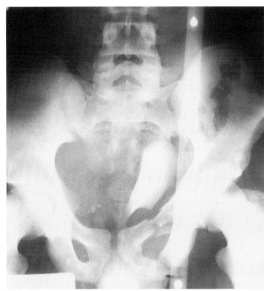

Figure 1. Pelvic fracture caused by a motor vehicle accident. Note leftward displacement of the bladder by a pelvic hematoma.

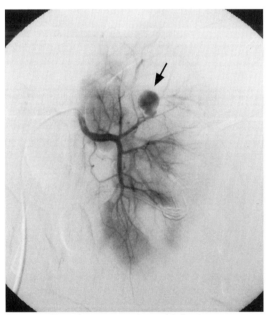

Figure 2. Pseudoaneurysm (arrow) following a percutaneous nephrostomy procedure.

TUTORIAL 18
EMBOLIZATION OF
ABDOMINAL TRAUMA
Michael D. Darcy, M.D.

Introduction

Between motor vehicle accidents **(Fig. 1)** and the increasingly common occurrence of knife- and gun-related trauma, it is not uncommon for radiologists to encounter post-traumatic bleeding. With the proliferation of "minimally invasive" procedures, iatrogenic trauma **(Fig. 2)** has also become a common cause of hemorrhage. Through diagnostic arteriography and embolotherapy, the radiologist can become an active member of the trauma team and can also manage some iatrogenic complications effectively. Since hemorrhage is a major cause of mortality in trauma patients, the radiologist must have sufficient training and understanding of embolization principles in order to perform embolotherapy quickly and efficiently. This tutorial will cover general and specific aspects of embolotherapy for abdominal trauma.

Benefits of Embolization

Embolotherapy provides several benefits in managing traumatic hemorrhage. First, bleeding can be terminated without subjecting the patient to a general anesthetic and a major operation. Embolization allows control of bleeding with minimal procedure-induced blood loss. Embolization also permits localization of bleeding sources that cannot be identified at surgery. For example, surgically opening a large pelvic retroperitoneal hematoma caused by pelvic fractures can cause massive blood loss and may not reveal the bleeding source, whereas embolotherapy can terminate bleeding **(Figs. 3, 4)** without removing the tamponading effect of the hematoma. Finally, embolization may permit greater preservation of tissue. For example, superselective renal embolization may infarct only a small percentage of a kidney **(Figs. 5–7)** whereas surgery for this same injury might lead to a heminephrectomy.

Initial Patient Evaluation

Patients must first be triaged based on their level of stability **(Fig. 8)**. A stable patient has been defined as one having a systolic blood pressure over 100 mm Hg with a pulse rate less than 110. Urine output and peripheral vasoconstriction can help gauge how well a patient is perfusing. Unstable patients are often best served by immediate surgical exploration; however, this decision needs to be made in the context of the type of injury. Although laparotomy is indicated in an unstable patient with a hepatic rupture, opening the abdomen in an unstable patient with a pelvic fracture can allow expansion of the retroperitoneal hematoma and cause the patient's condition to deteriorate. Computed tomography (CT) scanning can be used to triage the stable patient and pinpoint areas that need to be investigated **(Figs. 9, 10)**. Baron et al found that in stable patients with positive peritoneal lavages, laparotomy was avoided in 86% of cases when CT scanning and arteriography were used **(Fig. 11)**.

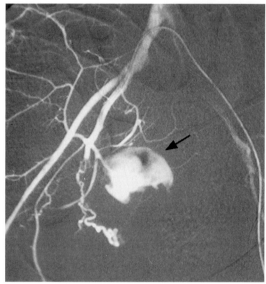

Figure 3. Massive retroperitoneal bleeding (arrow) from the right internal iliac artery in a trauma patient.

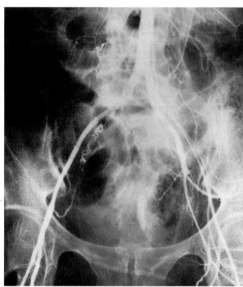

Figure 4. Postembolization image shows no extravasation.

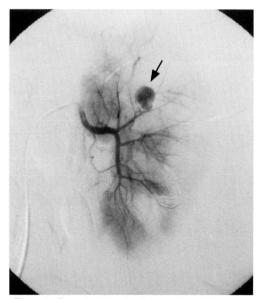

Figure 5. Pseudoaneurysm (arrow) following a percutaneous nephrostomy procedure.

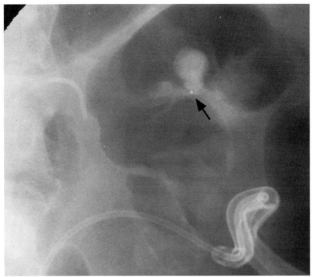

Figure 6. Same patient as in Figure 5. Microcatheter (arrow) advanced to the neck of the pseudoaneurysm.

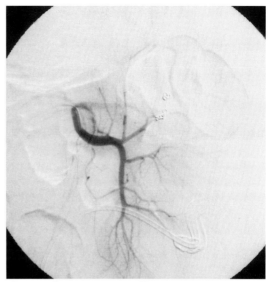

Figure 7. Same patient as in Figure 5. The post-embolization image shows minimal loss of renal parenchyma.

Triage Levels		
Level	*Patient Condition*	*Action*
1	Critically unstable	Immediate surgery
2	Unstable, but not critical	Needs surgery; rapid arteriography beneficial
3	Stable	May not need surgery

Figure 8.

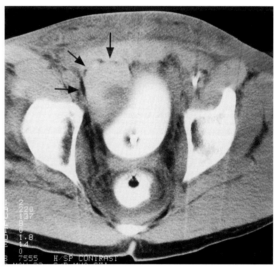

Figure 9. Right pelvic hematoma (arrows).

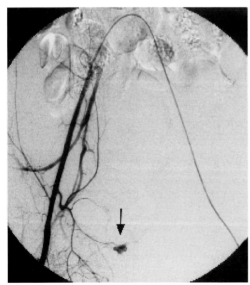

Figure 10. Injured right pelvic arterial branch (arrow).

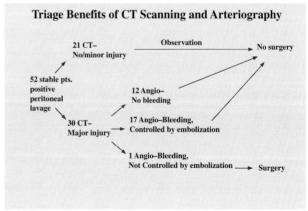

Figure 11.

291

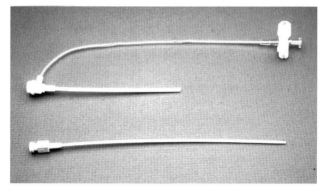
Figure 12. Vascular sheath.

Patient Preparation

Although trauma patients may not be able to provide much history, efforts should be made to determine if the patient has had prior surgery that might alter vascular anatomy, or if there are other medical conditions (eg, coronary disease) that might present problems during arteriography. Laboratory studies should be performed to determine if coagulation parameters and platelet count need to be optimized. Blood must be typed and cross-matched so that the patient can be transfused in the radiology suite to compensate for ongoing blood loss. During the embolization procedure, the patient should be fully monitored with electrocardiography, pulse oximetry, and automated blood pressure measurements. An arterial sheath **(Fig. 12)** should be placed in the access site. This not only makes it easier to perform rapid catheter exchanges but it also maintains vascular access should the angiographic catheter become obstructed by the embolic material.

Complete Arteriography

High-quality, complete arteriography is essential in order to determine the presence and extent of vascular injury. A nonselective flush aortogram is generally a good starting point for abdominal and pelvic trauma. Aside from providing a general road map for selective catheterization, an aortogram allows detection of injuries to the main arterial trunks before they are selectively catheterized. Since multiple arterial beds can be injured in severe trauma, aortography may also demonstrate associated injuries. **Figure 13** shows right renal pseudoaneurysms resulting from a car accident, but the flush aortogram **(Fig. 14)** also revealed extravasation from a lumbar artery. If no vascular injury is identified by aortography, selective studies of the most suspicious regions are indicated. This eliminates problems with vessel overlap. Additionally, the more selective injection of contrast material will make extravasation more apparent **(Figs. 15–18)**.

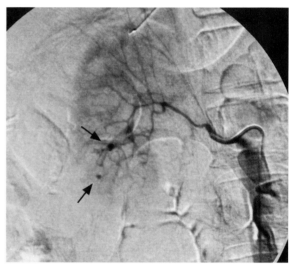
Figure 13. Lower pole renal pseudoaneurysms (arrows).

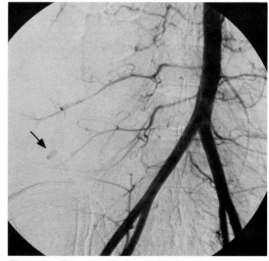
Figure 14. Extravasation from a lumbar artery (arrow).

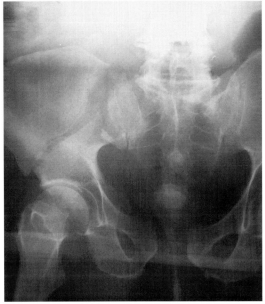

Figure 15. Pelvic fractures following a motor vehicle accident.

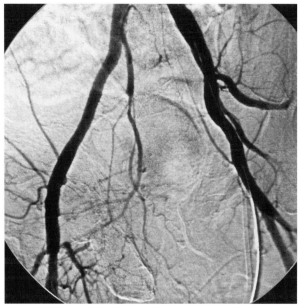

Figure 16. Nonselective study. Early phase image.

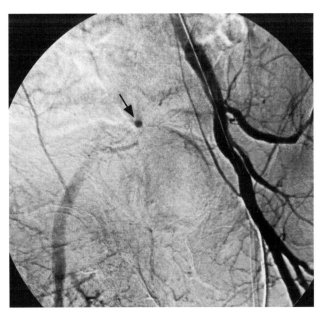

Figure 17. Later image demonstrates faint extravasation (arrow).

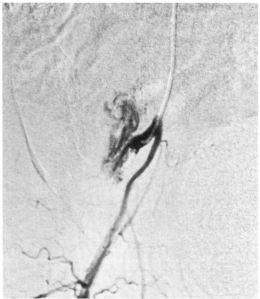

Figure 18. The extravasation is more evident on the selective internal iliac artery injection.

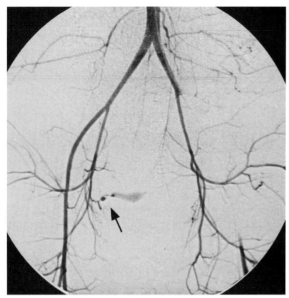

Figure 19. Injury (arrow) of the right internal iliac branch following a motor vehicle accident.

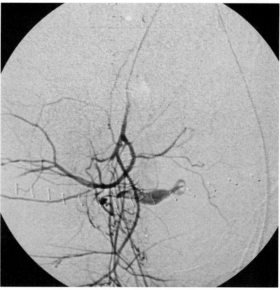

Figure 20. The arterial branch supplying the bleed is more obscured on the right posterior oblique (RPO) view.

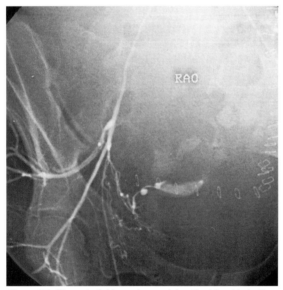

Figure 21. The arterial branch supplying the bleed is better defined on the right anterior oblique (RAO) view.

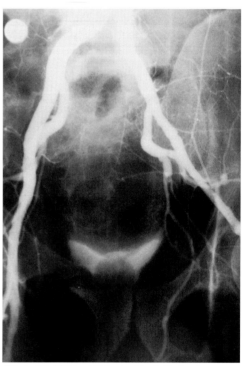

Figure 22. Motor vehicle accident. Early phase image.

Oblique views help to further define the specific site of injury. Oblique views can unravel overlapping vessels **(Figs. 19–21)** and they can also unmask subtle areas of extravasation that were hidden by bone or other densities. Film centering is always important, but with pelvic trauma the films must not be centered too cephalad, because scrotal **(Figs. 22, 23)** and other low pelvic branches can cause bleeding into the pelvis. If there is catheter-related iatrogenic bleeding in the liver or kidney, the tube itself may tamponade the bleeding and mask the injury. In order to see the vascular injury, it may be necessary to remove the tube over a guide wire just before obtaining the arteriogram to eliminate the tamponade effect **(Figs. 24–27)**.

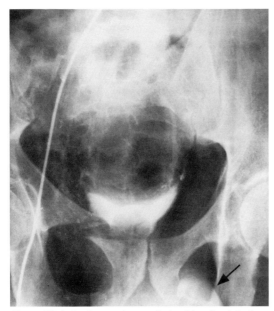

Figure 23. Later image demonstrates bleeding into the scrotum (arrow) from an internal pudendal artery injury.

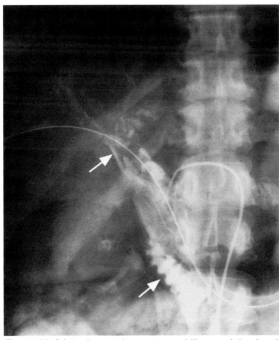

Figure 25. A later image demonstrates biliary and duodenal opacification (arrows).

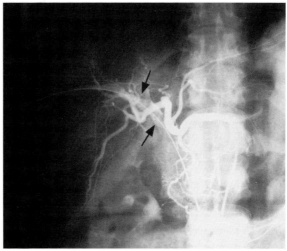

Figure 24. Hemobilia after a biliary drainage. The bile ducts (arrows) fill during hepatic arteriography.

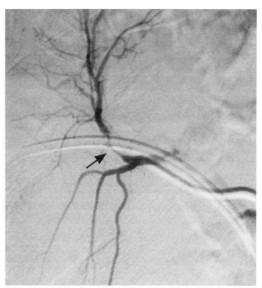

Figure 26. Selective hepatic arteriography shows arterial narrowing (arrow) but no extravasation.

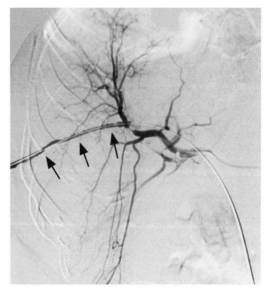

Figure 27. Arteriography with the biliary tube removed shows gross bleeding into the transhepatic track (arrows). The transhepatic guide wire remains in place during arteriography, allowing rapid replacement of the biliary catheter.

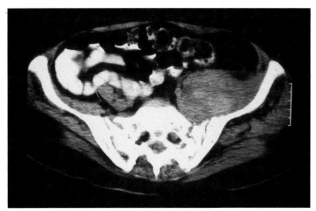

Figure 28. Left retroperitoneal hematoma following a motor vehicle accident.

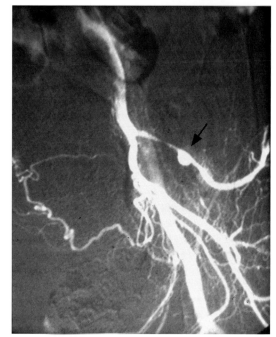

Figure 29. Magnified internal iliac arteriogram demonstrates a left superior gluteal pseudoaneurysm without extravasation (arrow).

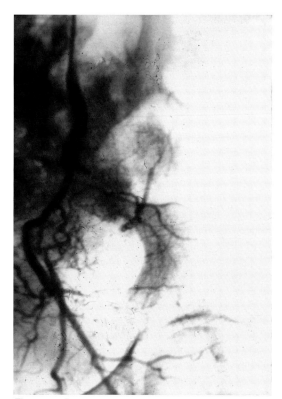

Figure 30. Postembolization film of the left superior gluteal artery.

Deciding to Embolize

What vascular injuries should be embolized? If bleeding or a potential source of bleeding is identified, embolization should be considered. A vessel with a pseudoaneurysm **(Figs. 28–30)**, or one that is transected but thrombosed, should be embolized even if there is no active extravasation, since this vessel may become a source of active bleeding after the spasm or the occluding thrombus has resolved. Whether the injured vessel can be embolized without undue risk to other tissues must also be determined. For example, this transected right internal iliac artery **(Figs. 31, 32)** could not be embolized without compromising the external iliac circulation. When contemplating embolization of a vital structure, the presence of patent collateral pathways should be evaluated in order to avoid tissue necrosis.

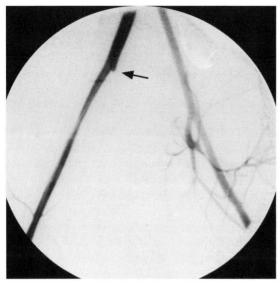

Figure 31. Transected right internal iliac artery (arrow).

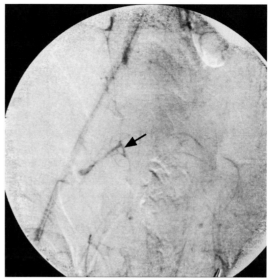

Figure 32. Later image demonstrates distal collateral reconstitution (arrow).

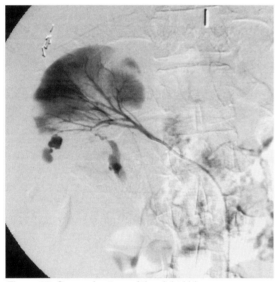

Figure 33. Severe fracture of the right kidney following a motor vehicle accident.

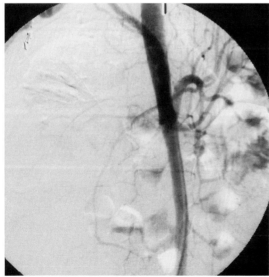

Figure 34. Postembolization film of the right renal artery.

Choosing the Level of Occlusion

With modern superselective catheter systems the ability to selectively catheterize the injured vessel is rarely an issue. The more frequent question is whether or not the vessel should be embolized selectively. Although embolization close to a point of extravasation is often desired, wider embolization (for example, a whole internal iliac artery) may be preferable if there are multiple bleeding sites or if the source of bleeding is unclear. The time required to do a superselective catheterization needs to be weighed against the need to quickly terminate bleeding in a potentially unstable patient. A realistic assessment as to whether or not the target tissue is worth preserving should also be done. **Figure 33** shows a severely fractured kidney in which selective embolization would not preserve a significant amount of functional parenchyma, so the entire renal artery was embolized **(Fig. 34)**.

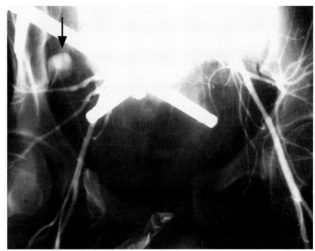
Figure 35. Right superior gluteal artery bleeding (arrow) following a pelvic fracture.

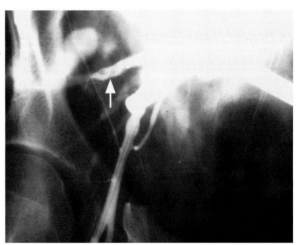
Figure 36. Continued flow into the superior gluteal artery despite coil embolization (arrow).

Embolic Agents

Gelfoam (Upjohn, Kalamazoo, MI) and coils are the most commonly used embolic agents in trauma. Alcohol or small Ivalon particles (Unipoint, High Point, NC) are usually not used because they cause tissue necrosis. Gelfoam is preferred when the goal is to ultimately have the vessel recanalize and restore perfusion to the tissue. For wide-field embolization, Gelfoam can be rapidly injected into multiple vessels. Gelfoam can also be flow-directed out to bleeding sites that cannot be reached with selective catheterization.

Coils are the best alternative in large, high-flow vessels or when precise placement of the embolic agent is needed. If coils fail to occlude the vessel **(Figs. 35, 36)**, their occlusive capabilities can be increased by soaking them in thrombin. If the injured vessel cannot be permanently sacrificed, a temporary balloon occlusion catheter can be used **(Fig. 37)**. This prevents exsanguination during preparation for surgical repair.

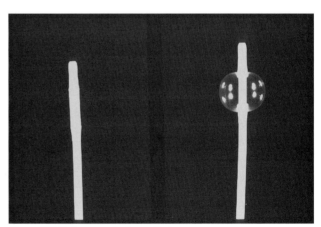
Figure 37. Balloon occlusion catheters.

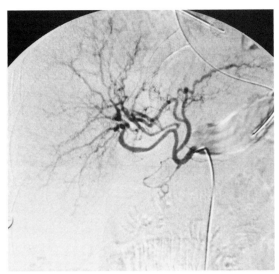

Figure 38. Hemobilia following a transjugular intrahepatic portosystemic shunting procedure.

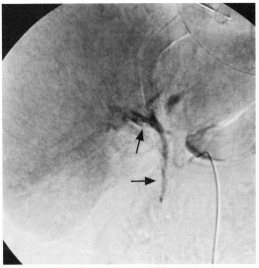

Figure 39. The bile duct (arrows) fills at hepatic arteriography.

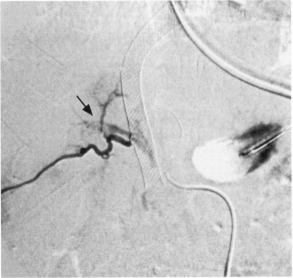

Figure 40. Superselective arteriography shows an arterial-biliary fistula (arrow).

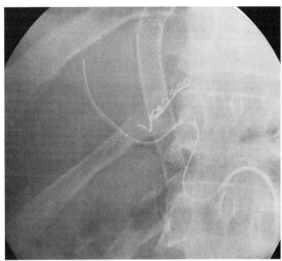

Figure 41. Superselective catheterization and microcoil embolization of the right hepatic artery with use of a coaxial microcatheter.

Methods of Delivering Embolic Agents

The equipment used to deliver embolic agents depends on the level of access needed. Standard angiographic catheters are adequate in most situations when access to the main trunk only is needed to embolize a whole arterial distribution (eg, whole internal iliac artery embolization). When embolization is performed from an arterial ostium, a balloon occlusion catheter can prevent reflux of emboli into non-target tissues. When more selective catheterization is needed, hydrophilic-coated catheters can often be advanced beyond the range of standard angiographic catheters. Superselective catheterization can be accomplished with microcatheter systems **(Figs. 38–41)** passed coaxially through standard diagnostic catheters. In patients with major bleeding, the need for rapid termination of the bleeding may outweigh the benefits of superselective catheterization.

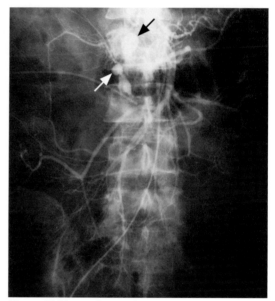

Figure 42. Traumatic pseudoaneurysms in the pancreatic head (arrows).

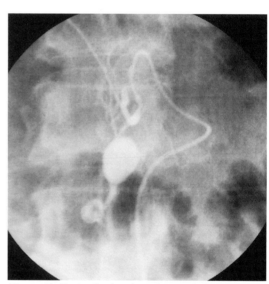

Figure 43. Gastroduodenal arteriogram before embolization.

Direct Percutaneous Puncture

Post-traumatic pseudoaneurysms may not be accessible via vascular catheterization, because of vessel tortuosity or occlusion. **Figures 42** and **43** show pseudoaneurysms in the pancreatic head that were embolized via the gastroduodenal artery (GDA). One of the pseudoaneurysms continued to fill from tiny superior mesenteric artery (SMA) branches. In this case, direct percutaneous puncture of the pseudoaneurysm provided access for embolization. The pseudoaneurysm was first opacified by SMA injections **(Figs. 44, 45)**. It was then percutaneously punctured **(Fig. 46)** with use of an 18-gauge needle. Contrast material injected through the needle confirmed the location of the needle tip **(Fig. 47)**. Coils were passed through the needle **(Fig. 48)**. Thrombin may also be injected to precipitate thrombosis. Repeat arteriography insured that the pseudoaneurysm no longer filled **(Fig. 49)**. Although there have been relatively few reports of this technique, it can yield success with low morbidity in difficult situations.

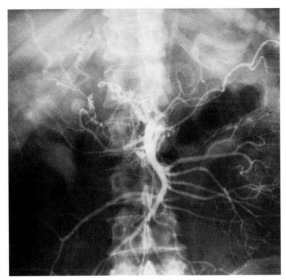

Figure 44. Postembolization film of the GDA.

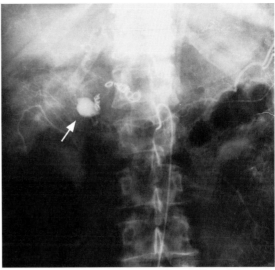

Figure 45. A later image shows continued filling of the pseudoaneurysm.

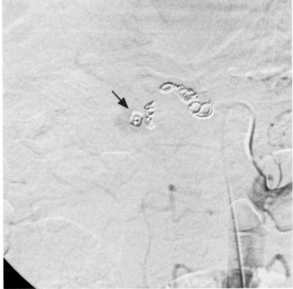

Figure 46. 18-gauge needle positioned end-on (arrow) over the pseudoaneurysm.

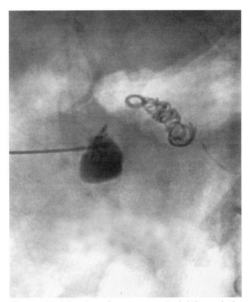

Figure 47. Injection of contrast material through the needle confirms its position in the pseudoaneurysm.

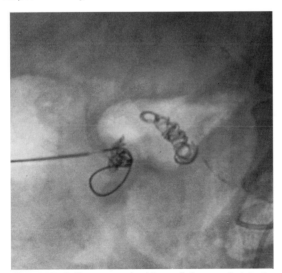

Figure 48. Coils were pushed through the needle into the pseudoaneurysm.

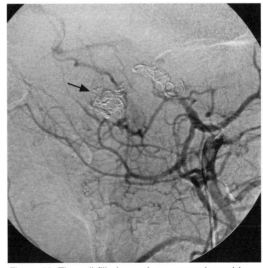

Figure 49. The coil-filled pseudoaneurysm (arrow) is thrombosed.

Postembolization Assessment

After completion of embolization, repeat arteriography is essential in order to ascertain that the vessel is effectively occluded and that collateral flow does not perfuse the injured segment. The patient must also be monitored clinically to confirm that the bleeding has stopped. This can be done by monitoring serial hematocrits and evaluating vital signs. When dealing with iatrogenic renal and biliary trauma, the output from the nephrostomy or biliary tubes can be monitored for blood. Serial CT scans or ultrasound studies may be used to evaluate for expansion of hematomas, persistent filling of pseudoaneurysms, or perfusion of an embolized organ. **Figures 50** and **51** show a fractured kidney for which the entire renal artery was embolized. A continued fall in the patient's hematocrit prompted a CT scan **(Fig. 52)**, which showed continued enhancement of the upper pole. This finding indicated collateral perfusion.

Addressing Other Problems

The success of a skillful embolization can be undermined by failure to pay attention to associated problems. Trauma patients frequently become coagulopathic very rapidly, and it is crucial to use plasma and platelet transfusions appropriately to achieve good hemostasis at the embolization site. Hypothermia also causes coagulopathy and should be corrected or prevented. The patient should be kept covered, and warmers should be used for blood or saline infusion whenever possible. Persistent blood loss may arise from concomitant venous bleeding rather than failure of the arterial embolization. This needs to be treated if possible, and, in the case of pelvic fractures, it can be effectively managed by orthopedic fixation.

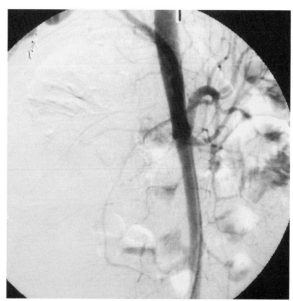

Figure 50. Severe fracture of the right kidney following a motor vehicle accident.

Figure 51. Postembolization film of the right renal artery.

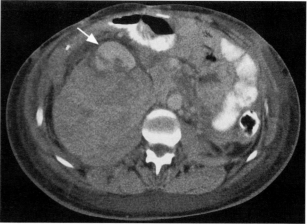

Figure 52. Right upper pole enhancement (arrow) after embolization indicates collateral perfusion.

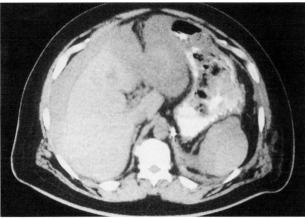
Figure 53. Splenic hematoma following a motor vehicle accident.

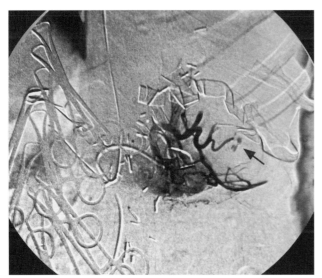
Figure 54. Extravasation from the spleen (arrow) indicating ongoing bleeding.

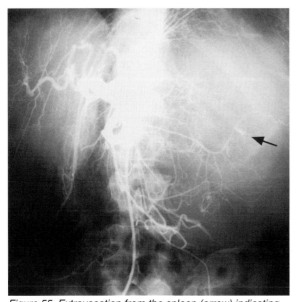
Figure 55. Extravasation from the spleen (arrow) indicating ongoing bleeding.

Splenic Trauma

In the past, splenectomy was routine for most splenic trauma; however, a conservative approach was adopted after it became apparent that these patients may develop overwhelming infections. CT scanning can demonstrate the presence of splenic trauma (Fig. 53), but it will not indicate whether there is ongoing bleeding. Arteriography is indicated when CT scanning suggests splenic injury. Extravasation of contrast material is the arteriographic finding indicating persistent bleeding (Figs. 54, 55). Mass effect (Fig. 56) or diffuse punctate enhancement of the spleen does not indicate active bleeding. The desired level of occlusion is debatable. Peripheral embolization (Figs. 57, 58) may be difficult due to splenic artery tortuosity and may also cause splenic infarction. Scalfani et al have recommended proximal embolization of the main splenic artery. This decreases the arterial pressure to the spleen but allows continued splenic perfusion via collaterals, thus preventing infarction.

Hepatic Trauma

Hepatic injury (Fig. 59) is one of main causes of mortality from abdominal trauma. The mortality of patients with liver trauma exceeds 10% and is generally due to exsanguination. Surgical therapy of hepatic trauma has been associated with mortality as high as 33%. Hepatic trauma differs from splenic or renal trauma in that the liver can not simply be removed; therefore, conservative therapy is relatively more important. Before embolization, patency of the portal vein should be determined. Superselective embolization can be done even in the face of portal occlusion, but main hepatic branch embolization in this setting would lead to excessive hepatic necrosis. Embolization is 88%–100% successful in terminating bleeding from hepatic trauma. Vessel tortuosity preventing catheterization of the injured branch is the main cause of technical failure.

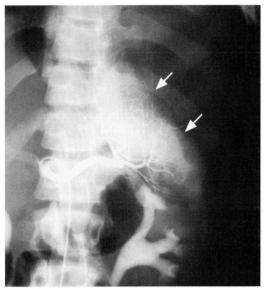

Figure 56. Splenic hematoma distorts the splenic contour without frank extravasation (arrows).

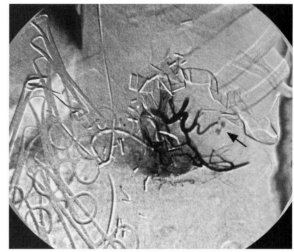

Figure 57. Pre-embolization splenic arteriogram.

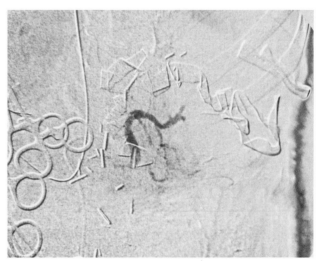

Figure 58. Postembolization splenic arteriogram.

Iatrogenic Hepatic Trauma

Hepatic arterial pseudoaneurysms caused by transhepatic biliary procedures are uncommon. They may be manifested by hemobilia, persistent bleeding through the biliary drainage tube, or bleeding out of the track during tube exchanges. One caveat is that the biliary tube itself may intermittently tamponade the bleeding. In order to obtain a correct diagnosis, arteriography may need to be performed after the biliary tube has been removed over a guide wire **(Figs. 24–27)**. It is essential to keep a guide wire across the transhepatic track so that the drainage catheter can be rapidly passed back after the arteriogram is obtained. This allows the drainage catheter to tamponade bleeding while the arterial branch is being selected for embolization. Superselective embolization with use of microcoils minimizes the arterial occlusion required. Depositing coils proximal and distal to the pseudoaneurysm is recommended to prevent backbleeding from intrahepatic collaterals.

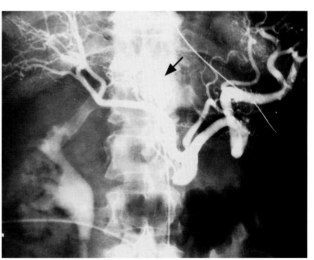

Figure 59. Post-traumatic hepatic pseudoaneurysm (arrow).

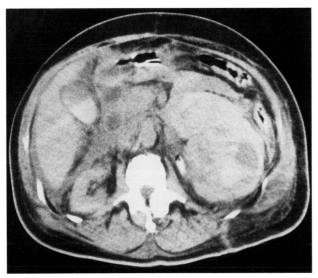

Figure 60. Left renal hematoma following nephrostomy.

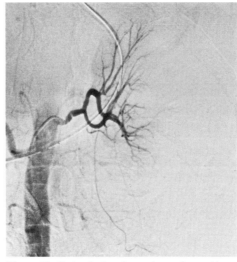

Figure 61. Abdominal aortography performed to assess renal trauma.

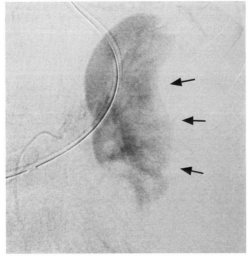

Figure 62. Mass effect (arrows) from hematoma but otherwise normal study. Part of the lower pole arteriographic nephrogram is incomplete.

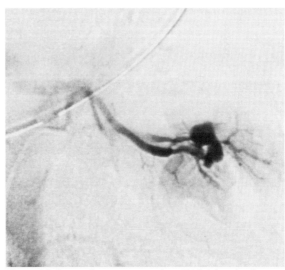

Figure 63. A pseudoaneurysm and an AV fistula arise from a separate lower pole artery.

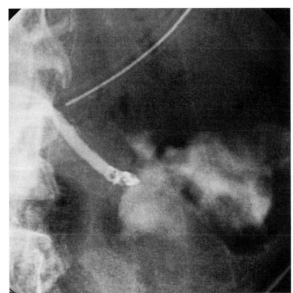

Figure 64. Postembolization arteriogram.

Renal Trauma

The degree and nature of renal damage is determined by the type of injury. Sharp penetrating trauma (knife wounds or iatrogenic injuries) often cause focal branch injuries such as pseudoaneurysms or arteriovenous (AV) fistulas with little parenchymal damage. Gun shot injuries and blunt trauma may cause more parenchymal damage. Blunt trauma can also damage the main renal artery by stretching the vascular pedicle. Abdominal aortography is a useful first step to assess the status of the main renal trunk and to ensure that accessory arteries are found **(Figs. 60–64)**. The type of embolization performed depends on the injury.

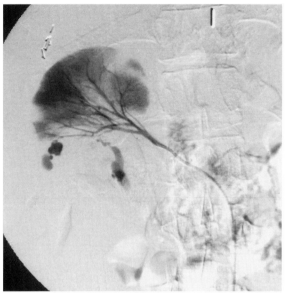

Figure 65. Severe fracture of the right kidney following a motor vehicle accident.

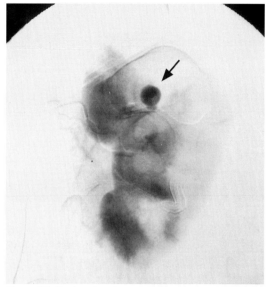

Figure 66. Postnephrostomy pseudoaneurysm (arrow).

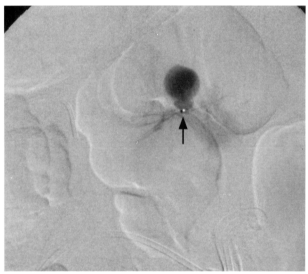

Figure 67. Microcatheter (arrow) advanced superselectively to the pseudoaneurysm.

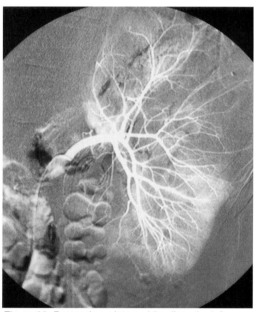

Figure 68. Postendopyelotomy bleeding; the left upper pole study shows no bleeding.

With extensive parenchymal damage and active bleeding **(Fig. 65)**, embolization of the entire kidney may be justified. Focal pseudoaneurysm and AV fistula due to iatrogenic trauma is the most common indication for renal trauma embolization. As with biliary tubes, nephrostomy tubes may also mask the injury and may need to be removed during arteriography in order to detect the injury. With focal lesions, the goal is to selectively occlude the injured branch vessel to allow greater preservation of renal tissue **(Figs. 66, 67)**. The use of 3-F catheters and microcoils is particularly helpful in this situation.

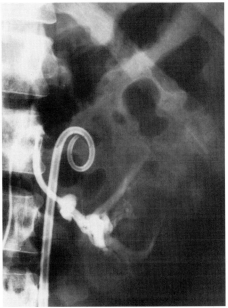

Figure 69. Selective lower pole arteriography shows a pseudoaneurysm and an arterio-venous fistula.

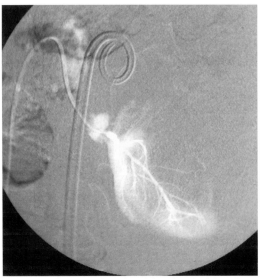

Figure 70. Catheter placed peripheral to the injury for alcohol ablation.

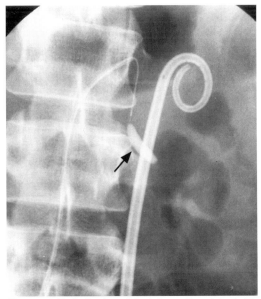

Figure 71. Embolization of the injury with a detachable balloon (arrow).

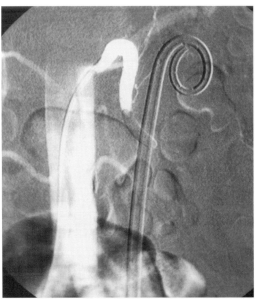

Figure 72. Postembolization left renal arteriogram with reflux into the abdominal aorta.

Although not well documented clinically, renal embolization carries the potential risk of causing hypertension due to ischemia of the tissue beyond the emboli. Alcohol ablation of the tissue beyond the vessel injury **(Figs. 68–72)** can be performed before the embolization to avoid this problem.

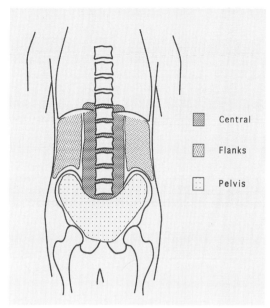

Figure 73. Zones of the retroperitoneum.

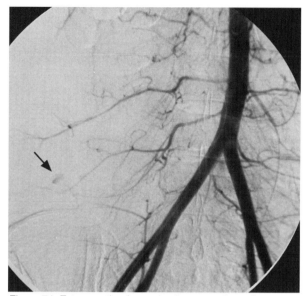

Figure 74. Extravasation from a lumbar artery (arrow).

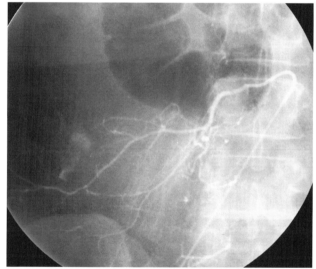

Figure 75. Improved visualization with selective injection.

Retroperitoneal Trauma

Traumatic retroperitoneal hemorrhage is a serious problem, with mortality of 18%–39%. Peritoneal lavage can be negative with hematomas contained in the retroperitoneum. CT scanning is useful for detection in these cases. Patients can be triaged based on the location of the hematomas **(Fig. 73)**. Central hematomas should be surgically explored because of the high incidence of injury to the major vascular structures in this region. Pelvic and flank hematomas should be treated arteriographically. For flank hematomas, selective catheterization of lumbar arteries **(Figs. 74, 75)** is indicated because injured lumbar arteries often opacify slowly and incompletely on nonselective studies. One must locate the artery of Adamkiewicz, which can arise from the upper lumbar arteries, and manipulate beyond its origin in order to embolize safely. Due to extensive collateral flow between lumbar branches, one may need to embolize multiple lumbar arteries. Gelfoam is the usual agent of choice for lumbar hemorrhage.

Mortality from Pelvic Fracture Based on Patient's Initial Status		
Hemodynamic Status of Patient Upon Arrival in ER	Stable	Unstable
Mortality	3.4%	42%

Figure 76.

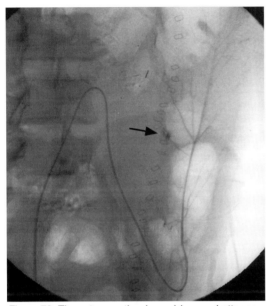

Figure 79. The extravasation (arrow) is seen better on an inferior epigastric arteriogram..

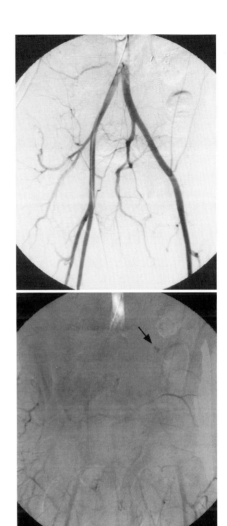

Figures 77 and 78. Faint focus of extravasation (arrow).

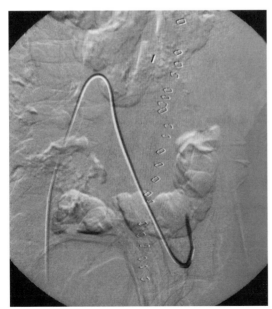

Figure 80. The postembolization film demonstrates successful arterial occlusion.

Pelvic Fractures

Patients with pelvic fractures have a high mortality, with the patient's stability upon arrival at the hospital being a key prognostic factor (Fig. 76). The type of fracture is important. Posterior disruptions of the pelvic ring are more often associated with significant vascular injury. Embolization should be attempted before surgical exploration because it can provide hemostasis without removing the tamponading effect of the pelvic hematoma. Superior gluteal, lateral sacral, and internal pudendal arteries are the most frequently injured branches. The femoral artery contralateral to the suspected injury should be used for access, since ipsilateral catheterization of these internal iliac branches can be difficult. Plain film or CT findings of fracture and hematoma location can indicate the most likely site of injury. For example, in Figures 77–80, the left inferior epigastric artery was studied because of CT findings of an anterior abdominal wall hematoma.

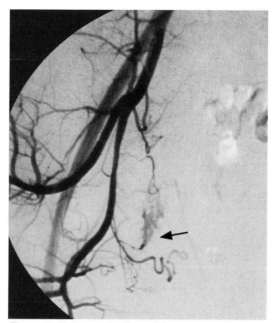

Figure 81. *Extravasation (arrow) from an anterior division branch of the internal iliac artery.*

Figure 82. *The postembolization film shows that most of the uninvolved internal iliac artery is preserved.*

Embolization for Pelvic Fractures

Selective embolization with use of 5-F or microcatheter systems can provide good hemostasis **(Figs. 81, 82)**. For multiple bleeding sites, or if the patient is unstable, embolization of the entire internal iliac artery may be warranted and can be done rapidly by flushing in Gelfoam pledgets. Embolization is superior to internal iliac artery ligation because it allows more peripheral occlusion and decreases the chance of collateral flow to the bleeding site. Success rates controlling bleeding of 87%–100% have been reported. Since bleeding after pelvic fractures is a combination of arterial, venous, and marrow bleeding, orthopedic fixation is important. Although the timing of fixation is somewhat controversial, it should probably be done after arteriography. Arteriography manages the more life-threatening arterial bleeding **(Figs. 83–86)**, whereas fixation handles lower pressure bleeding. Also, metallic fixation devices can obscure portions of the pelvis on arteriography.

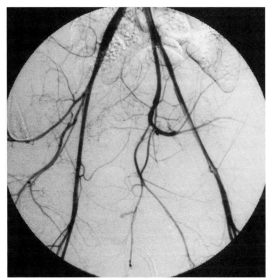

Figures 83. Pelvic bleeding following a motor vehicle accident.

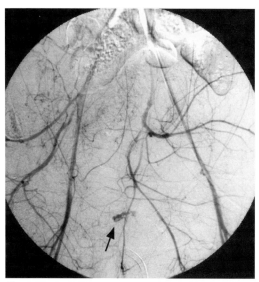

Figure 84. Later image demonstrates contrast material extravasation (arrow).

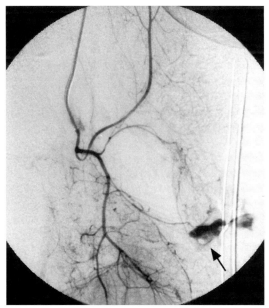

Figure 85. Active bleeding (arrow) from an obturator artery branch.

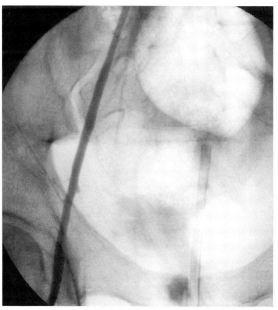

Figure 86. Postembolization arteriogram.

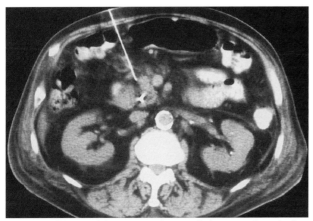

Figure 87. Biopsy of the pancreatic mass led to gastrointestinal hemorrhage.

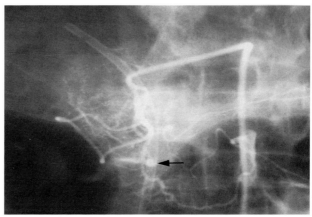

Figure 88. Gastroduodenal arteriogram shows gross bleeding (arrows).

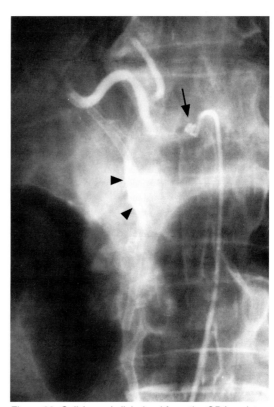

Figure 89. Coil (arrow) dislodged from the GDA up into the proper hepatic artery. The contrast material extravasation from the earlier GDA arteriogram remains visible (arrowheads).

Complications

Aside from the usual arteriographic complications (groin hematomas, etc) there are several complications unique to embolotherapy. Significant tissue necrosis is a very rare complication, with only a few case reports in the literature. Bladder necrosis after internal iliac artery embolization has been described. Sacral plexus nerve injury and impotence are two other uncommon problems seen after embolization therapy. Since the bony fractures themselves can cause these problems, it is difficult to determine when the embolization is the actual cause of these problems. Non-target embolization **(Figs. 87–89)** is another rare complication that can generally be avoided by paying careful attention to embolization technique. However, the need to treat life-threatening hemorrhage generally outweighs the small risk of these complications.

For further information on this topic, please see Teaching File Cases 15, 16, 60–63, and 67–69.

Selected Readings

Baron BJ, Scalea TM, Sclafani SJ, et al. Nonoperative management of blunt abdominal trauma: the role of sequential diagnostic peritoneal lavage, computed tomography, and angiography. Ann Emerg Med 1993; 22:1556–1562.

Ben-Menachem Y. Embolotherapy in pelvic trauma. In: Neal MP, Tisnado J, Cho SR, eds. Emergency interventional radiology. Boston: Little, Brown and Company, 1989; 91–106.

Ben-Menachem Y. Logic and logistics of radiography, angiography, and angiographic intervention in massive blunt trauma. Radiol Clin North Am 1981; 19:9–15.

Croce MA, Fabian TC, Spiers JP, Kudsk KA. Traumatic hepatic artery pseudoaneurysm with hemobilia. Am J Surg 1994; 168:235–238.

Goins WA, Rodriguez A, Lewis J, Brathwaite CE, James E. Retroperitoneal hematoma after blunt trauma. Surg Gynecol Obstet 1992; 174:281–290.

Hashimoto S, Hiramatsu K, Ido K, Yosii H, Motegi M, Yamamoto S. Expanding role of emergency embolization in the management of severe blunt hepatic trauma. Cardiovasc Intervent Radiol 1990; 13:193–199.

Matalon TS, Athanasoulis CA, Margolies MN, et al. Hemorrhage with pelvic fractures: efficacy of transcatheter embolization. AJR 1979; 133:859–864.

McLean GK, Stein EJ, Burke DR, Meranze SG. Steel occlusion coils: pretreatment with thrombin. Radiology 1986; 158:549–550.

Mucha P, Farnell MB. Analysis of pelvic fracture management. J Trauma 1984; 24:379–386.

Panetta T, Sclafani SJ, Goldstein AS, Phillips TF, Shaftan GW. Percutaneous transcatheter embolization for massive bleeding from pelvic fractures. J Trauma 1985; 25:1021–1029.

Routh WD, Tatum CM, Lawdahl RB, Rösch J, Keller FS. Tube tamponade: potential pitfall in angiography of arterial hemorrhage associated with percutaneous drainage catheters. Radiology 1990; 174:945–949.

Schwartz RA, Teitelbaum GP, Katz MD, Pentecost MJ. Effectiveness of transcatheter embolization in the control of hepatic vascular injuries. J Vasc Interv Radiol 1993; 4:359–65.

Sclafani SJ, Ben-Menachem Y. Embolotherapy in abdominal trauma. In: Neal MP, Tisnado J, Cho SR, eds. Emergency interventional radiology. Boston: Little, Brown and Company, 1989; 53–77.

Sclafani SJ, Florence LO, Phillips TF, et al. Lumbar arterial injury: radiologic diagnosis and management. Radiology 1987; 165:709–714.

Sclafani SJ, Weisberg A, Scalea TM, Phillips TF, Duncan AO. Blunt splenic injuries: nonsurgical treatment with CT, arteriography, and transcatheter arterial embolization of the splenic artery. Radiology 1991; 181:189–196.

Sieber PR. Bladder necrosis secondary to pelvic artery embolization: case report and literature review. J Urol 1994; 151:422.

TUTORIAL 19
DIAGNOSIS AND MANAGEMENT OF ARTERIOVENOUS MALFORMATIONS
Wayne F. Yakes, M.D.

Introduction

The subjects addressed in this tutorial include:
1. Classification of vascular malformations
2. Arteriographic evaluation of arteriovenous malformations
3. Indications for treatment of arteriovenous malformations
4. Ethanol endovascular management of arteriovenous malformations.

Introduction

Vascular malformations constitute some of the most difficult diagnostic and therapeutic enigmas that can be encountered in the practice of medicine. Arteriovenous malformations (AVMs) were first treated by surgeons. Proximal arterial ligation proved futile because neovascular recruitment reconstituted inflow to the AVM and worsened the clinical symptoms. Complete surgical removal of an AVM was very hazardous, so suboptimal partial resections were done. Because of the significant blood loss during surgery, embolotherapy became a useful preoperative adjunct; however, complete surgical extirpation of an AVM was still only rarely possible. In many cases, AVMs are in anatomically and surgically difficult or inaccessible areas. This has led to increased reliance on embolotherapy in the management of these patients. It must be plainly stated that radiation therapy (radiosurgery) has no role in the management of peripheral AVMs. The only role for radiosurgery is in treating small AVMs of the brain.

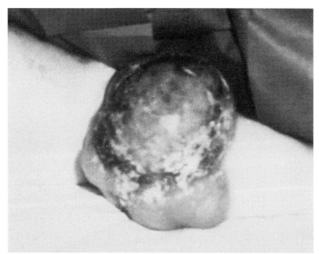

Figure 1. Hemorrhaging hemangioma of the left anterior thigh in a 4-month-old male.

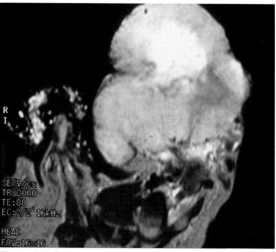

Figure 2. A T2-weighted magnetic resonance image shows increased signal in the mass consistent with hemangioma. Note the flow voids of the arteries and outflow veins within the mass.

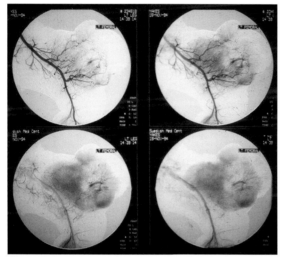

Figure 3. Left common femoral artery digital subtraction arteriogram. Note vascularity to the anterior thigh mass.

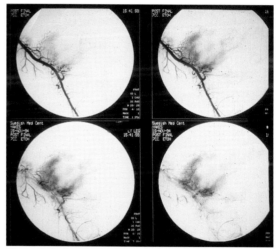

Figure 4. Left common femoral artery digital subtraction arteriogram after ethanol embolization. Note the devascularized portions of the tumor. The patient subsequently underwent surgical excision of the hemangioma.

Classification of Vascular Malformations and Hemangiomas

Pediatric hemangiomas are vascular tumors that manifest within the first month of life and exhibit a rapid growth phase in the first year. These tumors spontaneously regress to complete resolution by 7 years of age. Hemangiomas occur with a reported incidence of 1%–2.6%. Because of their natural history of spontaneous involution, hemangiomas rarely require treatment. When treatment is required for whatever reason, systemic steroid management and, failing this, alpha-interferon therapy can be employed. As a last resort, embolization with surgical resection is an option as well **(Figs. 1–4)**. Hemangiomas can be confused with AVMs in neonates. However, AVMs do not respond to steroid or alpha interferon management. Thus, it is important to distinguish between these two entities when evaluating the newborn patient with congestive heart failure secondary to a shunting vascular lesion.

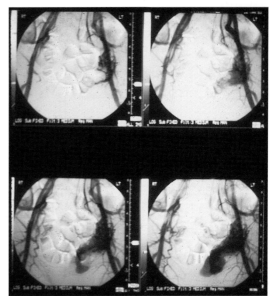

Figure 5. The anteroposterior (AP) digital subtraction arteriogram of the pelvis shows a left pelvic AVM shunting into the internal iliac veins.

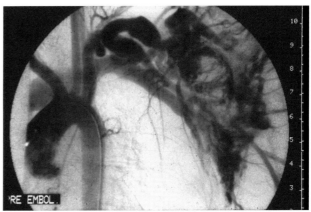

Figure 6. The right anterior oblique (RAO) digital subtraction arteriogram of the aortic arch shows a massive left shoulder AVM largely supplied by the left subclavian artery.

Arteriovenous Malformations

AVMs are congenital lesions typified by hypertrophied inflow arteries shunting through a nidus, and tortuous dilated outflow veins **(Figs. 5, 6)**. No intervening capillary bed is present. AVMs are high-flow lesions that demonstrate a shunt into a low-pressure venous system. Symptoms are usually related to the anatomic location of the AVM. Presenting symptoms can include pain, tissue ulceration, impairment of limb or organ function, hemorrhage, nerve deterioration or palsy, limiting claudication, and high-output cardiac consequences. When calculating hemodynamic parameters, most patients do demonstrate some element of increased cardiac output, increased cardiac index, and abnormally lowered systemic vascular resistance. AVMs may occur anywhere in the body and central nervous system.

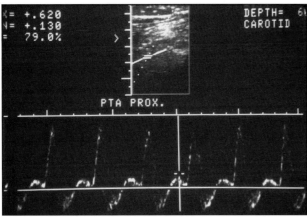

Figure 7. Spectral analysis shows a normal wave form consistent with normal systemic vascular resistance.

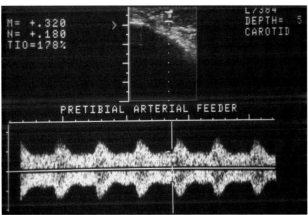

Figure 8. Spectral analysis shows an abnormal wave form consistent with lowered systemic vascular resistance because of arteriovenous shunting.

Baseline Work-up

The baseline imaging work-up prior to any therapy includes extensive arteriography, color Doppler imaging (CDI), and magnetic resonance (MR) scanning. Selective and superselective arteriography defines the angioarchitecture of the AVM and identifies dangerous anastomoses to normal structures, aneurysms within the lesion, the routes of venous drainage, and the potential routes for access for endosurgical ethanol ablative therapy. Furthermore, the baseline studies can be compared to follow-up studies to evaluate the efficacy of therapy. CDI is very useful in the baseline work-up as well as in follow-up. The most important parameters to evaluate are spectral analysis and calculated flow volume rates. Other parameters are helpful as well. Spectral analysis permits visualization of the wave form in order to determine if abnormally low resistance in the artery is present suggestive of arteriovenous shunting **(Figs. 7, 8)**. Calculated vascular flow volumes are important in the initial work-up because they can be compared to calculated flow volumes after therapy to document the decreased arteriovenous shunting.

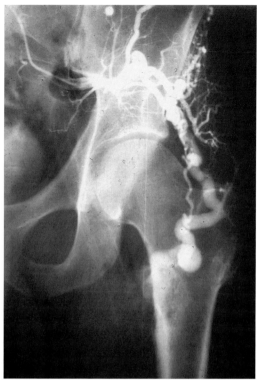

Figure 9. Digital subtraction arteriogram (AP view) of the left superior gluteal artery demonstrates a nonocclusive coil in a tortuous branch to an anterior thigh AVM.

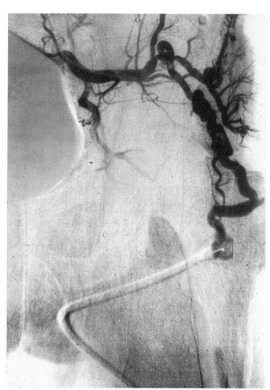

Figure 10. Direct puncture technique was used to circumvent catheterization obstacles and superselectively deliver ethanol into the AVM nidus. Note the absence of antegrade flow to the AVM.

Embolic Agents

Many embolic agents have been used to treat AVMs. Most agents can provide excellent palliation; however, follow-up procedures are usually required as recanalization and neovascular recruitment cause renewed symptoms. Arterial recanalization and neovascular recruitment are well-recognized phenomena occuring after the use of polyvinyl alcohol particles, metallic coils, Gelfoam (Upjohn, Kalamazoo, MI), acrylic tissue adhesives, and the like.

With the use of absolute ethanol, permanent occlusions have been documented at long-term follow-up, and the phenomena of vascular recanalization and neovascular recruitment have not been observed. However, ethanol is one of the most dangerous embolic agents that can be placed into the vascular tree, and significant skills in embolotherapy are required if use of ethanol is contemplated.

Superselective catheter placement in the AVM nidus itself is absolutely essential. When transcatheter techniques are impossible due to previous ligations or tortuosity, direct percutaneous puncture techniques can be used to circumvent catheterization obstacles **(Figs. 9–11)**. When superselective catheterization of the AVM nidus is not possible, the use of ethanol must be avoided. Inflow occlusion to achieve vascular stasis and maximize the thrombogenic effects of ethanol can be very helpful. The amount of ethanol used is titrated to the flow-volume characteristics of the AVM compartment being embolized.

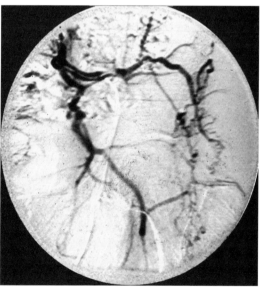

Figure 11. Digital subtraction arteriography (AP view) of the left superior gluteal artery at 2-year follow-up shows AVM occlusion.

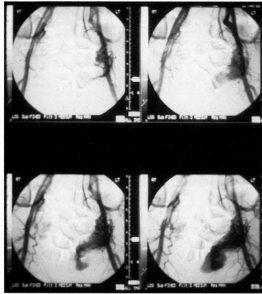

Figure 12. Pelvic arteriogram (AP view) shows a left pelvic AVM in a 40-year-old female which is causing pain.

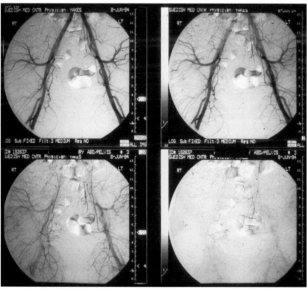

Figure 13. Pelvic arteriogram (AP view) shows cure of the AVM at 2-year follow-up with resolution of pain.

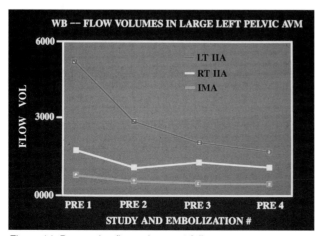

Figure 14. Decreasing flow volumes at follow-up.

Caveats on Ethanol Use

Because ethanol embolization can be extremely painful, some form of anesthesia is required. Intravenous sedation with a neuroleptic agent can be performed, but we prefer to use general anesthesia at our institution. Many patients presenting with AVMs are in the pediatric age group, so intravenous sedation is usually inadequate. Further, in larger lesions where larger amounts of ethanol may be used, a Swan-Ganz catheter and arterial line should be placed for monitoring and emergent management. A rare complication related to ethanol-induced pulmonary artery spasm is cardiopulmonary collapse. If a patient is already intubated and Swan-Ganz and arterial lines are in place, this complication can be managed adequately.

Ethanol Embolotherapy

AVMs can infiltrate multiple tissues and develop along major neurovascular distributions. Because of this, total surgical excision can cause severe morbidity and is therefore impossible in most cases. With superselective ethanol embolotherapy, the abnormal vascular elements can be obliterated while the normal vascular structures are maintained.

Absolute ethanol consistently affords a level of permanence in AVM occlusion that is seldom encountered with other agents. This is probably related to several factors. Ethanol, in and of itself, will cause thrombosis upon contact with various blood proteins. More importantly, ethanol completely destroys the endothelial cells lining the arterial wall and precipitates their protoplasm. Further, the vascular wall is fractured to the level of the internal elastic lamina. With the endothelial cell layer destroyed, angiogenesis factors stimulating neovascular recruitment and vascular recanalizations do not occur.

All other embolic agents merely form a plug within the vessel and do not affect the endothelium. This is the main reason that these other embolic agents usually provide only palliation of these lesions and seldom cure them.

Long-term Follow-up

The immediate result in AVM management is of no importance; what matters is the long-term result. Follow-up arteriography, CDI, and MR imaging are required, as well as clinic visits, to determine the efficacy of therapy. Long-term follow-up with arteriography is an invasive measure which is still required at this time (**Figs. 12–20**). CDI and MR imaging are important noninvasive modalities that may replace arteriography as a follow-up study. This possibility is currently being evaluated.

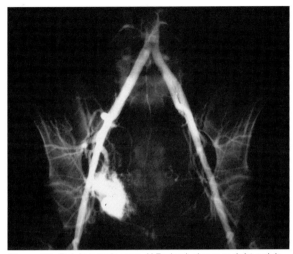

Figure 15. Pelvic arteriogram (AP view) shows a right pelvic AVM.

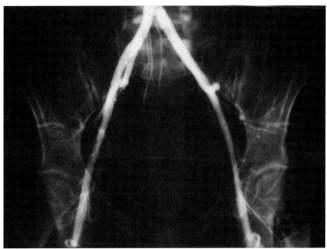

Figure 16. Pelvic arteriogram (AP view) at 3-year follow-up. Note the absence of the AVM.

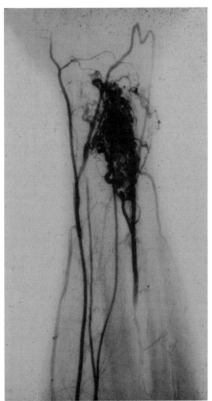

Figure 17. The left hand arteriogram (AP view) shows an AVM on the dorsal aspect of the wrist.

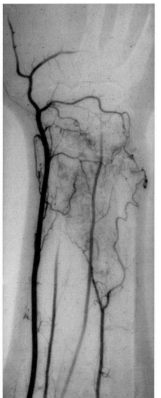

Figure 18. The left hand arteriogram (AP view) 4 months after embolization, documents AVM occlusion. At 7-year follow-up, no pain was present. No AVM recurrence was noted by CDI and clinical examination.

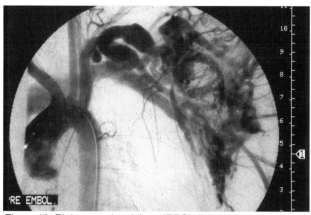

Figure 19. Right posterior oblique (RPO) digital subtraction arteriogram shows a massive left shoulder AVM.

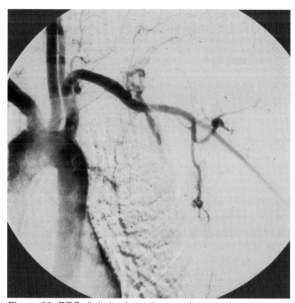

Figure 20. RPO digital subtraction arteriogram shows obliteration of the left shoulder AVM at 2-year follow-up.

Complications

A complication rate of 10% has been observed in our patient series. This includes all complications for AVMs in all anatomic locations. Complications such as tissue necrosis and neuropathy have been encountered. Because skin necrosis can occur, good wound care must be maintained to prevent superimposed infection and allow the tissues to heal. Sensory and motor nerve injuries can occur, although it is uncommon for a nerve injury to be permanent. The majority of these injuries recover to some degree over a period of several months or more.

Summary

Pediatric hemangiomas and AVMs pose some of the most significant challenges in the practice of medicine today. Clinical manifestations of these lesions are extremely variable, and attributing these symptoms to an AVM can be difficult for even the most experienced clinician. The rarity of these lesions augments the enormity of the problem because few people will ever gain enough experience to treat these lesions effectively. Patients with AVMs should be referred to centers where vascular malformations and the dilemmas they present are routinely managed. Only in this fashion can significant experience be gained, improved judgment in managing these lesions and the complications that occur develop, and definitive statements concerning their treatment evolve.

Selected Readings

Boxt LM, Levin DC, Fellows KE. Direct puncture angiography in congenital venous malformations. AJR 1983; 140:135–136.

Finn MC, Glowacki J, Mulliken JB. Congenital vascular lesions: clinical application of a new classification. J Pediatr Surg 1983; 18:894–900.

Geiser JH, Eversmann WW. Closed system venography in the evaluation of upper extremity hemangioma. J Hand Surg 1978; 3:173–178.

Glowacki J, Mulliken JB. Mast cells in hemangiomas and vascular malformations. Pediatrics 1982; 70:48–51.

Heiss JD, Doppman JL, Oldfield EH. Brief report: relief of spinal cord compression from vertebral hemangioma by intralesional injection of absolute ethanol. New Engl J Med 1994; 331:508–511.

Meyer JS, Hoffer FA, Barnes PD, Mulliken JB. Biological classification of soft-tissue vascular anomalies: MR correlation. AJR 1991; 157:559–564.

Mulliken JB, Glowacki J. Hemangiomas and vascular malformations in infants and children: a classification based on endothelial characteristics. Plast Reconstr Surg 1982; 69:412–420.

Mulliken JB, Young AE, eds. Vascular birthmarks: hemangiomas and malformations. Philadelphia: W.B. Saunders Company, 1988.

Mulliken JB, Zetter BR, Folkman J. In vitro characteristics of endothelium from hemangiomas and vascular malformations. Surgery 1982; 92:348–353.

Rak KM, Yakes WF, Ray RL, et al. MR imaging of symptomatic peripheral vascular malformations. AJR 1992; 159:107–112.

Reid MR. Studies on abnormal arteriovenous communications, acquired and congenital. I. Report of a series of cases. Arch Surg 1925; 10:601–638.

Upton J, Mulliken JB, Murray JE. Classification and rationale for management of vascular anomalies in the upper extremity. J Hand Surg 1985; 6:970–975.

Yakes WF. Extremity venous malformations: diagnosis and management. Semin Intervent Radiol 1994; 11:332–339.

Yakes WF, Haas DK, Parker SH, et al. Symptomatic vascular malformations: ethanol embolotherapy. Radiology 1989; 170:1059–1066.

Yakes WF, Luethke JM, Merland JJ, et al. Ethanol embolization of arteriovenous fistulas: a primary mode of therapy. J Vasc Interv Radiol 1990; 1:89–96.

Yakes WF, Luethke JM, Parker SH, et al. Ethanol embolization of vascular malformations. Radiographics 1990; 10:787–796.

Yakes WF, Parker SH. Diagnosis and management of vascular anomalies. In: Castaneda-Zuniga WR, Tadavarthy SM, eds. Interventional radiology. 2nd edition. Baltimore: Williams and Wilkins, 1992.

Yakes WF, Parker SH, Gibson MD, et al. Alcohol embolotherapy of vascular malformations. Semin Intervent Radiol 1989; 6:146–161.

Yakes WF, Pevsner P, Reed M, Donohue HJ, Ghaed N. Serial embolizations of an extremity arteriovenous malformation with alcohol via direct percutaneous puncture. AJR 1986; 146:1038–1040.

Yakes WF, Stavros AT, Parker SH, et al. Color Doppler imaging of peripheral high-flow vascular malformations pre and post ethanol embolo-therapy. Program of the 76th Scientific Assembly of the Radiological Society of North America. Chicago, IL 1990; 177:156.

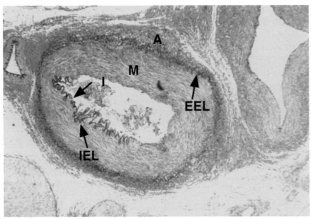

Figure 1. Histologic section of a small arteriole. I=intima; IEL=internal elastic lamina; M=media; EEL=external elastic lamina; A=adventitia.

TUTORIAL 20
SYSTEMIC VASCULITIDES

Donald L. Miller, M.D.,
Patricia E. Cole, Ph.D., M.D.,
Ian A. Sproat, M.D., FRCP(C), and
David M. Williams, M.D.

Introduction

The subjects addressed in this tutorial include:
1. Histology of the normal arterial wall
2. Schemes for classifying vasculitides
3. Clinical features, histopathology, and arteriographic findings of the more important vasculitides.

The vasculitides are uncommon disorders which produce inflammation of the walls of arteries or veins. These diseases may produce stenoses, occlusions, dissections, aneurysms or pseudoaneurysms. The arteriographic appearance of these disorders overlaps to some degree, but characteristic arteriographic features are often helpful in establishing a diagnosis.

The Normal Arterial Wall

The walls of all arteries and veins have three basic layers: the intima, the media, and the adventitia **(Fig. 1)**. The intima consists of a single layer of endothelial cells overlying a basement membrane and a layer of subendothelial connective tissue. The endothelial cell layer forms the luminal surface of the vessel, while the subendothelial connective tissue extends outward to the internal elastic lamina (IEL). The IEL is the dividing line between the intima and the media. The media extends outward from the outer surface of the IEL to the external elastic lamina (EEL), and consists of smooth muscle cells (SMC) and a connective tissue matrix with collagen fibrils and elastic fibers. The adventitia is the outer layer of the vessel wall, and contains nutrient blood vessels (the vasa vasorum), nerve fibers, and lymphatic channels.

Figure 2.

Types of Arteries

Three types of arteries are recognized. Elastic arteries are the largest in diameter (aorta, iliac arteries). They have the largest number of elastic fibers, which help maintain hydrostatic pressure due to recoil during diastole. Muscular arteries, such as the coronary, visceral, and peripheral arteries, regulate blood distribution. They have more SMCs and less elastic tissue than elastic arteries. Arterioles are the smallest in diameter. They regulate vascular tone and peripheral vascular resistance. Vasculitides usually affect only one or perhaps two of these artery types.

Classification Schemes for the Arteritides

There is no generally agreed upon classification scheme for the arteritides. These diseases have been grouped by etiology, by the nature of the underlying immunologic process, and by angiographic appearance. It is often convenient to classify arteritides based on the size of the artery most commonly involved. Large-vessel arteritides **(Fig. 2)** involve the aorta or its major branches. Small- and medium-vessel arteritides **(Fig. 3)** involve more peripheral branches of these arteries. Affected "small" arteries are large enough to be visible on arteriograms. Arteritides rarely involve both large and small vessels in the same patient. Many arteritides, such as Wegener's granulomatosis, principally produce lesions in vessels so small that they are not visible angiographically. These disorders are excluded from this classification.

Etiologic Classification of the Arteritides

Another common classification of arteritides is etiologic **(Fig. 4)**. While many of the arteritides are secondary to a well-defined disease process, others are idiopathic. Because recognition of the angiographic appearance of an idiopathic arteritis is often crucial for diagnosis, it is important to be familiar with these uncommon disorders. In this tutorial, the arteritides are grouped as either idiopathic or secondary, and are discussed in the order shown in **Figure 4**.

Angiographic Classification of Arteritis— Small- and Medium-Vessel Arteritides
Polyarteritis nodosa Buerger's disease (thromboangiitis obliterans) Kawasaki's disease Substance abuse vasculitis Arteritis associated with collagen-vascular disease Infection-related arteritis

Figure 3.

Etiologic Classification of Arteritis

Idiopathic Arteritides
    Polyarteritis nodosa
    Giant cell arteritides
        Takayasu's arteritis
        Temporal arteritis ("giant cell arteritis")
    Buerger's disease (thromboangiitis obliterans)
    Behçet's disease
 	
Secondary Arteritides
    Infection-related arteritis
    Vasculitis in collagen-vascular diseases—systemic lupus erythematosus, rheumatoid arthritis, scleroderma, ankylosing spondylitis, Reiter's syndrome, relapsing polychondritis, Sjögren's syndrome, dermatomyositis/polymyositis
    Substance-abuse vasculitis
    Kawasaki's disease
    Renal transplant vasculitis

Figure 4.

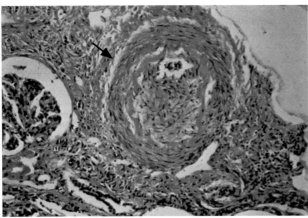

Figure 5. Healing polyarteritis in a renal arteriole (arrow). There is wall thickening and intimal fibrosis with clearing of inflammatory infiltrate. The lumen is nearly obliterated.

Polyarteritis Nodosa

Polyarteritis nodosa (PAN) is a rare disease (two cases/million/year) that affects medium and small arteries. It has a peak onset in the fifth decade of life and a male:female ratio of 2.5:1. Lesions are focal and segmental, with a predilection for vessel bifurcations. Its protean clinical manifestations reflect widely variable patterns of organ involvement. Systemic symptoms include fever, weight loss, and malaise. Renal abnormalities (hypertension, proteinuria, hematuria) are present in 70% of patients, musculoskeletal symptoms (myalgias, arthralgias) are present in 65% of patients, and gastrointestinal symptoms (pain, bleeding, bowel infarction) are observed in 45% of patients. The skin, heart, and central nervous system may also be involved.

Pathology of Polyarteritis Nodosa

Polyarteritis nodosa is a systemic, necrotizing vasculitis which progresses through three distinct histologic stages: acute, reparative, and chronic. All three stages commonly coexist in different portions of the same vessel. In the acute phase, polymorphonuclear leukocytes are seen throughout the arterial wall. The elastic lamina is destroyed and the media undergoes fibrinoid necrosis, characterized by fusion of the smooth muscle of the media and adjacent tissues into an amorphous, eosinophilic mass which stains for fibrin. Microaneurysms arise from weakened, necrotic portions of the arterial wall in the late acute phase. Small arteries may thrombose. In the reparative and chronic stages, fibroblast proliferation in the media and intima leads to wall thickening, narrowing of the lumen, and the development of acellular scar tissue. This results in fibro-obliterative occlusion and late ischemia **(Fig. 5)**.

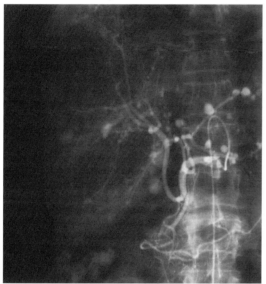

Figure 6. Common hepatic arteriogram in this 61-year-old female with polyarteritis nodosa demonstrates extensive, 1–12 mm saccular aneurysms of the hepatic, dorsal pancreatic, and pancreaticoduodenal arteries. Note scalloping of the liver edge and intraparenchymal lucency from subcapsular and intraparenchymal hemorrhage, respectively.

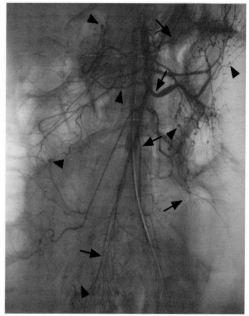

Figure 7. Polyarteritis nodosa. Superior mesenteric arteriogram in a 27-year-old male with abdominal pain. There are numerous microaneurysms characteristic of PAN (arrowheads) with multiple stenoses in both proximal and distal branches (arrows).

Arteriographic Findings in Polyarteritis Nodosa

Arteriographically, the hepatic (60%), renal (47%), and mesenteric (38%) artery territories are most commonly affected **(Figs. 6–11)**. The arteriographic characteristics of PAN are microaneurysms and stenoses or occlusions of small arteries. Microaneurysms are the arteriographic hallmark of the disease, but they are not always present, and they are *not* diagnostic. Microaneurysms are usually saccular and measure 1–5 mm in diameter (sometimes larger). Diseased areas are often located at bifurcations **(Fig. 8)**. They may resolve completely with therapy **(Figs. 9, 10)**. Microaneurysms and stenoses are present in more than 80% of patients with PAN, but a negative arteriogram does not exclude the disease. The risk of acute tubular necrosis following arteriography may be minimized by adequate preprocedure hydration and by limiting the contrast material load.

Differential Diagnosis and Treatment of Polyarteritis Nodosa

Polyarteritis nodosa is a diagnosis of exclusion. Neither the histologic nor the arteriographic appearance of PAN is pathognomonic. Both may be mimicked exactly by collagen-vascular disorders (especially systemic lupus erythematosus) or substance-abuse vasculitis **(Fig. 12)**. In addition, multiple small aneurysms may be seen in neurofibromatosis, Wegener's granulomatosis, Kawasaki's disease, fibromuscular dysplasia, and aneurysms due to septic emboli.

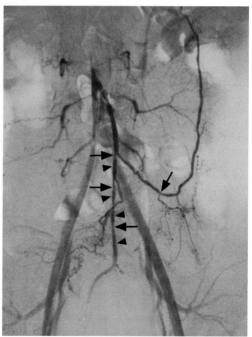

Figure 8. Polyarteritis nodosa in a 16-year-old female who has had PAN since childhood and had ischemic colonic ulcerations at colonoscopy. The inferior mesenteric arteriogram shows microaneurysms, stenoses, and narrow, irregular distal branches with occlusions. Note the alternating "skip" character of stenotic lesions (arrows) with normal arterial segments (arrowheads).

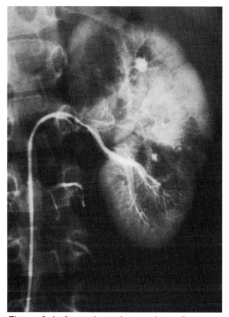

Figure 9. Left renal arteriogram in an 8-year-old patient. Small aneurysms and distal vessel stenoses and occlusions are present.

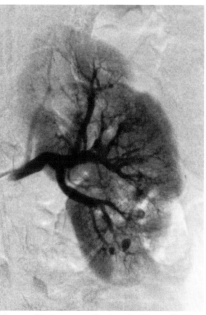

Figure 10. Same patient as in Figure 9. The repeat arteriogram at age16 shows interval healing of some aneurysms and the appearance of new aneurysms, illustrating the coexistence of acute and chronic lesions.

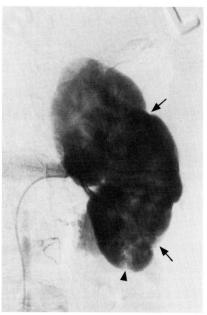

Figure 11. The nephrogram phase of the arteriogram at age 16 shows the "rat-bite" appearance of the renal contour. Cortical infarcts from vessel occlusions acutely produce lucent areas of hypoperfusion (arrowhead) and, chronically, scar retraction (arrows). Compare the contour in Figure 9.

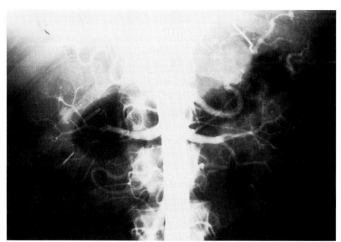

Figure 12. Cocaine-induced arteritis. Multiple microaneurysms are present in the renal, splenic, gastric, and hepatic arteries. The angiographic appearance is indistinguishable from that of PAN.

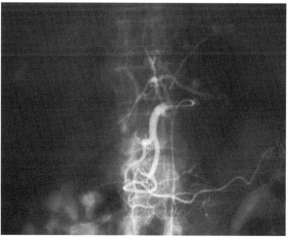

Figure 13. Same patient as in Figure 6. Hepatic arteriogram after embolization of the right hepatic artery following a PAN hemorrhage. A computed tomography scan had indicated right lobe hemorrhage but bleeding from a specific aneurysm was not identified angiographically. Gelfoam (Upjohn, Kalamazoo, MI) and coil embolization successfully controlled the hemorrhage.

Despite treatment with corticosteroids and cytotoxic drugs, 5-year survival in PAN is only 80%. Half of these deaths are due to renal failure and its complications. Gastrointestinal, peritoneal, retroperitoneal, hepatic, or renal hemorrhage may be catastrophic, requiring embolization or surgery **(Fig. 13)**. The precise bleeding point may not be visible, and embolization of the entire territory of the parent artery may be required.

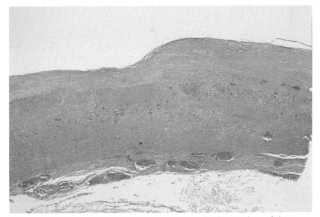

Figure 14. Temporal arteritis. A histopathologic section of the aorta reveals a thickened intima and media with a cellular inflammatory process at the intimomedial junction. The adventitia is relatively normal. The lumen is at the top of the image.

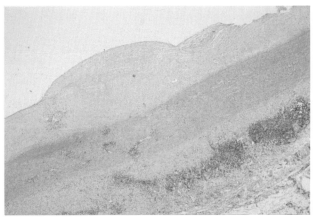

Figure 15. Takayasu's arteritis. A histologic cross section shows cellular infiltrate predominantly in the media and adventitia of the aorta plus intimal fibrous proliferation with some cells. Note the medio-adventitial dominance and greater wall thickness here in contrast with the temporal aortitis shown in Figure 14.

Giant Cell Arteritides

Takayasu's arteritis and temporal arteritis are both classified histopathologically as giant cell or granulomatous arteritides. Temporal arteritis is also called "giant cell arteritis," but we will refer to it as temporal arteritis to avoid confusion. Both Takayasu's arteritis and temporal arteritis are characterized by a granulomatous inflammatory infiltrate which begins in the media and fragments the IEL and, less commonly, the EEL. The infiltrate can extend into the adventitia and stimulates cellular proliferation in the intima (fibroblasts and myointimal cells). The acute infiltrate is lymphocyte-predominant and can be florid. Giant cells and occasionally granulomas are typically found in the region of the IEL and EEL. These giant cells are a nonspecific response to disrupted elastic tissue and can also be seen in syphilitic aortitis and atherosclerosis, although not to the same degree.

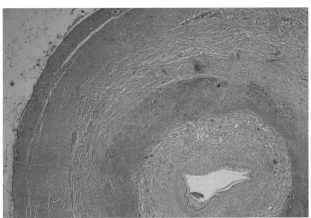

Figure 16. Takayasu's disease, chronic. A histologic section of the carotid artery shows extensive adventitial thickening with near obliteration of the lumen by intimal fibrosis.

The inflammation in temporal arteritis tends to be in the region of the inner media and IEL **(Fig. 14)**. In Takayasu's disease, inflammation is more prominent in the outer media and adventitia **(Fig. 15)**. Chronically, medial fibrosis, intimal fibrosclerosis, and diffuse sclerotic thickening of the adventitia occur. This causes thickening of the vessel wall and permanent stenoses or occlusions **(Figs. 16, 17)**. Aneurysms may also arise when disruption of the vessel wall and elastic fibers is extensive and there is inadequate production of supporting adventitial tissue.

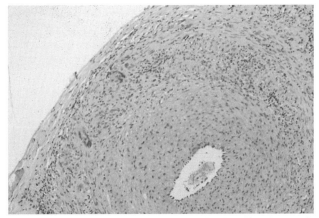

Figure 17. Temporal arteritis, subacute. Intimal proliferation nearly obliterates the lumen of this histologic section of the temporal artery. Note destruction of the elastic laminae.

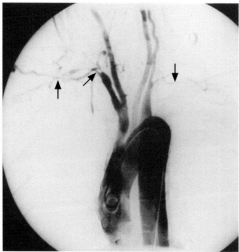

Figure 18. Biopsy-proven temporal arteritis in a 61-year-old female. There are severe stenoses in the axillosubclavian arteries and their branches (arrows). The origins of the great vessels are normal. This appearance is typical for temporal arteritis but not for Takayasu's arteritis. This patient is also older than the typical patient with Takayasu's arteritis.

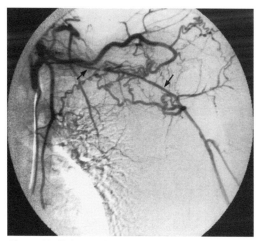

Figure 20. Takayasu's disease in a 22-year-old female with long, severe stenosis of the left postvertebral subclavian artery and axillary artery (arrows). Note the similarity to Figures 18 and 19. In this patient, the aortic arch and the great vessel origins were not involved.

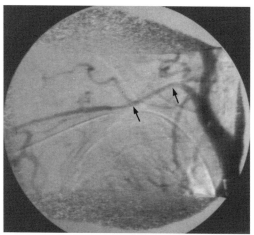

Figure 19. Temporal arteritis in a 65-year-old female. Intravenous digital subtraction arteriography shows a normal-sized brachiocephalic trunk with a long stenotic segment of the subclavian and axillary arteries (arrows).

Similarities Between Takayasu's Arteritis and Temporal Arteritis

Takayasu's arteritis and temporal arteritis are similar in other ways as well. Both occur most frequently in women. Both have associated constitutional symptoms (malaise, fever, anorexia, weight loss, myalgias, normocytic anemia). Both are treated in the same fashion, with corticosteroids and, if necessary, immunosuppressive therapy (azathioprine and cyclophosphamide). When the large arteries of the upper extremities are affected by temporal arteritis, the angiographic picture mimics Takayasu's arteritis **(Figs. 18–20)**. Both diseases occasionally involve the coronary arteries.

Takayasu's Arteritis

Also known as pulseless disease, middle aortic syndrome, and nonspecific aortoarteritis, Takayasu's arteritis is a chronic, recurrent, inflammatory, and fibrosing vasculitis. It affects the aorta and its major branches, and the pulmonary arteries. It is predominantly a disease of women in the reproductive age group, with a male:female ratio of 1:8 and an incidence of 2.6/million/year. Takayasu's arteritis is much more common in patients of Asian, Indian, South American, and African descent than in patients of northern European descent.

Takayasu's arteritis is one of the "great imitators." The diagnosis is based on both arteriographic findings and clinical features, which may include bruits, pulse deficits, headache, renovascular hypertension, and upper extremity and cerebral ischemia. Clinically, there are three phases: an early phase characterized by nonspecific systemic symptoms; an active inflammatory vascular phase with the development of arterial lesions; and a "burned-out" phase where symptoms are due to chronic vascular lesions. Ten-year survival is about 80%.

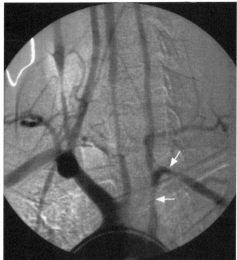

Figure 21. Right posterior oblique (RPO) aortic arch arteriogram of a 13-year-old female with Takayasu's arteritis. Proximal and postvertebral left subclavian artery segments are stenotic (arrows). The left vertebral artery origin is mildly stenotic. The right and left common carotid arteries have long moderate stenoses. The distal right brachiocephalic and proximal subclavian arteries are mildly dilated.

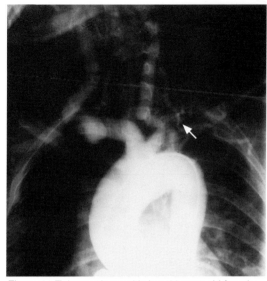

Figure 22. Takayasu's arteritis in a 20-year-old female. There is proximal aortic arch and right brachiocephalic artery dilatation with left subclavian stenosis (arrow).

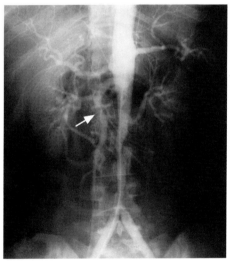

Figure 23. Same patient as in Figure 22. There is severe mid abdominal aortic stenosis with focal superior mesenteric artery (SMA) stenosis (arrow) and inferior mesenteric artery (IMA) origin occlusion.

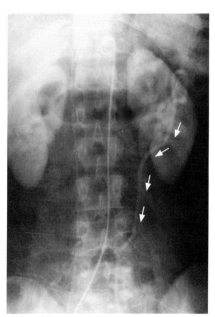

Figure 24. The late film from an abdominal aortogram shows reconstitution of the IMA supply via the arc of Riolan (arrows) filling from the middle colic artery. The middle colic artery arises proximal to the SMA stenosis.

Patterns of Arterial Involvement in Takayasu's Arteritis

The left subclavian artery is the most frequently involved aortic branch in patients with Takayasu's arteritis, but the other arch vessels and the renal arteries are also commonly involved, as is the aorta itself **(Figs. 21–25)**. Involvement of the external carotid artery or its branches is rare. Coronary arteries are not often involved (11%).

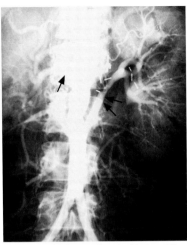

Figure 25. Takayasu's arteritis in a 28-year-old female with hypertension. Aortography shows areas of stenosis and dilatation in the abdominal aorta. The right renal artery origin is stenotic (single arrow). A left aortorenal bypass has already been performed (double arrow).

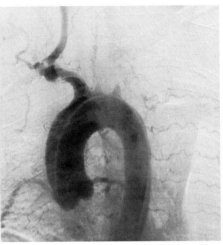

Figure 26. Type 1 Takayasu's arteritis in a 36-year-old female. The RPO thoracic aortogram reveals severe aortic arch disease ("bald arch"), left subclavian and carotid artery occlusions, and a right subclavian artery occlusion. Note the enlarged intercostal arteries on the left. No abnormalities were present distal to the arch.

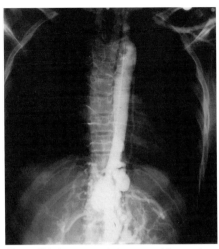

Figure 27. Aneurysmal changes of the aorta are seen at the thoracoabdominal junction in this 29-year-old female with Type 2 Takayasu's arteritis.

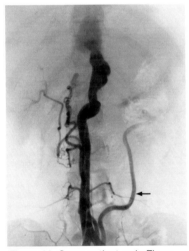

Figure 28. Same patient as in Figure 27. The abdominal aortogram reveals a tortuous and diffusely narrowed abdominal aorta with occlusions of all visceral vessels except for a dilated inferior mesenteric artery (arrow). The ascending aorta, arch, and great vessels were normal.

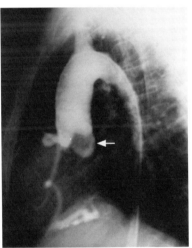

Figure 29. Type 4 Takayasu's arteritis in a 30-year-old female. The lateral thoracic aortogram demonstrates left coronary artery origin occlusion (arrow) (with reconstitution by a hypertrophied right coronary artery), left subclavian artery occlusion, and smooth long-segment stenoses of the descending thoracic aorta ("rat tail aorta").

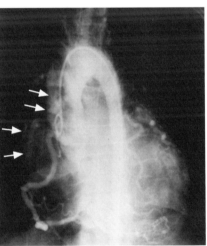

Figure 30. Same patient as in Figure 29. Contrast material fills the pulmonary arteries (arrows) via aortic collaterals in this patient with pulmonary artery involvement. The abdominal aorta was also diffusely narrowed (not shown).

Takayasu's arteritis has been classified into four types, based on the pattern of arterial involvement: type 1 **(Fig. 26)**, the aortic arch and its branches (8%); type 2 **(Figs. 27, 28)**, the descending thoracic aorta, abdominal aorta, and its branches (11%); type 3 **(Figs. 22–24)**, a combination of type 1 and type 2 (65%); and type 4 **(Figs. 29, 30)**, any of the above types with pulmonary artery involvement as well. The pulmonary arteries are affected in 25%–50% of patients.

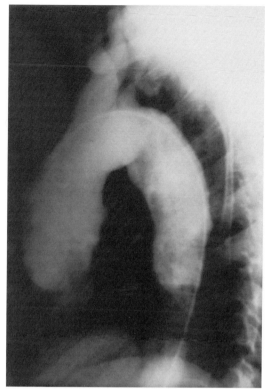

Figure 31. Takayasu's arteritis in a 22-year-old. Diffuse dilatation of the ascending and proximal descending aorta, aneurysmal dilatation of the right brachiocephalic artery, and left subclavian artery stenosis.

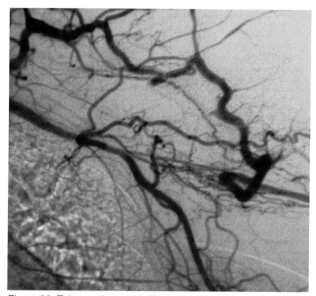

Figure 32. Takayasu's arteritis. There is a long, thread-like stenosis of the left axillary artery with prominent collaterals.

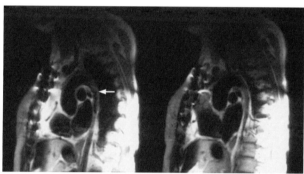

Figure 33. Takayasu's arteritis. There is marked aortic stenosis (arrow) and wall thickening on parasagittal T1-weighted images of the descending thoracic aorta.

Arterial Abnormalities in Takayasu's Arteritis

Arteriographic abnormalities in Takayasu's arteritis include stenoses, occlusions, aneurysmal dilatation, mural irregularity, and various combinations of these (**Figs. 23, 31**). Skip lesions are characteristic but not pathognomonic. The transition from diseased to normal vessel is abrupt as shown in **Figures 20** and **21**. Solitary or multiple stenoses are the most common abnormality. These may be short and segmental or long and diffuse and may progress to occlusion. Some are long and almost thread-like (**Fig. 32**). Takayasu's arteritis is the only primary vasculitis with aortic stenoses (**Figs. 33, 34; see also 23, 25, 28, 29**). Prominent collaterals are sometimes seen in the aortic wall. These are enlarged vasa vasorum in the adventitia (**Fig. 35**). Aneurysms are present in 10%–30% of patients with Takayasu's arteritis. They may be fusiform (**Fig. 36**); or saccular (**Fig. 37**), and range in size from several millimeters to several centimeters. Diffuse dilatation is more common in the ascending aorta (**Fig. 31**), while aneurysms, usually fusiform, are more common in the descending and abdominal aorta. Thickening of the aortic wall may be particularly prominent in Takayasu's arteritis (**Figs. 36, 33, 15**). Dissection is therefore rare, even in aneurysmal disease. Pulmonary artery disease is almost never aneurysmal in Takayasu's arteritis. Stenoses involve the main pulmonary artery and proximal branches with an upper lobe predominance and a propensity for bilaterality. Systemic collaterals provide collateral flow (**Fig. 30**).

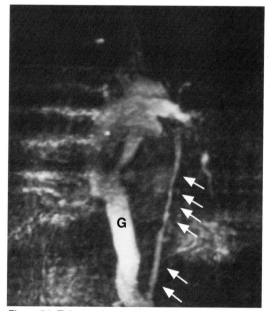

Figure 34. Takayasu's arteritis in a 33-year-old female. Maximum intensity projection images from a 2-D time of flight magnetic resonance arteriogram of the thoracoabdominal region. Note the long-segment aortic stenosis (arrows) just distal to the arch. A graft (G) has been placed and runs from the ascending aorta to the aortic bifurcation.

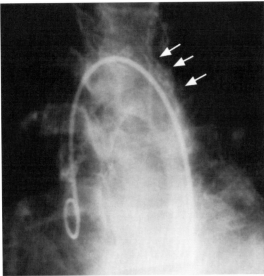

Figure 35. Takayasu's arteritis. There is adventitial vascularization due to hypertrophy of the vasa vasorum in the aortic wall acting as collaterals. Note that the collaterals parallel the catheter (arrows) and run in the wall.

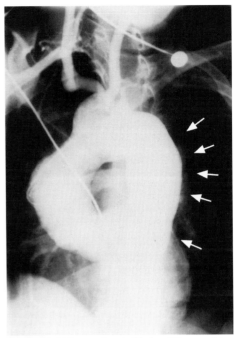

Figure 36. Takayasu's arteritis in a 25-year-old female. There is fusiform aneurysmal dilatation of the ascending and descending thoracic aorta. Note companion shadows of the thickened aortic wall (arrows). The left subclavian artery is occluded.

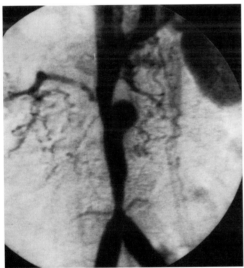

Figure 37. A saccular aneurysm arises from a severely stenotic portion of the abdominal aorta in a 20-year-old female with Takayasu's arteritis.

Dystrophic pencil-line calcification of the arterial media as well as secondary atherosclerotic calcification can occur in chronic lesions. Chest radiographs reveal aortic calcification in 10%–25% of patients. Areas most commonly involved are the arch, the descending thoracic aorta, and the brachiocephalic vessels. The ascending thoracic aorta is usually spared.

Arteriography and Interventions in Takayasu's Arteritis

Arteriographic evaluation of patients with Takayasu's arteritis should include aortography, with filming from the skull base to the common femoral arteries, including an oblique view of the aortic arch and a lateral view of the abdominal aorta. Serial arteriography is often used to evaluate disease progression. Once stenoses develop they do not resolve, and they may get worse. Ischemic steno-occlusive disease and aneurysms have traditionally been treated surgically **(Figs. 25, 34)**. Percutaneous transluminal angioplasty (PTA) is increasingly being used as an alternative for focal stenotic lesions. Occluded segments often contain thrombus within the arterial lumen, and thrombolysis may reveal an underlying stenosis amenable to PTA.

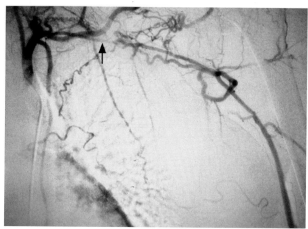

Figure 38. Takayasu's arteritis in a 22-year-old female with severe stenosis of the postvertebral subclavian artery (arrow) and proximal axillary artery before angioplasty.

Angioplasty has most often been used to treat lesions of the aorta, subclavian artery, and renal artery. There have been occasional reports of PTA of visceral and coronary lesions as well. In general, as with arterial lesions of other etiologies, the initial success and long-term patency rates are better for short stenoses than for long stenoses or occlusions, but longer lesions can be treated successfully **(Figs. 38, 39)**. Concentric lesions respond better than eccentric lesions. Initial success rates of 90%–100% have been reported for aortic lesions, with long-term patencies of 60% or better. In the renal arteries, an initial clinical success rate of 95% and a predicted 5-year patency rate of 70% have been reported. Overall clinical success rates in the subclavian artery are slightly lower (80%), but a cumulative patency rate of 100% has been reported for short stenoses.

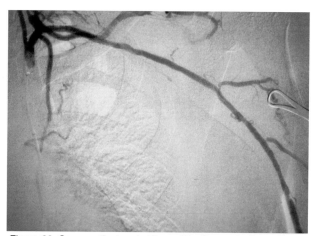

Figure 39. Same patient as in Figure 38, after angioplasty. The 5-year arteriographic follow-up demonstrated patent arteries.

Stenoses due to Takayasu's arteritis may be extremely difficult to dilate, and may require high-pressure balloons. Some interventional radiologists recommend graded dilation and limiting the balloon size to three times the diameter of the most stenotic portion of the artery in order to avoid vessel rupture. This technique is not standard practice. Acute arterial rupture as a result of percutaneous angioplasty appears to be an extremely rare event, even without use of this technique.

Neither PTA nor surgical bypass should be performed if there is clinical or laboratory evidence of active inflammation (elevated erythrocyte sedimentation rate or C-reactive protein). Arterial interventions performed in the presence of active inflammation may result in vessel occlusion or aneurysm formation **(Figs. 40–42)**.

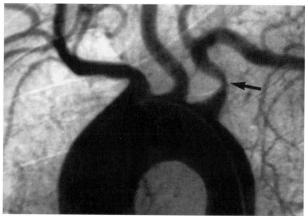

Figure 40. Takayasu's arteritis in a 35-year-old female with a focal stenosis (arrow) of the left subclavian artery.

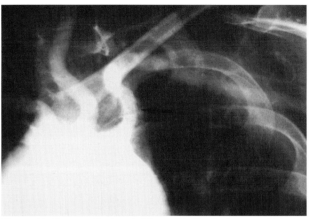

Figure 41. Same patient as in Figure 40. The lesion was dilated with a 6-mm balloon during active disease, with a good immediate result.

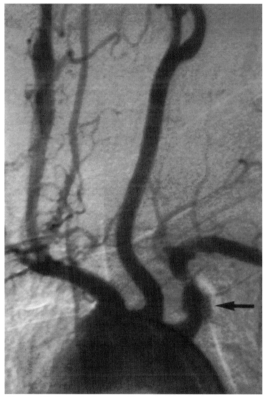

Figure 42. An arteriogram 5 weeks later reveals new aneurysmal dilatation at the site of the prior PTA (arrow).

Temporal Arteritis

Temporal arteritis is less common than Takayasu's arteritis, with an incidence of 1.7/million/year. The disease has two phases. The first phase is a flu-like syndrome with nonspecific systemic symptoms that may last several weeks. Patients usually do not present until the second phase, when arterial inflammation develops. Patients typically complain of temporal headaches, tender, reddened temporal arteries, and jaw claudication. Scalp tenderness and visual disturbances may also occur. All of these symptoms are due to involvement of branches of the external carotid artery. Polymyalgia rheumatica (PMR), aching stiffness in the proximal joints, is seen in 30%–40% of patients with temporal arteritis (but only 15% of patients with PMR have temporal arteritis). The diagnosis of temporal arteritis is normally established by biopsy of a symptomatic artery, typically an inflamed portion of the temporal artery.

Differences Between Temporal Arteritis and Takayasu's Arteritis

Temporal arteritis is principally distinguished from Takayasu's arteritis by epidemiology and the pattern of arterial involvement. Temporal arteritis occurs in patients older than 50 years, while Takayasu's arteritis is a disease of young adults. Temporal arteritis typically involves branches of the external carotid artery and other arteries of the head, neck, and upper extremities, but rarely involves visceral arteries. PMR and Raynaud's phenomenon do not occur with Takayasu's arteritis.

Aortic involvement may produce aneurysms in temporal arteritis, but this is much less common than in Takayasu's arteritis. Aortic stenoses are common in Takayasu's disease but do not occur in temporal arteritis. Pulmonary artery involvement is rare in temporal arteritis. The subclavian, axillary and brachial arteries are involved in only 3%–15% of patients with temporal arteritis. In temporal arteritis, involvement of upper extremity arteritis is more typically bilateral and extends more peripherally than in Takayasu's disease.

Raynaud's Phenomenon

Raynaud's phenomenon is due to episodic vasospasm of arterioles. It is characterized by the triad of: 1) episodic, self-limited attacks of reversible, white color changes of the fingers; 2) precipitation of the attacks by cold; and 3) symptoms of numbness, tingling, or pain on recovery. A classic three-phase color change (white to blue to red) is seen in a minority of patients. Raynaud's phenomenon may involve only one finger, but it may also affect the toes, earlobes, lips, and tip of the nose. Primary (idiopathic) Raynaud's phenomenon occurs in up to 11% of men and 19% of women. Raynaud's phenomenon may also be secondary to a variety of causes **(Fig. 43)**. Arterial stenoses and occlusions should improve with the administration of intra-arterial vasodilators if they are due to Raynaud's phenomenon, but not if they are due to vasculitis.

Buerger's Disease

Buerger's disease (thromboangiitis obliterans) is a medium- to small-vessel vasculitis characterized by inflammatory segmental occlusions of arteries and veins of the distal upper and lower extremities. It is classically seen in male smokers younger than 40 years, but the disease is becoming more common in women. The male:female ratio, once 49:1, is now 4:1. The small vessels of the calf and foot are most commonly involved in patients with Buerger's disease, with less frequent involvement of the popliteal and superficial femoral arteries. In the upper extremity, the ulnar, radial, palmar and digital arteries are most commonly involved. Fifty percent of patients have involvement of the lower extremities alone, 40% have involvement of both lower and upper extremities, and 10% have only upper extremity involvement.

Diagnosis of Buerger's Disease

The most common presentation is lower extremity claudication or rest pain, occasionally with tissue loss. Proximal pulses are normal, and pedal pulses are absent or diminished. The erythrocyte sedimentation rate is often normal. Most patients have a history of regular cigarette smoking. Cessation of smoking arrests the disease, but up to 30% of patients require leg amputation because there are no adequate distal vessels for surgical bypass. Buerger's disease is a clinical syndrome with four major diagnostic criteria: 1) onset of ischemic symptoms before age 45; 2) tobacco abuse; 3) normal arteries proximal to the popliteal and brachial arteries; and 4) exclusion of other etiologies (including hypercoagulable states). Minor criteria include Raynaud's phenomenon (30%) and migratory superficial phlebitis (40%). Arteriography is usually essential for diagnosis.

Causes of Raynaud's Phenomenon

Idiopathic
Systemic rheumatic disorders
 Scleroderma, systemic lupus erythematosus, polymyositis/dermatomyositis, Sjögren's syndrome, rheumatoid arthritis
Vasculitis
 Buerger's disease, temporal arteritis
Occupational
 Rock drillers, lumberjacks, grinders, riveters, pneumatic hammer operators
Drugs
 ß-blockers, ergot, methysergide, vinblastine, bleomycin, imipramine, bromocriptine, clonidine, cyclosporine A, vinyl chloride
Arterial occlusive disease
 Embolic/thrombotic occlusions, carpal tunnel syndrome, thoracic outlet syndrome

Figure 43.

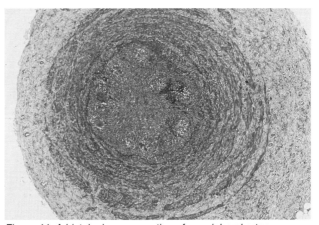

Figure 44. A histologic cross section of a peripheral artery demonstrates luminal obliteration with microabscesses from Buerger's disease. The layers of the arterial wall are preserved and the IEL is intact.

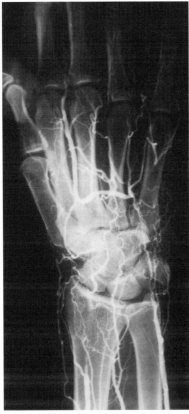

Figure 45. Buerger's disease in a 29-year-old male smoker with digital ischemia. The left hand arteriogram demonstrates abrupt occlusions of the ulnar and multiple metacarpal arteries. Note also the tree root-like tapering of the radial artery to occlusion. Corkscrew collaterals are well demonstrated beyond the radial, ulnar, and metacarpal artery occlusions.

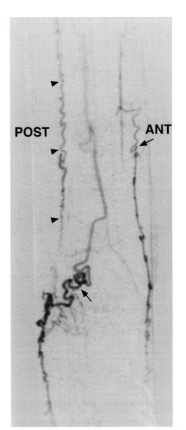

Figure 46. Left lower extremity arteriogram, lateral view, in a young male smoker with Buerger's disease. Note the corrugated corkscrew collaterals (arrows) providing flow around the occluded posterior perforator branch of the peroneal artery and distal anterior tibial arteries. The collateral following the original course of the posterior tibial artery illustrates a direct collateral within the recanalized lumen, representing Martorell's sign (arrowheads).

Pathology of Buerger's Disease

In contrast to other vasculitides, the architecture of the arterial wall remains histologically intact in the acute lesions of Buerger's disease. Polymorphonuclear leukocytes infiltrate all layers of the vessel wall, but there is no necrosis or destruction of the internal elastic lamina. Luminal thrombi, when present, are hypercellular and harbor microabscesses **(Fig. 44)**. Multinucleated giant cells within the microabscesses are pathognomonic for Buerger's disease. The adjacent vein and nerve may be affected along with the artery. In chronic lesions, scattered inflammatory cells are present. Perivascular and intimal fibrosis develop, and luminal thrombi recanalize. The layers of the arterial wall are preserved.

Arteriographic Findings in Buerger's Disease

At arteriography, vascular involvement is segmental, with an abrupt transition from the normal vessel to the diseased segment and involvement of multiple segments, giving the appearance of skip lesions **(Fig. 45)**. Distal arteries may demonstrate irregular tapering proximal to the occlusion, with a "tree-root" appearance. More proximal vessels are normal. Recanalization of previously occluded segments—direct collaterals—may occur in up to 80% of patients (Martorell's sign). Collateral vessels arising at occlusions are "corkscrew," "ripple-like," or corrugated **(Figs. 45, 46)**. These findings are typical, but not diagnostic.

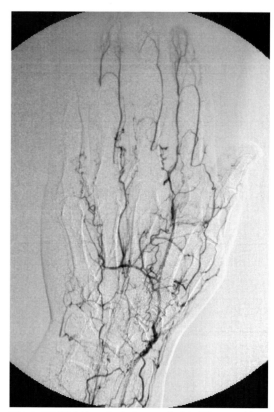

Figure 47. *Right hand arteriogram in this 50-year-old diabetic with digital ischemia reveals multiple arterial occlusions and corkscrew-like collaterals which mimic those seen in Buerger's disease.*

Similar arteriographic findings may be seen with arterial emboli, other arteritides, atherosclerosis, diabetes, hyperlipidemia, and hypercoagulable states **(Fig. 47)**. In the lower extremities of otherwise healthy young patients, the differential diagnosis also includes popliteal entrapment with distal emboli and adventitial cystic disease of the popliteal artery. The differential diagnosis in the upper extremity includes repetitive microtrauma ("hammer" syndrome) and emboli from thrombi or aneurysms due to entrapment syndromes such as thoracic outlet syndrome and quadrilateral space syndrome.

Behçet's Disease

This disorder is a multisystem disease, most common in the Mediterranean, Middle East, and Japan. The disease usually begins in the third or fourth decade. The male:female ratio is 2:1. The classic clinical triad includes oral and genital ulcers and relapsing iridocyclitis, but patients may present with a wide variety of symptoms and signs, including gastrointestinal tract ulcerations, skin lesions, arthralgias, meningoencephalitis, and vascular lesions. Vasculitis is responsible for all of these clinical manifestations and may affect vessels of any size. Both arteries and veins may be affected. Because of the protean nature of the disease and the lack of diagnostic laboratory tests, the diagnosis is made on clinical criteria alone.

Pathology of Behçet's Disease

Behçet's disease is a nonspecific panvasculitis, characterized by an inflammatory infiltrate of lymphocytes or plasma cells in the adventitia and media, fragmentation of the elastic lamina and elastic fibers, and obliterative endarteritis of the vasa vasorum. These pathological changes produce weakness and dilatation of the vessel wall, aneurysm formation, and pseudoaneurysms. Aneurysm rupture occurs in 10% of patients, and is the major cause of death in this disease.

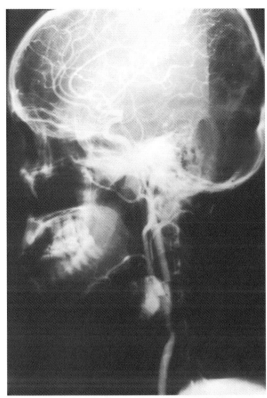

Figure 48. Behçet's disease in a 25-year-old Korean female with bilateral pulsating neck masses and a lower abdominal mass with bruit. Right common carotid artery angiography demonstrates a saccular, partially thrombosed aneurysm of the common carotid artery.

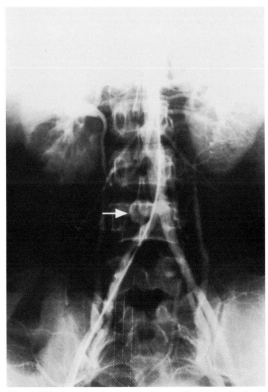

Figure 49. Same patient as in Figure 48. Abdominal aortography reveals a 2-cm saccular aneurysm arising from the right side of the distal abdominal aorta (arrow).

Vascular Abnormalities in Behçet's Disease

Vascular lesions are present in 7%–29% of patients with Behçet's disease. Venous lesions, usually occlusions, are more common than arterial lesions. Aneurysms of medium and large systemic and pulmonary arteries are the most common arterial manifestations. Two thirds of arterial lesions are aneurysms, and one third are occlusions **(Figs. 48, 49)**. Pseudoaneurysms may develop at arterial puncture sites and at bypass graft anastomoses. There have been several reports of aortic involvement, with aneurysms of the ascending aorta and aortic valvular insufficiency. Behçet's disease is the only known primary vasculitis which produces aneurysms in the pulmonary arteries.

Infection-Related Arteritis

Infectious inflammation of arteries may be due to bacteria, fungi, spirochetes, viruses, *Mycobacteria,* or *Rickettsia*. Large arteries are prone to perforation, and aneurysm or pseudoaneurysm formation. These aneurysms may be true or false, and are often saccular. Their angiographic appearance is nonspecific. Inflammation of small arteries may produce occlusion or thrombosis.

The nomenclature for infection-related arteritis is confusing and not consistently applied. The term "mycotic aneurysm" was originally used by Osler to describe all arterial infections, both bacterial and fungal, arising from endocarditis-related septic emboli. "Mycotic aneurysm" has also been used to indicate fungal infection specifically. "Microbial arteritis" usually refers to nonembolic infection. "Mycotic aneurysm" is sometimes used to indicate all infections and all mechanisms.

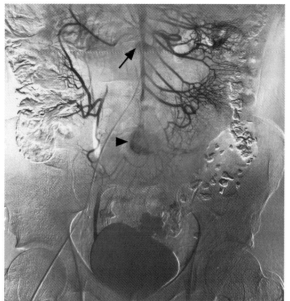

Figure 50. Young male with fever, abdominal pain, a prosthetic aortic valve, and mycotic aneurysms from septic emboli from Candida albicans. Superior mesenteric arteriography demonstrates a small lobulated aneurysm (arrow) occluding the ileocecal branch and a large saccular aneurysm (arrowhead) occluding several ileal branches which reconstitute distally by collateral flow.

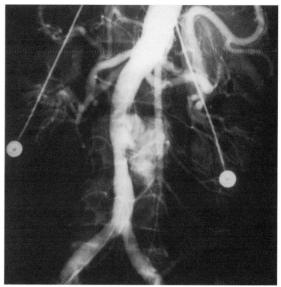

Figure 51. Infection-related arteritis in a 65-year-old female with Group A Streptococcus endocarditis. The early film from an abdominal aortogram shows a saccular pseudoaneurysm of the infrarenal abdominal aorta.

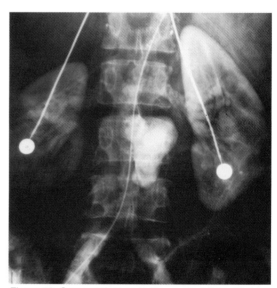

Figure 52. Same patient as in Figure 51. A later film shows delayed washout of contrast material from the pseudoaneurysm.

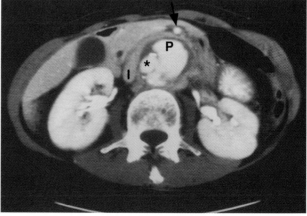

Figure 53. Same patient as in Figure 51. The left renal vein and the superior mesenteric artery (arrow) are displaced anteriorly by the pseudoaneurysm (P). The true aortic lumen (asterisk) sits immediately to the left of the inferior vena cava (I).

Routes of Infection in Patients with Infection-Related Arteritis

Vessels may be affected by a number of mechanisms: emboli, hematogenous seeding, contiguous invasion, and direct injury with contamination. Emboli tend to lodge at vessel branch points or in the vasa vasorum of large arteries **(Figs. 50–53)**. Hematogenous seeding occurs from either the luminal surface or vasa vasorum. It is often due to distant abscesses or infections, but the source is occult in 50% of patients. Blood-borne microbes lodge in underlying abnormalities in the vessel wall caused by pre-existing atherosclerosis, aneurysms, coarctation, or a vascular anastomosis **(Figs. 54, 55)**. Contiguous invasion by direct extension or lymphangitic spread from an abscess, osteomyelitis, adenopathy, or a phlegmon leads to aneurysm or perforation. Arteritis due to a contaminated arterial injury may be iatrogenic, iatrogenically-introduced, caused by penetrating trauma or open fractures, or related to intravenous drug abuse.

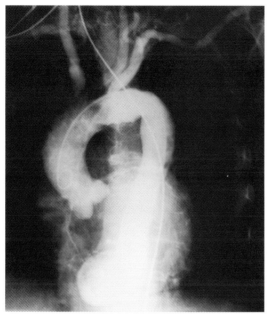

Figure 54. Infection-related arteritis in a 74-year-old female with underlying severe atherosclerosis. The RPO thoracic aortogram reveals a large saccular aneurysm at the thoracoabdominal junction.

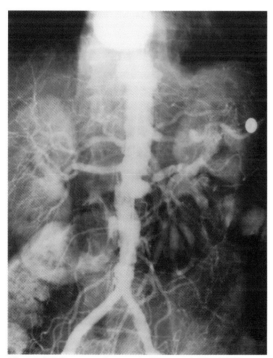

Figure 55. Same patient as in Figure 54. The antero-posterior (AP) abdominal aortogram demonstrates the thoracic aneurysm as well as a smaller aneurysm at the origin of the left renal artery. Both aneurysms were due to Staphylococcus aureus.

Infectious Aortitis

Some infectious agents show a predilection for aortic involvement, due to either septic emboli to the vasa vasorum, direct extension, or hematogenous spread. Rubella can cause aortic and pulmonary stenosis, but most other infections result in aneurysms which enlarge rapidly and will rupture if not treated. Infectious aortitis is classically caused by *Salmonella*, but *Staphylococcus* and *Streptococcus* infections are more common **(Figs. 51–55)**. Other infectious diseases with a predilection for aortic involvement include tuberculosis and syphilis.

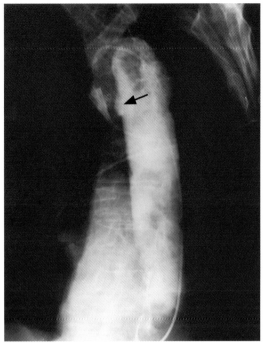

Figure 56. RPO thoracic aortogram in a 79-year-old male with Salmonella arteritis shows a small focal aneurysm (arrow) at the upper anastomosis of a descending thoracic aortic graft. Note the corrugated wall of the graft.

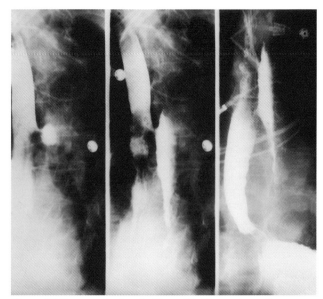

Figure 57. Same patient as in Figure 56. The gastrografin esophagram demonstrates a fistula between the esophagus and aortic graft. Note the corrugation of the graft seen in relief against the linear area of extravasated contrast material on the far right image.

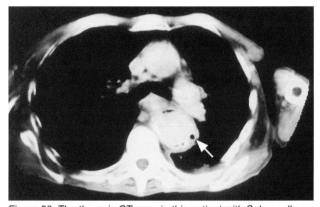

Figure 58. The thoracic CT scan in this patient with Salmonella arteritis shows air around the descending aortic graft (arrow).

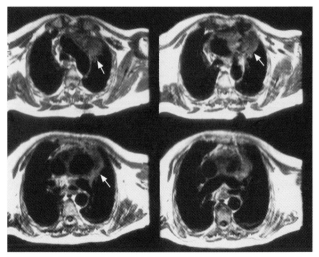

Figure 59. Elderly male with a pseudoaneurysm of the proximal arch due to Salmonella. The aneurysm has a significant amount of thrombus (arrows) and there is marked edema of the mediastinal fat on the T1-weighted axial MR examination.

Salmonella Aortitis

Salmonella aortitis produces aneurysms of the thoracic (20%) and abdominal aorta (80%). Thoracic aneurysms carry a higher mortality. Most patients are older than 60 years and have pre-existing atherosclerosis, a pre-existing aortic aneurysm, or a graft (Fig. 56). Thirty percent have diabetes. Eighty percent to 85% of patients present with fever, an elevated white blood cell count, and chest, back, or abdominal pain. Aneurysms may develop rapidly. Perforation may occur with an aneurysm (Fig. 57), or even in the absence of an aneurysm. The aortic wall may be thickened on computed tomography (CT) scans, and may enhance (Fig. 58). Magnetic resonance (MR) images demonstrate similar findings, both without (Figs. 59, 60) and with gadolinium (Figs. 61, 62). The overall mortality rate is 53%, but increases to 95% if patients are treated with antibiotics alone, without prompt surgery. Extra-anatomic bypass may be needed for recurrent infections.

Syphilitic Aortitis

Syphilitic (luetic) aortitis is a manifestation of tertiary syphilis and is initiated by hematogenous seeding of spirochetes into the vasa vasorum. It is characterized histologically by destruction of the smooth muscle and elastic tissue of the media, with its replacement by fibrous connective tissue (Fig. 63). The vasa vasorum are obliterated by a perivascular infiltrate of lymphocytes, plasma cells, and fibrosis.

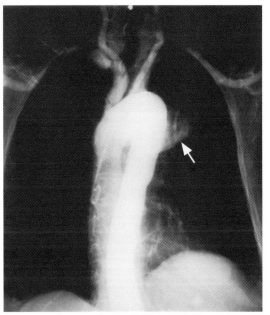

Figure 60. Same patient as in Figure 59. Thoracic aortography demonstrates the lumen of a focal pseudoaneurysm (arrow).

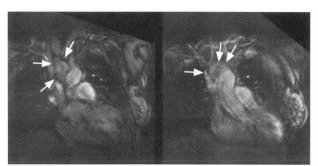

Figure 61. Magnetic resonance arteriogram of an infected pseudoaneurysm of the right brachiocephalic artery (arrows).

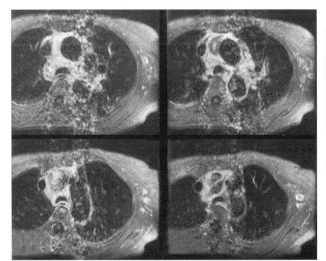

Figure 62. Same patient as Figure 61. There is intense enhancement throughout the mediastinum and even within the pseudoaneurysm following administration of gadolinium. Note particularly the wall of the right brachiocephalic artery and compare it to the distal arch and descending aorta.

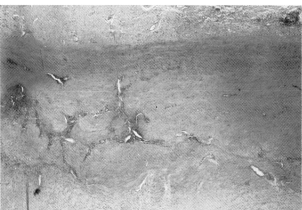

Figure 63. Histologic section of the aorta, with a typical neovascularized fibrous scar within the media in a patient with tertiary syphilis and aortic involvement.

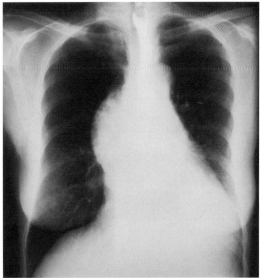

Figure 64. Elderly female with a large fusiform aneurysm of the ascending aorta. Note the linear calcification in the ascending aorta and the rightward mediastinal bulge. This is classic chest radiography of a syphilitic aneurysm.

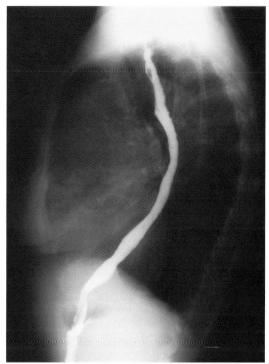

Figure 65. Same patient as in Figure 64. The lateral chest radiograph shows the aneurysm, etched in calcification, filling the retrosternal window and displacing the esophagus.

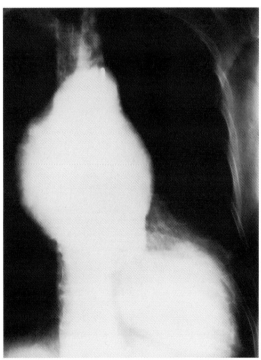

Figure 66. Same patient as in Figure 64. The AP thoracic aortogram demonstrates the fusiform aneurysm, the distorted aortic annulus, and aortic insufficiency.

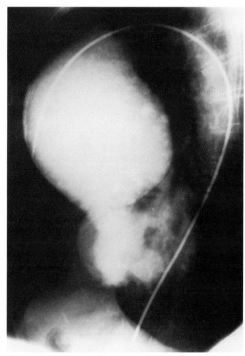

Figure 67. Same patient as in Figure 64. Lateral thoracic aortogram.

The ascending aorta and aortic arch are most commonly involved. There are four types of aortic disease: aortitis without aneurysm; aortitis with aneurysm (which is prone to rupture) **(Figs. 64, 65)**; aortic valvulitis with or without valvular incompetence **(Figs. 66, 67)**; and coronary ostial stenoses. Linear calcification is present in the aorta in 70% of cases (dystrophic, linear calcification in the scarred intima and media plus the degenerative chunky calcification of secondary atherosclerosis in the intima). Diagnosis may be difficult because there may be no reliable history of syphilis and serologic studies may be negative. These patients are elderly, and ubiquitous atherosclerotic changes may dominate the arteriographic picture.

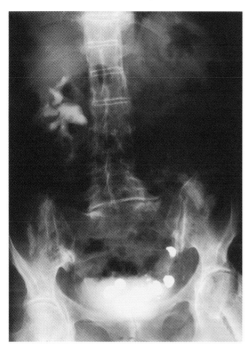

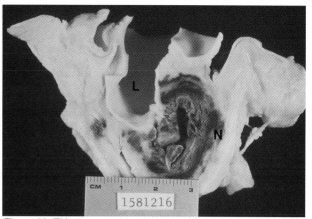

Figure 69. This 11-year-old male with undiagnosed tuberculosis died suddenly. Erosion of the ascending aorta was caused by tuberculous infection in adjacent hilar nodes (N). L=aortic lumen.

Figure 68. A nonfunctioning left "putty" kidney filled with caseating granulomas, spinal fusion, and bilateral calcified psoas abscesses from tuberculous spondylitis could all contribute to the development of a tuberculous aneurysm in this 77-year-old female.

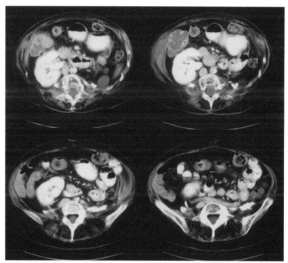

Figure 71. Same patient as in Figure 68. This block of CT images reveals the hypertrophic right kidney, tuberculous spondylitic changes, and bilateral calcified psoas abscesses. Note that the rest of the abdominal aorta is smaller in diameter than the 3-cm aneurysm in Figure 70, which itself is not very striking in size.

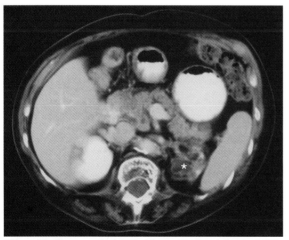

Figure 70. Same patient as in Figure 68. An abdominal CT section demonstrates a focal oval-shaped 3 x 1.5-cm abdominal aortic aneurysm and the left-sided tuberculous pyelonephritis (asterisk).

Tuberculous Aortitis

Tuberculous aortitis is characterized by granulomatous inflammation due to infection with acid-fast bacilli. It arises via direct spread from a tuberculous focus, such as tuberculous spondylitis **(Fig. 68)**, para-aortic adenopathy **(Fig. 69)** or pulmonary infection, or via hematogenous spread to the aortic wall through the vasa vasorum. Contiguous extension is more common. Tuberculous aortitis may itself cause hematogenous spread of the infection. Tuberculous aortitis erodes the aortic wall and leads to a true aneurysm or, more commonly, a false one. These aneurysms are typically saccular **(Figs. 70, 71)** and involve the descending thoracic or abdominal aorta. Dissection or rupture may occur, even with small aneurysms, because of septic destruction of the aortic wall. A Rasmussen's aneurysm is a pulmonary artery aneurysm which occurs in the wall of a tuberculous cavity.

345

Arteritis Due to Collagen-Vascular Diseases

Vasculitis is often associated with systemic lupus erythematosus (SLE), is sometimes associated with rheumatoid arthritis, and is occasionally seen with scleroderma. It may also be present in patients with Sjögren's syndrome, polymyositis/dermatomyositis, relapsing polychondritis, ankylosing spondylitis, and Reiter's syndrome. It is uncommon in psoriatic arthritis. Raynaud's phenomenon is seen in more than 80% of patients with scleroderma, up to 30% of patients with SLE, and in some patients with poly-myositis/dermatomyositis.

Systemic Lupus Erythematosus

Systemic lupus erythematosus may be accompanied by a hypersensitivity vasculitis characterized by intimal fibrosis of small arteries. Occasionally, PAN-like arteritis of small and medium arteries occurs, with microaneurysms. Narrowing and occlusion of digital arteries, mesenteric artery branch occlusions, and PAN-type microaneurysms of the viscera and central nervous system may be demonstrable arteriographically **(Figs. 72, 73)**. Because hyperco-agulability is common in patients with SLE due to the presence of lupus anticoagulant and anticardiolipin antibodies, arterial occlusions may be due to vasculi-tis or to in situ thrombosis. The two etiologies may be indistinguishable arteriographically.

Rheumatoid Arthritis

Arteritis develops in a small number of patients with long-standing, severe rheumatoid arthritis. One or all of several histologic appearances may be present—leukocytoclastic, PAN, and granulomatous arteritis. Histologically, granulomatous arteritis demonstrates classic rheumatoid granulomas with necrosis. Occlusion of digital arteries, nerve sheath arterioles, and mesenteric arterial branches leads to digital ischemia, peripheral neuropathy, and bowel infarc-tion. Granulomatous involvement of the myocardium and aortic valve may produce aortic valvular insufficiency.

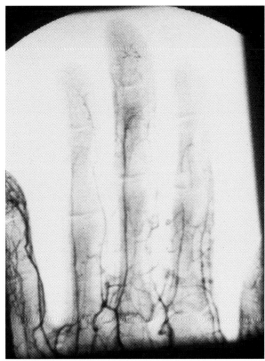

Figure 72. The hand arteriogram in a patient with SLE demonstrates irregular digital arteries with stenoses and occlusions. Collaterals tend to be more prominent in Buerger's disease (compare with Figure 45).

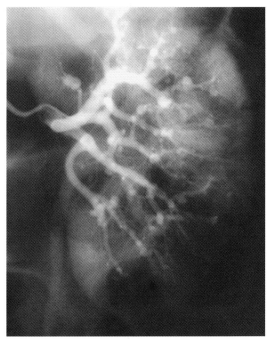

Figure 73. The left renal arteriogram demonstrates multiple small intraparenchymal artery aneurysms in a young female with SLE. The angiographic appearance is indistinguishable from PAN (compare with Figure 10).

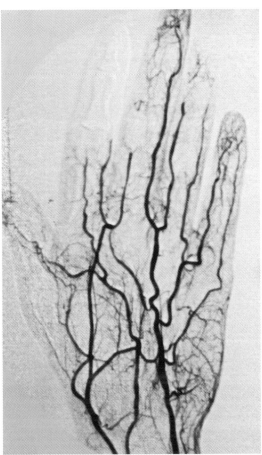

Figure 74. The hand arteriogram in this 37-year-old female with scleroderma demonstrates irregular narrowing and occlusion of multiple digital arteries unresponsive to vasodilation therapy with Priscoline. Rheumatoid vasculitis, SLE (compare with Figure 72), and obliterative atherosclerosis can have similar appearances.

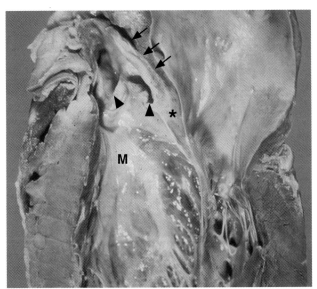

Figure 75. Ankylosing spondylitis. This gross specimen of the heart demonstrates fibrosis extending into the aortic valve with shortening and thickening of the valve cusps (arrowheads). Fibrosis also extends into the membranous portion of the ventricular septum (M) as well as the anterior leaflet of the mitral valve, producing a bump (asterisk). The aortic thickening extends only a few centimeters into the tubular aorta (arrows).

Scleroderma and Ankylosing Spondylitis

In scleroderma, occluded small arteries are seen arteriographically in the kidneys, heart, digits **(Fig. 74)**, mesenteric arterial bed, and occasionally in the pulmonary arteries. Typically, this is due to noninflammatory intimal proliferation, but these patients sometimes develop a necrotizing vasculitis which is similar histologically to PAN. Over 80% of patients have Raynaud's phenomenon. Up to 10% of patients with ankylosing spondylitis have characteristic involvement of the aortic valve and aortic root **(Fig. 75)**, with thickening of the valve cusps, the aortic root, and the first several centimeters of the ascending aorta. This is due to chronic inflammatory infiltrates and fibrosis, and often produces aortic valvular insufficiency. The coronary ostia and anterior leaflet of the mitral valve are often involved, but usually without clinical mitral valve disease.

Relapsing Polychondritis

Relapsing polychondritis is marked by intermittent destructive inflammation of the cartilaginous tissues of the respiratory tract, joints, ears, and nose. Focal destruction of the media, fragmentation of elastic tissue, and a mononuclear cell infiltrate lead to weakening of the arterial wall. Aortitis results in aortic aneurysms in 10% of patients, and is seen most often in the ascending aorta. Aortic valvular insufficiency and occasionally aortic dissection may occur. Aortic aneurysms may be multiple and may involve the abdominal aorta **(Fig. 76)**. Medium and small peripheral arteries are also occasionally involved.

Arteritis in Other Collagen-Vascular Diseases

Reiter's syndrome is characterized by nongonococcal urethritis, conjunctivitis, and arthritis. Cardiovascular abnormalities are seen in up to 50% of patients, with a pattern of involvement similar to that of ankylosing spondylitis. Sjögren's syndrome is marked by dry mouth and dry eyes. The vasculitis in these patients usually involves microscopic cutaneous arteries, but some patients with Sjögren's syndrome develop a necrotizing vasculitis with occlusion of small central nervous system arteries and the medium and small arteries of the gastrointestinal tract. Vasculitis of small vessels occurs in up to 25% of children with polymyositis/dermatomyositis, but vasculitis is uncommon in adults with this disease.

Substance-Abuse Vasculitis

This disorder may arise from the use of prescribed or illicit drugs. Most cases are associated with the use of amphetamine, methamphetamine, heroin, cocaine, phenylpropanolamine (PPA), ephedrine, or methylphenidate. PPA is a component of over-the-counter diet pills, nasal sprays, and decongestants. Symptoms may appear within minutes to hours after drug use, or may be delayed for days. The disease involves both small and medium arteries, with a predilection for bifurcations. Intracranial arteries are the most commonly involved vessels. Histologically, substance-abuse vasculitis may mimic PAN exactly. Giant cells are absent, in contrast to primary granulomatous vasculitis of the central nervous system, temporal arteritis, and neurosarcoidosis.

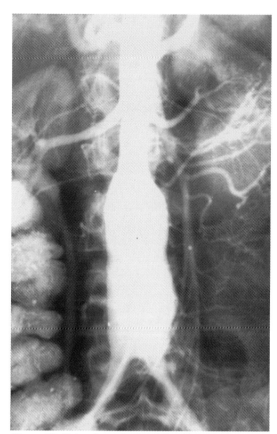

Figure 76. Relapsing polychondritis. Abdominal aortography demonstrates a large fusiform aneurysm of the abdominal aorta.

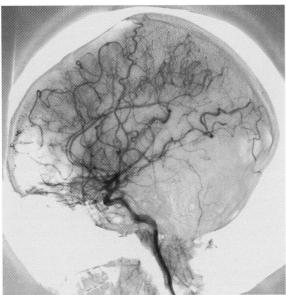

Figure 77. Substance-abuse vasculitis in a 39-year-old female with severe headache and a history of taking cold medications containing PPA. The right internal carotid arteriogram shows multifocal beading and segmental narrowing of small intracranial branches. This appearance is nonspecific and can be mimicked by almost any central nervous system vasculitis (SLE vasculitis, idiopathic, cocaine-abuse, etc).

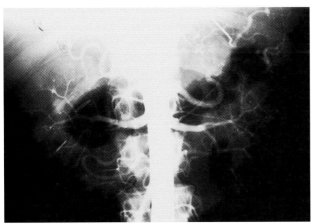

Figure 78. Cocaine-induced arteritis. The angiographic appearance is indistinguishable from PAN.

Arteriographic Findings in Substance-Abuse Vasculitis

The arteriographic appearance of substance-abuse vasculitis is nonspecific. Radiographic findings may include segmental areas of stenosis and dilatation with a "beaded" or "sausage" pattern, occlusion of small arteries, microaneurysms, and vasospasm **(Fig. 77)**. Most vasculitides affecting the central nervous system can have a similar appearance. In the visceral arteries, substance-abuse vasculitis mimics PAN **(Fig. 78)**.

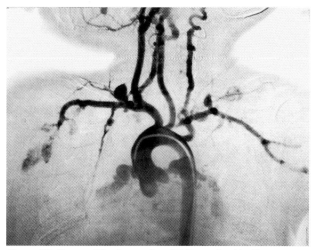

Figure 79. Kawasaki's disease in a 5 1/2-month-old with extensive arterial involvement including fusiform and saccular aneurysms of coronary, subclavian, carotid, vertebral, and internal mammary arteries. Most vessels are irregular in caliber as well. The axillary arteries are occluded by large aneurysms. Iliac, visceral, and lumbar arteries were also involved (not shown).

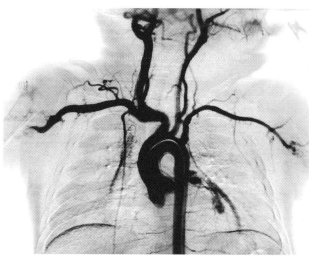

Figure 80. Same patient as in Figure 79 at 11 months of age after therapy. There has been interval regression of numerous aneurysms (compare costocervical trunk origins, internal mammary and coronary arteries). The right axillary artery aneurysm continued to expand (not shown).

Kawasaki's Disease

This disorder, also known as mucocutaneous lymph node syndrome, is an acute febrile illness of infants and young children. It is occasionally seen in young adults. Coronary arteritis is probably present in all patients. Kawasaki's disease is initially a small-vessel vasculitis which may progress to a PAN-type arteritis of medium-sized arteries. Inflammation initially produces aneurysms, while healing results in mural fibrosis and stenoses **(Fig. 79)**. Aneurysms are fusiform or saccular, usually smaller than 3 mm, and may regress with time or therapy **(Fig. 80)**. About 5% of patients have one or more systemic aneurysms, most commonly in the axillary or iliac arteries, and less often in the renal, internal mammary, mesenteric, or bronchial arteries or in the aorta.

Renal Transplant Vasculitis

Transplant rejection is the result of both humoral and cellular immune mechanisms. Acute endothelial cell damage leads to chronic fibro-intimal hyperplasia. Arteriography may demonstrate irregular intrarenal vessels with segmental stenoses and occlusions **(Fig. 81)** The number of occlusions increases with time. Poor cortical filling is evident in affected arterial territories, with poor definition of the corticomedullary junction. Arterial washout is normal or delayed. Arteriovenous shunting is sometimes present. Tubular stenosis of the postanastomotic portion of the main renal artery may be due to rejection, but flow turbulence hyperplasia and iatrogenic injury to the intima or vasa vasorum at the time of surgery should also be considered.

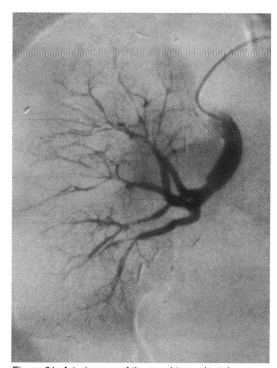

Figure 81. Arteriogram of the renal transplant demonstrates multiple intraparenchymal arterial stenoses and vessel irregularity. Peripheral branches are attenuated. The findings are consistent with chronic rejection 2 years after the transplant.

Summary

There are a number of different ways to classify the clinically diverse group of diseases which cause vasculitis. An etiologic classification is useful for learning about these diseases, while classification by the size of the affected vessels is useful for determining the differential diagnosis. Even though there is substantial overlap in the angiographic appearance of many of these disorders, arteriography plays an important role in their diagnosis, especially for the idiopathic (primary) vasculitides. The clinical features of these disorders may be extremely variable because the symptoms and signs are usually due to the vascular abnormalities, and these diseases may affect a number of different vessels in a variety of patterns and to a variable extent.

For further information on this topic, please see Teaching File Cases 7, 20, and 25–27.

Selected Readings

Churg J, Churg A. Idiopathic and secondary vasculitis: a review. Mod Pathol 1989; 2:144–160.

Cipriano PR, Alonso DR, Baltaxe HA, Gay WA Jr, Smith JP. Multiple aortic aneurysms in relapsing polychondritis. Am J Cardiol 1976; 37:1097–1102.

Evans JM, O'Fallon WM, Hunder GG. Increased incidence of aortic aneurysm and dissection in giant cell (temporal) arteritis: a population-based study. Ann Intern Med 1995; 122:502–507.

Forman HP, Levin S, Stewart B, Patel M, Feinstein S. Cerebral vasculitis and hemorrhage in an adolescent taking diet pills containing phenylpropanolamine: case report and review of the literature. Pediatrics 1989; 83:737–741.

Gersony WM. Diagnosis and management of Kawasaki disease. JAMA 1991; 265:2699–2703.

Gravallese EM, Corson JM, Coblyn JS, Pinkus GS, Weinblatt ME. Rheumatoid aortitis: a rarely recognized but clinically significant entity. Medicine 1989; 68:95–106.

Hagen B, Lohse S. Clinical and radiologic aspects of Buerger's disease. Cardiovasc Intervent Radiol 1984; 7:283–293.

Hekali P, Kajander H, Pajari R, Stenman S, Somer S. Diagnostic significance of angiographically observed visceral aneurysms with regard to polyarteritis nodosa. Acta Radiol 1991; 32:143–148.

Jennette JC, Falk RJ, Andrassy K, et al. Nomenclature of systemic vasculitides: proposal of an international consensus conference. Arthritis Rheum 1994; 37:187–192.

Joseph S, Mandalam KR, Rao VR, et al. Percutaneous transluminal angioplasty of the subclavian artery in nonspecific aortoarteritis: results of a long-term follow-up. J Vasc Interv Radiol 1994; 5:573–580.

Kerr GS, Hallahan CW, Giordano J, et al. Takayasu arteritis. Ann Intern Med 1994; 120:919–929.

Klein RG, Hunder GG, Stanson AW, Sheps SG. Large artery involvement in giant cell (temporal) arteritis. Ann Intern Med 1975; 83:806–812.

Klippel JH. Raynaud's phenomenon: the French tricolor. Arch Intern Med 1991; 151:2389–2393.

Lande A, Berkman MY. Aortitis: pathologic, clinical and arteriographic review. Radiol Clin North Am 1976; 14:219–240.

Lapointe JS, Nugent RA, Graeb DA, Robertson WD. Cerebral infarction and regression of widespread aneurysms in Kawasaki's disease: case report. Pediatr Radiol 1984; 14:1–5.

Lie JT. Nomenclature and classification of vasculitis: plus ça change, plus c'est la même chose. Arthritis Rheum 1994; 37:181.

Liu Y-Q, Jin BL, Ling J. Pulmonary artery involvement in aortoarteritis: an angiographic study. Cardiovasc Intervent Radiol 1994; 17:2–6.

Marks C, Kuskov S. Pattern of arterial aneurysms in acquired immunodeficiency syndrome. World J Surg 1995; 19:127–132.

Ninet JP, Bachet P, Dumontet CM, Du Colombier PB, Stewart MD, Pasquier JH. Subclavian and axillary involvement in temporal arteritis and polymyalgia rheumatica. Am J Med 1990; 88:13–20.

Oskoui R, Davis WA, Gomes MN. Salmonella aortitis: a report of a successfully treated case with a comprehensive review of the literature. Arch Intern Med 1993; 153:517–525.

Park JH, Han MC, Bettmann MA. Arterial manifestations of Behçet's disease. AJR 1984; 143:821–825.

Rao SA, Mandalam KR, Rao VR, et al. Takayasu arteritis: initial and long-term follow-up in 16 patients after percutaneous transluminal angioplasty of the descending thoracic and abdominal aorta. Radiology 1993; 189:173–179.

Subramanyan R, Joy J, Balakrishnan KG. Natural history of aortoarteritis (Takayasu's disease). Circulation 1989; 80:429–437.

Tunaci A, Berkmen YM, Gökmen E. Thoracic involvement in Behçet's disease: pathologic, clinical, and imaging features. AJR 1995; 164:51–56.

Wilson SE, van Wagenen P, Passaro E Jr. Arterial infection. Current Probl Surg 1978; 15:1–89.

Yamada I, Shibuya H, Matsubara O, et al. Pulmonary artery disease in Takayasu's arteritis: angiographic findings. AJR 1992; 159:263–269.

Yamato M, Lecky JW, Hiramatsu K, Kohda E. Takayasu's arteritis: radiographic and angiographic findings in 59 patients. Radiology 1986; 161:329–334.

End Notes

The opinions expressed herein are those of the authors and do not necessarily reflect the views of the United States Navy or the Department of Defense.

Figures 5, 7, 8, 9–11, 20, 25, 38–42, and 73 are U.S. Government works and are in the public domain.

Figure 6 courtesy of K. Laffey, Ph.D., M.D., New York, NY.

Figures 16, 44, 69, and 75 courtesy of the Armed Forces Institute of Pathology, Washington, D.C.

Figures 32, 47, and 74 courtesy of T. Vesely, M.D., St. Louis, MO.

Figures 46 and 80 courtesy of S. Lossef, M.D., Washington, D.C.

Figures 48 and 49 courtesy of J.H. Park, Seoul, Korea. From Park JH, Han MC, Bettmann MA. Arterial manifestations of Behçet's disease. AJR 1984; 143:823. Used with permission.

Figure 76 courtesy of P. Cipriano, Palo Alto, CA.

Figure 77 courtesy of W.R.K. Smoker, Richmond, VA.

Figures 78 and 79 courtesy of J.S. Lapointe, Vancouver. From Lapointe JS, Nugent RA, Graeb DA, Robertson WD. Cerebral infarction and regression of widespread aneurysms in Kawasaki's disease: case report. Pediatr Radiol 1984; 14:3. Used with permission.

TEACHING FILE CASES

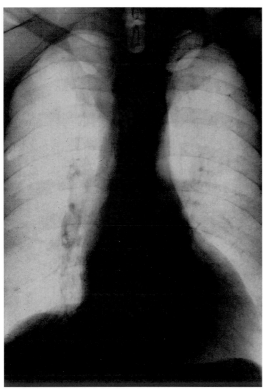

Figure 1. Admission chest radiograph.

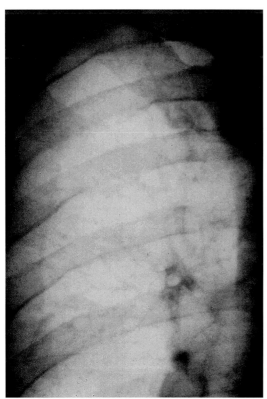

Figure 2. Coned-down view of the right upper chest from the admission film.

TEACHING FILE CASE 1
David Sacks, M.D.

History

A 51-year-old man with chronic severe hypertension and coronary artery disease was being evaluated for severe, bilateral lower extremity claudication and symptomatic carotid artery disease. His admission chest radiograph is provided **(Fig. 1)** with a coned-down view of the right upper chest **(Fig. 2)**.

What is your diagnosis?

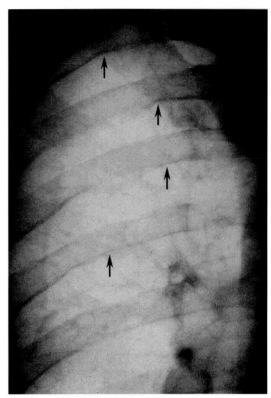

Figure 3. Notching of the undersurface of multiple ribs (arrows).

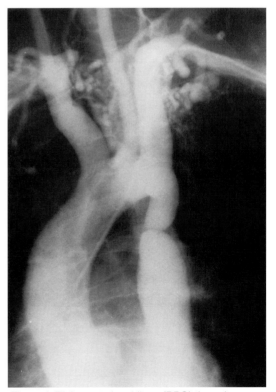

Figure 4. Right posterior oblique (RPO) thoracic arteriogram.

Radiographic Findings

There is mild cardiomegaly but no evidence of congestive heart failure. There is notching of the undersurface of multiple ribs bilaterally **(Fig. 3)**.

Although the femoral pulses were diminished, arteriography was attempted from the groin; however, the catheter could not be advanced to the aortic arch. Through a left axillary approach, an arch aortogram was obtained **(Fig. 4)**.

What is your diagnosis now?

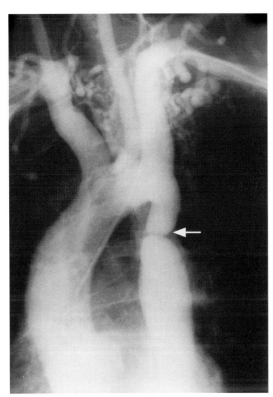

Figure 5. RPO thoracic aortogram shows a focal web-like stenosis (arrow) present in the proximal descending aorta.

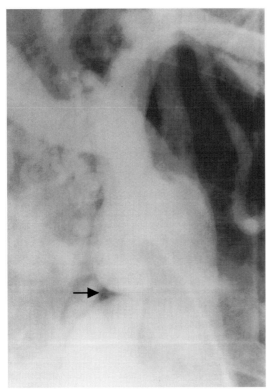

Figure 6. Left posterior oblique thoracic arteriogram shows the stenosis in profile.

There is a focal diaphragm-like narrowing of the thoracic aorta distal to the left subclavian artery **(Fig. 5)**. The left posterior oblique view shows the eccentric invagination of the aorta to better advantage **(Fig. 6)**. This forward displacement of the stenotic area has been attributed to tethering by the ductus ligament. Note that the left subclavian artery is double the size of the left carotid artery. Multiple large collateral vessels descend from the subclavian arteries to the lower chest, including bilaterally enlarged internal mammary arteries and costocervical trunks.

The first posterior intercostal artery is large and fills in a retrograde fashion as seen on a left subclavian artery injection performed at a different time (Figs. 7, 8). There was a 50-mm-Hg peak systolic pressure gradient across the aortic stenosis.

Diagnosis
Coarctation of the thoracic aorta.

Management
Surgical management of childhood coarctations has excellent results, although restenosis and aneurysms can occur. Balloon dilation can be effective in treatment of restenosis. Balloon dilation of native coarctations has also been performed in both children and adults with mixed results.

The Valvuloplasty and Angioplasty of Congenital Anomalies Registry reported data on 141 native coarctation balloon angioplasty procedures. Approximately 90% of patients had the pressure gradient across the coarctation reduced to less than 20 mm Hg. The complication rate was 17%, including six cases of aneurysm formation at the angioplasty site. In a smaller series of eight adults with native coarctations, balloon dilation was successful in seven out of eight patients, including a patient aged 49. Five of the patients had intimal tears noted at transesophageal echocardiography, one of whom had a type 3 dissection present at 6-month follow-up.

Although intimal tears are expected from balloon dilation, the association of cystic medial necrosis with coarctation may contribute to the risk of dissection after dilation. Covered or uncovered arterial stents may be useful in preventing restenosis, aneurysms, and aortic dissections, but favorable results are currently limited to animal experiments.

The patient in this teaching file was not considered a candidate for primary surgical repair of his coarctation because of his cerebral and coronary artery disease. It was elected to treat this patient with an axillobifemoral graft.

Discussion
Coarctation of the thoracic aorta is usually detected in childhood. Upper extremity hypertension and diminished femoral pulses are present. Half of the patients with coarctation will have additional cardiovascular abnormalities such as patent ductus arteriosus, bicuspid aortic valve, subaortic stenosis, ventricular or atrial septal defects, mitral stenosis or regurgitation, or atrioventricular canal. In severe cases, infants can present with hypoplastic left heart syndrome. Adults may present with nosebleeds, headaches, and coldness or pain in the legs.

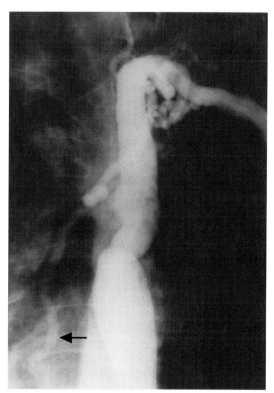

Figure 7. RPO left subclavian arteriogram reveals an enlarged left internal mammary artery (arrow).

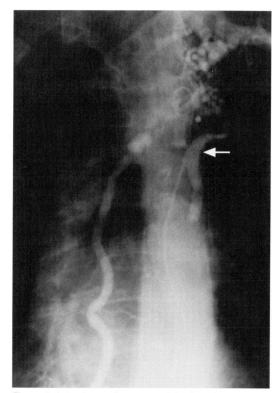

Figure 8. Later image from same injection shown in Figure 7. The left first posterior intercostal artery can also be seen (arrow).

The chest radiographic findings include indentation of the aortic contour below the aortic notch, dilatation of the ascending aorta, dilatation of the left subclavian artery, enlargement of the internal mammary arteries causing an undulating substernal soft tissue density on the lateral chest film, and rib notching.

Many of these findings are due to the presence of enlarged collaterals from the upper to lower aorta. The internal mammary arteries supply the anterior intercostal arteries, which then flow posteriorly into the distal thoracic aorta. These hypertrophied and occasionally aneurysmal intercostal arteries erode the undersurface of the ribs causing the characteristic notched appearance. In this case the intercostals fill so late that they are not opacified on the arteriogram. The internal mammary arteries also supply the superior epigastric vessels which then join the inferior epigastric vessels. Collaterals may also arise from the vertebral arteries through the anterior spinal artery, from the thyrocervical trunk through the transverse scapular and cervical arteries, from the costocervical trunk through the first and second intercostal arteries, and through the thoracoacromial trunk and the descending scapular artery.

For further information on this topic, please see Tutorial 1.

Selected Readings

Abrams HL, Jonsson G. Coarctation of the aorta. In: Abrams HL, ed. Abrams angiography: vascular and interventional radiology. 3rd edition. Boston: Little, Brown and Company, 1983; 388–412.

Bass JL, Rocchini AP. Catheter-directed interventional procedures in children. In: Castaneda-Zuniga WR, Tadavarthy SM, eds. Interventional radiology. 2nd edition. Baltimore: Williams and Wilkins, 1992.

Erbel R, Bednarczyk I, Pop T, et al. Detection of dissection of the aortic intima and media after angioplasty of coarctation of the aorta. An angiographic, computer tomographic, and echocardiographic comparative study. Circulation 1990; 81:805–814.

Tynan M, Finley JP, Fontes V, Hess J, Kan J. Balloon angioplasty for the treatment of native coarctation: results of valvuloplasty and angioplasty of congenital anomalies registry. Am J Cardiol 1990; 65:790–792.

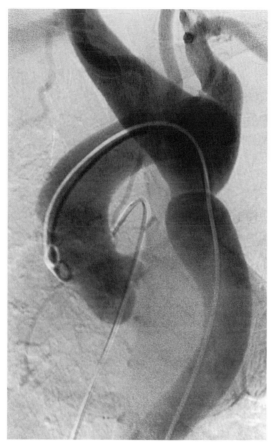

Figure 1. Thoracic aortogram, right posterior oblique (RPO) projection.

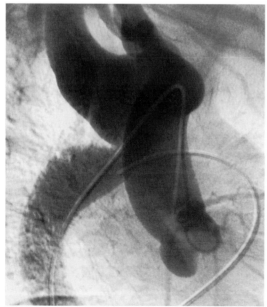

Figure 2. Thoracic aortogram, right anterior oblique (RAO) projection.

TEACHING FILE CASE 2
Joseph Krysl, M.D.

History
A 47-year-old woman came to the hospital with a history of cough and occasional mild shortness of breath. Previous magnetic resonance imaging evaluation of the chest had raised a question of a patent ductus arteriosus as well as an aortic coarctation or pseudocoarctation. At the time of cardiac catheterization she was found to have pulmonary hypertension. Thoracic arteriography was performed (Figs. 1, 2).

What is your diagnosis?

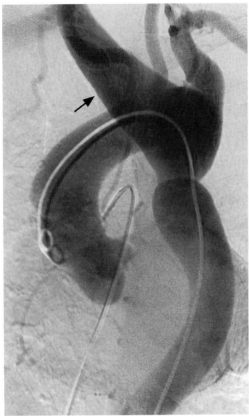

Figure 3. RPO thoracic aortogram demonstrates the aberrant right subclavian artery (arrow) with the dilated origin indicative of a diverticulum of Kommerell.

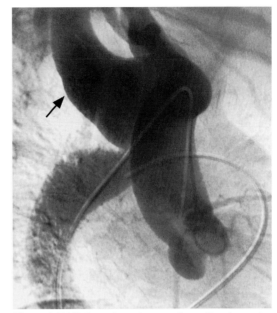

Figure 4. RAO thoracic aortogram shows the aberrant right subclavian artery with the diverticulum of Kommerell in profile (arrow).

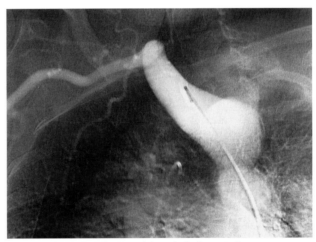

Figure 5. Selective aberrant right subclavian arteriogram demonstrates the diverticulum of Kommerell.

Radiographic Findings

The thoracic arteriogram **(Figs. 3, 4)** demonstrates an aberrant right subclavian artery originating distal to the left subclavian artery. The origin and proximal portion of the right subclavian artery are markedly dilated as it courses posteriorly. In addition, there is an abnormal configuration of the descending thoracic aorta with a "kink" in this region. No collaterals are present. No pressure gradient was noted across this area.

Diagnosis

1. Aberrant right subclavian artery with a diverticulum of Kommerell.
2. Aortic pseudocoarctation.

Management

A selective injection of the origin of the aberrant right subclavian artery was performed which demonstrated the dilated origin and proximal portion of the right subclavian artery. The selective injection was performed with a 5-F pigtail catheter due to the large origin of the vessel **(Fig. 5)**.

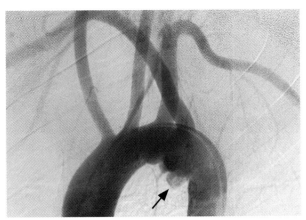

Figure 6. Thoracic aortogram depicts a normal sized aberrant right subclavian artery. A mycotic aneurysm on the inferior aspect of the aortic arch, separate from the origin of the right subclavian artery, is present (arrow).

Discussion

Aberrant right subclavian artery occurs in approximately 0.5% of the population and represents one of the most common arch anomalies. The subclavian artery courses posteriorly to the esophagus in most cases (80%); in 15% of cases the artery passes between the esophagus and the trachea, and in 5% of cases it is anterior to the trachea.

The origin of the aberrant subclavian artery is usually normal in size but may occasionally be dilated. The dilatation can be related to persistence of the dorsal aortic root leading to a diverticulum of Kommerell at the origin of the aberrant subclavian artery. Alternatively, the origin of the artery may be dilated because of atherosclerotic disease. It may be difficult to distinguish between these two entities angiographically. **Figure 6** demonstrates an aberrant right subclavian artery of normal caliber. This patient had a mycotic aneurysm of the aorta near the origin of the aberrant right subclavian artery. This may have been due to turbulent flow in this region.

Multiple symptoms have been attributed to the dilated origin of an aberrant right subclavian artery. These include dysphagia (also called dysphagia lusoria), dyspnea, and chest discomfort or pain. In addition, rupture of the aneurysmal origin has been described.

The "kink" noted in the descending thoracic aorta represents a pseudocoarctation of the aorta. There was no pressure gradient across this region, a finding corroborated by the absence of collaterals. Although pressure gradients have been described with pseudocoarctation of the aorta, more typically no gradient is identified. The etiology of pseudo-coarctation remains unclear; it may be due to elongation and tortuosity of the thoracic aorta or may be related to failure of regression of the right aortic arch with its incorporation into the distal left aortic arch.

For further information on this topic, please see Tutorial 1.

Selected Readings

Abrams, HL. Additional applications of thoracic aortography. In: Abrams HL, ed. Abrams angiography: vascular and interventional radiology. 3rd edition. Boston: Little, Brown and Company, 1983.

Knight GC, Codd JE. Anomalous right subclavian artery aneurysm: report of three cases and review of the literature. Tex Heart Inst J 1991; 18:209–218.

Stone WM, Brewster DC, Moncure AC, Franklin DP, Cambria RP, Abbott WM. Aberrant right subclavian artery: varied presentations and management options. J Vasc Surg 1990; 11:812–817.

Vega A, Ortiz A, Longo JM, Pagola MA. CT of ruptured aneurysm of aberrant right subclavian artery. Cardiovasc Intervent Radiol 1987; 10:13–15.

Walker TG, Geller SC. Aberrant right subclavian artery with a large diverticulum of Kommerell: a potential for misdiagnosis. AJR 1987; 149:477–478.

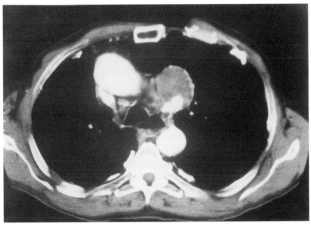

Figure 1. Contrast-enhanced CT scan of the upper thorax in a 69-year-old man with dysphagia and an abnormal chest radiograph.

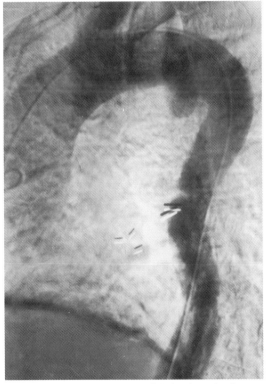

Figure 2. Thoracic aortogram, digital subtraction image.

TEACHING FILE CASE 3
Robert Principato, D.O.

History

A 69-year-old man came to the hospital with dysphagia and had an abnormal chest radiograph. A computed tomography (CT) scan was performed and showed a vascular mass in the aortopulmonary window extending from the aortic arch (Fig. 1). An aortogram was subsequently obtained (Fig. 2).

What is your diagnosis?

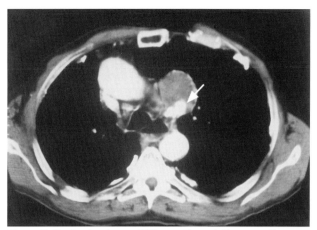

Figure 3. Contrast-enhanced CT scan through the upper thorax shows a 6-cm mass within the aortopulmonary window. Dense contrast extends into the dorsal aspect of the mass (arrow).

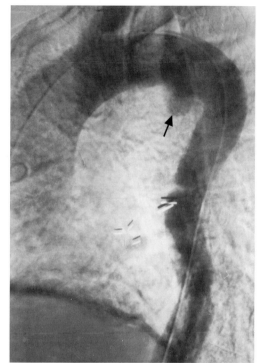

Figure 4. Subtraction image from the thoracic aortogram shows an aneurysmal outpouching (arrow) from the caudal surface of the transverse aorta.

Radiographic Findings

The CT scan demonstrates a 6-cm mass in the area of the aortopulmonary window with a small central area of contrast enhancement **(Fig. 3)**. The thoracic aortogram subtraction image shows a nipple-like communication from the caudal aspect of the transverse aorta **(Fig. 4)**. Note how difficult this was to visualize on the unsubtracted film **(Fig. 5)**.

Diagnosis

Aneurysm of the ductus diverticulum.

What treatment would you recommend?

Discussion

These aneurysms are very uncommon and are usually managed surgically. Surgical repair can be technically challenging and may require cardiac bypass. In the future, endovascular treatment with the placement of a covered stent may be feasible.

As with most aortic aneurysms, cross-sectional imaging with CT scanning or magnetic resonance imaging provides valuable anatomic information, accurately depicting the size of the aneurysm. Angiography often underestimates the size of an aneurysm due to the presence of thrombus.

For further information on this topic, please see Tutorials 1 and 2.

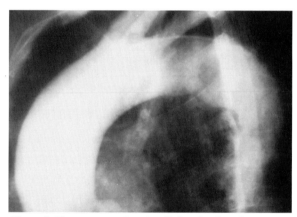

Figure 5. The aneurysm is not well visualized on the unsubtracted image.

Selected Readings

Goodman PC, Jeffrey RB, Minagi H, Federle MP, Thomas AN. Angiographic evaluation of the ductus diverticulum. Cardiovasc Intervent Radiol 1982; 5:1–4.

Hattori T, Hirata K, Shimizu S. Aneurysm of the diverticulum of the ductus arteriosus. Nippon Kyobu Geka Gakkai Zasshi 1994; 42:150–155.

Mitchell RS, Seifert FC, Miller DC, Jamieson SW, Shumway NE. Aneurysm of the diverticulum of the ductus arteriosus in the adult: successful surgical treatment in five patients and review of the literature. J Thorac Cardiovasc Surg 1983; 86:400–408.

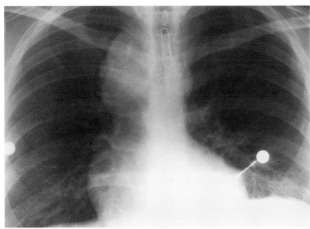

Figure 1. Chest radiograph of a 27-year-old man following a high-speed motor vehicle accident.

TEACHING FILE CASE 4
Eric W. Olcott, M.D.

History

A 27-year-old man was brought to the emergency department following a high-speed motor vehicle accident. He was hypotensive upon admission and aggressive resuscitation was initiated. A chest radiograph was obtained **(Fig. 1)**. No prior films were available.

What is your diagnosis?

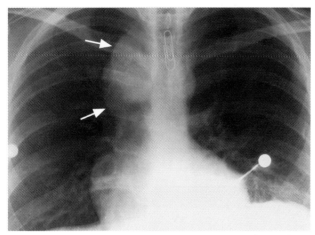

Figure 2. A widened superior mediastinum is present (arrows), predominantly to the right of the trachea.

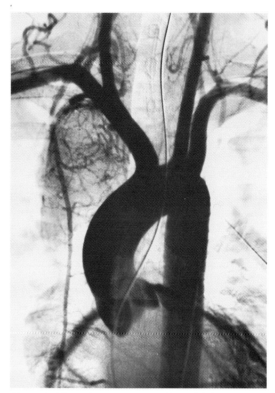

Figure 3. Thoracic aortogram, mid arterial phase.

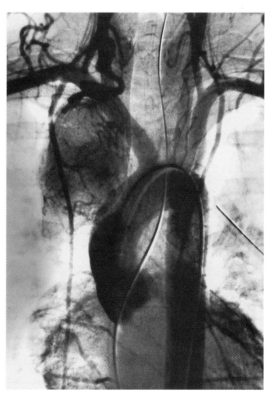

Figure 4. Thoracic aortogram, late arterial phase.

Radiographic Findings

The mediastinum is widened **(Fig. 2)**. In the setting of a high-speed deceleration event, an aortic injury is suspected. Additionally, one could question whether there is a right-sided aortic arch, or a double aortic arch.

Aortography was performed to rule out trauma to the aorta **(Fig. 3)**. Is there evidence of aortic injury?

Figure 4 is a later image from the same injection. No evidence of aortic injury is identified. Oblique projections also failed to show aortic injury. The aorta is left-sided and branches normally.

What is responsible for the mediastinal widening seen on the admission chest film?

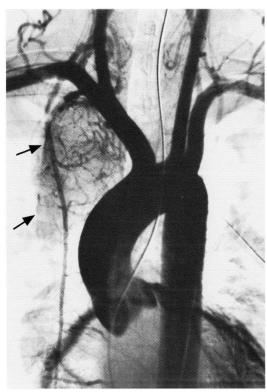

Figure 5. Thoracic aortogram shows a hypervascular right-sided mediastinal mass (arrows).

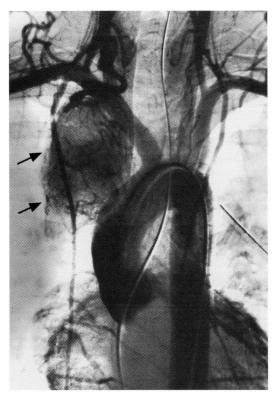

Figure 6. A later image from the thoracic aortogram reveals the right-sided mass (arrows) to be densely staining.

Diagnosis
Vascular mediastinal mass.

What management is appropriate at this point?

Management
A hypervascular mediastinal mass is present with a well-developed arterial supply **(Fig. 5)**. Additionally, no evidence of arterial injury is noted within the mass **(Fig. 6)**. Therefore, work-up of the lesion can proceed later, provided the patient remains stable.

Follow-up chest radiographs were unchanged from the initial film. The mass did not require immediate intervention.

Discussion

In the setting of a significant deceleration event with mediastinal widening, an aortic injury must be excluded. Aortography has traditionally been the procedure of choice. In some centers, spiral computed tomography with intravenous contrast material is being evaluated as a potential alternative.

Aortic injuries are life-threatening and can be readily diagnosed with aortography. Prompt surgical intervention can be life-saving when an aortic injury is present. In this patient, subsequent pathologic examination of the mass yielded a diagnosis of Castleman's disease (benign lymph node hyperplasia).

For further information on this topic, please see Tutorial 4.

Selected Readings

Marnocha KE, Maglinte DDT, Woods J, et al. Blunt chest trauma and suspected aortic rupture: reliability of chest radiograph findings. Ann Emerg Med 1985; 14:644–649.

Townsend RN, Colella JJ, Diamond DL. Traumatic rupture of the aorta: critical decisions for trauma surgeons. J Trauma 1990; 30:1169–1174.

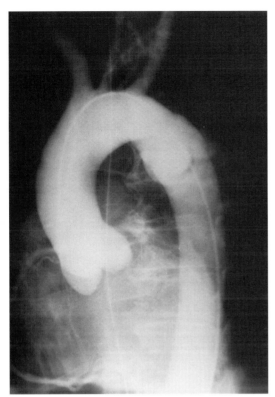

Figure 1. Right posterior oblique (RPO) cut film thoracic aortogram.

TEACHING FILE CASE 5
Niki Harris, M.D.

History
A 74-year-old man sustained a severe deceleration injury during a motor vehicle accident and came to the emergency department with a blood pressure of 130/74 mm Hg, a pulse of 86 beats per minute, and chest pain. A chest radiograph demonstrated a wide mediastinum and left apical capping. A thoracic aortogram was obtained **(Fig. 1)**.

What is your diagnosis?

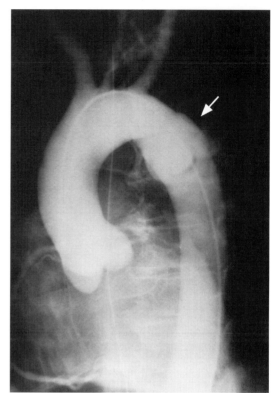

Figure 2. Thoracic arteriogram demonstrates a false aneurysm distal to the left subclavian artery origin (arrow). The remainder of the thoracic aorta is normal.

Radiographic Findings

The thoracic arteriogram demonstrates a contained leak distal to the left subclavian artery origin **(Fig. 2)**. The remainder of the thoracic aorta is normal.

Diagnosis

Aortic transection.

Management

Immediate open surgical repair.

Discussion

More than 90% of aortic transections seen on thoracic aortography occur in the region of the aortic isthmus. Fewer than 10% are seen at the aortic root or distal descending thoracic aorta. The diagnosis must be made quickly because a significant percentage of these patients will die within 24 hours if the transection is not surgically repaired. **Figures 3–7** provide examples of differential diagnosis of contour abnormalities of the aortic isthmus. Spiral computed tomography is currently thought to be a sensitive screening modality for the evaluation of mediastinal hematoma suggesting aortic injury, but it has not yet been proven to be specific or accurate enough to direct surgical repair with positive results.

For further information on this topic, please see Tutorial 4.

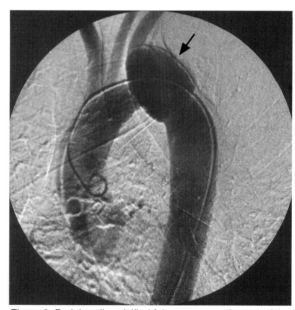

Figure 3. Peripherally calcified false aneurysm (arrow) of the aortic isthmus consistent with a chronic post-traumatic false aneurysm.

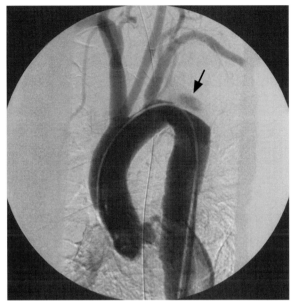

Figure 4. Focal intramural dissection (arrow) which communicates with the true lumen of the aorta. This injury represents avulsion of an intercostal artery which occurred during a motor vehicle accident.

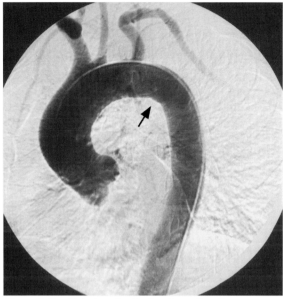

Figure 5. Small ductus diverticulum (arrow) on the anteromedial aspect of the aorta; this finding is of no clinical significance.

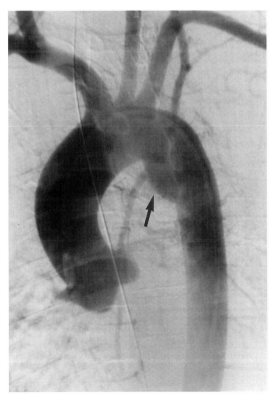

Figure 6. Larger ductus diverticulum (arrow) or "ductus bump" which is also of no clinical significance. No intimal flap, irregularity, or lateral margin defect is seen to suggest aortic injury.

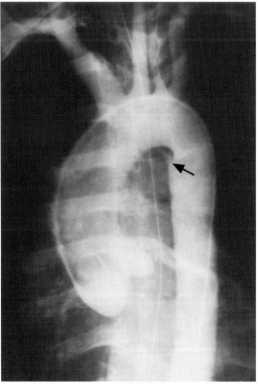

Figure 7. The origin of the right bronchial artery (arrow) can give a disturbing appearance to the medial aspect of the descending aorta.

Selected Readings

Heystraten FM, Kingma LM, Lacquet LK, Rosenbusch G.
Chronic post-traumatic aneurysm of the thoracic aorta:
surgically correctable occult threat. AJR 1986; 146:303–308.

Stark P. Traumatic rupture of the thoracic aorta: a review. Crit
Rev Diagn Imaging 1984; 21:229–255.

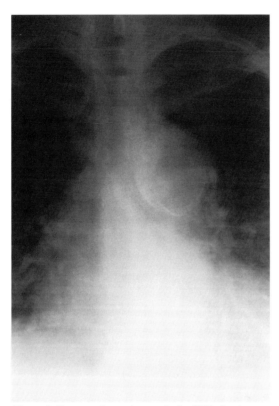

Figure 1. Preoperative anteroposterior (AP) chest radiograph.

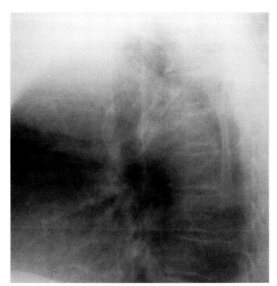

Figure 2. Preoperative lateral chest radiograph.

TEACHING FILE CASE 6
Jeet Sandhu, M.D.

History

A preoperative chest radiograph was obtained in an asymptomatic 44-year-old woman **(Figs. 1, 2)**.

What is your diagnosis?

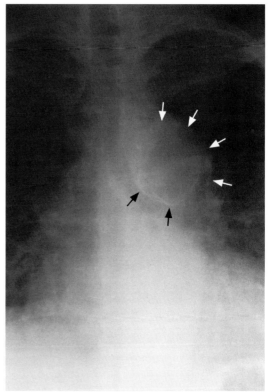

Figure 3. Frontal chest radiograph demonstrates calcification and enlargement of the transverse and proximal descending portions of the thoracic aorta (arrows).

Radiographic Findings

On the AP film **(Fig. 3)** an area of curvilinear calcification contiguous with the wall of the aorta is identified, associated with focal aortic dilatation at that level. There are no visible calcifications elsewhere in the thoracic aorta. In addition, the edges of the aortic arch are not well defined. The lateral film **(Fig. 4)** indicates that the mass with peripheral calcification originates from the anterior and inferior surface of the proximal descending thoracic aorta. Magnetic resonance (MR) imaging **(Figs. 5, 6)** shows focal dilatation of the aorta with an extraluminal flow void that is continuous with the aorta.

This saccular aneurysm of the aorta originates immediately distal to the left subclavian artery. The patient had surgical resection of this aneurysm with aortic reconstruction. Upon further questioning, the patient indicated that she had been involved in a motor vehicle accident 10 years ago for which she never sought any medical attention; this was the likely cause of the traumatic injury to the aorta.

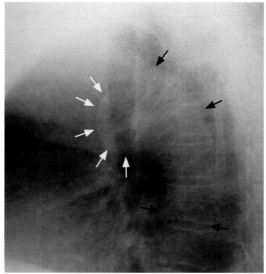

Figure 4. Lateral chest radiograph demonstrates a mass with curvilinear calcification contiguous with the anterior and inferior surfaces of the aorta (white arrows). Black arrows outline the aorta.

Diagnosis

Post-traumatic pseudoaneurysm of the aorta.

Management

The patient underwent surgical repair of the aneurysm with aortic reconstruction.

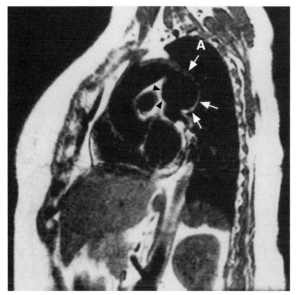

Figure 5. Sagittal MR scan shows a saccular aneurysm (arrows) contiguous with the aorta (A).

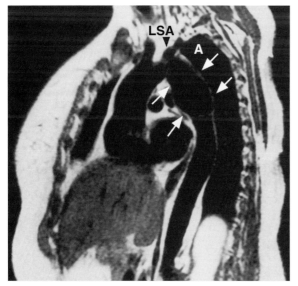

Figure 6. Sagittal MR scan of the thoracic aorta (A) shows focal dilatation (arrows) of the proximal descending aorta immediately distal to the left subclavian artery (LSA).

Differential Diagnosis of Calcified Mediastinal Masses	
Aneurysm	Cystic degeneration of a neurogenic
Lipoma	tumor
Bronchogenic cyst	Hemangioma (phleboliths)
Lymph nodes	Thymoma with cystic degeneration
Dermoid cyst/	Old hematoma
Teratoma	Thyroid goiter

Figure 7.

Discussion

There are numerous causes of mediastinal masses with calcifications **(Fig. 7)**. However, the only pathologic processes that commonly present with curvilinear calcifications are aneurysms and duplication cysts. The remainder will have irregular punctate or amorphous calcifications.

Although the plain films may have suggested a fusiform atherosclerotic aneurysm, the lack of calcifications elsewhere in the aorta and the eccentricity of the calcifications do not support this diagnosis. Moreover, the patient's young age does not favor an atherosclerotic aneurysm. A duplication cyst might be considered in the differential diagnosis, but because of the eccentricity, location, and contiguity with the aorta, the most likely diagnosis is a post-traumatic pseudoaneurysm.

Aortic pseudoaneurysms occur subsequent to disruption of the aortic wall and can develop as a complication of aortic and cardiac surgeries as well as blunt chest trauma. Rarely, pseudoaneurysms result from infection of the aortic wall or extension of infection from adjacent structures into the aorta. This latter mechanism will produce a mycotic aneurysm.

Aortic trauma can be caused by high-speed sudden deceleration injuries. The most commonly accepted hypothesis for the mechanism of injury is that sudden deceleration imposes the greatest stresses on the aorta at points of fixation, which include the aortic root, the aortic isthmus where it is tethered by the ligamentum arteriosum, and the aorta at the diaphragmatic hiatus.

With sudden deceleration, the non-tethered portions of the aorta continue with high-speed forward momentum while the fixed points suddenly stop, producing significant shear stresses that result in aortic tears that involve one or more layers of the vessel wall. In 60% of cases, the intima and media are both lacerated and the blood is contained by the adventitia. If all three layers are affected, the patient usually expires immediately from free rupture. If the patient survives, the blood will be contained by surrounding mediastinal structures. Although this is the most accepted hypothesis for post-traumatic aortic injury, other mechanisms have been proposed. An alternative explanation is that the aorta is injured by an "osseus pinch" mechanism.

The osseus pinch mechanism proposes that the aorta in the region of the ligamentum is compressed between the vertebral body and the anterior bony thoracic elements including the manubrium, the head of the clavicle, and the anterior first rib. With the massive force generally associated with aortic injuries, these bony elements are pushed inward and rotated about their posterior articulations until they impinge upon the vertebral body. Any structures between the anterior elements and vertebral bodies will be injured. Because of the fixed position of the proximal descending thoracic aorta, the isthmic portion of the aorta can be trapped and injured.

Regardless of the theories, aortic injuries are associated with high mortality rates. Pathologically, 20%–25% of injuries occur at the root of the aorta but the vast majority of these patients die immediately at the scene of the accident. As a result, the most common site of injury (>90%) seen clinically will be at the area of the ligamentum arteriosum **(Figs. 8, 9)**. Although the ductus diverticulum also occurs at this exact same location, the two entities can usually be distinguished radiographically. An aortic laceration or traumatic rupture will have acute margins with the aorta and an irregular surface. Moreover, with aortic lacerations, there is usually delayed transit of contrast material from the pseudoaneurysm lumen, and an intimal flap is often visualized. In contrast, a diverticulum will have obtuse margins, a smooth border, and there will be no hang-up of contrast material.

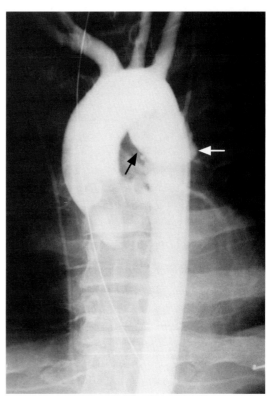

Figure 8. Thoracic aortogram shows a typical traumatic rupture at the ligamentum arteriosum (arrows).

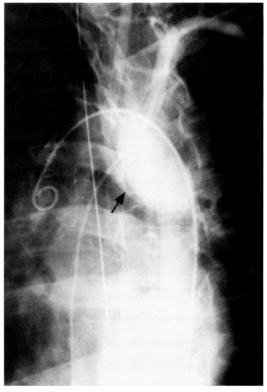

Figure 9. Thoracic aortogram, late arterial phase, shows delayed washout of contrast material contained within a traumatic aortic rupture (arrow).

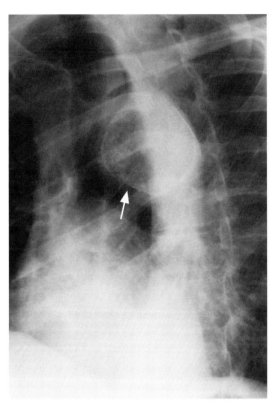

Figure 10. RPO plain film of another patient with a curvilinearly calcified post-traumatic aneurysm (arrow).

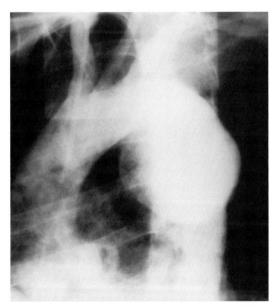

Figure 11. The aortogram confirms the presence of the pseudoaneurysm.

As noted earlier, 80%–90% of patients with an aortic injury will die immediately and 16% of immediate deaths from automobile accidents are due to traumatic laceration of the aorta. If the individual with an aortic rupture survives the initial injury, the long-term survival statistics are still grim. Without treatment, 30% of patients will die within 6 hours and an additional 20% will die within 24 hours. By 3 weeks, there is a 95%–98% mortality rate. Only 2%–5% of patients with aortic rupture will survive without treatment. It is within this group of patients that chronic post-traumatic pseudoaneurysms develop. Until 3 months after the initial injury, there is still a high chance of rupture and exsanguination. After 3 months, a layer of fibrous tissue may develop around the pseudoaneurysm and stabilize it, reducing the chances of sudden death.

Patients with chronic pseudoaneurysms may be asymptomatic or have a wide variety of symptoms including dyspnea, dysphagia, stridor, hoarseness, facial swelling, shoulder pain, diaphragmatic paralysis, and back pain. These symptoms are usually related to compression of adjacent mediastinal structures. If the pseudoaneurysm ruptures into the bronchus or esophagus, massive hemoptysis or hematemesis can result.

On plain films, the pseudoaneurysm can mimic mass lesions such as neoplasms. The most common plain film finding is an enlarged irregular contour of the transverse or proximal descending portion of the aorta. If curvilinear calcifications are noted (**Figs. 10, 11**), the suspicion for aortic pseudoaneurysm should increase dramatically. The diagnosis is usually confirmed with contrast-enhanced computed tomography or MR imaging.

The diagnosis of post-traumatic pseudoaneurysm is extremely important. The patient may have survived the initial insult, but the chances of rupture and death still exist because the pseudoaneurysm is never truly stable. In one series, 31 of 97 patients with chronic post-traumatic pseudoaneurysms died within 5 years. Another study showed that 20 of 60 patients with chronic post-traumatic pseudoaneurysm died from rupture. An additional series followed 105 patients with chronic pseudoaneurysm from traumatic aortic rupture. Sixty percent of these aneurysms showed clinical or radiographic signs of enlargement. Based on these studies, surgical resection should be considered for most patients with post-traumatic aneurysms.

For further information on this topic, please see Tutorial 4.

Selected Readings

Crass JR, Cohen AM, Motta AO, Tomashefski JF, Wiesen EJ. A proposed new mechanism of traumatic aortic rupture: the osseus pinch. Radiology 1990; 176:645–649.

Groskin SA. Selected topics in chest trauma. Radiology 1992; 183:605–617.

Petty SM, Parker LA, Mauro MA, Jaques PF, Mandell VS. Chronic post-traumatic aortic pseudoaneurysm: recognition before rupture. Postgrad Med 1991; 89:173–178.

Raptopoulos V. Chest CT for aortic injury: maybe not for everyone. AJR 1994; 162:1053–1055.

Razzouk A, Gundry S, Wang N, et al. Pseudoaneurysms of the aorta after cardiac surgery or chest trauma. Am Surg 1993; 59:818–823.

Woodring JH. The normal mediastinum in blunt traumatic rupture of the thoracic aorta and brachiocephalic arteries. J Emerg Med 1990; 8:467–476.

End Note

Figure 7 from Reeder MM, Felson B. Gamuts in radiology: comprehensive lists of roentgen differential diagnosis. Cincinnati: Audiovisual Radiology of Cincinnati, 1975; 412. Used with permission.

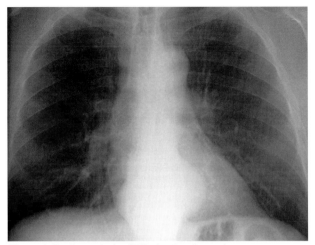

Figure 1. Posteroanterior (PA) chest radiograph.

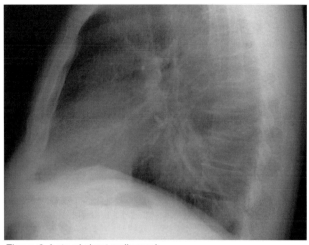

Figure 2. Lateral chest radiograph.

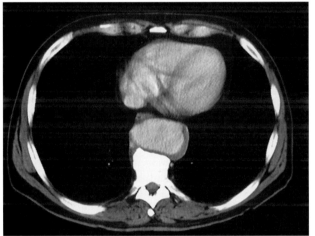

Figure 3. Contrast-enhanced thoracic CT scan.

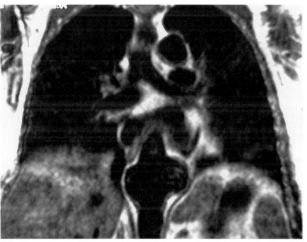

Figure 4. Coronal T1-weighted MR image through the chest and upper abdomen.

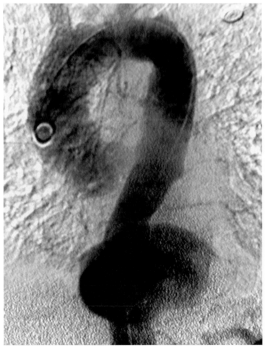

Figure 5. Thoracic aortogram.

TEACHING FILE CASE 7
Rajiv Sawhney, M.D., and
Susan D. Wall, M.D.

History
The patient is a 47-year-old man who has a fever of unknown origin. There is a history of intravenous drug abuse, but not of trauma. An abnormal chest radiograph **(Figs. 1, 2)** was followed up with a computed tomography (CT) study **(Fig. 3)**, a magnetic resonance (MR) exam **(Fig. 4)**, and an angiogram **(Fig. 5)**.

What is your diagnosis?

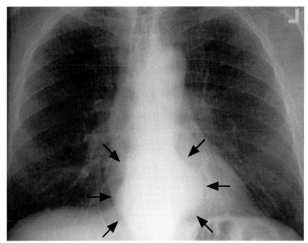

Figure 6. PA chest radiograph reveals a mass (arrows) in the caudal aspect of the thorax extending both to the left and right of the spine.

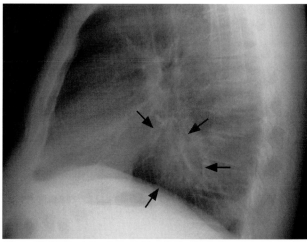

Figure 7. On the lateral chest film, the mass (arrows) is located anterior to the spine in the posterior mediastinum.

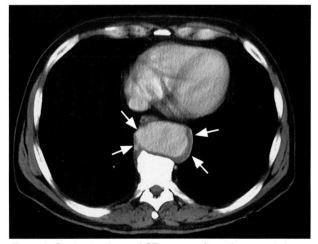

Figure 8. Contrast-enhanced CT scan confirms the mass to be a descending aortic aneurysm (arrows).

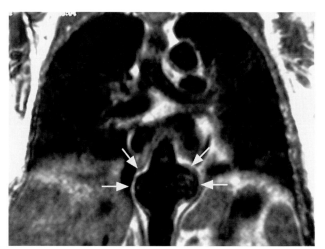

Figure 9. Coronal MR image depicts the aneurysm (arrows) to better advantage. The aneurysm extends both to the left and right of the anticipated aortic margin.

Radiographic Findings
Two views of the chest demonstrate an abnormal mass within the posterior mediastinum **(Figs. 6, 7)**. The CT, MR, and angiographic studies show a focal dilatation of the thoracic aorta representing a saccular aortic aneurysm **(Figs. 8–12)**.

Diagnosis
Mycotic aneurysm of the thoracic aorta.

How would you manage this patient?

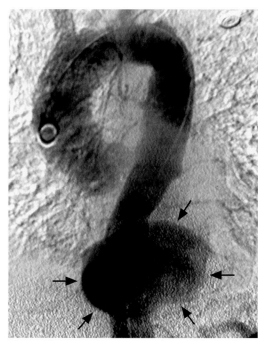

Figure 10. A saccular aneurysm (arrows) is clearly evident on aortography.

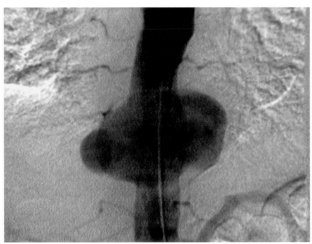

Figure 11. Magnification view of the distal thoracic aorta shows the aneurysm with better morphologic detail.

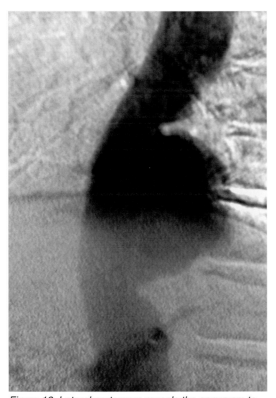

Figure 12. Lateral aortogram reveals the aneurysm to extend posteriorly from the normal aortic lumen.

Management

Patients with mycotic aneurysms of the thoracic aorta are treated surgically because these aneurysms can rapidly enlarge and rupture. This patient underwent resection of the aneurysm and aortic reconstruction.

Discussion

Although most frequently seen in the ascending aorta, mycotic aneurysms can occur in any artery. Patients who develop mycotic aneurysms usually have bacteremia or endocarditis. These aneurysms may also be seen following surgery or trauma. They arise because of destruction of the arterial wall layer by infectious agents, most commonly *Salmonella*, *Staphylococcus*, *Mycobacterium*, *E. coli*, and fungus. These agents seed pre-existing atheromatous lesions causing ongoing destruction. Spread from adjacent infected tissue into the arterial wall may also cause mycotic aneurysms, but this is rare because of the widespread use of antibiotics.

Mycotic aneurysms of the aorta are frequently seen in patients who use intravenous drugs. True aneurysms or false aneurysms develop depending on the extent of destruction. Angiographically, these aneurysms are saccular and eccentric in appearance. While post-traumatic aneurysms and occasionally atherosclerotic aneurysms can have this angiographic appearance, mycotic aneurysm should be strongly considered.

For further information on this topic, please see Tutorial 2.

Selected Readings

Edwards BS, Edwards JE. Localized aneurysms and dissecting hematomas of the thoracic aorta. In: Taveras JM, Ferrucci JT, eds. Radiology: diagnosis, imaging, intervention. Volume 2: Elliott LP, Buonocore E, eds. Cardiac vascular. Philadelphia: J.B. Lippincott Company, 1988; 1–8.

Guthaner DF. The plain chest film in assessing aneurysms and dissecting hematomas of the thoracic aorta. In: Taveras JM, Ferrucci JT, eds. Radiology: diagnosis, imaging, intervention. Volume 2: Elliott LP, Buonocore E, eds. Cardiac vascular. Philadelphia: J.B. Lippincott Company, 1988; 17.

Kadir S. Diagnostic angiography. Philadelphia: W.B. Saunders Company, 1986; 138–140.

Roberts AC, Kaufman JA, Geller SC. Angiographic assessment in peripheral vascular disease. In: Strandness DE Jr, van Breda A, eds. Vascular diseases: surgical and interventional therapy. New York: Churchill Livingstone, 1994; 210–211.

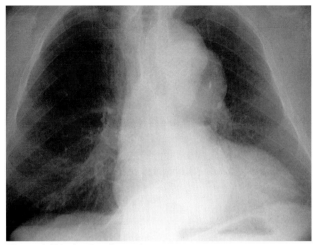

Figure 1. PA chest radiograph.

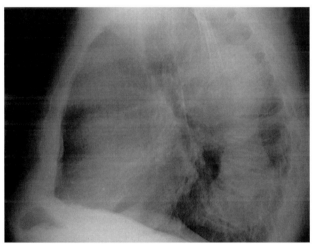

Figure 2. Lateral chest radiograph.

TEACHING FILE CASE 8

Rajiv Sawhney, M.D., and
Susan D. Wall, M.D.

History

A 75-year-old man complained of back pain. As part of his evaluation, posteroanterior (PA) and lateral chest radiographs were obtained **(Figs. 1, 2)**.

On the basis of the findings, what other diagnostic tests might be considered?

Radiographic Findings

The PA chest film **(Fig. 3)** shows diffuse enlargement of the thoracic aorta. The lateral view **(Fig. 4)** suggests that the aortic enlargement is principally confined to the descending thoracic aorta.

If the patient were unstable, transesophageal echocardiography would be useful to rapidly exclude aortic dissection involving the ascending aorta. In the stable patient, either magnetic resonance imaging or computed tomography (CT) scanning would be of value. This patient underwent CT scanning **(Fig. 5)**.

What is your diagnosis?

Diagnosis

Atherosclerotic aneurysm of the descending thoracic aorta **(Fig. 6)**.

How would you manage this patient?

Management

The decision to repair a thoracic aortic aneurysm is based upon the size of the aneurysm and the patient's age, symptoms, and overall medical condition. Aneurysms larger than 5 cm in diameter are considered for resection in patients who are reasonable candidates for surgery. Prior to surgery, arteriography is usually performed **(Figs. 7, 8)** for better anatomic delineation of the aneurysm. This patient underwent uneventful resection of the aneurysm with placement of an interposition graft.

Discussion

Atherosclerotic aneurysms occur due to weakening of the aortic wall. All layers of the arterial wall are involved. Turbulent blood flow and hypertension accelerate the process. Atherosclerotic aneurysms are usually fusiform in appearance; a saccular appearance is far less common. Atherosclerotic thoracic aortic aneurysms are seen in the descending aorta distal to the left subclavian artery and are less common than abdominal aortic aneurysms. Focal aneurysms of the proximal descending aorta are typical for chronic pseudoaneurysms due to trauma. Aneurysmal dilatation of the ascending aorta without involvement of the arch and with little calcification is seen in Marfan's or Ehlers-Danlos syndrome or may be idiopathic.

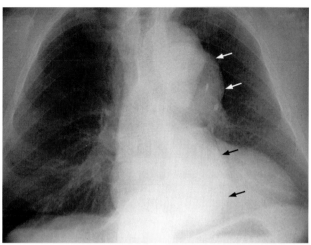

Figure 3. The thoracic aorta is diffusely dilated (arrows).

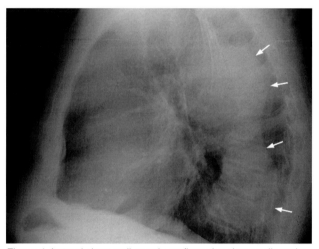

Figure 4. Lateral chest radiograph confirms the abnormality to be an enlarged descending aorta (arrows).

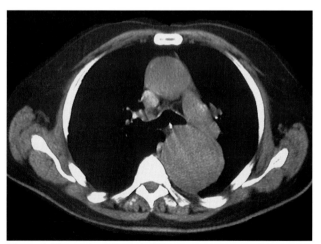

Figure 5. Noncontrast thoracic CT scan.

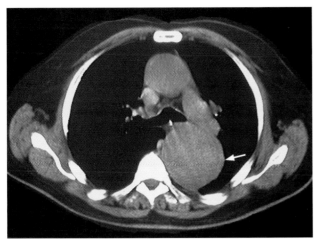

Figure 6. Thoracic CT scan reveals a descending thoracic aortic aneurysm (arrow). Subsequent to bolus intravenous contrast material injection there was no evidence of aortic dissection.

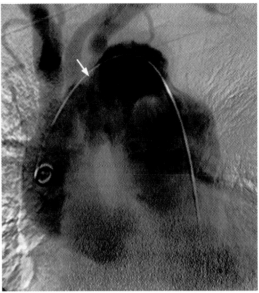

Figure 7. Right posterior oblique digital subtraction thoracic aortogram shows that the aneurysm begins just beyond the origin of the left subclavian artery (arrow).

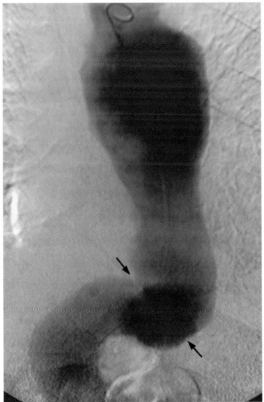

Figure 8. PA thoracic aortogram demonstrates the caudal extent of the aneurysmal lumen at the thoracoabdominal junction (arrows).

At arteriography, the lumen of the atherosclerotic aneurysm may be aneurysmal or normal in caliber because of the presence of mural thrombus. A widened soft tissue margin or mural calcification may help predict the lumen diameter. CT or magnetic resonance imaging will reveal the true diameter.

The prognosis for thoracic aortic aneurysms is worse than for abdominal aortic aneurysms, with a higher rate of rupture. These patients are treated with elective surgical repair because there is a significant difference in the mortality rate of patients who undergo elective surgery versus emergent surgery after rupture has occurred. Recently, a few centers have been treating selected cases with aortic stent-grafts using endovascular techniques.

For further information on this topic, please see Tutorial 2.

Selected Readings

Dake MD, Miller DC, Semba CP, Mitchell RS, Walker PJ, Liddell RP. Transluminal placement of endovascular stent-grafts for the treatment of thoracic descending aortic aneurysms. New Engl J Med 1994; 331:1729–1734.

Durham JD, Kaufman JA. Imaging of acquired thoracic and abdominal aortic disease. In: Strandness DE Jr, van Breda A, eds. Vascular diseases: surgical and interventional therapy. New York: Churchill Livingstone, 1994; 237–249.

Kadir S. Diagnostic angiography. Philadelphia: W.B. Saunders Company, 1986; 134–138.

Mitchell RS, Dake MD, Semba CP, et al. Endovascular stent-graft repair of thoracic aortic aneurysms. J Thorac Cardiovasc Surg 1996; 111:1054–1062.

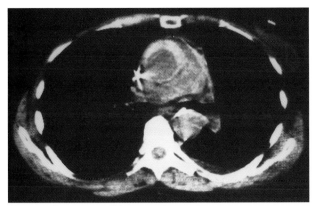

Figure 1. Precontrast CT scan at the aortic root.

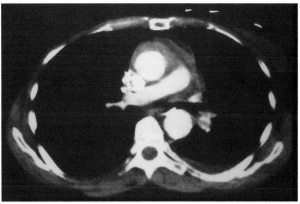

Figure 2. Post-contrast CT scan at the aortic root.

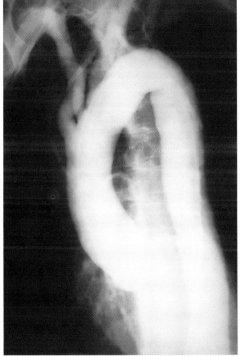

Figure 3. Right posterior oblique (RPO) thoracic aortogram.

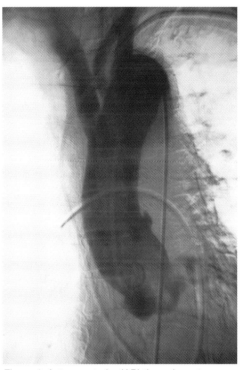

Figure 4. Anteroposterior (AP) thoracic aortogram, subtraction image.

TEACHING FILE CASE 9
Donald J. Ponec, M.D.

History
The patient is a 70-year-old female who was brought to the emergency department in shock. Pericardiocentesis yielded nonclotting blood and resulted in hemodynamic stability. The patient underwent computed tomography (CT) scanning of the thoracic aorta with repeated scanning at a single level during administration of a contrast material bolus at each of three levels (aortic root, arch, and descending aorta). Representative images at the level of the aortic root are shown in **Figures 1** and **2**. The CT study was followed by arch aortography **(Figs. 3, 4)**.

What is your diagnosis?

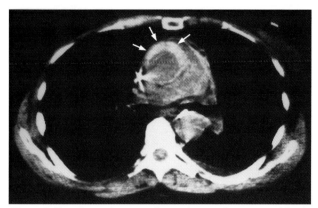

Figure 5. Precontrast image at the aortic root. A crescent of fresh clot surrounds the anterior aortic margin (arrows).

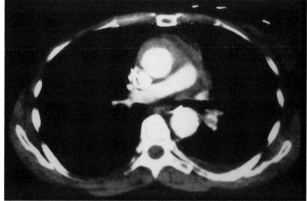

Figure 6. The post-contrast image at the aortic root reveals no dissection flap or deformity of the lumen.

Radiographic Findings

A precontrast CT image **(Fig. 5)** at the aortic root demonstrates a high-density crescent along the anterior margin of the ascending aorta, which was presumed to be clot. During a contrast bolus the lumen of the ascending aorta appears normal **(Fig. 6)**. The RPO aortogram appears normal **(Fig. 7)**. The AP subtracted aortogram reveals a focal ulceration involving the aortic root **(Fig. 8)**.

Diagnosis

Penetrating atherosclerotic ulcer with focal dissection and rupture into the pericardium (surgically proven).

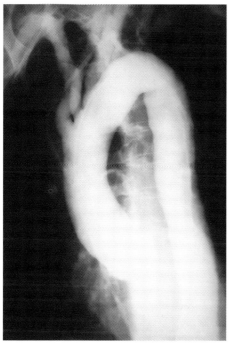

Figure 7. The RPO arch aortogram reveals no dissection flap.

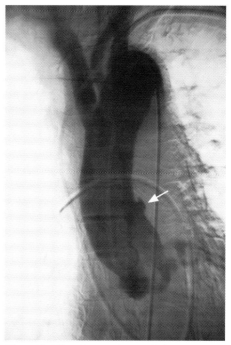

Figure 8. AP aortogram demonstrates a penetrating ulcer (arrow) that involves the ascending aorta.

Management

The appropriate management of a penetrating atherosclerotic ulcer is determined largely by the clinical presentation. In this case, the lesion resulted in a focal dissection that caused pericardial tamponade. The initial management consists of diagnostic imaging and treatment of hypertension. This case was ultimately managed surgically as a type A aortic dissection with replacement of the diseased aortic segment with graft material.

Discussion

Penetrating atherosclerotic ulcer of the aorta is a poorly understood entity that can have a variety of presentations. These lesions are associated with focal thickening of the aortic wall and may present with chest or back pain, distal embolization, intramural hematoma, dissection, saccular aneurysm formation, and aortic rupture. The diagnosis is usually made arteriographically, although CT and magnetic resonance imaging can rule out dissection and, in many cases, identify the area of abnormality.

For further information on this topic, please see Tutorial 2 and Teaching File Case 10.

Selected Readings

Ando Y, Minami H, Muramoto H, Narita M, Sakai S. Rupture of thoracic aorta caused by penetrating aortic ulcer. Chest 1994; 106:624–626.

Dake MD, Miller DC, Semba CP, Mitchell RS, Walker PJ, Liddell RP. Transluminal placement of endovascular stent-grafts for the treatment of thoracic descending aortic aneurysms. New Engl J Med 1994; 331:1729–1734.

Harris JA, Bis KG, Glover JL, Bendick PJ, Shetty A, Brown OW. Penetrating atherosclerotic ulcers of the aorta. J Vasc Surg 1994; 19:90–98.

Williams DM, Kirsh MM, Abrams GD. Penetrating athero-sclerotic aortic ulcer with dissecting hematoma: control of bleeding with percutaneous embolization. Radiology 1991; 181:85–88.

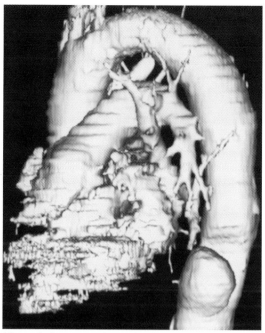

Figure 1. Contrast-enhanced spiral CT scan of the thorax, left lateral view, shaded-surface display.

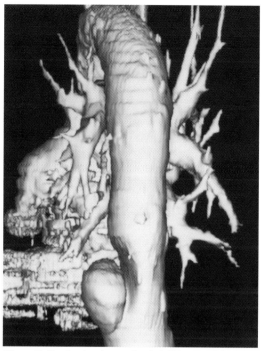

Figure 2. Contrast-enhanced spiral CT scan of the thorax, posterior view, shaded-surface display.

TEACHING FILE CASE 10

Charles P. Semba, M.D., and
Michael D. Dake, M.D.

History

The patient is a 66-year-old man with a history of severe chronic obstructive pulmonary disease who came to the hospital with the acute onset of mid thoracic back pain. A spiral computed tomography (CT) arteriogram was obtained **(Figs. 1, 2)**.

What is your diagnosis?

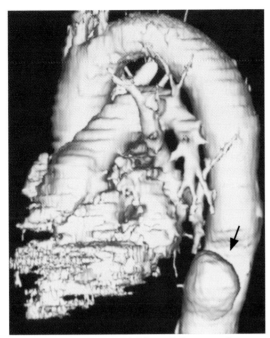

Figure 3. Spiral CT scan, left lateral view, reveals an eccentric accumulation of contrast material extending into the aortic wall (arrow).

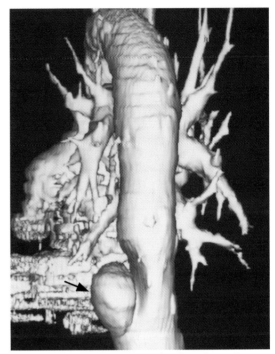

Figure 4. Spiral CT scan, posterior view, shows the luminal abnormality in profile (arrow).

Radiographic Findings
The three-dimensional spiral CT arteriogram shaded-surface displays show a focal penetrating aortic ulcer at the level of the diaphragm in the descending thoracic aorta **(Figs. 3, 4)**. The intraoperative arteriogram **(Fig. 5)** shows ulceration above the celiac trunk.

Diagnosis
Focal penetrating ulcer of the descending thoracic aorta.

How would you manage this patient?

Figure 5. Thoracic aortogram confirms the presence of a penetrating aortic ulcer along the left lateral descending aortic margin (arrow).

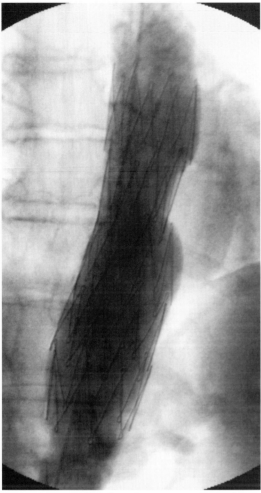

Figure 6. Descending thoracic aortogram obtained following deployment of a stent-graft shows successful exclusion of the penetrating aortic ulcer.

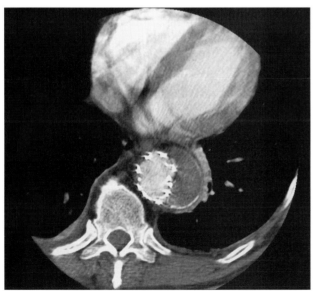

Figure 7. Contrast-enhanced CT scan confirms successful thrombosis of the aortic ulceration.

Management

Traditional management for this lesion has been open surgical resection and placement of an interposition graft. However, stent-grafts are emerging as an experimental alternative for this type of lesion.

In this patient, the ulcer was repaired with use of a 36-mm diameter self-expanding stent-graft constructed from modified Z-stents (Cook, Bloomington, IN) covered with a polyester graft and deployed via a right femoral arteriotomy **(Fig. 6)**. Follow-up spiral CT scanning shows complete exclusion of the ulcer sac by the stent-graft endoprosthesis **(Fig. 7)**.

Discussion

Endovascular repair of thoracic aneurysms is technically possible using self-expanding stent-grafts. This patient would have required a thoracoabdominal incision so that proximal and distal control of the aorta could be obtained; furthermore, he probably would not have survived the operation because of his severe lung disease. Stent-graft techniques may offer a solution for these otherwise high-risk patients in which the aneurysm is located distal to the left subclavian and above the celiac trunk. Focal penetrating aortic ulcers can clinically mimic acute dissections or myocardial infarctions and can spontaneously rupture if left untreated. The etiology of these lesions is controversial; they probably arise from focal inflammatory ulceration of a pre-existing atherosclerotic plaque.

For further information on this topic, please see Tutorial 2 and Teaching File Case 9.

Selected Readings

Dake MD, Miller DC, Semba CP, Mitchell RS, Walker PJ, Liddell RP. Transluminal placement of endovascular stent-grafts for the treatment of descending thoracic aortic aneurysms. New Engl J Med 1994; 331:1729–34.

Harris JA, Bis KG, Glover JL, et al. Penetrating atherosclerotic ulcers of the aorta (ab). Radiology 1994; 192:590.

Mitchell RS, Dake MD, Semba CP, Fogarty TJ, Zarins CK, Liddel RP, Miller DC. Endovascular stent-graft repair of thoracic aortic aneurysms. J Thorac Cardiovasc Surg 1996; 111:1054–62.

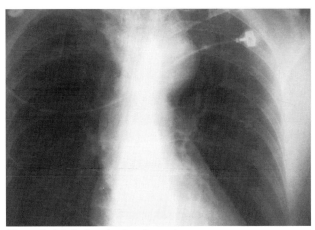

Figure 1. Admission chest radiograph.

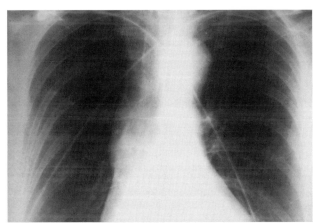

Figure 2. Chest radiograph obtained 3 months earlier.

TEACHING FILE CASE 11
Donald J. Ponec, M.D.

History

This 62-year-old man came to the emergency department with substernal chest pain and nausea. He was admitted to the hospital with a presumptive diagnosis of myocardial ischemia. He had been admitted 3 months earlier with similar complaints, at which time he suffered a small myocardial infarction. An upright portable chest radiograph was obtained **(Fig. 1)** and compared to a film obtained at the last admission **(Fig. 2)**.

What is your diagnosis?

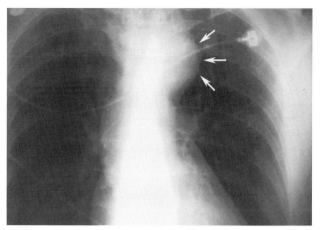

Figure 3. Chest radiograph reveals slight widening of the aortic knob (arrows).

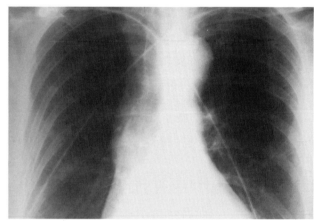

Figure 4. Chest radiograph obtained 3 months earlier shows a less prominent aortic knob.

Radiographic Findings

The chest radiograph **(Fig. 3)** reveals interval widening of the aortic arch compared to the previous examination **(Fig. 4)**. A "dissection protocol" computed tomography (CT) scan of the chest was performed (dynamic scanning at single position during a contrast bolus) demonstrating a type A dissection **(Figs. 5–7)**. Thoracic aortography demonstrates a complex dissection of the ascending and descending aorta with extension into the left subclavian artery **(Figs 8, 9)**.

Diagnosis

Type A aortic dissection.

Management

Control of hypertension is critical for patients with an aortic dissection, regardless of type. In the case of type A lesions, most surgeons advocate emergency surgical repair as soon as the diagnosis is confirmed. This usually involves placement of an ascending aortic graft.

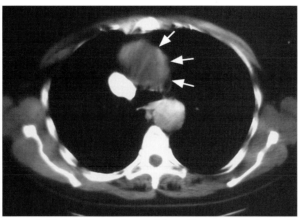

Figure 5. Early CT image from a "dissection protocol" study with dense opacification of the superior vena cava and a prominent ascending aorta (arrows).

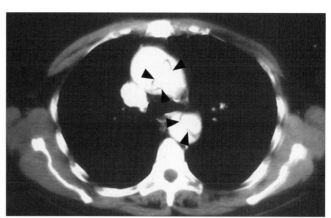

Figure 6. CT image at the same level as that in Figure 5, approximately 12 seconds later, demonstrates the intimal flap (arrowheads).

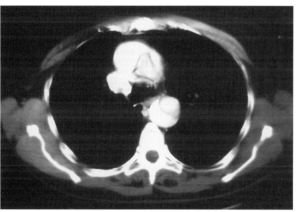

Figure 7. Slightly later image, now showing differential opacification of the false and true lumens.

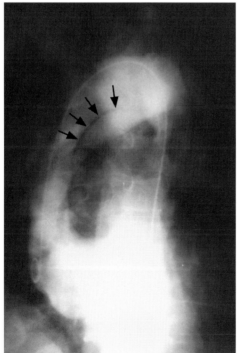

Figure 8. Arch aortogram, early arterial phase, shows ascending aortic dissection (arrows). Note the catheter position in the true lumen relative to the outer margin of the false lumen.

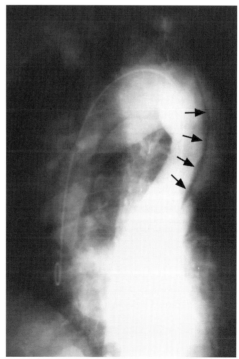

Figure 9. Later film from the aortogram demonstrates the intimal flap in the descending thoracic aorta (arrows).

Discussion

Acute aortic dissection is the most common lethal condition of the aorta, occurring twice as often as ruptured abdominal aortic aneurysm. Most occur in patients between the ages of 40 and 70 with a 2–3:1 male predominance. Hypertension is the most common risk factor; other risk factors include aortic valve stenosis, coarctation, bicuspid aortic valve, connective tissue disorders, trauma (including iatrogenic, ie, coronary artery bypass graft) and pregnancy.

Dissections are usually described in accordance with the Stanford classification system into type A or type B. Type A dissections involve the ascending and/or transverse aorta and usually extend into the descending aorta. Type B dissections begin distal to the origin of the left subclavian artery and involve the descending thoracic and abdominal aorta. Approximately two thirds of dissections are type A.

Chest film findings in aortic dissection include a widened mediastinum, cardiomegaly, displaced intimal calcification, and pleural effusion; however, 6% of patients with dissection have a normal chest radiograph. CT scanning using a dissection protocol is thought to be approximately 95% sensitive. Imaging findings of dissection include displacement of intimal calcification **(Fig. 10)**, visualization of the dissection flap or thrombosed false lumen, differential opacification of two lumens, and branch involvement **(Fig. 11)**. Transesophageal echocardiography and magnetic resonance imaging are also highly sensitive for aortic dissection.

For further information on this topic, please see Tutorial 3 and Teaching File Case 12.

Selected Readings

DeSanctis RW, Doroghazi RM, Austen WG, Buckley MJ. Aortic dissection. New Engl J Med 1987; 317:1060–1067.

Thorsen MK, San Dretto MA, Lawson TL, Foley WD, Smith DF, Berland LL. Dissecting aortic aneurysms: accuracy of computed tomographic diagnosis. Radiology 1983; 148:773–777.

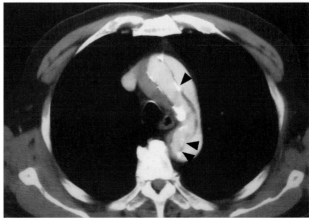

Figure 10. CT scan of a different patient with type A dissection. There is displacement of intimal calcification (arrowheads).

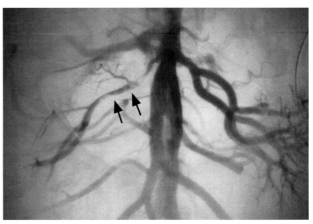

Figure 11. Abdominal aortogram from a patient with a type A dissection demonstrates involvement of the right renal artery (arrows).

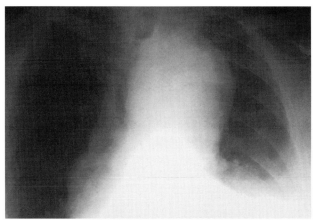

Figure 1. Chest radiograph.

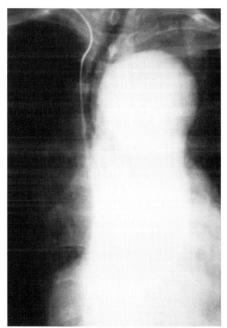

Figure 3. Thoracic aortogram, late arterial phase.

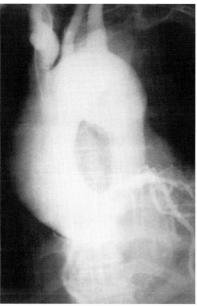

Figure 2. Thoracic aortogram, early arterial phase.

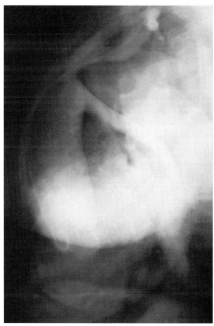

Figure 4. Lateral aortogram.

TEACHING FILE CASE 12
Donald J. Ponec, M.D.

History

A 63-year-old obese woman came to the hospital with a history of chest pain over the past few weeks which had become more severe in the past 24 hours. She had no history of trauma or recent surgery. She was hemodynamically stable but her femoral pulses were reduced. The electrocardiogram was normal. A portable upright posteroanterior (PA) chest radiograph was obtained **(Fig. 1)** followed by a thoracic aortogram **(Figs. 2–4)**.

What is your diagnosis?

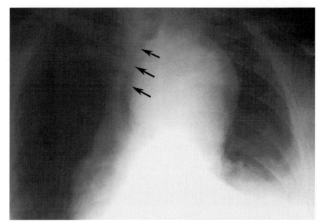

Figure 5. Chest radiograph reveals widening of the superior mediastinum and compression of the trachea (arrows).

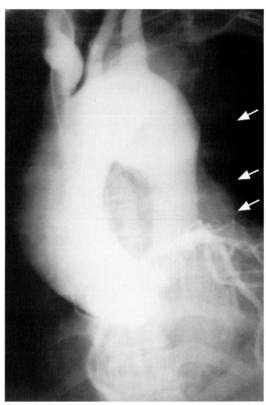

Figure 6. Injection of contrast material into the ascending aorta reveals opacification of the true lumen of a type B dissection and the margin of a large unopacified false lumen (arrows).

Radiographic Findings

The chest radiograph reveals widening of the superior mediastinum with compression of the trachea. There is marked enlargement of the aortic arch **(Fig. 5)**. The AP arch aortogram obtained via a right axillary approach reveals a dissection involving the descending aorta **(Fig. 6)** with delayed filling of the false lumen **(Fig. 7)**. A lateral aortogram reveals compression of the true lumen by a large false lumen **(Fig. 8)**.

Diagnosis

Chronic Stanford type B aortic dissection.

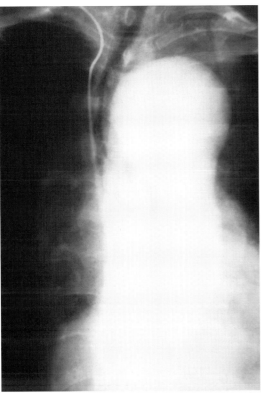

Figure 7. Later image from the same injection shown in Figure 6 demonstrates partial filling of a complex false lumen.

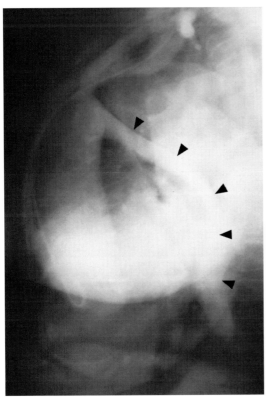

Figure 8. Lateral aortogram reveals the intimal flap (arrowheads) and compression of the true lumen.

Management

Many Stanford type B aortic dissections are managed with antihypertensives only. Surgical treatment is indicated when pain or hypertension cannot be controlled, when significant peripheral ischemia is present (renal/mesenteric/limb), or when a sizable false lumen aneurysm is present. This patient underwent surgical repair because of her ongoing chest pain and the large false lumen diameter.

Discussion

Dissections are arbitrarily classified as chronic if they present greater than 14 days from the onset of symptoms. Unlike type A dissections, many patients (~60%) will survive an undiagnosed type B dissection at 1 month. The most common cause of death in type B dissections is intrathoracic rupture. Surgical treatment is recommended in all symptomatic chronic dissections and in asymptomatic chronic dissections with a diameter of 7 cm or greater, or in cases where there is documented enlargement of smaller dissections.

For further information on this topic, please see Tutorial 3 and Teaching File Case 11.

Selected Readings

DeSanctis RW, Doroghazi RM, Austen WG, Buckley MJ. Aortic dissection. New Engl J Med 1987; 317:1060–1067.

Moreno-Cabral CE, Miller DC. Surgical treatment for acute and chronic thoracic aortic dissections. In: Ernst CB, Stanley JC, eds. Current therapy in vascular surgery. 2nd edition. Philadelphia: B.C. Decker, 1987; 341–346.

Neya K, Omoto R, Kyo S, et al. Outcome of Stanford type B acute aortic dissection. Circulation 1992; 86:111–117.

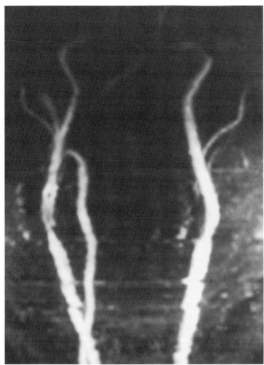

Figure 1. MR arteriogram of the neck.

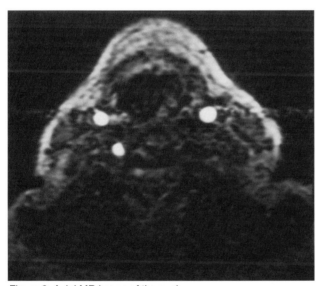

Figure 2. Axial MR image of the neck.

TEACHING FILE CASE 13
John A. Kaufman, M.D.

History

A 61-year-old woman experienced an episode of confusion and disorientation while she was lecturing. Upon closer questioning, she also described several episodes of dizziness when turning her head to the left while driving, as well as some left arm claudication. The left arm symptoms occurred independently of any neurological symptoms. The physical examination showed no neck bruits, and there was a 50 mm Hg difference in blood pressure between the left and right arms. A cranial computed tomography (CT) scan, electroencephalogram, Holter monitor recording, and duplex carotid ultrasound were normal. The vertebral arteries were not studied. The patient underwent magnetic resonance (MR) arteriography of the neck **(Figs. 1, 2)**.

What is your diagnosis?

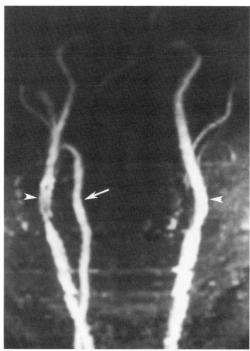

Figure 3. MR arteriogram of the neck shows normal flow in both carotid arteries (arrowheads) and the right vertebral artery (arrow).

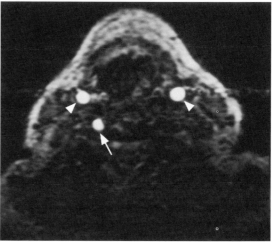

Figure 4. Axial MR image depicts bilateral common carotid (arrowheads) and right vertebral (arrow) arteries. The left vertebral artery is not identified.

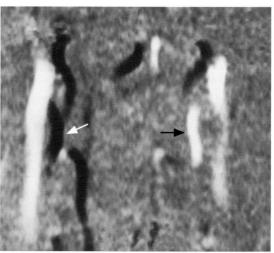

Figure 5. Coronal phase contrast study shows the left vertebral artery (black arrow) and the right vertebral artery (white arrow).

Radiographic Findings

The coronal maximum intensity projection (MIP) from the two-dimensional time of flight (2-D TOF) study shows normal flow in both carotid arteries and in the right vertebral artery (**Fig. 3**). There is absence of signal in the left vertebral artery on both the MIP and a representative axial source image (**Fig. 4**). Can you exclude the diagnosis of subclavian steal?

Not on the basis of this study. The absence of signal in the left vertebral artery could be due to occlusion of the vessel, but remember that a superior saturation slab is used in 2-D TOF MR carotid arteriography to eliminate signal from the jugular veins. Abnormal arterial flow (such as reversed flow in a vertebral artery) entering the slice from above will also be saturated. In order to determine the etiology of signal loss in the left vertebral artery, the saturation band can simply be reversed, or a sequence specifically designed to look for flow in a superior to inferior direction could be utilized. In this case the latter was done with a coronal 2-D phase contrast (PC) study (**Fig. 5**) using 10-mm-thick slices and with the velocity encoding set for 80 cm/second. Notice that the left vertebral artery is now visible, and appears white (as do the jugular veins), indicative of superior to inferior flow. The right vertebral artery is black, consistent with flow in the normal (inferior to superior) direction.

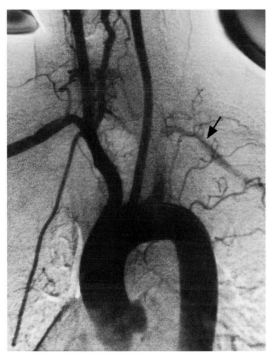

Figure 6. Thoracic aortogram reveals faint filling of the left subclavian artery (arrow).

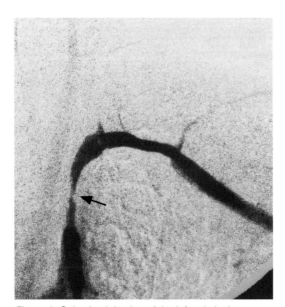

Figure 8. Selective injection of the left subclavian artery depicts atherosclerotic stenosis (arrow).

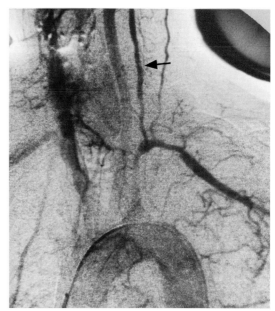

Figure 7. Delayed image shows reversal of flow in the left vertebral artery (arrow).

Diagnosis
Subclavian steal syndrome with retrograde flow in the left vertebral artery.

How would you manage this patient?

Management
The MR study of the neck does not provide information about the proximal left vertebral artery or the left subclavian artery. The patient subsequently underwent conventional contrast arteriography. There is faint filling of the left subclavian artery from the arch injection **(Fig. 6)**. Delayed filming was necessary in order to visualize the reversal of flow in the left vertebral artery **(Fig. 7)**. Selective injection of the left subclavian artery confirmed severe proximal atherosclerotic stenosis **(Fig. 8)**. The carotid arteries were normal, and no abnormalities of the intracranial collateral pathways were identified (not shown). Based upon the patient's impressive symptoms and radiographic findings, a left carotid to subclavian bypass was performed. The patient became asymptomatic after the surgery, with normalized blood pressures in the left arm.

Discussion
Reversal of flow in a vertebral artery is common in the presence of a hemodynamically significant proximal subclavian artery stenosis, but it is usually asymptomatic. The low resistance of the vascular bed of the upper arm results in recruitment of the vertebral artery as a source of collateral blood supply. Vertebral flow may be only intermittently reversed, or to-and-fro, depending on the degree of subclavian artery stenosis and the demand of the upper extremity.

The presentation of symptomatic subclavian steal is varied. Patients may report vertigo or blurred vision related to upper arm activity, reflecting transient posterior circulation ischemia. Other patients may not be able to associate arm activity with neurologic symptoms. True arm claudication may occur without neurologic symptoms.

Hemispheric or global neurologic symptoms suggest the presence of additional lesions, such as internal carotid artery stenosis. Rarely, patients with internal mammary bypass grafts distal to a subclavian artery stenosis may present with angina (graft steal).

Because true symptomatic subclavian artery steal is rare, patients with neurologic symptoms and evidence that suggests subclavian steal should be carefully evaluated for other neurovascular lesions such as carotid bifurcation disease, as well as cardiac arrythmias and otological disorders. A number of vascular imaging modalities can be used. Reversal of vertebral artery flow can be detected on noninvasive carotid ultrasound studies, and transcranial Doppler interrogation of the basilar artery and the circle of Willis can outline intracranial collateral circulation. MR arteriography is well suited for the evaluation of the carotid and vertebral arteries, and the circle of Willis.

The natural history of subclavian artery steal syndrome is somewhat uncertain. One study suggests that most patients can be managed conservatively, because symptoms abate spontaneously in 50% of cases. However, bilateral subclavian artery steal is highly predictive of posterior circulation ischemic events and should be managed aggressively. When nonhemispheric neurologic symptoms persist in the absence of compromised internal carotid arteries or circle of Willis (as in this patient), mechanisms to consider are microembolization or disturbances in autoregulation of intracranial circulation. A complete evaluation to exclude other etiologies should be performed in patients with subclavian artery steal and neurologic symptoms prior to intervention.

For further information on this topic, please see Tutorial 7 and Teaching File Case 14.

Selected Readings

Ackermann H, Diener HC, Seboldt H, Huth C. Ultrasonographic follow-up of subclavian stenosis and occlusion: natural history and surgical treatment. Stroke 1988; 19:431–435.

Bornstein NM, Norris JW. Subclavian steal: a harmless haemodynamic phenomenon? Lancet 1986; 2:303–305.

Delaney CP, Couse NF, Mehigan D, Keaveny TV. Investigation and management of subclavian steal syndrome. Br J Surg 1994; 81:1093–1095.

Drutman J, Gyorke A, Davis WL, Turski PA. Evaluation of subclavian steal with two-dimensional phase contrast and two-dimensional time-of-flight MR angiography. Am J Neuroradiology 1994; 15:1642–1645.

Hennerici M, Klemm C, Rautenberg W. The subclavian steal phenomenon: a common vascular disorder with rare neurologic deficits. Neurology 1988; 38:669–673.

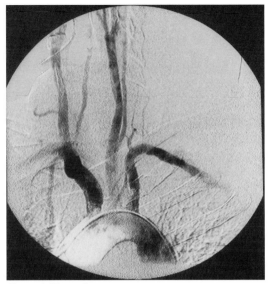

Figure 1. Thoracic aortogram.

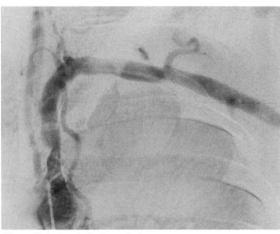

Figure 2. Left subclavian arteriogram.

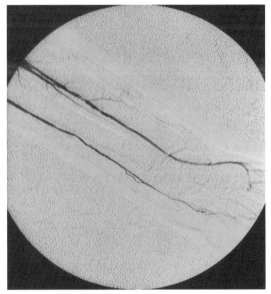

Figure 3. Left forearm arteriogram.

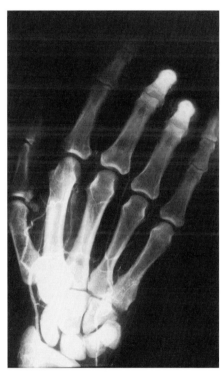

Figure 4. Left hand arteriogram.

TEACHING FILE CASE 14
Matthew S. Johnson, M.D.

History

A 47-year-old man with diabetes and end stage renal disease came to the hospital with a painful, swollen left index finger. Examination of the affected digit revealed an ischemic area along the radial border of the proximal phalanx. Doppler examination of the left upper extremity demonstrated triphasic brachial, radial, and ulnar wave forms. There was faint signal in the palmar arch and no signal in the digital arteries. Arteriography of the aortic arch and arteries of the left upper extremity was performed **(Figs. 1–4)**.

What is your diagnosis?

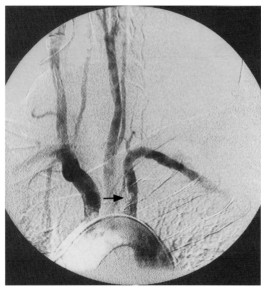

Figure 5. Thoracic aortogram. An eccentric stenosis of the proximal left subclavian artery is present (arrow).

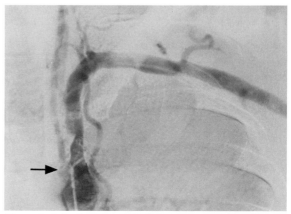

Figure 6. Selective left subclavian arteriogram with reflux of contrast material into the aortic arch. The left vertebral artery (arrow) originates from the aortic arch.

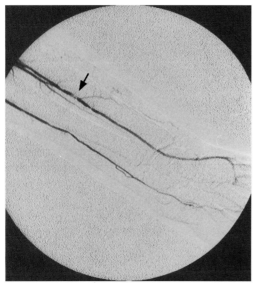

Figure 7. Image of the distal forearm arteries reveals a filling defect in the radial artery (arrow).

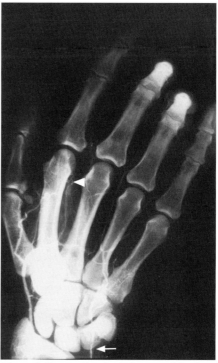

Figure 8. Conventional arteriogram of the hand shows a narrowed distal ulnar artery (arrow) and occlusion of the distal common digital artery (arrowhead).

Radiographic Findings

The arch arteriogram **(Fig. 5)** demonstrates an eccentric stenosis of the proximal left subclavian artery (SCA). Selective injection of the left SCA **(Fig. 6)** also shows the stenosis more clearly. There is a filling defect in the radial artery **(Fig. 7)**. The radial artery supplies the palmar arch, which is incomplete. There are multiple digital occlusions **(Fig. 8)** with no opacification of any vessel distal to the proximal interphalangeal joint of the index finger.

Diagnosis

Subclavian artery stenosis with distal embolization.

How would you manage this patient?

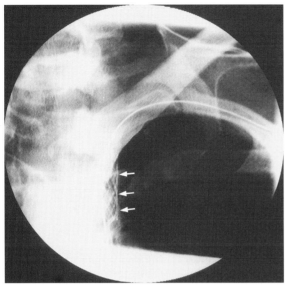

Figure 9. Unsubtracted digital image of the proximal left subclavian artery stent (arrows) prior to contrast material injection. The tip of the injection catheter is at the origin of the subclavian artery. The guide wire extends through the stent into the brachial artery.

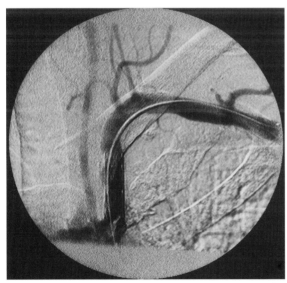

Figure 10. DSA image of the left SCA following stent placement. There is no residual stenosis.

Management

Because of this patient's debilitated status, percutaneous intervention was performed. The left SCA had been cannulated for the diagnostic arteriogram. An exchange guide wire was advanced through this catheter into the brachial artery. The diagnostic catheter was removed and heparin was administered. A long 10-F sheath was unavailable; therefore, the indwelling 5-F sheath was replaced with a short 10-F sheath. A Palmaz P308 stent (Johnson & Johnson Interventional Systems, Warren, NJ) was crimped onto an 8-mm x 3-cm balloon catheter. The catheter was advanced over the guide wire until the middle of the stent was at the level of the stenosis. The stent was dilated to 8 mm, and the balloon catheter was removed. A 10-mm balloon was used to fully dilate the stent. With the guide wire in place, a 5-F angled catheter was introduced through the 10-F sheath, over a second guide wire, into the origin of the left SCA, and digital subtraction images were obtained **(Figs. 9, 10)**. After the procedure, the patient had no further episodes of embolization.

Discussion

Atheroembolization may result in limb loss or organ failure. The embolic source is most often an unstable plaque in the aorta or iliac arteries. Atheroembolism arising from a subclavian plaque is much less common. Medical management alone, usually with aspirin or warfarin, results in a very high recurrence rate. Therefore, surgical therapy, ie, direct arterial replacement, endarterectomy and patch angioplasty, or extraanatomic bypass with exclusion of the source, is the accepted treatment for atheroembolization. However, in selected patients, including those with contraindications to surgical intervention such as this patient, arterial stent placement may be a suitable alternative.

For further information on this topic, please see Tutorial 7 and Teaching File Case 13.

Selected Readings

Baumann DS, McGraw D, Rubin BG, Allen BT, Anderson CB, Sicard GA. An institutional experience with arterial atheroembolism. Ann Vasc Surg 1994; 8:258–265.

Keen RR, McCarthy WJ, Shireman PK, et al. Surgical management of atheroembolism. J Vasc Surg 1995; 21:773–781.

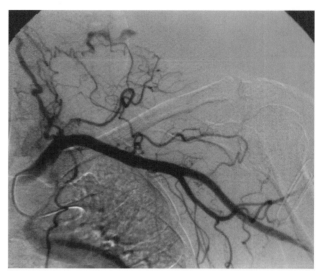
Figure 1. Left subclavian arteriogram.

TEACHING FILE CASE 15

Brian A. Solomon, M.D., and
Ziv J. Haskal, M.D.

History

A 73-year-old man sustained a stab wound to the left supraclavicular region and had persistent bleeding from the wound site despite surgical packing. A left subclavian arteriogram was obtained **(Fig. 1)**.

What is your diagnosis?

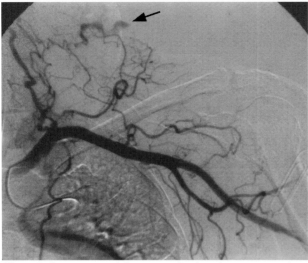

Figure 2. Contrast material extravasation into the suprascapular soft tissues (arrow) from a branch of the suprascapular artery is present.

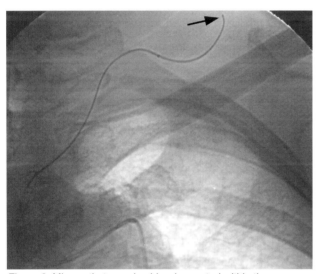

Figure 3. Microcatheter and guide wire seated within the suprascapular branch of the left thyrocervical trunk (arrow).

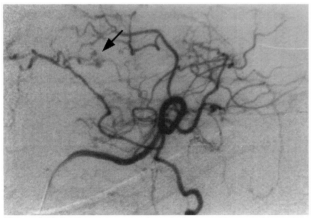

Figure 4. Selective suprascapular arteriogram shows extravasation (arrow) from a small, muscular branch.

Radiographic Findings
Figure 2 demonstrates extravasation of contrast material from a branch of the suprascapular artery into the suprascapular soft tissues.

Diagnosis
Traumatic disruption of the suprascapular branch of the left thyrocervical trunk.

How would you proceed?

Management
The affected branch of the thyrocervical trunk was selectively catheterized with a 3-F microcatheter which was inserted coaxially through an H-1-H catheter. The microcatheter was heated over steam in order to shape its leading tip into a curve that matched the course of the bleeding artery. This greatly facilitated vessel catheterization **(Fig. 3)**. Digital subtraction arteriography performed through the microcatheter demonstrated disruption of a branch of the suprascapular artery, a division of the thyrocervical trunk **(Fig. 4)**.

With the custom-shaped microcatheter seated in the suprascapular artery, selective embolization was performed. Gelfoam slurry (Upjohn, Kalamazoo, MI) was injected through the microcatheter, followed by three 3-mm x 30-mm coils and one 4-mm x 30-mm coil **(Fig. 5)**. The microcatheter was removed and digital subtraction arteriography was performed through the left subclavian catheter. This demonstrated adequate embolization of the suprascapular branch vessel. No extravasation of contrast material was observed and there was no collateral filling at the site of the vessel laceration **(Fig. 6)**.

Discussion

Surgical interventions for deep traumatic vascular injuries are often difficult. Lesions are either surgically inaccessible (as in a post-traumatic renal arteriovenous fistula), or the surgical intervention fails (as in this case with failed surgical packing). In these cases the radiologist can use arteriographic techniques to superselect and subsequently embolize small tortuous vessels.

When heated over a steam bath, these microcatheters quickly become very pliable and can be curved to match the course of a tortuous vessel **(Fig. 7)**. A guide wire must be placed within the catheter while shaping to prevent the lumen from collapsing.

In visceral and thoracic arteriography, coaxial microcatheters can be used in any situation that requires superselection of small branch arteries: liver chemoembolization, embolization of renal and spinal arteriovenous malformations, localization of bowel angiodysplasia, embolization of hepatic artery pseudoaneurysms, and bronchial artery embolization.

For further information on this topic, please see Tutorial 13.

Selected Readings

Beaujeux R, Saussine C, al-Fakir A, et al. Superselective endovascular treatment of renal vascular lesions. J Urol 1995; 153 (1):14–17.

Hibbard M, Holmes DR. The Tracker catheter: a new vascular access system. Cathet Cardiovasc Diag 1992; 27:309–316.

Kadir S. Diagnostic angiography. Philadelphia: W.B. Saunders Company, 1986.

Zuckerman DA, Gaz RD, Catheter-guided intraoperative localization of a jejunal angiodysplasia using a Tracker-18 coaxial catheter system: case report. Cardiovasc Intervent Radiol 1991; 14(6): 358–359.

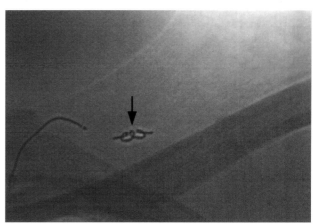

Figure 5. A single embolization microcoil has been deployed within the suprascapular artery (arrow).

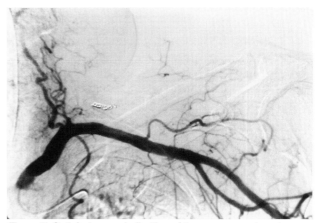

Figure 6. Satisfactory embolization of the suprascapular artery. No collateral filling of the lacerated vessels is present. The embolization coils are faintly visible.

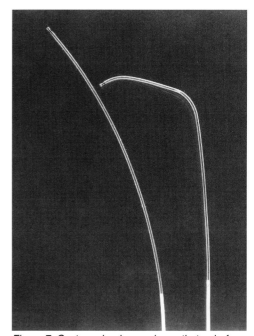

Figure 7. Custom-shaping a microcatheter, before and after heating over steam. The shape can match the vessel of interest.

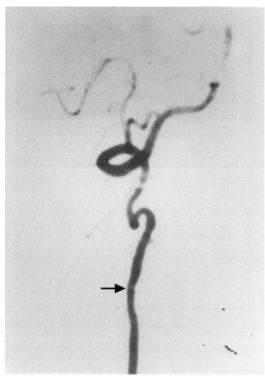

Figure 1. Right vertebral arteriogram demonstrates a mild, focal narrowing (arrow).

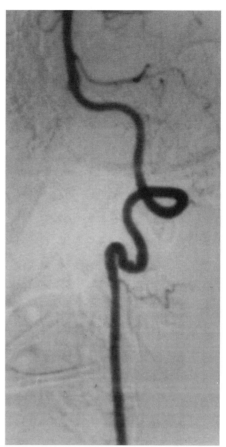

Figure 2. Left vertebral arteriogram.

TEACHING FILE CASE 16
Robert Principato, D.O.

History

A 21-year-old man who had attempted suicide was brought to the trauma center. The patient had profuse bleeding from a stab wound to the right side of the neck. He was immediately transported to the operating room, where the neck wound was explored and packed. After surgery, the patient was taken to interventional radiology for an arteriogram.

The selective right vertebral arteriogram demonstrated a mild narrowing at the level of the C3 vertebral body **(Fig. 1)**. There was no extravasation of contrast material from this site. The left vertebral artery was also injected **(Fig. 2)**. When the patient was moved from the angiography table for catheter removal, there was marked bleeding from the neck. The patient was moved back onto the angiography table and the right vertebral arteriogram was repeated **(Fig. 3)**.

What is your diagnosis?

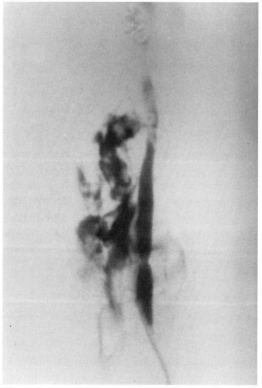

Figure 3. Repeat right vertebral arteriogram.

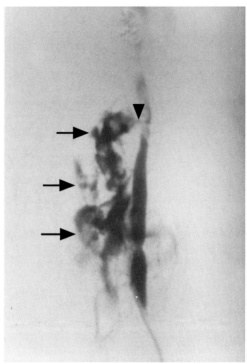

Figure 4. Right vertebral arteriogram shows extravasation (arrows) from an arterial laceration (arrowhead).

Radiographic Findings

The selective right vertebral arteriogram **(Fig. 4)** reveals extensive extravasation from an arterial laceration. The vertebral artery distal to the laceration is not well opacified.

Diagnosis

Laceration of the right vertebral artery.

What treatment would you recommend?

Management

There are several treatment options available for a laceration of the right vertebral artery. Surgical repair of the artery is a possibility; however, surgical exposure of this area is extremely difficult due to overlying bone. Another option would be surgical ligation of the vertebral artery at its origin from the subclavian artery. However, the possibility of retrograde filling from the left vertebral artery makes this an unattractive option. Alternatively, the right vertebral artery could be occluded with embolization coils.

Embolization was elected for this patient. Coils were placed above and below the laceration **(Fig. 5)**. A right vertebral arteriogram following the embolization confirmed successful occlusion of the artery **(Fig. 6)**.

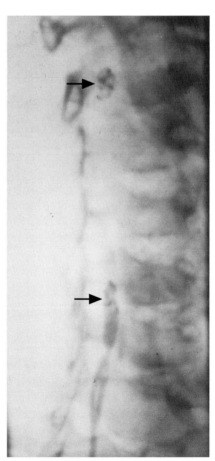

Figure 5. Stainless steel coils (arrows) have been deposited distal and proximal to the arterial laceration.

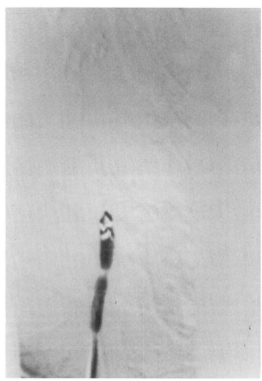
Figure 6. Postembolization right vertebral arteriogram shows successful occlusion of the artery.

Discussion

Injury to the vertebral arteries can be caused by blunt trauma, chiropractic manipulation, fractures and dislocations of the cervical spine, as well as by penetrating trauma. The clinical sequelae range from none to death depending upon intracranial extension of an intimal flap, the formation of emboli, and the status of the contralateral vertebral artery and circle of Willis. Wallenberg's syndrome (ataxia, dysphagia, dysarthria, and nystagmus) has been reported due to occlusion of the ipsilateral posterior inferior cerebellar artery.

Treatment is directed toward controlling hemorrhage and includes both open surgical and transcatheter techniques. When embolization is used to stop hemorrhage, it is imperative that coils be placed both proximal and distal to the arterial defect. This prevents continued hemorrhage from collateral flow. Particles are never used to embolize the vertebral artery, as this treatment would almost certainly lead to brain infarction.

For further information on this topic, please see Tutorial 13.

Selected Readings

Deen HG Jr, McGirr SJ. Vertebral artery injury associated with cervical spine fracture: report of two cases. Spine 1992; 17:230–234.

Garg P, Singh JP. Vertebral artery injury: management by packing. J Indian Med Assoc 1991; 89:171–172.

Garrett TJ, Hubbard SA. Vertebral artery thrombosis due to motor vehicle accident. Ann Emerg Med 1993; 22:1064–1066.

Ghurye M, McQuillan PJ, Madden GJ, Smith GB, Taylor BL. Acute upper airway obstruction due to a ruptured vertebral artery caused by minor cervical trauma. Injury 1992; 23:424–425.

Glauser J, Hastings OM, Mervart M, Volk MA, Bahntge M. Dissection of the vertebral arteries: case report and discussion. J Emerg Med 1994; 12:307–315.

Halvach VV, Higashida RT, Dowd CF, et al. Endovascular treatment of vertebral artery dissections and pseudoaneurysms. J Neurosurg 1993; 79:183–191.

Hamann G, Felber S, Haas A, et al. Cervicocephalic artery dissections due to chiropractic manipulations. Lancet 1993; 341:764–765.

Nakamura CT, Lau JM, Polk NO, Popper JS. Vertebral artery dissection caused by chiropractic manipulation. J Vasc Surg 1991; 14:122–124.

Olteanu-Nerbe V, Bauer M, Vogl T, Marguth F. Endovascular treatment of traumatic arteriovenous fistulas of the vertebral artery. Neurosurg Rev 1993; 16:267–273.

Parent AD, Harkey HL, Touchstone DA, Smith EE, Smith RR. Lateral cervical spine dislocation and vertebral artery injury. Neurosurgery 1992; 31:501–509.

Pikielny R, Parera IC, Micheli F. Wallenberg's syndrome secondary to bullet injury of the vertebral artery. Stroke 1993; 24:141–142.

Schwarz N, Buchinger W, Gaudernak T, Russe F, Zechner W. Injuries to the cervical spine causing vertebral artery trauma: case reports. J Trauma 1991; 31:127–133.

Song WS, Chiang YH, Chen CY, Lin SZ, Liu MY. A simple method for diagnosing traumatic occlusion of the vertebral artery at the craniovertebral junction. Spine 1994; 19:837–839.

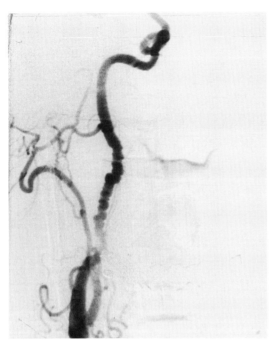

Figure 1. Right common carotid arteriogram, posteroanterior (PA) view.

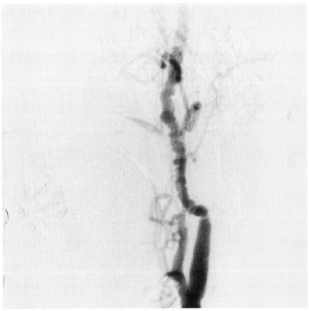

Figure 2. Right common carotid arteriogram, lateral view.

TEACHING FILE CASE 17
Tom Livingston, M.D., Frank Rivera, M.D., and Chet Rees, M.D.

History
A 68-year-old woman came to the hospital with a 2-month history of a disabling audible bruit in her right ear. A right carotid arteriogram was obtained **(Figs. 1, 2)**.

What is your diagnosis?

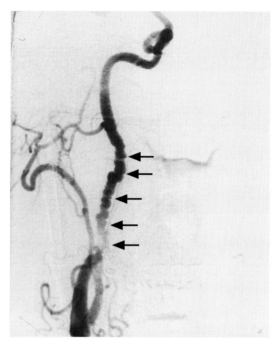

Figure 3. PA right common carotid arteriogram shows the typical beaded appearance of fibromuscular dysplasia (arrows) within the proximal right internal carotid artery.

Radiographic Findings

The right carotid arteriogram demonstrates irregularly spaced constrictions of the cervical internal carotid artery alternating with luminal dilatation from fibrous bands, giving the typical "string of beads" appearance of fibromuscular dysplasia **(Figs. 3, 4)**.

Diagnosis

Fibromuscular dysplasia of the right internal carotid artery.

What are the management options?

Management

Because this bruit was disabling to the patient and prevented her from sleeping, a therapeutic intervention was determined to be appropriate. The options were an open surgical procedure or a percutaneous endovascular intervention. Though carotid angioplasty must be considered experimental, this patient with fibromuscular dysplasia appeared to be an ideal candidate. After discussing the options with the primary physician, the vascular surgeon, and the patient, it was decided to attempt percutaneous transluminal angioplasty.

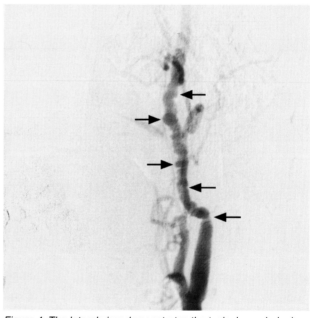

Figure 4. The lateral view demonstrates the typical morphologic changes of fibromuscular dysplasia (arrows).

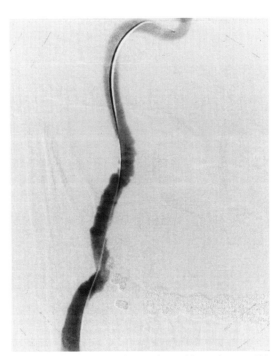

Figure 5. Selective right internal carotid arteriogram, PA view, following balloon angioplasty shows improvement in the degree of arterial lumen irregularity.

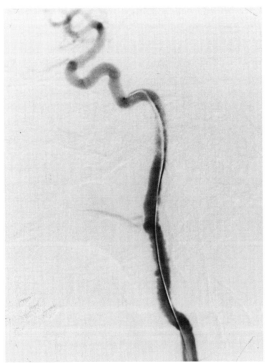

Figure 6. Selective right internal carotid arteriogram (lateral view) following balloon angioplasty.

After the patient received heparin intravenously and nifedipine sublingually, the right common carotid artery was catheterized with a 5-F catheter through a 5-F sheath. The lesion was traversed with a 4-F, 5-mm angioplasty balloon over an 0.018-inch Nitinol wire. Care was taken to exclude air bubbles from the balloon and not to exceed 4 atm pressure. The patient was no longer able to hear a bruit immediately after the angioplasty was performed. A postangioplasty arteriogram demonstrated improvement in the luminal diameter of the internal carotid artery **(Figs. 5, 6)**.

Discussion

Of the five basic histologic types of fibromuscular dysplasia, 80% of the lesions are of the medial fibroplasia type producing the typical "string of beads" appearance. Fibromuscular dysplasia is an angiopathy of unknown pathogenesis. The overall incidence is approximately 0.6% in the cerebral vessels. Though the renal arteries are most commonly affected, the internal carotid arteries are the second most common site. Both carotid arteries are involved in approximately 65% of cases. This disease is nine times more frequent in women. The peak occurrence is the fifth decade.

Bruits audible to the patient are much more commonly associated with fibromuscular dysplasia than with atherosclerotic lesions because fibromuscular dysplasia usually involves the upper cervical carotid artery, closer to the ear than atherosclerotic lesions. The risks of transluminal angioplasty relate to the possibility of distal embolus or creation of a subintimal dissection that could lead to an occlusion or stroke. The use of safety occluding balloons during angioplasty to prevent embolic stroke has been described, but this technique is controversial because it lengthens the procedure and may increase the complication rate.

Surgical transluminal angioplasty done through an open procedure has also been described. No treatment should be instituted for a nondisabling bruit.

For further information on this topic, please see Tutorial 7 and Teaching File Case 18.

Selected Readings

Sundt TM Jr. Carotid bruit audible to the patient. JAMA 1991; 265:121.

Theron J, Raymond J, Casasco A, Courtheoux F. Percutaneous angioplasty of atherosclerotic and postsurgical stenosis of carotid arteries. Am J Neuroradiology 1987; 8:495–500.

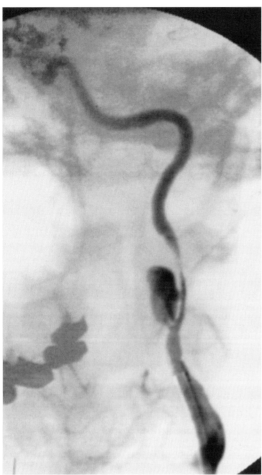

Figure 1. Selective left internal carotid arteriogram.

TEACHING FILE CASE 18
Charles P. Semba, M.D., and
Michael D. Dake, M.D.

History
The patient is a 53-year-old woman who was found to have a subarachnoid hemorrhage. The initial work-up revealed an aneurysm of the right anterior communicating artery which was subsequently clipped. The patient was asymptomatic after surgery and later underwent routine postoperative arteriography **(Fig. 1)**.

What is your diagnosis?

Radiographic Findings

Selective arteriography of the left internal carotid artery reveals a large saccular pseudoaneurysm with compressive stenosis of the adjacent artery **(Fig. 2)**. There are also vascular changes which may be secondary to fibromuscular dysplasia.

Diagnosis

Pseudoaneurysm of the internal carotid artery (secondary to fibromuscular dysplasia?)

How would you manage this patient?

Management

Proximal internal carotid artery stenoses have been traditionally treated with open surgical procedures. Recently, considerable interest has emerged in treating carotid vascular disease with endovascular techniques. This approach is experimental and extremely controversial for the treatment of typical atherosclerotic stenoses of the proximal internal carotid artery.

However, the location of this patient's aneurysm and stenosis near the base of the skull make an open surgical procedure unattractive in comparison to the endovascular therapeutic alternatives. Therefore, it was elected to treat this lesion by deployment of a 6-mm-diameter Palmaz stent (Johnson & Johnson Interventional Systems, Warren, NJ) **(Fig. 3)**.

Discussion

This patient probably developed a small, spontaneous dissection of the internal carotid artery that progressed to a pseudoaneurysm due to fibromuscular disease. While a covered stent-graft may have been ideal for this case, the interventionalists felt that an uncovered stent would be effective in changing the hemodynamics of the native carotid artery and obliterating the neck of the pseudoaneurysm. Before the stent was placed, a test occlusion of the carotid artery was performed after systemic anticoagulation with heparin. Some interventionalists advocate the use of self-expanding stents to avoid potential crushing of the balloon-expandable stent during normal neck motion or external trauma.

For further information on this topic, please see Tutorial 7 and Teaching File Case 17.

Selected Readings

Becker GJ. Should metallic vascular stents be used to treat cerebrovascular occlusive diseases? Radiology 1994; 191:309–312.

Marks MP, Dake MD, Steinberg GK, Norbash AM, Lane B. Stent placement for arterial and venous cerebrovascular disease: preliminary experience. Radiology 1994; 191:441–446.

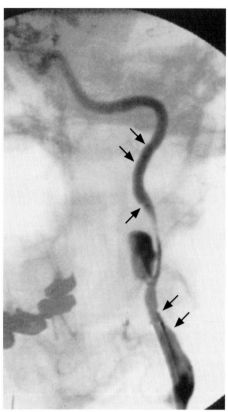

Figure 2. Selective left internal carotid arteriogram shows a saccular aneurysm extending from the medial aspect of the vessel compressing the adjacent lumen. Mild irregularity of the arterial lumen is present (arrows) which may be secondary to fibromuscular dysplasia.

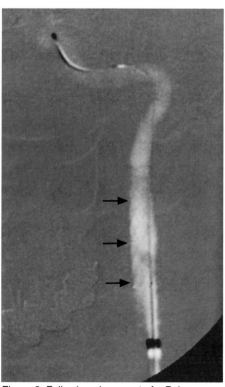

Figure 3. Following placement of a Palmaz stent (arrows), the aneurysm is excluded and the luminal caliber is normal.

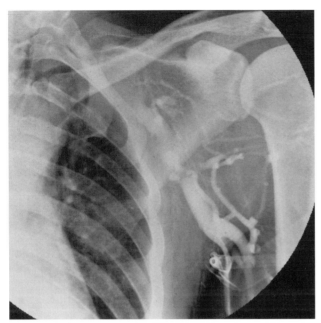
Figure 1. Left upper extremity venogram.

TEACHING FILE CASE 19
Richard Duszak, Jr., M.D., and
Ziv J. Haskal, M.D.

History
A 46-year-old house painter came to the hospital with 3 days of left upper extremity swelling. There was no history of central venous catheterization. Of note, the patient reported a period of similar symptoms in the other arm many years ago, which spontaneously resolved after 1 week.

Although some radiologists might evaluate acute upper extremity swelling with duplex sonography, venography was requested. **Figure 1** is a representative film from an upper extremity venogram.

What is your diagnosis?

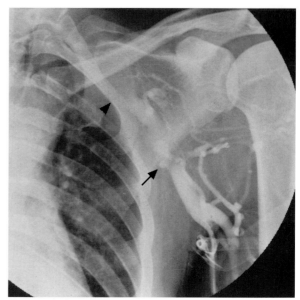

Figure 2. Left upper extremity venogram reveals a filling defect in the left axillary vein (arrow) and occlusion of the left subclavian vein (arrowhead).

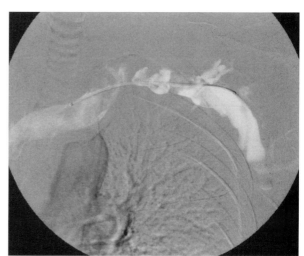

Figure 3. 5-F multiple-side-hole catheter has been advanced through the thrombus for urokinase infusion.

Radiographic Findings
A filling defect is present within the axillary vein **(Fig. 2)** and there is abrupt occlusion of the subclavian vein. Several collateral veins are seen.

Diagnosis
Primary axillosubclavian venous thrombosis.

What intervention could you offer?

Management
Using antecubital vein access, a hydrophilic guide wire was used to traverse the clot. A 5-F multiple-side-hole catheter was placed across the thrombus **(Fig. 3)**.

Over the next 5 hours, 250,000 U of urokinase were infused. At this time, repeat venography showed near complete thrombolysis **(Fig. 4)**.

Are there any provocative maneuvers you might perform to evaluate the etiology of the thrombosis?

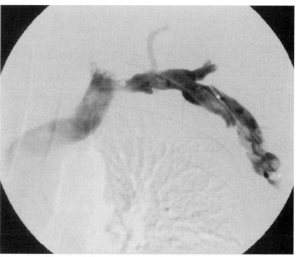

Figure 4. Repeat left upper extremity venogram following urokinase infusion shows a patent left subclavian vein.

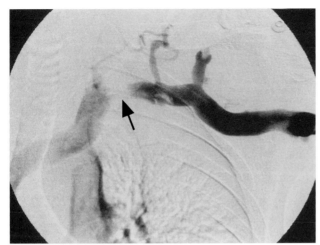

Figure 5. Left upper extremity venogram with the arm abducted discloses a high-grade narrowing of the medial left subclavian vein (arrow).

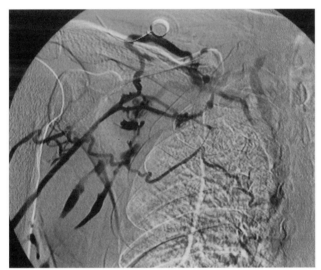

Figure 6. Right upper extremity venogram. The right subclavian vein is occluded.

Venography was repeated with the arm in abduction, revealing marked narrowing of the left subclavian vein **(Fig. 5)**. Remember, this segment of vein appeared to be normal when the arm was in adduction.

Additionally, venography of the contralateral upper extremity reveals occlusion of the axillary and subclavian veins and well-formed collateral vessels **(Fig. 6)**, suggesting that a similar occlusion on this currently asymptomatic side occurred in the distant past.

The etiology of the patient's venous thrombosis is thoracic outlet syndrome, causing extrinsic venous compression and leading to spontaneous subclavian and axillary vein thrombosis.

Discussion

Although many individuals refer to thoracic outlet syndrome as a single entity, it can appear clinically as a spectrum of symptoms related to compression on the brachial plexus, the subclavian artery, and the subclavian vein. Symptoms of brachial plexus involvement are the most common, accounting for 97% of patients with this syndrome. Thus, only a minority of patients with thoracic outlet syndrome are referred to an interventional radiologist.

Venous compression sometimes presents a confusing clinical picture, often manifesting as positional discoloration and swelling of the upper extremity. The extrinsic venous compression, most commonly in the costoclavicular space, may lead to thrombosis with repetitive activity or heavy lifting. This idiopathic or spontaneous axillary vein thrombosis, as seen in this case, is called Paget-Schroetter syndrome. Although there is typically an acute presentation of symptoms, some authors have postulated that the axillary and subclavian vein thrombosis occurs more insidiously but becomes acutely symptomatic with propagation of thrombosis into collateral veins (most commonly the cephalic vein).

A majority of patients with spontaneous axillary and subclavian vein thrombosis will have chronic postphlebitic symptoms despite conventional conservative management with elevation, short-term intravenous heparin, and long-term anticoagulation with warfarin.

Because of these disappointing results, some interventionalists have successfully used thrombolysis to treat acute thrombosis. After thrombolysis, surgical decompression of the thoracic outlet offers more definitive treatment of the underlying anatomic abnormality.

An additional example of a patient with a thoracic impingement syndrome is shown in **Figures 7** and **8**. This 19-year-old man complained of numbness and weakness whenever he lifted his arm.

A thoracic aortogram was obtained **(Fig. 7)**, demonstrating a normal left subclavian artery with the arm in adduction. With abduction, however, there is marked focal narrowing of the subclavian artery **(Fig. 8)**.

In thoracic impingement syndromes, three potential sites of compression can be demonstrated angiographically:

1. The interscalene triangle is formed by the anterior and middle scalene muscles and the first rib. This is the most common location for arterial narrowing. Because the subclavian vein passes anteriorly to the anterior scalene muscle, venous compression is not seen in this location.

2. The costoclavicular space is formed superiorly by the clavicle and subclavius muscle and inferiorly by the first rib. This is the most common location for venous compression.

3. Narrowing at the pectoralis minor tunnel is least commonly seen, with compression occurring between the pectoralis minor tendon and the coracoid process.

Treatment usually entails surgical decompression by resection of the anterior aspect of the first rib, scalenectomy, and lysis of any compromising fibrotic bands.

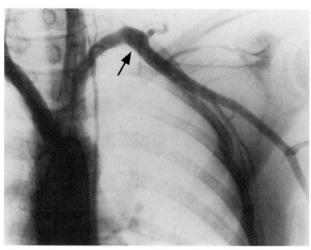

Figure 7. Thoracic aortogram with the left arm adducted shows a slight dilatation of the left subclavian artery (arrow), but is otherwise unremarkable.

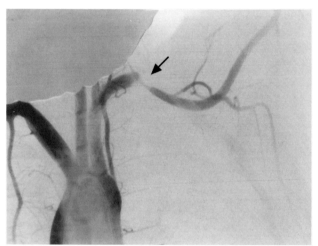

Figure 8. Thoracic aortogram with the left arm abducted reveals a high-grade compression of the left subclavian artery (arrow).

Selected Readings

Becker GJ, Holden RW, Rabe FE, et al. Local thrombolytic therapy for subclavian and axillary vein thrombosis: treatment of the thoracic inlet syndrome. Radiology 1983; 149:419–423.

Kadir S. Diagnostic angiography. Philadelphia: W.B. Saunders Company, 1986.

Kobinia GS, Olbert F, Russe OJ, Denck H. Chronic vascular disease of the upper extremity: radiologic and clinical findings. Cardiovasc Intervent Radiol 1980; 3:25–41.

Lang EK. Arteriography and venography in the assessment of thoracic outlet syndromes. South Med J 1972; 65:129–136.

Roos DB. Thoracic outlet syndromes: update 1987. Am J Surg 1987; 154:568–573.

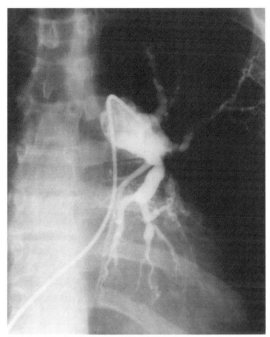

Figure 1. Left pulmonary arteriogram.

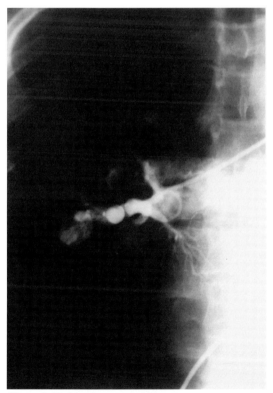

Figure 2. Right pulmonary arteriogram.

TEACHING FILE CASE 20

Erik Insko, M.D., and
Ziv J. Haskal, M.D.

History

A 19-year-old male came to the emergency department with dyspnea, chest pain, and hemoptysis. The patient had a 2-year history of shortness of breath. Emergent pulmonary arteriography was performed. Selective left and right pulmonary arteriograms are shown in **Figures 1** and **2**. The mean pulmonary artery pressure was 57 mm Hg and the mean right ventricular pressure was 46 mm Hg.

What is your diagnosis?

Radiographic Findings

The left pulmonary arteriogram **(Fig. 3)** demonstrates the residua of chronic pulmonary emboli with multiple strictures and dilatations in both the upper and lower lobe vessels. The lingular pulmonary artery is completely occluded. The right pulmonary arteriogram **(Fig. 4)** reveals complete occlusion of the lower and middle lobe pulmonary arteries.

Diagnoses

1. Chronic and possibly acute pulmonary emboli.
2. Pulmonary hypertension.
3. Hypercoagulability (in this case due to antiphospholipid syndrome).

How would you manage this patient?

Management

The patient was anticoagulated with heparin to treat the chronic deep venous thrombosis (DVT) discovered in both lower extremities and to minimize the risk of further pulmonary emboli. A vena caval filter was placed to maximize prophylaxis against future emboli. The next day the patient underwent surgical pulmonary thromboendarterectomy.

Discussion

This case illustrates the severity of thromboembolic disease that can occur in patients with a hypercoagulable syndrome. Antiphospholipid syndrome (APS), also known as lupus anticoagulant or anticardiolipin antibody syndrome, is associated with deep venous thrombosis, stroke, fetal loss, visceral thromboembolic disease, and arterial occlusions. **Figures 5–8** illustrate other manifestations of APS. Compared to other syndromes of hypercoagulability, APS results in a greater number of arterial thromboembolic events. These events commonly recur at the same site or within the same vascular system (venous versus arterial) as the primary thromboembolic event.

A catastrophic occlusive syndrome can occur in patients with APS that resembles diffuse intravascular coagulation without the hallmark consumption of clotting factors. Anticoagulation alone has been shown to reduce the number of recurrent thromboembolic events in APS patients. Corticosteroids have demonstrated no therapeutic benefit in patients with this disorder.

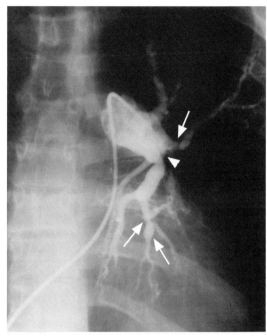

Figure 3. Left pulmonary arteriogram demonstrates the residua of chronic pulmonary emboli with multiple strictures and dilatations in both the upper and lower lobe vessels (arrows). The lingular pulmonary artery is completely occluded (arrowhead).

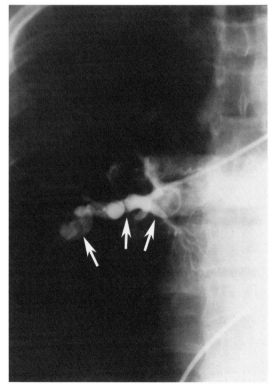

Figure 4. Right pulmonary arteriogram reveals complete occlusion of the lower and middle lobe pulmonary arteries (arrows).

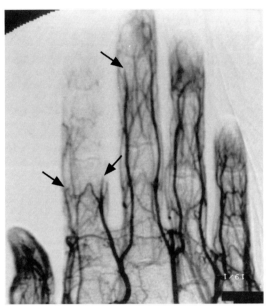

Figure 5. Hand arteriogram in a 19-year-old male with APS and acute pain and cyanosis of his index and middle fingers. The digital arteries supplying these fingers are occluded (arrows). His symptoms slowly improved with anticoagulation.

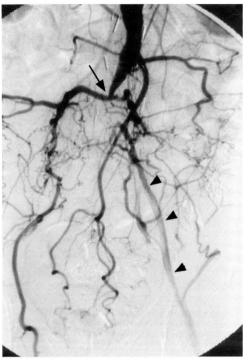

Figure 6. Abdominal aortogram in a 35-year-old man with APS reveals chronic occlusion of the distal aorta (arrow). The left external iliac artery reconstitutes through pelvic collaterals (arrowheads). This patient had unexplained back and leg pain for over 1 year. After thrombosis of six different surgical bypass grafts, he underwent bilateral above-the-knee amputations.

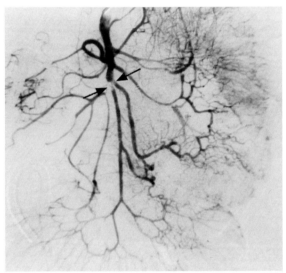

Figure 7. Superior mesenteric arteriogram in a 46-year-old patient with APS and acute abdominal pain demonstrates an embolus (arrows) in a branch of the superior mesenteric artery. The infrarenal aorta was occluded (not shown).

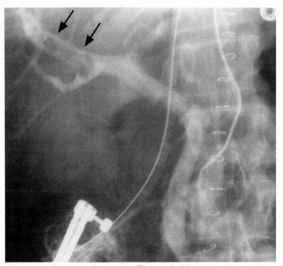

Figure 8. Same patient as in Figure 6. Venous phase of the superior mesenteric arteriogram shows partial right portal vein thrombosis (arrows). A left hemicolectomy was performed for treatment of ischemic bowel.

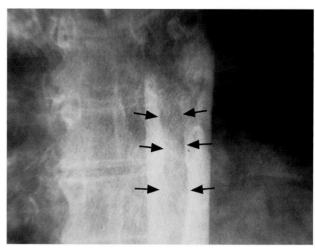

Figure 9. Antithrombin III deficiency. Anteroposterior descending thoracic aortogram reveals an elongated intraluminal thrombus (arrows).

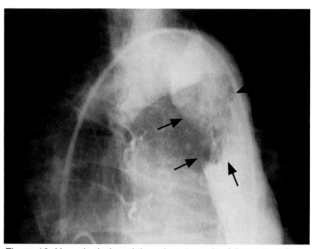

Figure 10. Heparin–induced thrombocytopenia. A large mural thrombus is present (arrows) in the proximal descending aorta.

Other hypercoagulable states which are occasionally encountered include antithrombin III deficiency **(Fig. 9)**, heparin-induced thrombocytopenia **(Fig. 10)**, dysfibrinogenemia, homocystinuria, protein C deficiency, and protein S deficiency. An evaluation for a hypercoagulable state should be performed in patients who have recurrent thromboembolism, unexplained in situ arterial thrombosis, or require unusual doses of anticoagulants to achieve a therapeutic level.

Selected Readings

Khamashta MA, Cuadrado MJ, Mujic F, Taub NA, Hunt BJ, Hughes GR. The management of thrombosis in the antiphospholipid-antibody syndrome. New Engl J Med 1995; 332:993–997.

Lockshin MD. Antiphospholipid antibody syndrome. Rheum Dis Clin North Am 1994; 20:45–59.

Nachman RL, Silverstein R. Hypercoagulable states. Ann Intern Med 1993; 119:819–827.

Perler BA. Hypercoagulability and the hypercoagulability syndromes. AJR 1995; 164:559–564.

Perler BA. Review of hypercoagulability syndromes: what the interventionalist needs to know. J Vasc Interv Radiol 1991; 2:183–193.

Rosove MH, Brewer PM. Antiphospholipid thrombosis: clinical course after the first thrombotic event in 70 patients. Ann Intern Med 1992; 117:303–308.

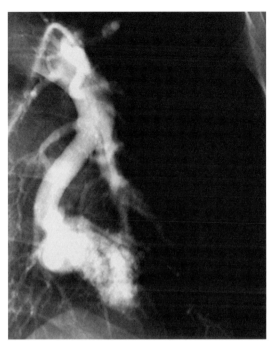

Figure 1. Left pulmonary arteriogram, early arterial phase.

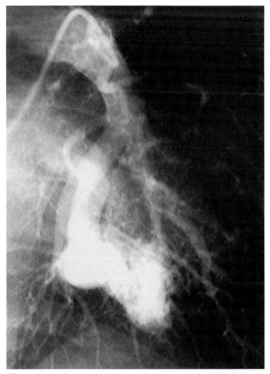

Figure 2. Left pulmonary arteriogram, mid arterial phase.

TEACHING FILE CASE 21
Rajiv Sawhney, M.D., and
Susan D. Wall, M.D.

History
The patient is a 43-year-old male with dyspnea and hypoxia. Chest films demonstrated a round, somewhat lobulated mass in the left lower lobe. Because of the suggestive appearance of the mass and the patient's history, a pulmonary arteriogram was obtained **(Figs. 1, 2)**.

What is your diagnosis?

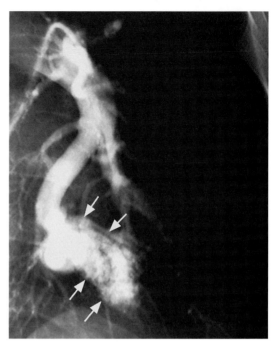

Figure 3. Left pulmonary arteriogram shows abnormally dilated vascular structures at the left base (arrows).

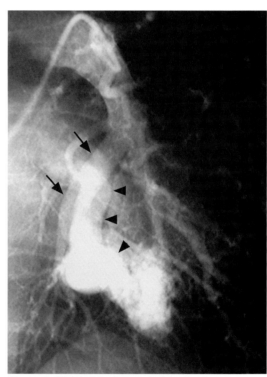

Figure 4. Slightly later image depicts simultaneous opacification of the dilated pulmonary artery (arrows) and pulmonary vein (arrowheads).

Radiographic Findings

The left pulmonary artery injection **(Fig. 3)** demonstrates a tangle of vessels in the left lower lobe which is fed by two dilated left lower lobe arteries. The same injection **(Fig. 4)** shows early draining enlarged pulmonary veins.

Diagnosis

Pulmonary arteriovenous malformation (PAVM).

Management

This patient was treated by percutaneous transcatheter coil embolization of the PAVM. The catheter was advanced selectively into the feeding vessels and coils were deployed beyond branches to normal lung tissue. An injection following coil embolization **(Figs. 5, 6)** demonstrates occlusion of the feeding vessels. Following embolization, no draining venous structures are seen.

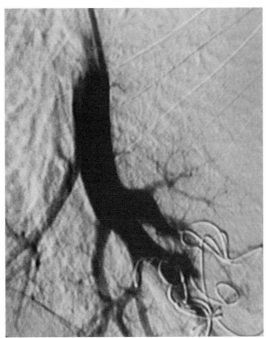

Figure 5. Following deposition of coil spring emboli, the malformation no longer fills.

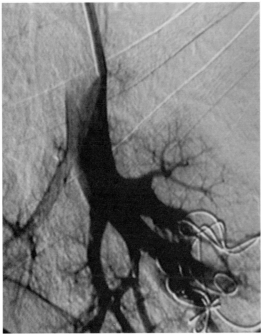

Figure 6. Later image confirms successful occlusion of the malformation.

Discussion

PAVMs may be sporadic or associated with hereditary hemorrhagic telangiectasia (Rendu-Osler-Weber syndrome). PAVMs are usually congenital, and enlarge over time. PAVMs may also be acquired as a result of trauma, ruptured aneurysms, and infection. PAVMs may be asymptomatic, or associated with a variety of clinical problems.

Symptoms such as dyspnea, cyanosis, clubbing, and hemoptysis can usually be anticipated by the size and number of PAVMs. Moreover, because of the right to left shunt, paradoxical emboli occur and cerebrovascular accidents and brain abscesses can be seen.

On chest films, the PAVMs appear as oval or round, lobulated opacities with feeding and draining vessels sometimes seen. Angiographically, two types of PAVMs have been described. The simple type (80% of cases) has a direct communication between the artery and vein. The draining vein is characteristically dilated. The complex type (20% of cases) have a tangle of tortuous vascular structures bridging the feeding artery (or arteries) and draining veins.

Percutaneous transcatheter embolization has emerged as a first-line treatment option in patients with PAVMs. It is usually recommended that PAVMs with feeding arteries greater than 3 mm in size be embolized by positioning a catheter within the feeding artery or arteries distal to branches that supply normal lung tissue and then deploying coils and/or detachable balloons. Obviously, the correct sized coil should be chosen to avoid the risk of systemic embolization or too proximal occlusion.

For further information on this topic, please see Tutorial 5.

Selected Readings

Dutton JA, Jackson JE, Hughes JM, et al. Pulmonary arteriovenous malformations: results of treatment with coil embolization in 53 patients. AJR 1995; 165:1119–1125.

Kadir S. Diagnostic angiography. Philadelphia: W.B. Saunders Company, 1986; 603, 608–610.

White RI. Pulmonary arteriovenous malformations: how do we diagnose them and why is it important to do so? Radiology 1992; 182:633–635.

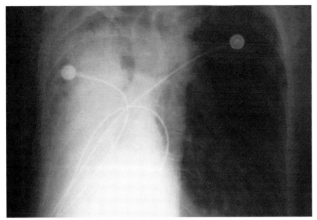
Figure 1. Posteroanterior (PA) upright chest radiograph.

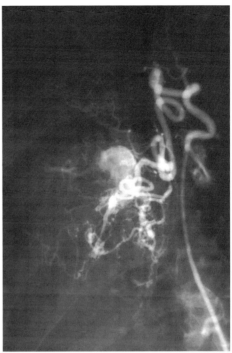
Figure 2. Right bronchial arteriogram.

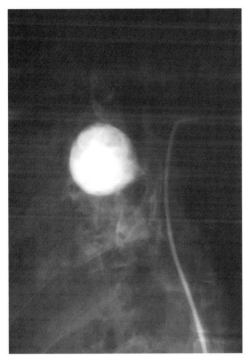
Figure 3. Right bronchial arteriogram, delayed image.

TEACHING FILE CASE 22
Donald J. Ponec, M.D.

History

The patient is a 64-year-old woman who underwent "collapse" therapy for pulmonary tuberculosis at age 16. She has a 1-year history of coughing up blood-streaked sputum. She now presents with massive hemoptysis (more than 300 mL in 24 hours). A chest radiograph was obtained **(Fig. 1)**. Bronchial arteriography was then performed **(Figs. 2, 3)**.

What is your diagnosis?

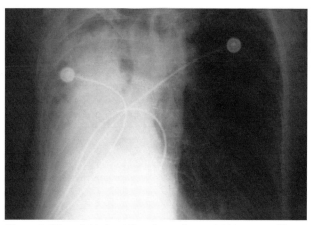

Figure 4. PA upright chest film shows dense right lung opacification and volume loss.

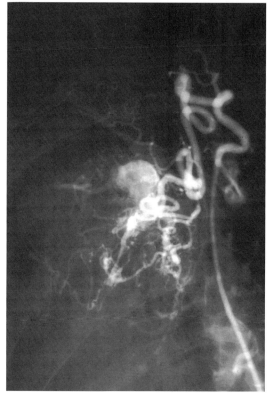

Figure 5. Right bronchial/intercostal trunk injection demonstrates hypervascularity.

Radiographic Findings

The chest film reveals volume loss in the right lung and shift of mediastinal structures. Dense opacification of the right thorax suggests extensive fibrosis **(Fig. 4)**. The bronchial arteriogram revealed a hypervascular mass in the right hilar region and opacification of the right pulmonary artery **(Figs. 5, 6)**.

Diagnosis

Massive hemoptysis from the right lung secondary to old tuberculosis.

Management

The most common causes of hemoptysis are bronchiectasis, tuberculosis, and cystic fibrosis. Bronchial artery embolization is indicated in patients with massive hemoptysis who have not responded to medical management. Bronchoscopic localization of the bleeding segment or lobe can be quite useful because active bronchial bleeding is rarely visualized angiographically. Common radiographic signs are an enlarged bronchial artery, bronchopulmonary artery communication, or peribronchial hypervascularity. Arterial pseudoaneurysms of the bronchial or pulmonary arteries may form in association with a necrotizing process (Rasmussen's aneurysm) but these are relatively uncommon. Bronchial arteries are the most common bleeding source but pulmonary and nonbronchial systemic arteries can also be the source of hemoptysis.

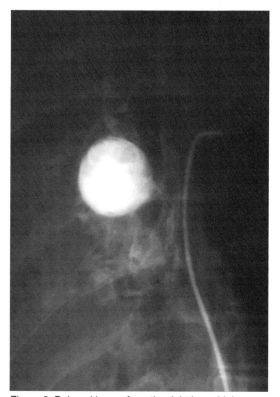

Figure 6. Delayed image from the right bronchial injection demonstrates a large round structure which is presumed to be a pulmonary artery versus a pseudoaneurysm.

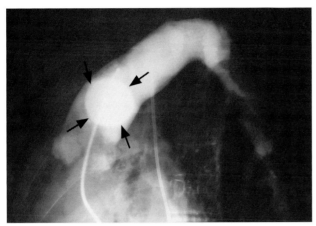

Figure 7. Pulmonary arteriogram demonstrates the same structure as seen in Figure 6 (arrows).

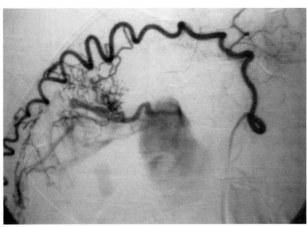

Figure 8. Right fifth intercostal artery injection with transpleural supply to the presumed bleeding site.

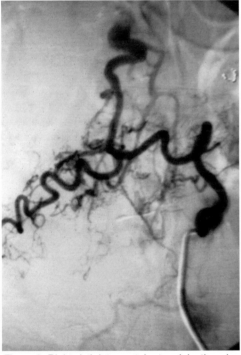

Figure 9. Right sixth intercostal artery injection also demonstrates transpleural feeders to the presumed bleeding site.

The choice of embolic agent depends on the lesion. Small particulate material (~0.5 mm) is generally satisfactory for systemic vessels, while coils or detachable balloons are utilized in the pulmonary arteries. Ethanol is contraindicated. Care must be taken to identify and avoid embolization of spinal arteries.

Discussion

The round structure opacified on this bronchial arteriogram proved to be the stagnant right pulmonary artery, seen end-on **(Fig. 7)**, and was not a Rasmussen's aneurysm. The right bronchial artery was selectively embolized with use of a microcatheter and polyvinyl alcohol particles.

The patient's bleeding continued, and study of the intercostal, internal mammary, and phrenic vessels revealed multiple nonbronchial systemic sources of bleeding **(Figs. 8, 9)**. Once these were embolized, the bleeding ceased and the patient become hemodynamically stable.

For further information on this topic, please see Tutorial 6.

Selected Readings

Cremaschi P, Nascimbene C, Vitulo P, et al. Therapeutic embolization of bronchial artery: a successful treatment in 209 cases of relapse hemoptysis. Angiology 1993; 44:295–299.

McPherson S, Routh WD, Nath H, Keller FS. Anomalous origin of bronchial arteries: potential pitfall of embolotherapy for hemoptysis. J Vasc Interv Radiol 1990; 1:86–88.

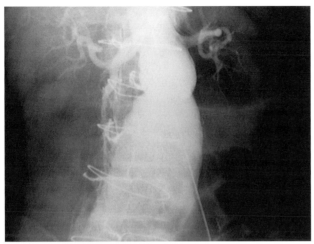

Figure 1. Anteroposterior (AP) abdominal aortogram.

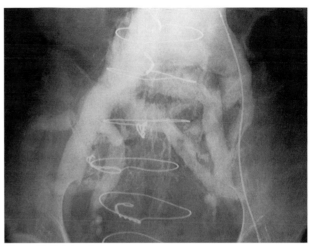

Figure 2. Pelvic arteriogram.

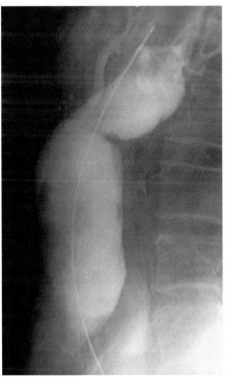

Figure 3. Lateral abdominal aortogram.

TEACHING FILE CASE 23
Robert K. Kerlan, Jr., M.D., and
Mark W. Wilson, M.D.

History
A 67-year-old man underwent an attempted urologic surgery. Upon opening the abdomen, bleeding was encountered which required termination of the procedure. The patient was taken to the angiography suite where an abdominal aortogram **(Figs. 1–3)** was performed.

What is your diagnosis?

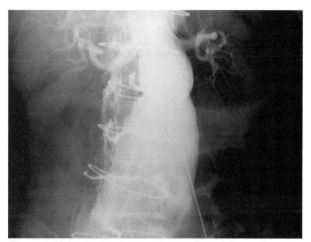

Figure 4. Abdominal aortogram shows a large infrarenal abdominal aortic aneurysm.

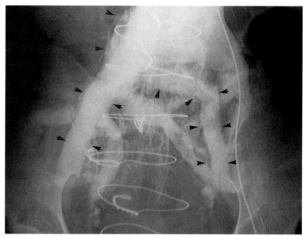

Figure 5. Pelvic arteriogram reveals simultaneous opacification of the iliac veins (arrowheads), the distal aorta, and the proximal iliac arteries.

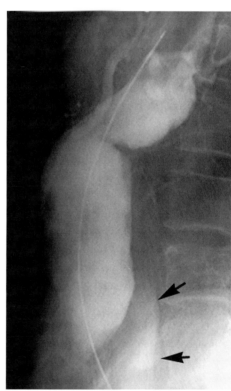

Figure 6. On the lateral view, early filling of the inferior vena cava (arrows) is evident.

Radiographic Findings

The AP abdominal aortogram **(Fig. 4)** shows an infrarenal abdominal aortic aneurysm (AAA) which becomes considerably larger approximately 5 cm below the origin of single non-stenotic renal arteries. The appearance of this aneurysm proximally is not atypical. The views obtained over the pelvis **(Fig. 5)** to determine the caudal extent of the aneurysm, however, are quite unusual. This view shows a greater number of opacified vascular structures than is usually encountered during abdominal aortography, with simultaneous visualization of both iliac arteries and iliac veins.

The lateral aortogram **(Fig. 6)** delineates the proximal neck of the aneurysm and reveals opacification of the caudal aspect of the inferior vena cava.

Diagnosis

Atherosclerotic infrarenal abdominal aortic aneurysm which has ruptured into an iliac vein. The precise point of communication is not revealed on this study.

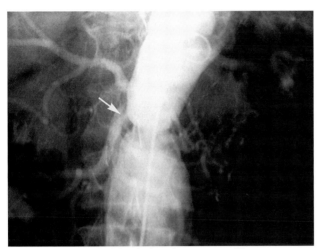

Figure 7. Juxtarenal abdominal aortic aneurysm. The aneurysm extends immediately caudal to the origin of the right renal artery (arrow).

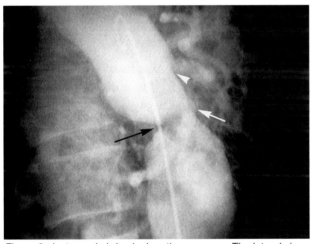

Figure 8. Juxtarenal abdominal aortic aneurysm. The lateral view is usually the best projection to delineate the aneurysmal neck (black arrow). The relationship of the neck to the origin of the right renal artery (white arrow) and superior mesenteric artery (arrowhead) is well demonstrated.

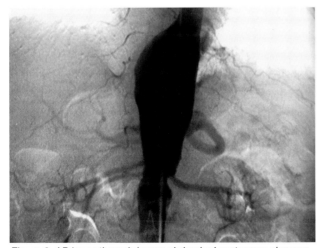

Figure 9. AP lower thoracic/upper abdominal aortogram shows a thoracoabdominal aneurysm spanning the diaphragm.

Discussion

Rupture of abdominal aortic aneurysms into the iliac venous system or inferior vena cava is rare but well recognized, comprising somewhere between 1% and 10% of all ruptures. Rather than presenting with hypovolemic shock, patients with aortic rupture into the systemic venous system have symptoms related to high-output congestive heart failure, renal failure, and peripheral edema. Though the case depicted in this teaching file is unusual, the diagnosis and treatment of problems related to abdominal aortic aneurysmal disease are extremely common in daily practice.

An aortic aneurysm is defined as a focal 50% or greater increase from the anticipated normal aortic diameter. In the abdominal aorta, a diameter of 3 cm or greater is usually considered an aneurysm. Abdominal aortic aneurysms are estimated to occur in 1%–5% of the population, with a 2:1 male:female predominance, and account for approximately 15,000 deaths per year in the United States. The mortality of a ruptured abdominal aneurysm is 80%–90%, compared to an approximate 5% mortality rate related to elective surgical repair.

Though aneurysms of all different etiologies including infection and dissection can be encountered in the abdominal aorta, the vast majority are related to atherosclerosis. The precise mechanism of the formation of atherosclerotic aneurysms is unknown, but is presumably multifactorial. In human coronary arteries, the abdominal aorta, and superficial femoral arteries (but not the thoracic aorta), plaque deposition is accompanied by arterial enlargement, likely as a compensatory mechanism to minimize luminal narrowing. As this enlargement progresses, there is thinning of the media. Concomitantly, an infiltration of inflammatory cells occurs which may release proteolytic enzymes, further damaging the structural integrity of the media and leading to the formation of an aneurysm. A genetic predisposition appears to exist, making certain individuals more prone to develop aneurysms under these circumstances.

Over 95% of abdominal aortic aneurysms are infrarenal in position, allowing for the surgical placement of a vascular clamp and the creation of an anastomosis to an interposition graft below the origins of the renal arteries. A juxtarenal aneurysm **(Figs. 7, 8)** extends to the origin of the renal arteries, requiring the placement of a suprarenal clamp for surgical repair. In a pararenal AAA, at least one renal artery takes its origin from the aneurysmal lumen. A thoracoabdominal aneurysm **(Fig. 9)** involves the distal thoracic aorta as well as the origin of the visceral vessels.

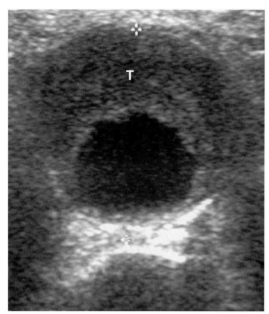

Figure 10. Transverse abdominal ultrasound image reveals a 6-cm abdominal aortic aneurysm. The majority of the lumen ventrally is filled with thrombus (T).

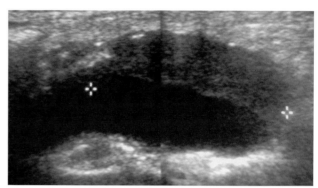

Figure 11. Same patient as in Figure 10. The morphology of the aneurysm is more apparent on this longitudinal view.

Risk of Rupture Based on Aneurysm Diameter	
Aneurysm Size	*5-year Rupture Risk*
< 4.0 cm	2%
4.0 cm–5.0 cm	3%–12%
>5.0 cm	25%–41%

Figure 12.

Most abdominal aortic aneurysms are detected by physical examination in asymptomatic patients. Abdominal ultrasound **(Figs. 10, 11)** is usually used to confirm the diagnosis and accurately determine the aneurysmal size. Aneurysmal size is the most important factor in predicting the risk of rupture; size is therefore crucial in deciding which patients should undergo aneurysm repair. The risk of rupture according to maximal aneurysm diameter measured from the aortic wall (including thrombus material) is shown in **Figure 12**. Because of the risk of rupture, it is generally agreed that abdominal aortic aneurysms greater than 5 cm in diameter should be resected, unless the patient is an extremely poor surgical risk. Some surgeons recommend surgical repair for aneurysms 4.0–5.0 cm in size in younger, otherwise healthy patients.

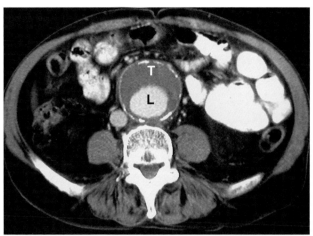

Figure 13. Typical appearance of an infrarenal abdominal aortic aneurysm on contrast-enhanced computed tomography. The calcified aortic wall, thrombus material (T), and patent aortic lumen (L) are clearly depicted.

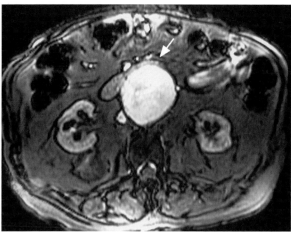

Figure 14. Axial gradient echo magnetic resonance imaging has similar resolution as computed tomography. Note the left renal vein in the normal position ventral to the aorta (arrow).

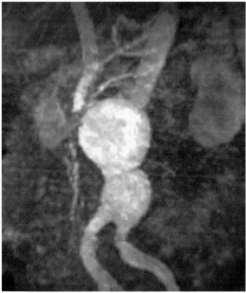

Figure 15. Coronal magnetic resonance image demonstrates an infrarenal AAA extending to the aortic bifurcation, but not into the iliac arteries.

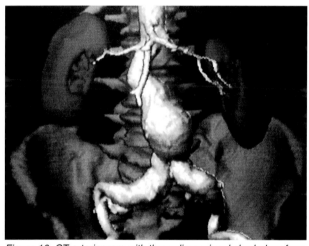

Figure 16. CT arteriogram with three-dimensional shaded-surface display reveals an infrarenal AAA extending into both common iliac arteries.

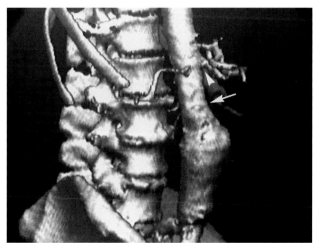

Figure 17. CT arteriogram graphically depicts the length of the aneurysm neck (arrow) and its relationship to the origin of the superior mesenteric artery (arrowhead).

Once the decision has been made to repair an abdominal aortic aneurysm, the necessity of obtaining additional imaging studies or arteriography is controversial. However, most surgeons do prefer some form of preoperative imaging to define the proximal and distal extent of the aneurysm, and to delineate abnormalities of the renal arteries or left renal vein. These features can be determined noninvasively with computed tomography (CT) **(Fig. 13)** or magnetic resonance (MR) imaging **(Fig. 14)**. Moreover, using computer-generated reconstructions, two- and three-dimensional images **(Figs. 15–17)** from both CT and MR imaging may be rendered, providing a more detailed anatomic picture for the referring surgeon. With use of these techniques, accessory renal arteries and significant renal, visceral, and iliac stenoses may be detected.

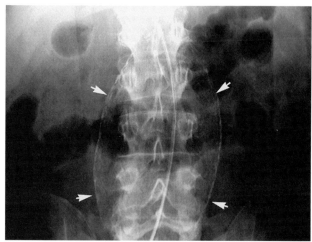

Figure 18. Scout film prior to abdominal aortography shows curvilinear calcifications (arrows) typical of a large atherosclerotic aortic aneurysm.

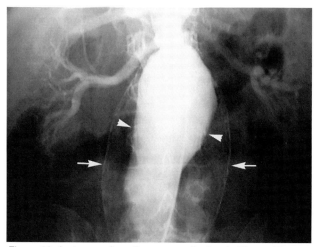

Figure 19. Aortogram from the same patient as in Figure 18 shows the patent lumen (arrowheads) of this juxtarenal aneurysm to be substantially smaller than the aneurysm itself (arrows).

If there is reason to suspect that the proximal extent of an aneurysm may involve the renal and/or visceral vessels, or if there is clinical evidence of coexistent occlusive disease involving the visceral, renal, or iliac arteries, arteriography may be required for more precise anatomic delineation. Though arteriography gives the most morphologic detail of the aortic branches, only the patent aortic lumen is visualized, which may severely underestimate the true size of the aneurysm. However, calcifications within the arterial wall are usually present **(Figs. 18, 19)**, giving a more accurate estimation of the external aortic contour.

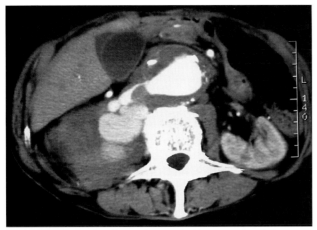

Figure 20. Contrast-enhanced computed tomography. Active extravasation of contrast media into the retroperitoneum is present from a ruptured abdominal aorta aneurysm.

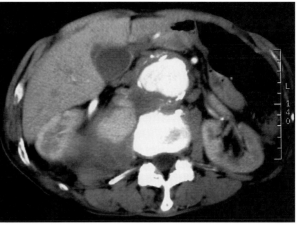

Figure 21. Contrast-enhanced computed tomography. A massive retroperitoneal hematoma displaces the right kidney.

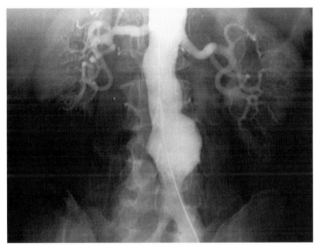

Figure 22. Abdominal aortogram, early arterial phase, shows a typical infrarenal AAA.

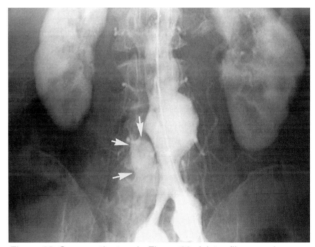

Figure 23. Same patient as in Figure 20. A later film reveals extravasation of contrast material (arrows) into the para-aortic retroperitoneal tissues indicative of rupture. The patient did not survive.

Rupture of an abdominal aortic aneurysm is associated with a mortality rate of 80%–90%. If a moderate or high degree of clinical suspicion for a ruptured aortic aneurysm exists, the patient should undergo emergent open surgical exploration without arteriography or other imaging procedures. In stable patients with equivocal clinical findings, computed tomography can be an important diagnostic tool in establishing this diagnosis. CT findings of ruptured abdominal aortic aneurysm include retroperitoneal hematoma (Fig. 20), abnormal soft tissue collections along the posterior border of the aneurysm, indistinctness of the aortic wall, renal displacement (Fig. 21), and extravasation of iodinated contrast material. Arteriography (Figs. 22, 23) should never be performed when there is suspicion of a ruptured aneurysm.

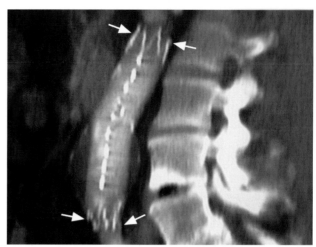

Figure 24. Maximum intensity projection from a CT arteriogram demonstrates the metallic markers and the proximal and distal metallic fixation stents (arrows) from a covered stent-graft. The device which was inserted through a right femoral cutdown successfully excludes flow from the AAA.

Elective repair of a non-ruptured abdominal aortic aneurysm has traditionally been performed by open surgical placement of a prosthetic interposition graft. The surgical mortality varies from 3% in patients under 60 years of age to 12% in patients more than 80 years old. Because of the associated surgical mortality, considerable interest has been generated in finding a less invasive method of treatment. The placement of covered stent-grafts with endovascular techniques **(Fig. 24)** has become a realistic alternative. Though currently only performed in controlled experimental trials, the initial results of endovascular therapy for abdominal aortic aneurysms has been encouraging, with technical and functional success in more than 80% of treated patients. Several designs of covered stent-grafts are currently being evaluated, and technologic refinements will be necessary if the procedure is to gain widespread clinical acceptance.

Selected Readings

Blum U, Langer M, Spillner G, et al. Abdominal aortic aneurysms: preliminary technical and clinical results with transfemoral placement of endovascular self-expanding stent-grafts. Radiology 1996; 198:25–31.

Chuter TA, Green RM, Ouriel K, Fiore WM, DeWeese JA. Transfemoral endovascular aortic graft placement. J Vasc Surg 1993; 18:185–197

Ghilardi G, de Monti M, Longhi F, Scorza R. Aorto-iliac aneurysms rupturing into the iliac veins. Vasa 1995; 24:290–294.

Miani S, Giorgetti PL, Arpesani A, Giuffrida GF, Biasi GM, Ruberti U. Spontaneous aorto-caval fistulas from ruptured abdominal aortic aneurysms. Eur J Vasc Endovasc Surg 1994; 8:36–40.

Murphy KD, Richter GM, Henry M, Encarnacion CE, Le VA, Palmaz JC. Aortoiliac aneurysms: management with endovascular stent-graft placement. Radiology 1996; 198:473–480.

End Notes

Figures 20 and 21 courtesy of Central Oregon Radiology Associates, Saint Charles Medical Center, Bend, OR.

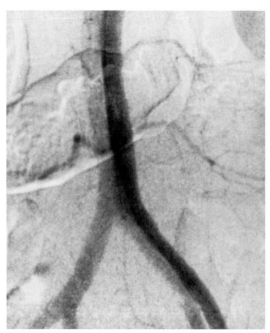

Figure 1. Digital subtraction abdominal aortogram.

TEACHING FILE CASE 24
Charles P. Semba, M.D., and
Michael D. Dake, M.D.

History
A 51-year-old woman with prolonged hypertension came to the hospital with the acute onset of mid thoracic back pain that evolved into abdominal pain over the next several hours. She had a weak right femoral pulse and a normal left femoral pulse. Transesophageal echocardiography showed a type B dissection, and the patient was sent to the intensive care unit for control of blood pressure. Because of persistent right leg ischemia, diagnostic arteriography was performed via the left femoral approach **(Fig. 1)**.

What is your diagnosis?

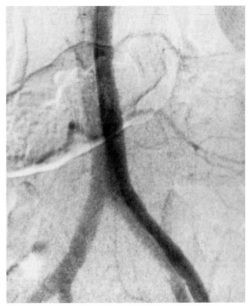

Figure 2. Abdominal aortogram confirms the presence of a dissection flap extending into the left iliac artery. The right iliac system is suboptimally opacified.

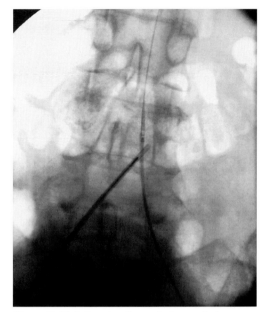

Figure 3. Digital spot radiograph demonstrates an intravascular ultrasound probe inserted from the left common femoral artery and a Colapinto needle inserted from the right common femoral artery.

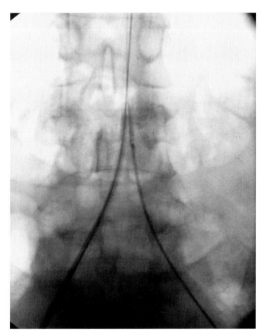

Figure 4. A Colapinto needle is advanced through the intimal flap under ultrasound guidance.

Radiographic Findings

The left common femoral artery was catheterized and the injection was performed with the pigtail catheter in the false lumen. The abdominal aortic arteriogram shows a longitudinal dissection flap and poor opacification of the true lumen and right iliac artery **(Fig. 2)**.

Diagnosis

Acute type B dissection with extension into the abdominal aorta and compromised perfusion of the right lower extremity.

How would you manage this patient?

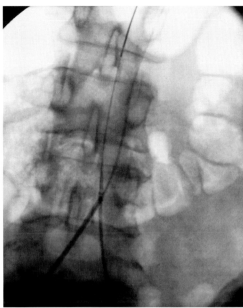

Figure 5. The Colapinto needle is removed and a guide wire inserted.

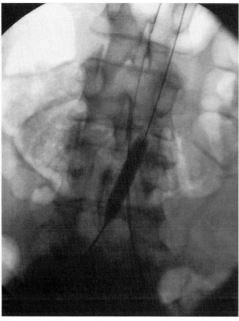

Figure 6. A 10-mm diameter angioplasty balloon has been inflated across the fenestration.

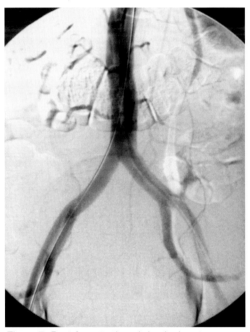

Figure 7. Post-fenestration abdominal aortogram shows improved opacification of the right iliac system.

Management

Traditional management would require open surgical revascularization of the right lower extremity. Due to the complexity of revascularization procedures in the presence of intimal dissection, interest has been generated in developing endovascular techniques to fenestrate the dissection flap. At the present time, these techniques are not generally accepted and must be considered experimental.

In this patient, percutaneous fenestration was performed **(Figs. 3–7)**. The right femoral artery was catheterized, permitting access to the true lumen. A Colapinto needle was placed over a guide wire into the right iliac artery and an intravascular ultrasound probe was placed into the left iliac artery **(Fig. 3)**. With use of combined fluoroscopic and ultrasound guidance, the needle was advanced toward the ultrasound probe, creating a tear across the dissection flap **(Fig. 4)**. The needle was removed over a guide wire **(Fig. 5)** and the tear was enlarged with use of a large diameter angioplasty balloon **(Fig. 6)**. The completion arteriogram from the false lumen shows improved perfusion of the true lumen and right iliac artery **(Fig. 7)**. Pressure tracings show no residual gradient.

Discussion

Peripheral vascular complications occur in 20%–30% of acute aortic dissections. Management typically consists of emergent surgery for type A dissections and aggressive medical management of both type A and B dissections to reduce hypertension. Mortality rates for patients with both mesenteric and renal ischemia is 40%–60% despite control of blood pressure. The ischemia is caused by occlusion of the vessels by the dissection flap and cannot be reversed with medical treatment alone.

Surgical mortality in the setting of mesenteric and renal ischemia is 40%–80%; therefore, endovascular treatments may offer a strategic advantage. In the Stanford series, 22 patients underwent percutaneous interventions for peripheral vascular ischemic complications, and there were no procedure-related deaths. Twenty-one of the 22 patients were alive at 1-year follow-up (one patient died of unrelated causes).

In this teaching file case, the patient had limb ischemia only. Commonly, the femoral artery with the weaker pulse communicates with the smaller compromised true lumen, as in this case. Fenestrations can also be performed across the dissection plane in the supraceliac or infra-inferior mesenteric aorta.

For further information on this topic, please see Tutorial 3.

Selected Reading

Slonim SM, Nyman U, Semba CP, Miller DC, Mitchell RS, Dake MD. Aortic dissection: percutaneous management of ischemic complications with endovascular stents and balloon fenestration. J Vasc Surg 1996; 23:241–253.

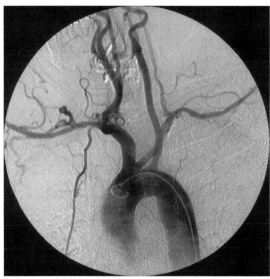

Figure 1. Thoracic aortogram.

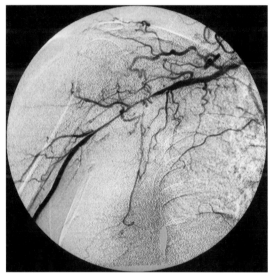

Figure 2. Right subclavian/axillary arteriogram.

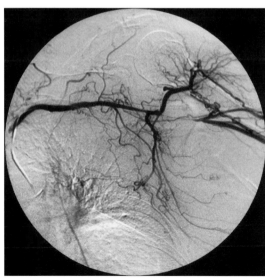

Figure 3. Left subclavian/axillary arteriogram.

TEACHING FILE CASE 25
Timothy J. Carmody, M.D., and
Scott O. Trerotola, M.D.

History
A 67-year-old woman came to the hospital with complaints of bilateral upper extremity muscular weakness, paresthesias, and intermittent claudication. On physical examination, the pulses were diminished in both upper extremities and no audible bruits were apparent. Review of systems revealed an equivocal history of myalgias, headaches, and visual disturbances. Laboratory studies revealed an erythrocyte sedimentation rate of 105 mm/hour. An arteriogram was obtained **(Figs. 1–3)**.

What is your diagnosis?

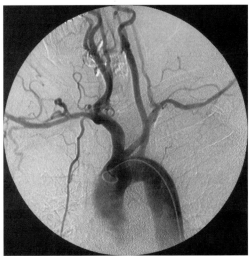

Figure 4. Thoracic aortogram shows no origin disease in the great vessels and mild narrowing of the postvertebral subclavian arteries bilaterally. There is bovine origin of the left common carotid artery.

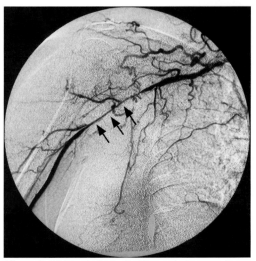

Figure 5. Right subclavian/axillary arteriogram shows marked long-segment smooth narrowing (arrows) of the axillary and proximal brachial arteries.

Radiographic Findings

A thoracic aortogram **(Fig. 4)** demonstrates no significant atherosclerotic disease of the arch or origins of the great vessels, and a common (bovine) origin of the innominate and left common carotid arteries. Mild symmetric stenoses of the proximal postvertebral subclavian arteries are present. Selective right and left subclavian arteriograms **(Figs. 5, 6)** demonstrate nearly symmetric long, smooth tapered narrowings of the right axillary and both proximal brachial arteries with near occlusion on the left and extensive development of collateral circulation bilaterally. Ulcerations and plaque are noticeably absent. The location and morphology of these lesions in this clinical setting is characteristic of giant cell arteritis (GCA). The primary differential diagnostic consideration would be Takayasu's arteritis, but this usually involves slightly larger vessels.

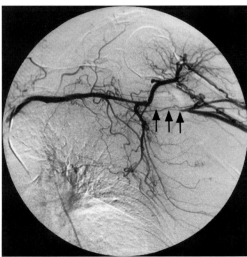

Figure 6. Left subclavian/axillary arteriogram shows marked long-segment smooth narrowing (arrows) of the proximal brachial artery. There is also mild axillary artery narrowing.

Diagnosis

Bilateral axillary artery stenoses secondary to giant cell arteritis.

How would you manage this patient?

Management

Nearly all patients with narrowing of the subclavian, axillary, or brachial arteries caused by GCA and symptoms of ischemia will show clinical improvement with initiation of corticosteroid therapy. No defined role for transcatheter therapy in this disease exists to date. Surgical intervention with bypass procedures has an equally limited role and is considered only in those patients whose ischemic symptoms persist despite adequate steroid therapy.

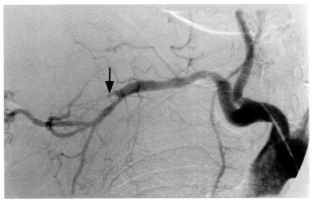

Figure 7. Right subclavian/axillary arteriogram reveals occlusion (arrow) of the axillary artery after a short segment of smooth tapering.

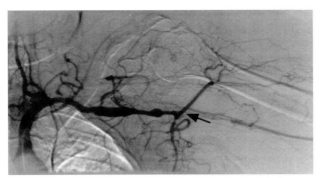

Figure 8. Left subclavian/axillary arteriogram shows occlusion (arrow) of the distal axillary artery with reconstitution of the brachial artery via collaterals. The subclavian and proximal axillary arteries show alternating areas of dilatation and stenosis.

Discussion

Giant cell arteritis is an idiopathic, generalized vasculitis that affects medium- and large-sized arteries. It occurs in patients over 50 years of age, with a female predominance. Classically, it presents as "temporal arteritis" with symptoms of headache, scalp tenderness, jaw claudication, and visual disturbances. However, it can also present with constitutional symptoms only (fever, weight loss, fatigue, and anorexia) or as in this case, with vascular symptoms as the first manifestation. GCA often coexists with polymyalgia rheumatica (PMR), a syndrome of proximal muscle aching and stiffness. The majority (50%–90%) of patients with GCA present with or develop PMR, and up to 33% of patients with PMR have a positive temporal artery biopsy for GCA. Blindness, stroke, myocardial infarction, and bowel ischemia are the infrequent but catastrophic sequelae of GCA when vessels to these end organs are affected.

The angiographic appearance of the lesions in combination with the clinical presentation allows for a confident angiographic diagnosis of GCA. Atherosclerotic stenoses typically involve the origins of the great vessels and are short-segment abnormalities. Arterial stenoses from trauma or thoracic outlet syndrome can give a similar appearance. Relevant history of trauma or the presence of a cervical rib should be investigated. Macroembolism from the heart, a proximal pseudoaneurysm, or an occluded axillofemoral graft can also cause stenosis or short-segment occlusion of the axillobrachial region. Radiation-induced arterial occlusive disease is rare, but it can be seen as early as 10 years after radiotherapy for malignancies in this region (breast cancer, lymphoma).

Figures 7 and **8** demonstrate bilateral axillary artery occlusion in another patient with known GCA. Multifocal areas of short-segment narrowing alternating with areas of mild dilatation involve the subclavian and proximal axillary arteries bilaterally; this is better seen in the left upper extremity **(Fig. 7)**. Distinguishing GCA from atherosclerotic disease in a vessel with this degree of luminal irregularity can be difficult in older patients; however, bilaterality is often seen in GCA.

Recent studies suggest that patients with GCA are 17.3 times more likely to develop thoracic aortic aneurysms and 2.4 times more likely to develop isolated abdominal aortic aneurysms than unaffected persons of the same age and sex.

For further information on this topic, please see Tutorial 20.

Selected Readings

Bengtsson BA, Andersson R. Giant cell and Takayasu's arteritis. Curr Opin Rheumatol 1991; 3:15–22.

Evans JM, O'Fallon WM, Hunder GG. Increased incidence of aortic aneurysm and dissection in giant cell (temporal) arteritis. Ann Intern Med 1995; 122:502–507.

Hellmann DB. Immunopathogenesis, diagnosis, and treatment of giant cell arteritis, temporal arteritis, polymyalgia rheumatica, and Takayasu's arteritis. Curr Opin Rheumatol 1993; 5:25–32.

Klein RG, Hunder GG, Stanson AW, Sheps SG, et al. Large artery involvement in giant cell (temporal) arteritis. Ann Intern Med 1975; 83:806–812.

Ninet JP, Bachet P, Dumontet CM, Du Colombier PB, Stewart MD, Pasquier JH. Subclavian and axillary involvement in temporal arteritis and polymyalgia rheumatica. Am J Med 1990; 88:13–20.

Schumacher HR Jr, ed. Primer on the rheumatic diseases. 9th edition. Atlanta: Arthritis Foundation, 1988.

Strandness DE Jr, van Breda A, eds. Vascular diseases: surgical and interventional therapy. New York: Churchill Livingstone, 1994.

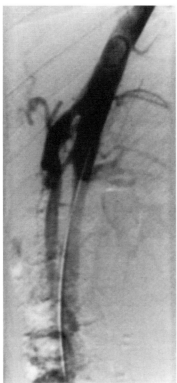

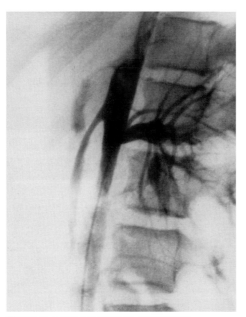

Figure 2. Lateral aortogram, later phase.

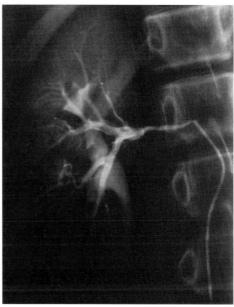

Figure 3. Right renal arteriogram.

Figure 1. Lateral aortogram.

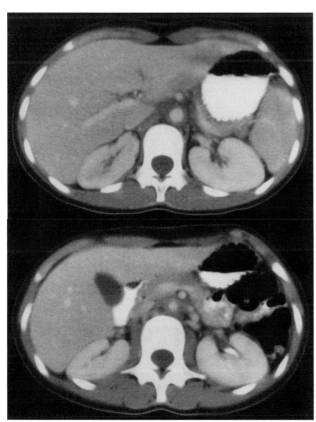

Figure 4. Images from a contrast-enhanced CT scan of the abdomen.

TEACHING FILE CASE 26
Timothy J. Carmody, M.D., and
Scott O. Trerotola, M.D.

History
A 16-year-old female came to the hospital with a recurrent history of intermittent fever, malaise, myalgias/arthralgias, and rash. On the most recent visit to her physician, her blood pressure was recorded at 132/95 mm Hg. Her physical examination revealed findings consistent with pulmonary edema, and an audible abdominal bruit was noted. Peripheral pulses were symmetric. The erythrocyte sedimentation rate was elevated at 45 mm/hour. The lateral aortogram (Figs. 1, 2), a selective right renal arteriogram (Fig. 3), and images from an enhanced abdominal computed tomography (CT) scan (Fig. 4) are shown.

What is your diagnosis?

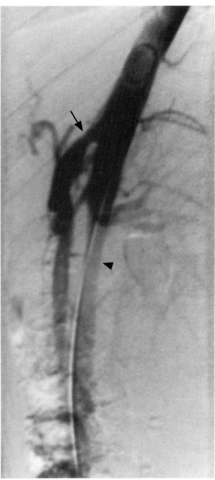

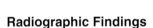

Figure 5. Lateral aortogram shows stenosis of the celiac artery (arrow) and narrowing of the infrarenal aorta (arrowhead).

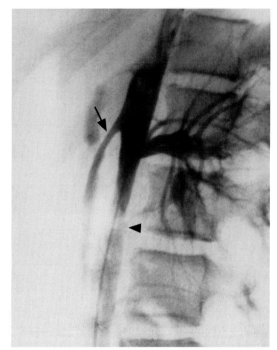

Figure 6. Later phase of the lateral aortogram shows stenosis of the superior mesenteric artery (arrow) and narrowing of the infrarenal aorta (arrowhead).

Radiographic Findings

The lateral abdominal aortogram **(Figs. 5, 6)** demonstrates segmental stenoses of the celiac and superior mesenteric arteries just beyond their origins. Short-segment stenosis of the infrarenal abdominal aorta is also present. Selective injection of the right renal artery **(Fig. 7)** demonstrates severe stenosis involving the proximal 2 cm of the vessel, including the origin. The CT scan at the level of the infrarenal aorta **(Fig. 8)** confirms concentric aortic wall thickening with compromise of the luminal diameter. These findings confirm the suspected diagnosis of Takayasu's arteritis.

Diagnoses

1. Takayasu's arteritis.
2. Aortic and mesenteric branch stenoses.
3. Right renal artery stenosis with secondary hypertension.

How would you manage this patient?

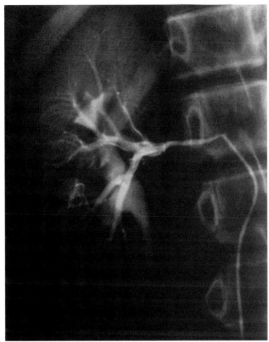

Figure 7. Selective right renal arteriogram shows long-segment stenosis of the renal artery. Intrarenal vessels are normal.

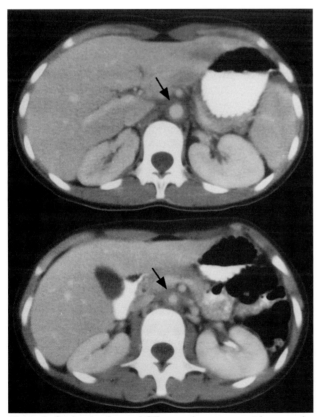

Figure 8. Contrast-enhanced CT scan shows concentric narrowing of the abdominal aorta (arrows) corresponding to that seen in Figures 5 and 6. There is thickening of the aortic wall.

Management

Corticosteroids are the first line of therapy for these patients, with cytotoxic agents available to those who fail to respond to steroids alone. Surgical bypass and endovascular therapy are options in those patients who have progressive vascular involvement. Nonemergent endovascular or surgical intervention should be performed during periods of clinical disease quiescence. Arteriography cannot distinguish the vascular narrowing of acute inflammation from the chronic fibro-occlusive sequelae of the disease, and clinical assessment may also be misleading. Up to 44% of surgical specimens taken during bypass procedures in patients deemed clinically "inactive" showed histological evidence of ongoing inflammation.

Technical success rates as high as 95% for renal artery percutaneous transluminal angioplasty (PTA) have been reported, but long-term patency varies with the clinical course of the disease. The rate of restenosis is higher for male patients, for lesions affecting the origin of the vessel, and for postangioplasty residual stenoses of more than 20%. Overall patency for subclavian stenoses following angioplasty is approximately 65% at 26 months mean follow-up. Aortic stenoses have been successfully treated with PTA; however, those lesions with eccentric wall thickening are at higher risk for intimal dissection.

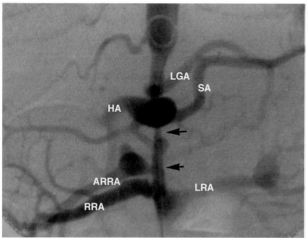

Figure 9. Abdominal aortogram from another patient with Takayasu's aortitis. Marked narrowing of the abdominal aorta (arrows) is present. LGA=left gastric artery; HA=hepatic artery; SA=splenic artery; LRA=left renal artery; RRA=right renal artery; ARRA=accessory right renal artery. The superior mesenteric artery is not opacified.

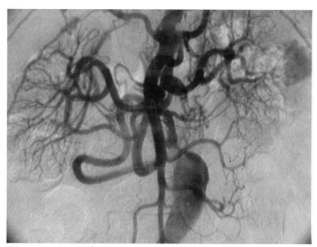

Figure 10. Abdominal aortogram. Takayasu's aortitis with marked narrowing of the perivisceral abdominal aorta.

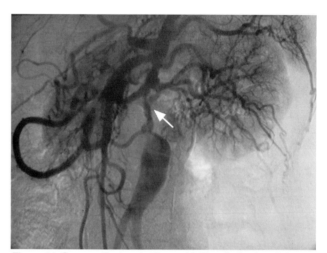

Figure 11. Same patient as in Figure 10. The diminutive abdominal aorta is more clearly visualized (arrow) on the right posterior oblique view.

Discussion

Takayasu's arteritis **(Figs. 9–11)** is a chronic, idiopathic inflammatory disease occurring predominantly in females (>95%) during their reproductive years. It primarily affects the aorta and its major branches. There is a wide spectrum of clinical presentation, disease severity, and pace of progression. Vascular findings are the hallmark of this disease, manifesting as bruits, claudication, hypertension, or diminished pulses at some time during the course of the disease in nearly 100% of patients. Neurologic symptoms (visual aberrations, light-headedness, transient ischemic attack), musculoskeletal complaints (53%: myalgias/arthralgias), constitutional abnormalities (43%: fever, malaise, weight loss), and cardiac involvement (38%: aortic regurgitation, coronary artery disease) represent the other manifestations of this disease.

Arteriography remains the gold standard to confirm the diagnosis and evaluate the extent of vascular involvement. Inflammatory aortitis from other causes (other rheumatic diseases, infectious agents, connective tissue disorders, neurofibromatosis **(Fig. 12)**, ergotism) can usually be excluded on the basis of clinical criteria and serologic studies. The arteriographic morphology is classically described as noncalcified long-segment stenoses or occlusions involving the thoracoabdominal aorta (65%–76%), or the subclavian (56%–93%), renal (38%–68%), carotid (58%), vertebral (35%), innominate (27%), axillary (20%), mesenteric (18%), or iliac (17%) arteries. The pulmonary arterial system is involved up to 15% of the time, and may be asymptomatic. Aneurysms also occur, but are 3.6 times less common than stenoses.

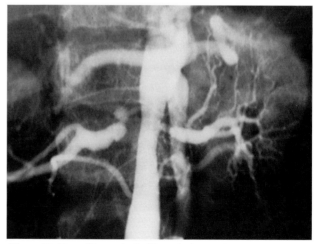

Figure 12. Neurofibromatosis. Though the aortic narrowing and renal artery stenoses mimic Takayasu's disease, the patient had extensive clinical stigmata of neurofibromatosis.

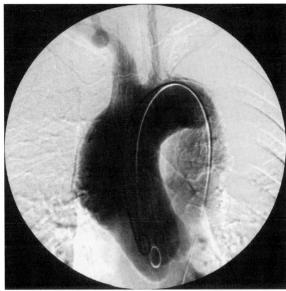

Figure 13. Thoracic aortogram shows a dilated ascending aorta. The left subclavian artery is not seen.

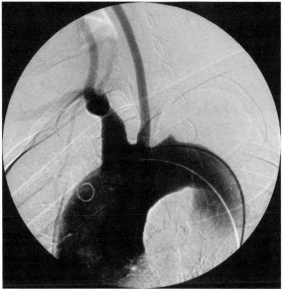

Figure 14. Same patient as in Figure 13. Right posterior oblique projection demonstrates the subclavian occlusion more clearly.

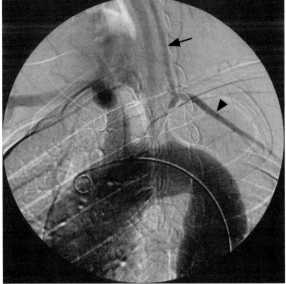

Figure 15. Same patient as in Figure 13. A later image shows reconstitution of the left subclavian artery (arrowhead) via the left vertebral artery (arrow).

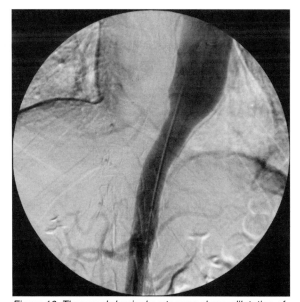

Figure 16. Thoracoabdominal aortogram shows dilatation of the lower thoracic aorta with return to normal caliber below the diaphragm.

Figures 13–16 show a more classic angiographic appearance of this disease in a 35-year-old woman with absent left upper extremity pulses. The thoracic aortogram demonstrates fusiform aneurysmal dilatation of the thoracic aorta and innominate artery, with occlusion of the left subclavian artery. **Figure 15** demonstrates reconstitution of the subclavian artery from retrograde flow through the vertebral system. **Figure 16** demonstrates the transition from the aneurysmal descending thoracic aorta to the more normal appearing upper abdominal aorta.

For further information on this topic, please see Tutorial 20.

Selected Readings

Joseph S, Mandalam KR, Rao VR, et al. Percutaneous transluminal angioplasty of the subclavian artery in nonspecific aortoarteritis: results of long-term follow-up. J Vasc Interv Radiol 1994; 5:573–580.

Kerr GS, Hallahan CW, Giordano J, et al. Takayasu's arteritis. Ann Intern Med 1994; 120:919–929.

Park JH, Chung JW, Im JG, Kim SK, Park YB, Han MC. Takayasu's arteritis: evaluation of mural changes in the aorta and pulmonary artery with CT angiography. Radiology 1995; 196:89–93.

Schumacher HR Jr, ed. Primer on the rheumatic diseases. 9th edition. Atlanta: Arthritis Foundation, 1988.

Sharma S, Shrivastava S, Kothari SS, Kaul U, Rajani M. Influence of angiographic morphology on the acute and longer-term outcome of percutaneous transluminal angioplasty in patients with aortic stenosis due to nonspecific aortitis. Cardiovasc Intervent Radiol 1994; 17:147–151.

Sharma S, Thatai D, Saxena A, Kothari SS, Guleria S, Rajani M. Renovascular hypertension resulting from nonspecific aortoarteritis in children: midterm results of percutaneous transluminal renal angioplasty and predictors of restenosis. AJR 1996; 166:157–162.

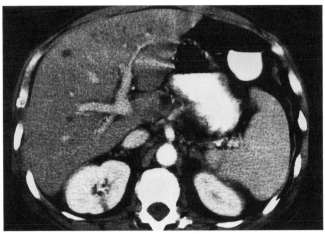

Figure 1. Contrast-enhanced abdominal CT scan.

TEACHING FILE CASE 27
Eric W. Olcott, M.D.

History

A 45-year-old man came to the hospital complaining of 4 days of abdominal pain with intermittent nausea and vomiting. The patient was moderately febrile and his abdomen was diffusely tender. He did not appear to be markedly ill. Laboratory studies disclosed leukocytosis (13,600/µL) and elevated hepatic transaminases. Alkaline phosphatase was mildly elevated. The patient's sexual partner was a hepatitis B virus carrier and was seropositive for human immunodeficiency virus (HIV). The referring clinicians suspected an intraabdominal abscess, and a computed tomography (CT) scan was performed **(Fig. 1)**.

What is your diagnosis?

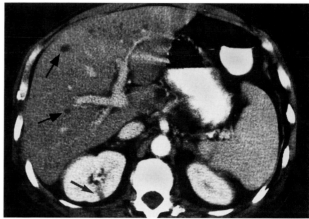

Figure 2. Contrast-enhanced CT scan shows focal subcentimeter parenchymal hypodensities (arrows) in the liver and right kidney.

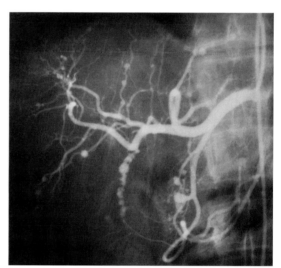

Figure 3. Selective common hepatic arteriogram.

Radiographic Findings

The contrast-enhanced CT scan shows multiple hypodense lesions in the liver and kidney **(Fig. 2)**. Hypodense abnormalities were present in the pancreas as well. The initial differential diagnosis advanced for this patient at risk for HIV disease was visceral candidiasis. However, in light of the lack of severe clinical symptoms, vasculitis was also considered. Accordingly, visceral arteriography was performed. The common hepatic arteriogram is shown in **Figure 3**.

What is your diagnosis now? Are there any other arterial territories which are likely to be affected?

Diagnosis

Polyarteritis nodosa (PAN).

In addition to the hepatic arterial involvement **(Fig. 4)**, this disease also involved the renal **(Fig. 5)** and superior mesenteric **(Fig. 6)** arterial territories.

What treatment would be appropriate?

464

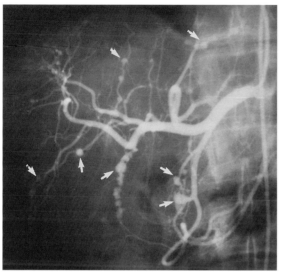

Figure 4. Common hepatic arteriogram shows multiple, small saccular aneurysms (arrows) most compatible with an inflammatory vasculitis.

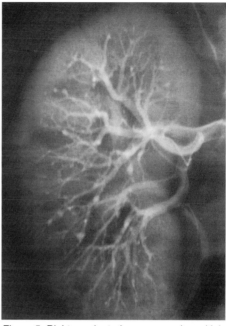

Figure 5. Right renal arteriogram reveals multiple small saccular aneurysms typical of PAN.

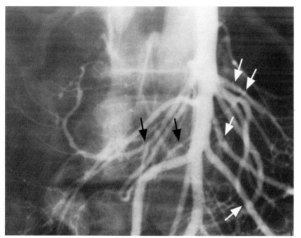

Figure 6. Multifocal arterial irregularities and narrowings (arrows) typical of PAN are evident on the superior mesenteric arteriogram.

Management

Arteriography can play a key role in the diagnosis of PAN. Treatment usually consists of medical management. Corticosteroids and cytotoxic drugs currently are the therapeutic agents of choice. Plasma exchange therapy may also be beneficial. Interventional embolization of a hemorrhagic aneurysm in the setting of PAN has been reported, and should be considered when clinically appropriate.

Discussion

Polyarteritis nodosa, also known as periarteritis nodosa, is a necrotizing vasculitis. Patients are frequently in their forties and male. Symptoms often include fever, malaise, and abdominal pain. Other clinical features may include myalgias, arthralgias, hypertension, and mononeuritis multiplex. Leukocytosis with elevation of hepatic transaminases and alkaline phosphatase may be noted. An association with hepatitis B surface antigen seropositivity has been documented.

Arteriography characteristically reveals numerous small aneurysms involving medium-size and small arteries. Nonspecific findings of vasculitis may be present, such as vascular pruning and narrowing. Renal, visceral, and muscular arteries may be involved, as may cerebral vessels. The differential diagnosis of multiple aneurysms of small and medium-size vessels includes vasculitis secondary to methamphetamine abuse. In addition, multiple aneurysms have been described secondary to Wegener's granulomatosis.

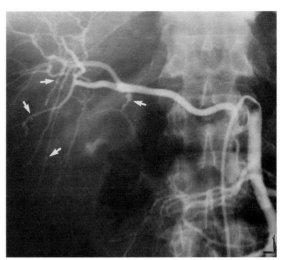

Figure 7. Superior mesenteric arteriogram reveals a replaced right hepatic artery. Small aneurysms typical of PAN are present in intrahepatic branches of the replaced right hepatic artery (arrows).

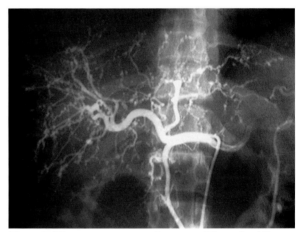

Figure 8. Microaneurysms are also present throughout the hepatic arterial system.

The diagnosis of polyarteritis nodosa may also be made by biopsy of the affected tissues such as muscles, testes, and nerves. The arterial aneurysms may hemorrhage and regress following treatment. Arteriograms of other patients with PAN are included in **Figures 7–9**.

Imaging studies performed during the diagnostic work-up may reveal hepatic infarcts, hepatic bile lakes, and evidence of infarction or ischemia in other organs. The pattern of small hypodense hepatic lesions on contrast CT has been reported recently.

For further information on this topic, please see Tutorial 20.

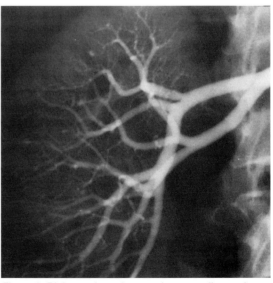

Figure 9. Right renal arteriogram shows small saccular aneurysms secondary to PAN.

Selected Readings

Hekali P, Kajander H, Pajari R, Stenman S, Somer T. Diagnostic significance of angiographically observed visceral aneurysms with regard to polyarteritis nodosa. Acta Radiol 1991; 32:143–148.

Herskowitz MM, Flyer MA, Sclafani SJ. Percutaneous transhepatic coil embolization of a ruptured intrahepatic aneurysm in polyarteritis nodosa. Cardiovasc Intervent Radiol 1993; 16:254–256.

Jennette JC, Falk RJ, Andrassy K, et al. Nomenclature of systemic vasculitides. Proposal of an international consensus conference. Arthritis Rheum 1994; 37:187–192.

Olcott EW, Openshaw KL. Polyarteritis nodosa mimicking hepatic candidiasis on postcontrast CT. J Comput Assist Tomogr 1994; 18:305–307.

End Note

Figures 3 and 4 from Olcott EW, Openshaw KL. Polyarteritis nodosa mimicking hepatic candidiasis on postcontrast CT. J Comput Assist Tomogr 1994; 18:306. Used with permission.

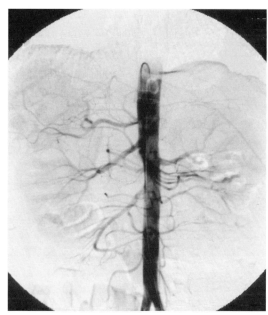

Figure 1. Abdominal aortogram, early arterial phase.

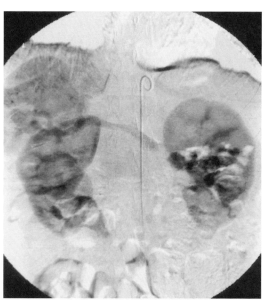

Figure 2. Abdominal aortogram, venous phase.

TEACHING FILE CASE 28
Ian D. Timms, M.D., and
Michael A. Amygdalos, M.D.

History

A 35-year-old woman suffered a colonic injury during cesarean section, and anomalous anatomy was encountered at surgery. A repeat operation for lysis of adhesions was needed and the general surgeon requested a preoperative visceral arteriogram to better define the anatomy. An aortogram **(Figs. 1, 2)**, selective superior mesenteric arteriogram **(Figs. 3, 4)** and selective inferior mesenteric arteriogram **(Fig. 5)** were obtained. A chest radiograph was also obtained **(Fig. 6)**.

What is your diagnosis?

468

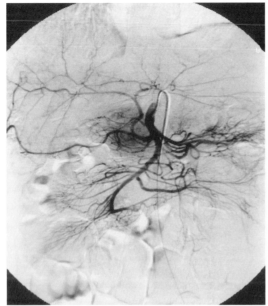

Figure 3. Superior mesenteric arteriogram, mid arterial phase.

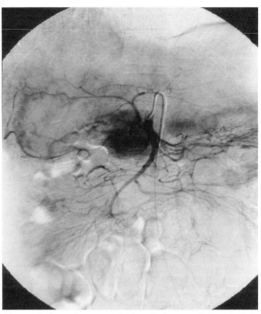

Figure 4. Superior mesenteric arteriogram, late arterial phase.

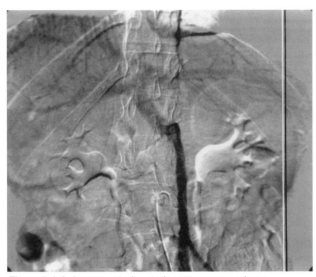

Figure 5. Inferior mesenteric arteriogram, venous phase.

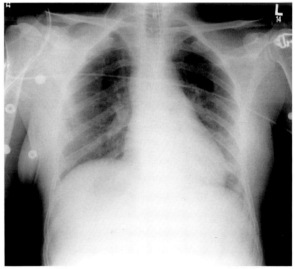

Figure 6. Chest radiograph.

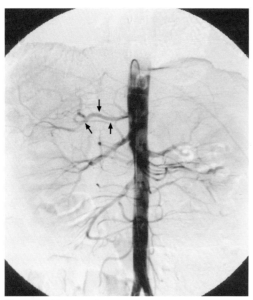

Figure 7. Abdominal aortogram demonstrates an artery taking origin from the aorta extending into the right upper quadrant (arrows).

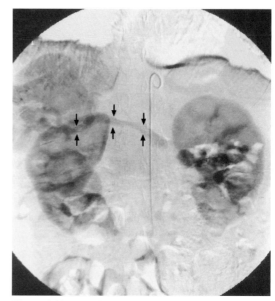

Figure 8. Venous phase of the abdominal aortogram shows a vein (arrows) draining the right upper quadrant structure toward the midline.

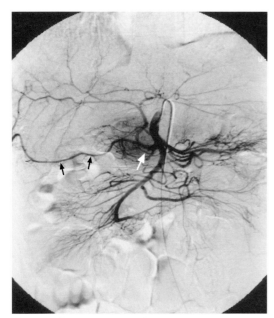

Figure 9. Superior mesenteric arteriogram shows an anomalous common hepatic artery (white arrow) and gastroepiploic artery (black arrows).

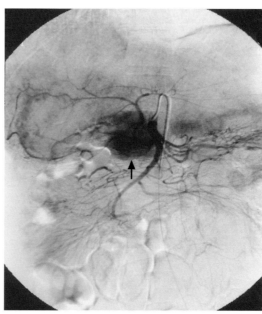

Figure 10. Superior mesenteric arteriogram, late arterial phase. A densely staining structure (arrow) is present adjacent to the SMA.

Radiographic Findings

The aortogram demonstrates a vascular structure in the right upper quadrant of the abdomen supplied by a single artery directly arising from the aorta **(Fig. 7)** with a prominent draining vein **(Fig. 8)**. This vein drains into the portal system. The selective superior mesenteric artery (SMA) injection **(Figs. 9, 10)** demonstrates a replaced common hepatic artery (CHA) and a gastroepiploic artery (GE) supplying a right-sided stomach. Note the unusual horizontal and midline distribution of the hepatic arterial circulation, indicating a symmetric liver.

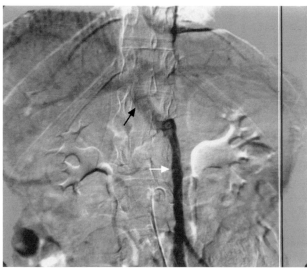

Figure 11. Inferior mesenteric arteriogram, venous phase, depicts the inferior mesenteric vein (white arrow) and portal vein (black arrow).

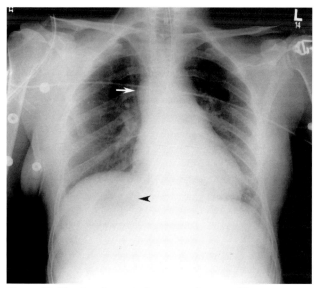

Figure 12. Chest radiograph shows prominence of the azygos vein (arrow) compatible with azygos continuation of the inferior vena cava. The gastric air bubble can be faintly seen in the right upper quadrant (arrowhead).

A second hypervascular structure is present adjacent to the SMA. The venous phase of the inferior mesenteric artery injection **(Fig. 11)** demonstrates the portal venous anatomy and the hepatic symmetry. The chest radiograph **(Fig. 12)** confirms the right-sided location of the stomach and demonstrates azygos continuation of the inferior vena cava.

Diagnosis
Situs ambiguus (heterotaxy syndrome) with polysplenia.

Discussion
Heterotaxy syndromes are characterized by a failure of lateralization of the thoracic and abdominal viscera into a pattern of either situs solitus ("normal" situs) or situs inversus (the mirror image of "normal" situs). Heterotaxy syndromes are associated with either polysplenia (multiple spleens located on either side of the abdomen) or asplenia (complete absence of splenic tissue). Those patients with asplenia uniformly have a severe, specific type of congenital heart disease and rarely survive beyond infancy. In contrast, patients with polysplenia may not have clinically significant associated congenital anomalies, and they may survive into adulthood asymptomatic and undetected. Characteristics of situs ambiguus with polysplenia exemplified by this patient include a right-sided stomach, multiple splenules (the enhancing structures seen on the arteriograms), hepatic symmetry, and azygos continuation of the inferior vena cava.

For further information on this topic, please see Tutorial 9.

Selected Readings

Gedgaudas E, Moller JH, Castaneda-Zuniga WR, Amplatz K. Cardiovascular radiology. Philadelphia: W.B. Saunders Company, 1985.

Spindola-Franco H, Fish BG. Radiology of the heart: cardiac imaging in infants, children, and adults. New York: Springer-Verlag, 1985.

Strife JL, Bisset GS. Cardiovascular system. In: Kirks DR, ed. Practical pediatric imaging: diagnostic radiology of infants and children. 2nd edition. Boston: Little, Brown and Company, 1991; 326–399.

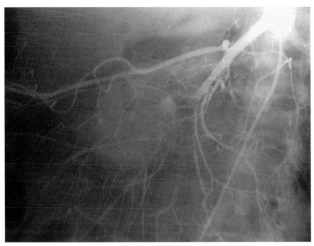
Figure 1. Superior mesenteric arteriogram.

TEACHING FILE CASE 29
*Rajiv Sawhney, M.D., and
Susan D. Wall, M.D.*

History
The patient is a 55-year-old who came to the emergency department with severe abdominal pain and diarrhea. There is a history of atrial fibrillation. Abdominal plain films were unrevealing. A mesenteric arteriogram was obtained **(Fig.1)**.

What is your diagnosis?

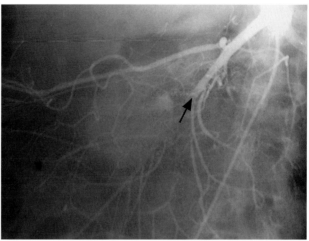

Figure 2. The superior mesenteric artery abruptly terminates in its mid portion (arrow). The lack of well-defined collaterals indicates that the occlusion is acute.

Radiographic Findings

A selective injection of the superior mesenteric artery (SMA) **(Fig. 2)** demonstrates an occlusion of the SMA approximately 7–8 cm distal to its origin.

Diagnosis

Superior mesenteric artery embolus.

Management

The patient's large SMA embolus was treated by surgical embolectomy.

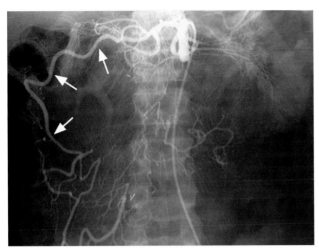

Figure 3. Superior mesenteric arteriogram shows a chronic occlusion as evidenced by the large middle colic collateral (arrows).

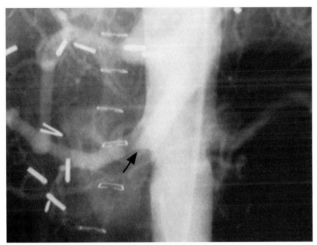

Figure 5. Acute SMA occlusion (arrow) due to inadvertent surgical ligation during a Whipple procedure.

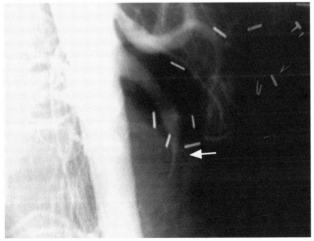

Figure 6. Lateral view from the same patient as in Figure 5. There is abrupt termination of the SMA (arrow).

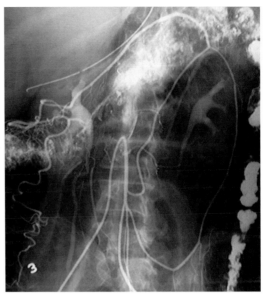

Figure 4. Inferior mesenteric arteriogram shows filling of middle and right colic arteries in a patient who has chronic occlusion of the SMA.

Discussion

SMA embolus is a common cause of acute mesenteric ischemia, accounting for 30%–50% of cases. The embolus is usually cardiac in origin with arrhythmias, especially atrial fibrillation, as the underlying cause. The characteristic filling defect or abrupt vessel termination is usually seen at narrowed segments of the SMA distal to the origins of major branches such as the inferior pancreatic duodenal and middle colic arteries. Mesenteric arteriography serves as the main diagnostic test; plain films are usually only helpful to rule out other causes of abdominal pain.

Because of the vascular insult, patients clinically present with sudden severe abdominal pain. Typically there is a history of heart disease (arrhythmias, myocardial infarction). Peritoneal signs are usually not present unless intestinal infarction has already occurred. Patient prognosis depends on the level of occlusion, the timing of the diagnosis, and the prompt initiation of appropriate treatment. The usual treatment is surgical thromboembolectomy. Sometimes patients with small, nonocclusive emboli can be treated nonsurgically with fibrinolytic infusion. However, the safety of this treatment strategy has not been unequivocally established. Patients with significant abdominal discomfort usually require surgical exploration to exclude necrotic bowel.

Other examples of SMA occlusions are shown in **Figures 3–6**.

For further information on this topic, please see Tutorials 9 and 10.

Selected Readings

Bech FR, Giewertz BL. Pathophysiology of intestinal ischemia. In: Strandness DE Jr, van Breda A, eds. Vascular diseases: surgical and interventional therapy. New York: Churchill Livingstone, 1994; 745–746.

Durham JD, Flinn WR. Surgical management of acute mesenteric ischemia. In: Strandness DE Jr, van Breda A, eds. Vascular diseases: surgical and interventional therapy. New York: Churchill Livingstone, 1994; 776–777.

Kadir S. Diagnostic angiography. Philadelphia: W.B. Saunders Company, 1986; 353–354.

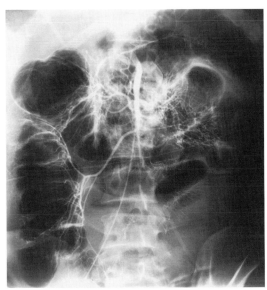

Figure 1. Superior mesenteric arteriogram, mid arterial phase.

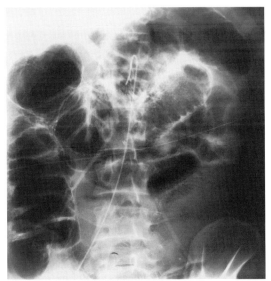

Figure 2. Superior mesenteric arteriogram, venous phase.

TEACHING FILE CASE 30
Keith M. Horton, M.D.

History

A 46-year-old prison inmate was found unresponsive on the floor of his cell. He was subsequently revived and sent to the emergency department. Upon arrival at the hospital the patient complained of crampy abdominal pain. The patient was afebrile and had a systolic blood pressure of 100 mm Hg and a pulse of 110 beats per minute. The physical examination revealed abdominal distention and diffuse tenderness without guarding or rebound. The patient's white blood cell count was 15,000 cells/μL. Stool guaiac was negative. Plain films failed to demonstrate intestinal obstruction or perforation. The patient was sent for an arteriogram (Figs. 1, 2).

What is your diagnosis?

Radiographic Findings
Selective injection of the superior mesenteric artery (SMA) shows diffuse vasoconstriction of the distal branches of the SMA **(Figs. 3, 4)**. This pattern is commonly referred to as the "pruned" appearance of the mesenteric branches.

Diagnosis
Nonocclusive mesenteric ischemia secondary to cocaine abuse.

How would you manage this patient?

Management
The patient was treated initially with intraarterial papaverine via the SMA catheter. The patient had persistent peritoneal signs despite the infusion and was taken to surgery for exploration. There was no evidence of infarcted bowel and the patient was subsequently observed in the intensive care unit. Twenty-four hours later a repeat arteriogram was performed **(Figs. 5, 6)** which showed marked improvement in bowel perfusion. The papaverine infusion was switched to saline for 30 minutes and the catheter was then removed.

Discussion
This case represents part of the spectrum of entities that comprise nonocclusive mesenteric ischemia. Nonocclusive mesenteric ischemia is defined as "intestinal gangrene in the presence of a patent arterial tree." It is a relatively uncommon disorder characterized by splanchnic vasoconstriction usually resulting from systemic hypotension. Nonocclusive mesenteric ischemia is responsible for an estimated 20%–30% of cases of acute mesenteric ischemia. This condition is primarily seen in elderly patients who have cardiac disease.

Arteriographic findings usually include diffuse vasoconstriction of the mesenteric branches (usually the SMA), increased aortic reflux, spasm of the intestinal arcades, and diminished arterial and venous flow. By definition there is no major occlusive lesion.

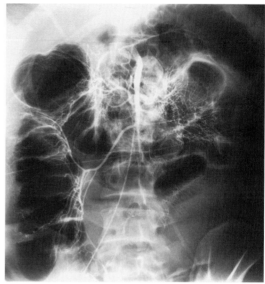

Figure 3. Superior mesenteric arteriogram shows diffuse vasoconstriction of the distal branches of the SMA. Arterial branches supplying bowel in the left lower quadrant are not visualized.

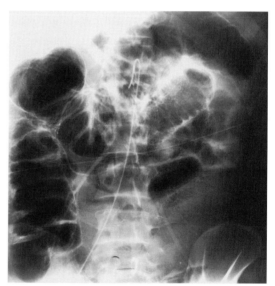

Figure 4. Venous phase of the superior mesenteric arteriogram shows sparse venous opacification and small bowel distention.

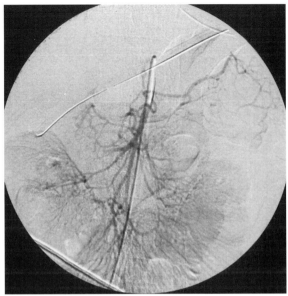

Figure 5. SMA injection after exploratory laparotomy shows improved filling of the distal branches.

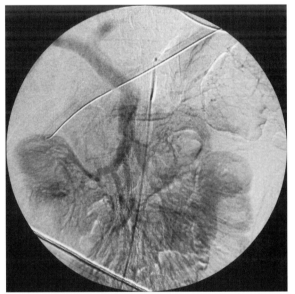

Figure 6. The venous phase of the same injection as Figure 5 now reveals opacification of the superior mesenteric and portal veins.

Nonocclusive mesenteric ischemia is best treated nonsurgically if there is no sign of intestinal infarction. Papaverine is generally prepared as a drip and infused via the selectively placed angiographic catheter. This may sometimes be preceded by a bolus of the drug as well. The infusion is usually continued for 24 hours but can be prolonged up to 5 days. When the patient becomes asymptomatic the infusion is changed to saline for 30 minutes, and repeat arteriography is then performed. If there is no vasoconstriction, the infusion is discontinued and the catheter is removed.

If peritoneal signs develop, prompt surgical exploration is indicated to rule out bowel infarction. The drip should be continued during surgery and throughout the recovery period to maximize bowel perfusion.

Abdominal pain and leukocytosis are seen in 75%–85% of patients who have acute mesenteric ischemia. The absence of pain is more commonly seen in patients with nonocclusive ischemia. Prompt diagnosis of this disorder is necessary in order to prevent infarction, sepsis, and death, which are seen in a high proportion of these patients.

For further information on this topic, please see Tutorial 10.

Selected Readings

Brandt LJ, Boley SJ. Nonocclusive mesenteric ischemia. Annu Rev Med 1991; 42:107–117.

Haglund U, Lundgren O. Nonocclusive acute intestinal vascular failure. Br J Surg 1979; 66:155–158.

Kaleya RN, Sammartano RJ, Boley SJ. Aggressive approach to acute mesenteric ischemia. Surg Clin North Am 1992; 72:157–182.

Siegelman SS, Sprayregen S, Boley S. Angiographic diagnosis of mesenteric arterial vasoconstriction. Radiology 1974; 112:533–542.

Wilcox M, Howard TJ, Plaskon LA, Unthank JL, Madura JA. Current theories of pathogenesis and treatment of nonocclusive mesenteric ischemia. Dig Dis Sci 1995; 40:709–716.

End Notes

Images contributed by Scott Trerotola, M.D., Indiana University Medical Center, Indianapolis, IN.

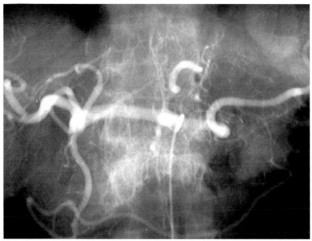

Figure 1. Celiac arteriogram.

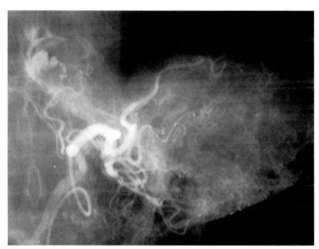

Figure 2. Left gastric arteriogram.

TEACHING FILE CASE 31
Harjit Singh, M.D., and
Anthony Venbrux, M.D.

History
A 76-year-old man came to the emergency department complaining of dizziness and three episodes of hematemesis. Emergent endoscopy revealed active bleeding at the gastroesophageal (GE) junction. Celiac arteriography was performed **(Figs. 1, 2)**.

What is your diagnosis?

Radiographic Findings

Celiac arteriography **(Fig. 3)** reveals normal vascular anatomy. No extravasation of contrast material is seen on the celiac injection. Subselective injection of the left gastric artery demonstrates contrast material extravasation at the GE junction **(Fig. 4)**. After transcatheter embolotherapy using Gelfoam pledgets (Upjohn, Kalamazoo, MI), a repeat injection of the left gastric artery shows no further extravasation **(Fig. 5)**.

Diagnosis

Mallory-Weiss tear.

Discussion

Gastrointestinal hemorrhage seen in alcoholic patients with a recent history of heavy drinking was first described by Mallory and Weiss in 1929. Post mortem examination in four patients in the original series described fissure-like linear mucosal tears arranged circumferentially around the GE junction. More recently, with the routine use of endoscopy to evaluate patients with upper gastrointestinal hemorrhage, a better understanding of the etiology and natural history of these lesions has helped guide therapy.

As a cause of upper gastrointestinal hemorrhage, Mallory-Weiss tears account for 5%–15% of cases. Greater than 80% of the tears are found along the lesser curvature of the stomach at the level of the GE junction. In 17% of cases, there are multiple tears. Although patients with a history of alcohol ingestion are commonly thought of as the typical patient with a Mallory-Weiss tear, other causes include nonsteroidal anti-inflammatory drug ingestion, acute pancreatitis, and gravida emesis associated with pregnancy. One third of patients may not have the classic history of emesis.

Before the use of endoscopy became widespread, physicians turned to arteriography for identification of the source of bleeding. Arteriography is now considered a therapeutic alternative if conservative and/or endoscopic treatment have failed.

Previously, vasopressin infusions were commonly used to control upper gastrointestinal hemorrhage. Though effective, these infusions required prolonged arterial catheterization and were associated with complications including hypertension, hyponatremia, and peripheral and myocardial ischemia. Moreover, catheter dislodgment can occur, rendering the infusion ineffective. Therefore, embolotherapy has replaced vasopressin infusion in most centers for the management of bleeding from celiac axis branches.

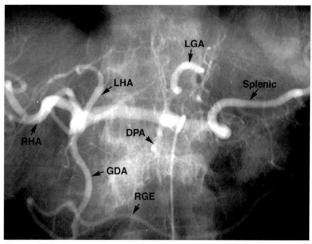

Figure 3. Celiac arteriogram demonstrates normal vascular anatomy. LHA=left hepatic artery; RHA=right hepatic artery; LGA=left gastric artery; GDA=gastroduodenal artery; DPA=dorsal pancreatic artery; RGE=right gastroepiploic artery.

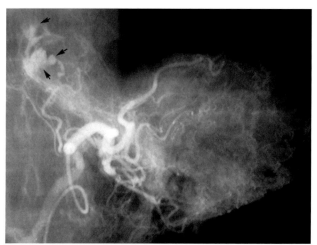

Figure 4. Left gastric artery injection shows contrast material extravasation (arrows) at the GE junction.

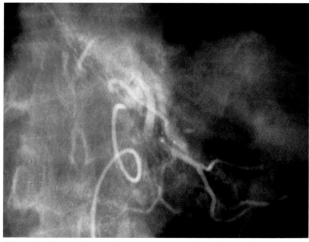

Figure 5. Postembolization arteriogram. No further extravasation is identified.

A selective celiac arteriogram should be performed followed by a selective left gastric artery (LGA) injection. The LGA will supply the bleeding site more than 85% of the time. When active extravasation is identified, transcatheter therapy to control the bleeding should be performed.

Gelfoam is the most common agent used for left gastric arterial embolization. Once embolization has been accomplished, repeat arterio-graphy with gentle contrast material injection should be performed to confirm successful occlusion of the selected vessel.

Complications of transcatheter embolotherapy include non-target organ infarction (spleen, etc) and bowel ischemia. Fortunately, clinically significant complications are rare following this procedure.

More than 90% of patients with Mallory-Weiss tears and gastrointestinal hemorrhage respond to conservative measures. Those who do not respond to conservative means frequently respond to endoscopic therapeutic measures such as cautery. Should these fail, transcatheter embolotherapy will be successful in more than 85% of the remaining cases.

For further information on this topic, please see Tutorials 13 and 14, and Teaching File Cases 32 and 33.

Selected Readings

Bataller R, Llach J, Salmeron JM, et al. Endoscopic sclerotherapy in upper gastrointestinal bleeding due to Mallory-Weiss syndrome. Am J Gastroenterol 1994; 89:2147–2150.

Harris JM, DiPalma JA. Clinical significance of Mallory-Weiss tears. Am J Gastroenterol 1993; 88:2056–2058.

Keller F, Routh W. Treatment of Mallory-Weiss tears. In: Kadir S, ed. Current practice of interventional radiology. St. Louis: Mosby Year Book, 1991.

Steffes C, Fromm D. The current diagnosis and management of upper gastrointestinal bleeding. Adv Surg 1992; 25:331–361.

End Note

Case courtesy of Sally E. Mitchell, M.D., The Johns Hopkins Medical Institutions, Baltimore, MD.

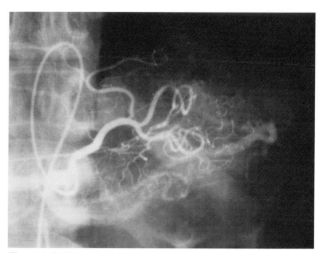

Figure 1. Left gastric arteriogram.

TEACHING FILE CASE 32
Jeet Sandhu, M.D.

History

A 42-year-old woman with a long history of alcohol abuse came to the emergency department with hematemesis. Endoscopy was performed and revealed a bleeding Mallory-Weiss tear. This was sclerosed endoscopically with epinephrine injection, and the bleeding stopped. She had another episode of bleeding the next day for which she underwent repeat endoscopic treatment. The patient was stable for 2 more days until she began bleeding again, with a decrease in her hematocrit from 46 to 23. Angiography was requested to identify the bleeding site given the presence of continued bleeding. A selective left gastric arteriogram was performed **(Fig. 1)**.

What is your diagnosis?

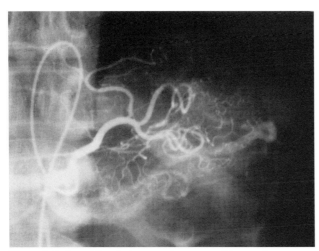

Figure 2. Left gastric arteriogram shows no evidence of extravasation.

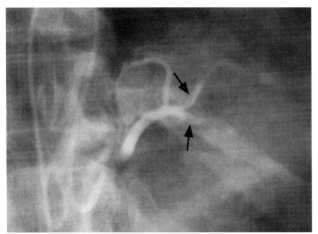

Figure 3. Left gastric arteriogram after embolization with Gelfoam slurry and torpedoes (black arrows).

Radiographic Findings

The selective left gastric arteriogram **(Fig. 2)** is normal with conventional anatomy. Selective injections of the hepatic, splenic, and superior mesenteric arteries were also performed to exclude any other foci of bleeding. None were shown. There was no evidence of extravasation, pseudoaneurysm, or arteriovenous fistula from the left gastric artery.

Diagnosis

Endoscopically evident Mallory-Weiss tear. No evidence of active bleeding.

How would you manage this patient?

Management

With no specific bleeding source identified, the options are to do nothing unless the patient bleeds again, to send the patient to surgery for repair of the tear, or to perform an empiric embolization.

Because the patient had already had two severe episodes of bleeding, an empiric embolization was performed with a Gelfoam slurry (Upjohn, Kalamazoo, MI) and pledgets **(Fig. 3)**. Although surgery is an option, it is much more invasive and has greater morbidity than embolization. The patient's condition stabilized and she was discharged without any further episodes of bleeding.

Discussion

Mallory-Weiss tears account for 5%–15% of all cases of acute upper gastrointestinal bleeding. The Mallory-Weiss tear is a mucosal laceration along the lesser curve of the gastric cardia or gastroesophageal junction induced classically by prolonged violent vomiting or retching, often in alcoholics after a recent binge. Tears have also been associated with blunt trauma, defecation, coughing, asthma, heavy lifting, seizures, primal scream therapy, cardiopulmonary resuscitation, and iatrogenic causes such as endoscopy or nasogastric tube passage. However, in a substantial number of patients with Mallory-Weiss tears, a causative factor cannot be identified.

Pathophysiologically, the Mallory-Weiss tear appears to occur from large pressure differences between the thoracic and abdominal cavities induced by emesis or any activity which increases intraabdominal pressures significantly. If the gastroesophageal junction slides above the level of the diaphragm while the lower esophageal sphincter is closed, the gastroesophageal junction dilates when the intraluminal pressure of the stomach increases. When the intraluminal pressure quickly rises to a high level, the rapid dilation may result in mucosal tears of the cardia or gastroesophageal junction. If the tear extends into a vessel, hematemesis results.

Historically, it was thought that these tears were relatively benign and that the bleeding would cease spontaneously in 90% of cases. However, recent studies indicate that Mallory-Weiss tears can be much more serious. Mortality rates of up to 12% have been documented secondary to the multi-organ failure induced by the bleeding. Morbidity and mortality are much worse in patients with underlying portal hypertension. If bleeding or a visible vessel is identified at the time of initial endoscopy (noted in 25% of patients with Mallory-Weiss tears), endoscopic sclerotherapy should be initiated. If no bleeding or visible vessel is present, the patient can be treated conservatively. Refractory hemorrhage should prompt angiographic evaluation and possible embolization, with surgery reserved for embolization and endoscopic failures.

The presence of pneumo- or hydrothorax on the chest radiograph should raise the concern of esophageal perforation, and surgical consultation should be obtained. If angiography is performed to evaluate bleeding from a Mallory-Weiss tear, a celiac arteriogram should be obtained initially to evaluate the overall anatomy. If the celiac injection shows no evidence of bleeding, selective left gastric arteriography should be performed. If the left gastric arteriogram shows no extravasation, a complete selective upper gastrointestinal arteriogram (including splenic, gastroduodenal, and superior mesenteric artery injections) should be obtained to identify an occult bleeding source. If there is no angiographic evidence of bleeding, it is safe and reasonable to do an empiric embolization of the left gastric artery since the risks are minimal and this artery supplies the bleeding site in 90%–95% of cases.

The embolic material of choice is Gelfoam. Either small pledgets or a slurry should be used initially to obtain hemostasis of the distal branches, followed by larger pledgets or torpedoes to occlude the more proximal larger branches. Because the Mallory-Weiss tear is a nonmalignant lesion that heals rapidly, a resorbable agent should be employed that will allow the vessel to recanalize once the acute tear has resolved. Some interventionalists also use metallic coils. It should be noted, however, that a coil in the proximal left gastric artery will limit access for future embolizations.

For further information on this topic, please see Tutorials 13 and 14, and Teaching File Cases 31 and 33.

Selected Readings

Bataller R, Llach J, Salmerón J, et al. Endoscopic sclerotherapy in upper gastrointestinal bleeding due to Mallory-Weiss syndrome. Am J Gastroenterol 1994; 89:2147–2150.

Carsen GM, Casarella W, Spiegel R. Transcatheter embolization for treatment of Mallory-Weiss tears of the esophagogastric junction. Radiology 1978; 128:309–313.

Harris JM, DiPalma JA. Clinical significance of Mallory-Weiss tears. Am J Gastroenterol 1993; 88:2056–2058.

Katz PO, Salas L. Less frequent causes of upper gastrointestinal bleeding. Gastroenterol Clin North Am 1993; 22:875–889.

Keller FS, Rösch J. Embolization for acute gastric hemorrhage. Semin Intervent Radiology 1988; 5:25–31.

Steffes C, Fromm D. The current diagnosis and management of upper gastrointestinal bleeding. Adv Surg 1992; 25:331–361.

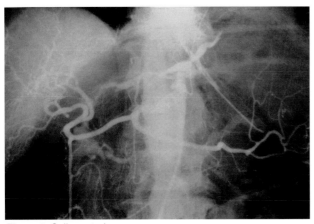

Figure 1. Celiac arteriogram.

TEACHING FILE CASE 33
Jeffrey L. Groffsky, M.D., and
Ziv J. Haskal, M.D.

History

A 53-year-old man came to the hospital with the acute onset of hematemesis. On evaluation in the emergency department, he was noted to be orthostatic, with a blood pressure of 85/50 mm Hg. There was no history of alcohol use or hepatic disease. At gastroscopy, active bleeding in the region of the lesser gastric curvature was identified. No varices were seen. Following unsuccessful attempts to treat the hemorrhage endoscopically, the patient was referred to the interventional radiology service. Celiac arteriography was performed **(Fig. 1)**.

What is your diagnosis?

Radiographic Findings

The arterial phase of the celiac arteriogram demonstrates a tubular, serpiginous structure, filled with contrast material, in the region of the lesser curvature of the stomach **(Figs. 2, 3)**. No other vascular abnormalities are present.

Diagnosis

Acute arterial gastric bleeding with a "pseudo-vein" sign of extravasation.

How would you manage this patient?

Management

The left gastric artery was embolized **(Fig. 4)** with a coaxial catheter system. The microcatheter was inserted through a Simmons catheter and guided into the left gastric artery. The tip of this catheter was positioned approximately 2 cm beyond the origin of the vessel. Gelfoam (Upjohn, Kalamazoo, MI) was initially administered, followed by placement of coils more proximally.

The postembolization arteriogram **(Fig. 5)** confirms successful occlusion of the left gastric artery distal to the coils. No extravasation is seen.

Discussion

The pseudo-vein sign is seen in approximately one third of patients with acute arterial hemorrhage identified on arteriography. The pseudo-vein sign is thought to represent extravasated, opacified blood which has accumulated within the crevices of a hematoma or along the edge of a viscera or peritoneal reflection. Its presence identifies the site of acute bleeding. It has been described in association with hemorrhage of a variety of etiologies, including duodenal or gastric ulcers, inflammatory bowel disease, gastritis, diverticulitis, post-gastrointestinal surgery or trauma, as well as in the setting of pelvic trauma. Knowledge of this entity will prevent confusion with a vascular malformation.

For further information on this topic, please see Tutorials 13 and 14, and Teaching File Cases 31 and 32.

Selected Readings

Abrams HL, ed. Abrams angiography: vascular and interventional radiology. 3rd edition. Boston: Litttle, Brown and Company, 1983; 1673.

Ring EJ, Athanasoulis CA, Waltman AC, Baum S. The pseudo-vein: an angiographic appearance of arterial hemorrhage. J Can Assoc Radiol 1973; 24:242–244.

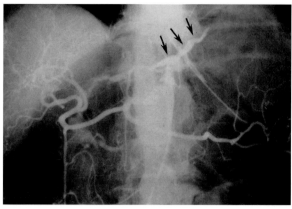

Figure 2. Extravasation is present along the lesser curvature of the stomach (arrows) with a "pseudo-vein" configuration.

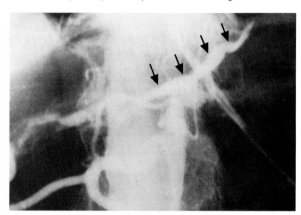

Figure 3. Magnification view of the left gastric pseudo-vein (arrows).

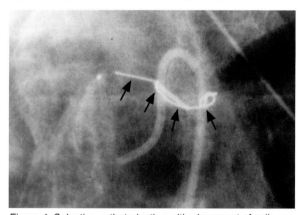

Figure 4. Selective catheterization with placement of coils (arrows) into the left gastric artery.

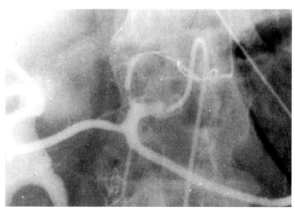

Figure 5. Postembolization arteriogram. The left gastric artery is occluded.

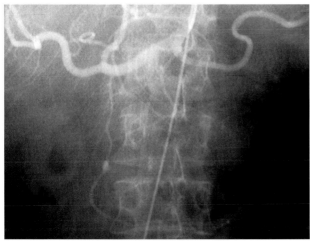

Figure 1. Celiac arteriogram.

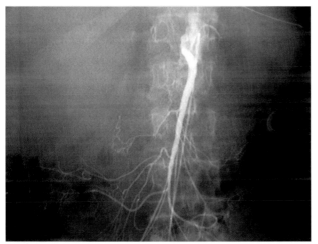

Figure 2. Superior mesenteric arteriogram.

TEACHING FILE CASE 34
Harjit Singh, M.D., and
Anthony Venbrux, M.D.

History
A 63-year-old woman previously diagnosed with stage III ovarian carcinoma underwent total abdominal hysterectomy with bilateral salpingo-oophorectomy, bowel resection, nephrostomy tube placement, and a complete course of chemotherapy. She was admitted with a 1-week history of anorexia and upper abdominal pain. During clinical evaluation, the patient developed repeated hematemesis. The patient was stabilized and emergent upper endoscopy was performed. Endoscopy revealed a duodenal bulb ulcer with adjacent clot. Arteriography was performed **(Figs. 1, 2)**.

What is your diagnosis?

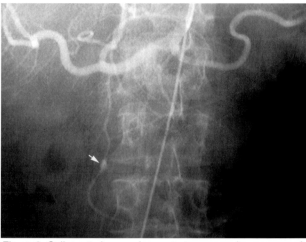

Figure 3. Celiac arteriogram demonstrates a pseudoaneurysm of the GDA (arrow).

Radiographic Findings
The selective celiac **(Fig. 3)** and superior mesenteric arteriograms **(Fig. 4)** demonstrate normal vascular anatomy. The gastroduodenal artery (GDA) is diminutive and reveals a pseudoaneurysm approximately 4 mm in diameter **(Fig. 3)**.

Diagnosis
Gastroduodenal artery pseudoaneurysm.

How would you manage this patient?

Management
The pseudoaneurysm and the adjacent portions of the GDA were embolized using a combination of coils and Gelfoam (Upjohn, Kalamazoo, MI). The postembolization arteriogram demonstrates complete hemostasis **(Fig. 5)**. One of the microcoils occludes a pancreaticoduodenal branch—the remainder occlude the right gastroepiploic artery, the GDA, and the pseudoaneurysm.

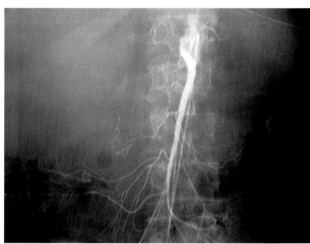

Figure 4. Superior mesenteric arteriogram shows no filling of the gastroduodenal artery through the IPD.

Discussion
There are several causes for upper gastrointestinal bleeding, the most common of which is peptic ulcer disease. Other causes include tumors, arteriovenous malformations, varices, and endoscopic instrumentation. A pseudoaneurysm of the GDA is an uncommon cause and may be secondary to peptic ulcer disease, tumor, or pancreatitis.

A pseudoaneurysm of the gastroduodenal artery is an ideal situation in which to use embolotherapy. Due to the extensive duodenal collateral network, occlusion of the vessel both proximal and distal to the arterial defect is essential. With use of relatively large particulates such as Gelfoam pledgets and coils, ischemic complications are extremely rare. Micropulverized agents such as Gelfoam powder should never be used to control gastrointestinal bleeding, due to the risk of causing bowel infarction.

For further information on this topic, please see Tutorials 13 and 14.

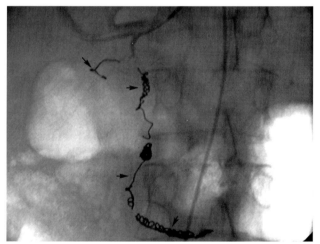

Figure 5. Postembolization arteriogram confirms successful occlusion of the gastroduodenal artery. Multiple coils (arrows) are identified within the gastroduodenal artery and its branches.

Selected Readings

Kadir S. Treatment of pyloroduodenal bleeding. In: Kadir S, ed. Current practice of interventional radiology. St. Louis: Mosby Year Book, 1991; 418–424.

Okazaki M, Higashihara H, Ono H, et al Embolotherapy of massive duodenal hemorrhage. Gastrointest Radiol 1992; 17:319–323.

Steffes C, Fromm D. The current diagnosis and management of upper gastrointestinal bleeding. Adv Surg 1992; 25:331–361.

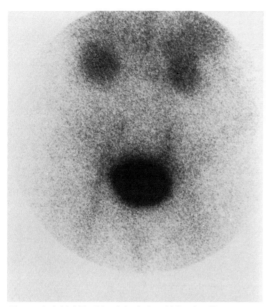

Figure 1. Initial Tc-99m labeled red blood cell scan.

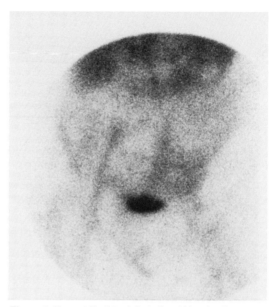

Figure 2. Repeat Tc-99m labeled red blood cell scan, early image.

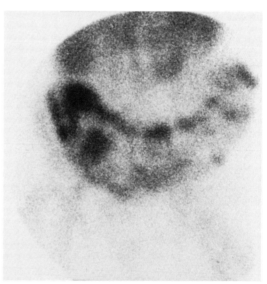

Figure 3. Repeat Tc-99m labeled red blood cell scan, late image.

TEACHING FILE CASE 35
David Sacks, M.D.

History

A 77-year-old woman had multiple episodes of intermittent gastrointestinal bleeding over several years. She had a prior negative endoscopy and laparotomy. She is now admitted with recurrent bleeding. A technetium-99m (Tc-99m) labeled red cell bleeding scan was performed **(Fig. 1)** and then repeated 5 days later **(Figs. 2, 3)**, followed by mesenteric arteriography **(Figs. 4–6)**.

What is your diagnosis?

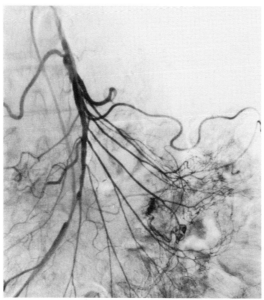

Figure 4. Superior mesenteric arteriogram, early arterial phase.

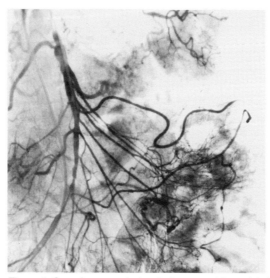

Figure 5. Superior mesenteric arteriogram, mid arterial phase.

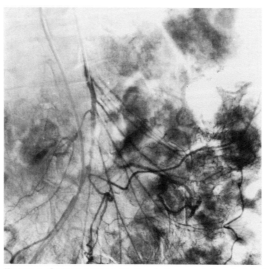

Figure 6. Superior mesenteric arteriogram, late arterial phase.

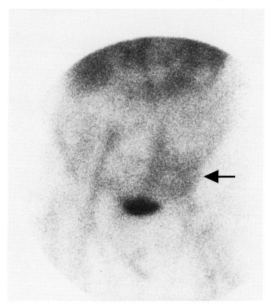

Figure 7. Repeat Tc-99m red blood cell scan shows evidence of bleeding in the left lower quadrant (arrow).

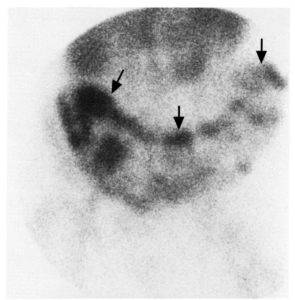

Figure 8. A later image from the study shown in Figure 7 reveals accumulation of tagged red blood cells within the colon (arrows).

Radiographic Findings

The initial bleeding scan is negative. The repeat scan shows bleeding in the left lower quadrant **(Fig. 7)** that fills the colon on the delayed image **(Fig. 8)**. The arteriogram shows a vascular malformation in the mid jejunum with abnormal vessels and an early draining vein **(Fig. 9)**. Multiple areas of vascular narrowing are also present, presumably due to arterial spasm.

Diagnosis

Vascular malformation of the small bowel.

What treatment would you recommend?

Management

The vessel feeding the malformation was superselectively catheterized with an injectable wire **(Figs. 10, 11)**. The patient was then taken to the operating room. When the bowel was exposed, the wire was injected with 0.5 mL of methylene blue dye to localize the malformation, and a short segment of bowel was resected **(Figs. 12, 13)**. The patient had had no further bleeding at 2-year follow-up.

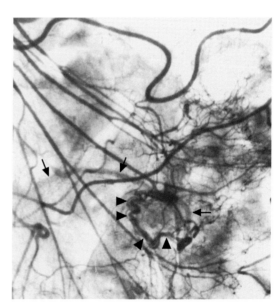

Figure 9. Magnification view of Figure 5 with a vascular malformation (arrowheads) and an early draining vein (arrows).

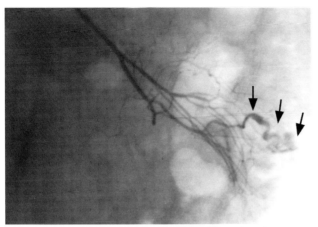

Figure 10. Subselective injection of a jejunal branch to the vascular malformation (arrows).

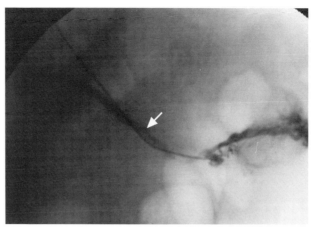

Figure 11. Superselective injection of the malformation. The draining vein (arrow) parallels the arterial course.

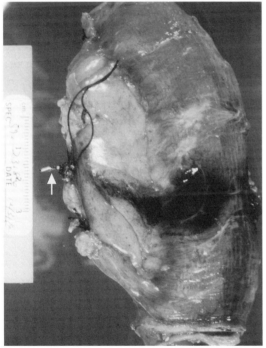

Figure 12. Resected jejunum with blue dye injection, serosal surface. Arrow marks the injectable wire.

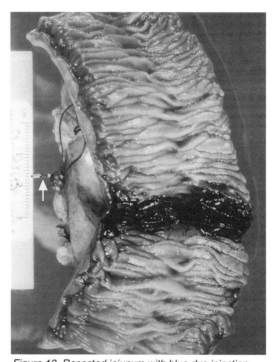

Figure 13. Resected jejunum with blue dye injection, mucosal surface. Arrow marks the injectable wire.

Discussion

Acute lower gastrointestinal bleeding is often evaluated with a nuclear medicine bleeding scan prior to arteriography. This not only localizes the bleeding to direct subsequent arteriography or surgery, but it also indicates that the patient is actively bleeding, which may be difficult to discern clinically. Delaying arteriography until the bleeding scan is positive markedly reduces the number of negative arteriograms. Spasmolytics, anti-coagulants, and thrombolytics are sometimes used to provoke bleeding during arteriography. The bleeding scan can also be useful in chronic bleeding if it can localize the site of bleeding, but arteriography will frequently detect an anatomic abnormality even in the absence of active extravasation.

Two other techniques helpful in evaluating occult gastrointestinal bleeding are enteroclysis and enteroscopy. Enteroclysis reportedly can find small bowel abnormalities in about 20% of patients. Enteroscopy has a higher sensitivity for detecting a bleeding source (about 50%), and is particularly useful in detecting arteriovenous malformations. In addition, enteroscopic cauterization of the bleeding site may be performed.

If arteriography is used to identify the source of hemorrhage, vasopressin or embolization can be used to control the bleeding. Vasopressin therapy has a substantial rate of rebleeding (up to 50%) and medical complications. Embolization has a higher success rate but with a risk of bowel infarction of up to 20%.

The patient in this case was medically stable and a good surgical candidate. After complete mesenteric arteriography excluded the presence of multiple vascular malformations, the solitary lesion was successfully resected. The injectable wire was placed immediately before surgery to avoid pericatheter clotting. The injection of methylene blue dye allowed precise resection of the involved bowel segment.

For further information on this topic, please see Tutorials 13 and 15, and Teaching File Case 36.

Selected Readings

Gomes AS, Lois JF, McCoy RD. Angiographic treatment of gastrointestinal hemorrhage: comparison of vasopressin infusion and embolization. AJR 1986; 146:1031–1037.

Moch A, Herlinger H, Kochman ML, Levine MS, Rubesin SE, Laufer I. Enteroclysis in the evaluation of obscure gastrointestinal bleeding. AJR 1994; 163:1381–1384.

Rollins ES, Picus D, Hicks ME, Darcy MD, Bower BL, Kleinhoffer MA. Angiography is useful in detecting the source of chronic gastrointestinal bleeding of obscure origin. AJR 1991; 156:385–388.

Rösch J, Keller FS, Wawrukiewicz AS, Krippaehne WW, Dotter CT. Pharmacoangiography in the diagnosis of recurrent massive lower gastrointestinal bleeding. Radiology 1982; 145:615–619.

Sebrechts C, Bookstein JJ. Embolization in the management of lower gastrointestinal hemorrhage. Semin Intervent Radiol 1988; 5:39–48.

Smith R, Copely DJ, Bolen FH. 99m-Tc RBC scintigraphy: correlation of gastrointestinal bleeding rates with scintigraphic findings. AJR 1987; 148:869–874.

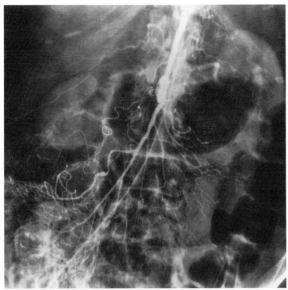

Figure 1. Superior mesenteric arteriogram, early arterial phase.

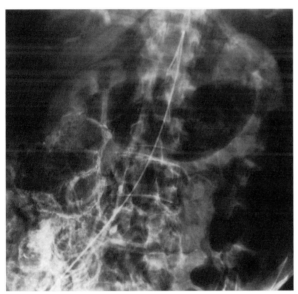

Figure 2. Superior mesenteric arteriogram, late arterial phase.

TEACHING FILE CASE 36
Scott J. Savader, M.D.

History
A 65-year-old woman had significant lower gastrointestinal hemorrhaging on three separate occasions which were all followed by negative angiographic evaluations. At the time of the fourth episode, heparin therapy at 1,000 units per hour was started and consultations with the medical intensive care unit and general surgeon were obtained. A nuclear medicine study suggested abnormal activity in the right lower quadrant, and an arteriogram was obtained **(Figs. 1, 2)**.

What is your diagnosis?

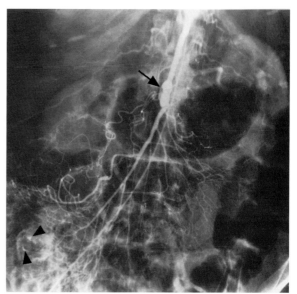

Figure 3. Superior mesenteric arteriogram demonstrates a fusiform aneurysm (arrow) about 8 cm beyond the vessel's origin. Contrast material extravasation (arrowheads) is present from small distal ileal branches.

Radiographic Findings

A superior mesenteric arteriogram demonstrates an aneurysm about 8 cm distal to the origin of the vessel (**Fig. 3**). Extravasation of contrast material is noted from ileal branches of the superior mesenteric artery (**Figs. 3, 4**).

Diagnosis

1. Arterial bleeding in the distal small bowel, etiology unknown.
2. Fusiform atherosclerotic aneurysm of the superior mesenteric artery.

Management

A 7-F guiding catheter was used to stabilize access at the superior mesenteric artery (SMA) origin. A 5-F catheter was advanced beyond the SMA aneurysm and positioned in the distal aspect of the artery. A selective injection (**Fig. 5**) was performed but no evidence of extravasation was seen. Priscoline, nitroglycerine, heparin, and urokinase were sequentially injected, followed by digital imaging after each pharmacologic provocation; however, the exact point of hemorrhage could not be delineated. Empiric embolization at the site of suspected bleeding was performed with microcoils delivered through a microcatheter (**Fig. 6**). The patient did well for 96 hours, at which time the bleeding recurred. At surgery, the microcoils were used to identify the site of hemorrhage which on pathologic examination proved to be a metastatic focus of spindle cell carcinoma.

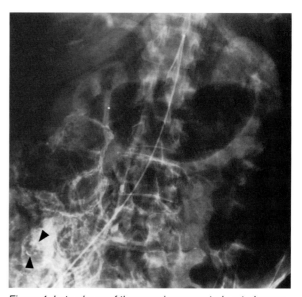

Figure 4. Late phase of the superior mesenteric arteriogram demonstrates continued extravasation (arrowheads) from the distal ileal branches.

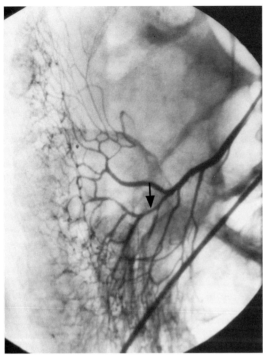

Figure 5. Magnified digital subtraction image obtained immediately after the cut film arteriogram reveals no evidence of continued bleeding. The arrow indicates the point of embolization.

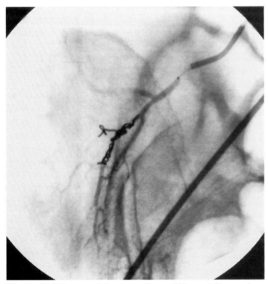

Figure 6. After careful comparison of the cut film and digital subtraction images, coil embolization was carried out at the arterial bifurcation (Fig. 5, arrow) just proximal to what was believed to be the point of hemorrhage.

Discussion

Multiple angiographic examinations in this patient were unable to identify the site of bleeding. Considering the patient's past failure rate with angiographic identification, it was decided that when her bleeding recurred, heparinization would be appropriate to improve the chances of a "positive" arteriogram. This requires both the consent of the patient and coordination between multiple services, including surgery for back-up. Coil embolization was performed at what was believed to be the appropriate site. The microcoils were "flushed" through the microcatheter positioned near the suspected site of the bleeding **(Fig. 5)**. Particle embolization was deferred because of the risk of small bowel infarction in this patient who was a poor surgical candidate. Although the patient's bleeding unfortunately recurred, the coils were detected at the time of surgery, making it possible to identify the small tumor responsible for the hemorrhage.

For further information on this topic, please see Tutorials 13, 15, and 18, and Teaching File Case 35.

Selected Readings

Encarnacion CE, Kadir S, Beam CA, Payne CS. Gastrointestinal bleeding: treatment with gastrointestinal arterial embolization. Radiology 1992; 183:505–508.

Guy GE, Shetty PC, Sharma RP, Burke MW, Burke TH. Acute lower gastrointestinal hemorrhage: treatment by superselective embolization with polyvinyl alcohol particles. AJR 1992; 159:521–526.

Koval G, Benner KG, Rösch J, Kozak BE. Aggressive angiographic diagnosis in acute lower gastrointestinal hemorrhage. Dig Dis Sci 1987; 32:248–253.

Makita K, Furui S, Irie T, et al. Embolization with steel coils using a saline flush technique. Br J Radiol 1991; 64:708–710.

Okazaki M, Furui S, Higashihara H, Koganemaru F, Sato S, Fujimitsu R. Emergent embolotherapy of small intestine hemorrhage. Gastrointest Radiol 1992; 17:223–228.

Rösch J, Keller FS, Wawrukiewicz AS, Krippaehne WW, Dotter CT. Pharmacoangiography in the diagnosis of recurrent massive lower gastrointestinal bleeding. Radiology 1982; 145:615–619.

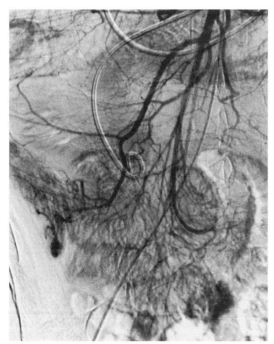

Figure 1. Superior mesenteric arteriogram.

TEACHING FILE CASE 37
Joseph Krysl, M.D.

History

The patient came to the hospital with the abrupt onset of lower gastrointestinal bleeding which was localized to the ileocecal region on nuclear medicine studies. She had undergone liver transplantation several weeks earlier. Superior mesenteric arteriography was performed **(Fig. 1)**.

What is your diagnosis?

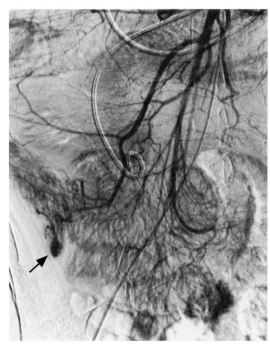

Figure 2. Superior mesenteric arteriogram demonstrates an abnormal area of blush in the right lower quadrant (arrow).

Radiographic Findings

The superior mesenteric arteriogram **(Fig. 2)** demonstrates an area of abnormal vascular blush in the right lower quadrant from a branch of the ileocolic artery. In addition, there is a prominent draining vein extending from this region. No other abnormalities are noted.

Diagnosis

Angiodysplasia in the ileocecal region.

How would you manage this patient?

Management

Management options for transcatheter therapy include vasopressin infusion and embolotherapy. The patient underwent superselective embolization of the bleeding vessel with polyvinyl alcohol particles (250–350 microns) followed by the deposition of two microcoils **(Fig. 3)**. The patient's bleeding stopped while she was on the angiography table, but she had recurrent bleeding the next day. The arteriogram was repeated, but no abnormalities were demonstrated. Follow-up at 3 months showed no further bleeding and no clinical evidence of ischemic change in the bowel.

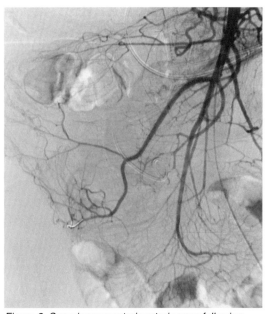

Figure 3. Superior mesenteric arteriogram following embolization of a bleeding angiodysplastic lesion in the ileocolic distribution. Embolization was achieved with polyvinyl alcohol particles and two microcoils.

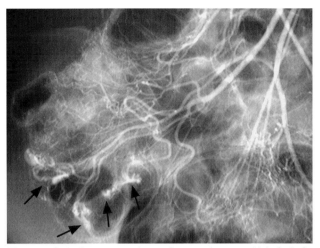

Figure 4. Superior mesenteric arteriogram shows multiple foci of angiodysplasia in the cecum (arrows).

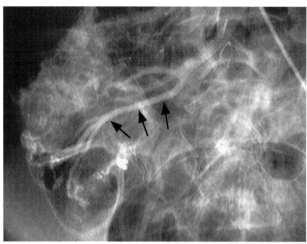

Figure 5. Same patient as in Figure 4. A mid arterial phase image shows dense opacification of an early draining vein (arrows).

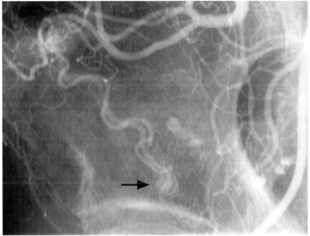

Figure 6. Superior mesenteric arteriogram. Magnification view of the cecum in another patient with angiodysplasia (arrow).

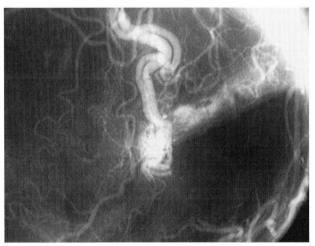

Figure 7. Injection of the surgical specimen resected from the patient shown in Figure 6 reveals the angiodysplastic morphology in better detail.

Discussion

Angiodysplasia is defined as a developmental lesion characterized by dilatation and ectasia of mucosal arteries and veins, usually associated with some degree of arteriovenous shunting. These lesions are extremely common, being found in 2% of the population in autopsy series. The lesions are much more prevalent in individuals more than 55 years of age and are associated with valvular aortic stenosis. Eighty percent of angiodysplasias are located in the cecum, 10% in the jejunum, and 5% in the ileum, with the remainder being found in the upper gastrointestinal tract and rectum.

Arteriographically **(Figs. 4–7)** these lesions are characterized by:
1. an abnormal tuft of vessels
2. an early draining vein
3. dense opacification of this vein late into the venous phase.

Lesions from angiodysplasia can be treated endoscopically. If endoscopic treatment is unsuccessful, surgical resection is generally performed. Transcatheter management is usually reserved for poor surgical candidates or as a temporizing measure prior to resection.

Transcatheter management of lower gastrointestinal bleeding includes vasopressin infusion therapy and embolization of the bleeding area. Vasopressin therapy has a relatively high success rate (up to 90%) but requires prolonged intraarterial infusion. There is also a risk of recurrent bleeding once the infusion is discontinued; this has been estimated to be as high as 20%. Furthermore, vasopressin infusion has a complication rate that has been reported to be as high as 43%.

Embolotherapy is an alternative treatment for patients with lower gastrointestinal bleeding. The use of microcatheters for superselective embolization has increased the effectiveness of this technique. A variety of embolic agents have been used including autologous clot, Gelfoam (Upjohn, Kalamazoo, MI), polyvinyl alcohol, and microcoils. Embolotherapy provides effective and, most often, immediate cessation of bleeding. Risks of bowel ischemia and infarction are present but can be minimized with judicious use of embolic material, using the least amount necessary to achieve hemostasis.

Controversy still exists as to when embolization for lower gastrointestinal bleeding should be considered a primary therapeutic technique.

For further information on this topic, please see Tutorials 13 and 15.

Selected Readings

Encarnacion CE, Kadir S, Beam CA, Payne CS. Gastrointestinal bleeding: treatment with gastrointestinal arterial embolization. Radiology 1992; 183:505–508.

Guy GE, Shetty PC, Sharma RP, Burke MW, Burke TH. Acute lower gastrointestinal hemorrhage: treatment by superselective embolization with polyvinyl alcohol particles. AJR 1992; 159:521–526.

Zuckerman DA, Bocchini TP, Birnbaum EH. Massive hemorrhage in the lower gastrointestinal tract in adults: diagnostic imaging and intervention. AJR 1993; 161:703–711.

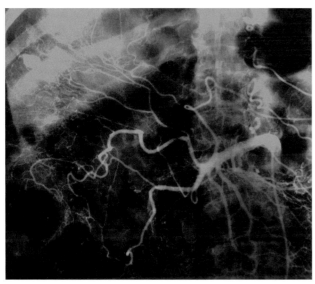

Figure 1. Superior mesenteric arteriogram.

TEACHING FILE CASE 38

Michael J. Flood, M.D., and
Richard R. Saxon, M.D.

History

An 80-year-old man with a history of lower gastrointestinal bleeding 6 months earlier returned with
bright red blood per rectum and a hematocrit of 10.8.
He was treated with a total of 5 units of packed cells.
Colonoscopy showed blood from the rectum to the
cecum but a focal bleeding site was not identified.
Colonic diverticula were present throughout the
colon. A visceral arteriogram was ordered
emergently to evaluate the bleeding **(Fig. 1)**.

What is your diagnosis?

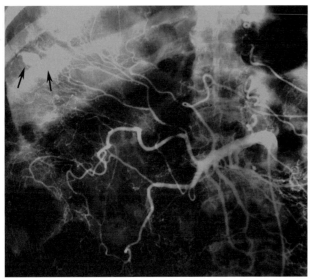

Figure 2. Active extravasation (arrows) is seen from the right colic branch during the early phase of the superior mesenteric artery injection.

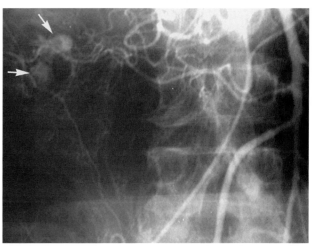

Figure 3. Extravasation of contrast material (arrows) reveals the location of bleeding in another patient with hepatic flexure diverticula.

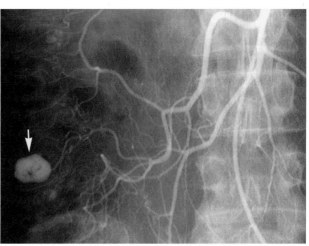

Figure 4. Superior mesenteric arteriogram shows extravasation into the cecum, indicative of brisk bleeding.

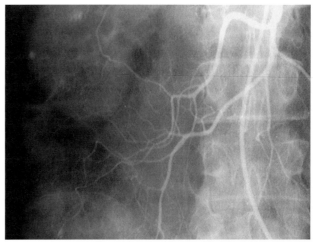

Figure 5. Same patient as in Figure 4. Following infusion of vasopressin, the bleeding has stopped.

Radiographic Findings

The superior mesenteric arteriogram demonstrates active extravasation from a right colic branch near the hepatic flexure (Fig. 2). Pooling of the contrast material in the lumen of the colon is noted.

Diagnosis

Lower gastrointestinal bleeding most likely from colonic diverticulosis.

Management

The patient's hemodynamic status became very unstable during the procedure. Because of this, the surgeons took the patient emergently to surgery and performed a subtotal colectomy with ileosigmoidostomy.

Discussion

Arteriography continues to play a very important role in the diagnosis and treatment of lower gastrointestinal bleeding. Extravasation of contrast material into a loop of bowel confirms the diagnosis (Fig. 3). The patient must be actively bleeding at the time of the examination at a rate of at least 0.5 mL per minute.

The most common cause of colonic bleeding is diverticular hemorrhage. Other causes include angiodysplasia, neoplasm, postpolypectomy, radiation, and colitis.

Transcatheter therapy for control of colonic bleeding has been shown to be very successful. Both vasopressin and embolotherapy play an important role in the management of colonic bleeding. Vasopressin infusion (Figs. 4, 5) can be effective in achieving hemostasis, but rebleeding may pose a problem. Vasopressin should not be used in patients with severe coronary artery disease.

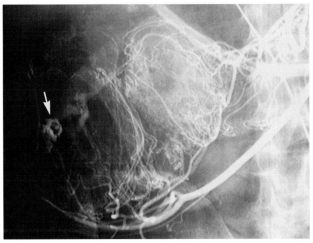

Figure 6. Superior mesenteric arteriogram from another patient. There is contrast material extravasation (arrow) in the cecum.

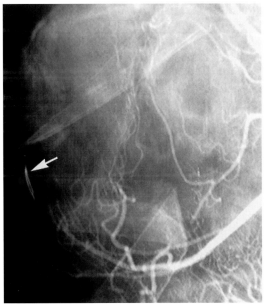

Figure 7. Same patient as in Figure 6. Platinum microcoils (arrow) have been used to occlude the bleeding artery. The patient experienced no further bleeding.

Embolotherapy **(Figs. 6, 7)** has a higher rate of hemostasis and a lower rate of rebleeding compared to vasopressin. Disadvantages include the requirement of subselective catheterization and the possibility of bowel ischemia or necrosis. In general, microcoils, polyvinyl alcohol particles (>250 microns), and Gelfoam pledgets (Upjohn, Kalamazoo, MI) are the most useful agents for subselective embolization. Gelfoam powder and absolute alcohol should not be used because of the risk of bowel necrosis.

The role of embolization in branches of the superior and inferior mesenteric arteries remains controversial. In most patients where the embolization is limited to a small area, no clinical evidence of bowel ischemia is observed. However, in a minority of patients, small bowel or colonic infarction develops, necessitating surgical resection. The incidence of infarction secondary to transcatheter embolization in the small bowel and colon is not known due to the limited number of reported cases. Rosenkrantz et al reported three cases of colonic mucosal infarction from twenty-three patients who underwent colonic embolization. Guy et al reported ten embolization procedures in nine patients (eight colon, one jejunum). Bleeding was controlled in all nine patients. One patient subsequently had severe mucosal ischemia which appeared to be unrelated to the embolization. Two additional asymptomatic patients had endoscopic evidence of ischemia in the region of the embolization which spontaneously resolved.

Currently, the decision to use superselective embolization or vasopressin infusion to control lower gastrointestinal bleeding depends on the experience and preference of the operator. This decision should be based upon the patient's overall medical condition as well as the specific anatomic location of the bleeding site.

For further information on this topic, please see Tutorials 13 and 15, and Teaching File Cases 37 and 39.

Selected Readings

Bennett JD, Kadir S. Treatment of colorectal bleeding. In: Kadir S, ed. Current practice of interventional radiology. St. Louis: Mosby Year Book, 1991; 428–436.

Guy GE, Shetty PC, Sharma RP, Burke MW, Burke TH. Acute lower gastrointestinal hemorrhage: treatment by superselective embolization with polyvinyl alcohol particles. AJR 1992; 159:521–526.

Rosen RJ, Sanchez G. Angiographic diagnosis and management of gastrointestinal hemorrhage: current concepts. Radiol Clin North Am 1994; 32(5):951–967.

Rosenkrantz H, Bookstein JJ, Rosen RJ, Goff WB, Healy JF. Postembolic colonic infarction. Radiology 1982; 142:47–51.

Sebrechts C, Bookstein JJ. Embolization in the management of lower gastrointestinal hemorrhage. Semin Intervent Radiol 1988; 5(1):39–48.

Walker TG, Waltman AC. Vasoconstrictive infusion therapy for management of arterial gastrointestinal hemorrhage. Semin Intervent Radiol 1988; 5(1):18–24.

Zuckerman DA, Bocchini TP, Birnbaum EH, Massive hemorrhage in the lower gastrointestinal tract in adults: diagnostic imaging and intervention. AJR 1993: 161:703–711.

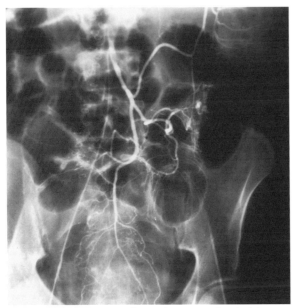

Figure 1. Inferior mesenteric arteriogram, early arterial phase.

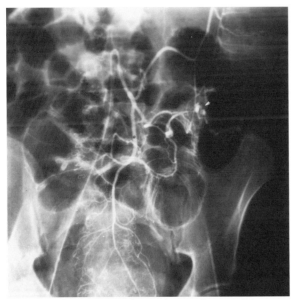

Figure 2. Inferior mesenteric arteriogram, late arterial phase.

TEACHING FILE CASE 39
Scott J. Savader, M.D.

History

A 36-year-old man with a history of Peutz-Jeghers disease underwent routine annual endoscopic evaluation of the large bowel. A suspicious polyp was noted at the junction of the sigmoid and descending colon. The polyp was removed endoscopically with a snare. Subsequently, the patient developed signifcant hemorrhage from the polypectomy site which could not be controlled endoscopically with cauterization. The patient was referred to the interventional radiology department. An inferior mesenteric artery (IMA) arteriogram was obtained **(Figs. 1, 2)**.

What is your diagnosis?

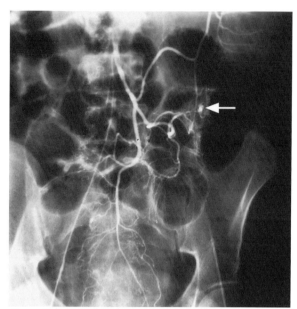

Figure 3. IMA arteriogram demonstrates a focal point of contrast material extravasation (arrow) along the medial border of the descending colon.

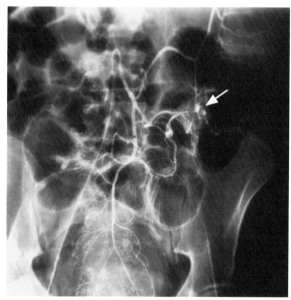

Figure 4. Late arterial phase demonstrates the extravasation more clearly (arrow).

Radiographic Findings

The IMA arteriogram **(Figs. 3, 4)** demonstrates the superior hemorrhoidal, sigmoid, and left colic branches of the IMA. Contrast material extravasation is present, arising from a sigmoid branch along the medial aspect of the proximal sigmoid colon.

Diagnosis

Postpolypectomy hemorrhage from the sigmoid branch of the inferior mesenteric artery.

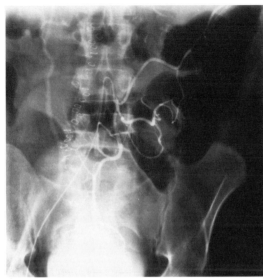

Figure 5. Arteriogram obtained 30 minutes after the initiation of vasopressin therapy. Contrast material extravasation is no longer identified.

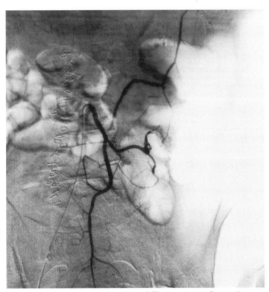

Figure 6. Subtraction image of Figure 5 confirms that the bleeding has stopped.

Management

The patient was young and had no other significant underlying health problems. The complexity of the arterial anatomy was thought to be such that focal embolization would be difficult. This would be an ideal situation for vasopressin therapy. Through the Simmons catheter, intraarterial vasopressin was initiated. The vasopressin infusion was continued for 30 minutes and the arteriogram repeated **(Figs. 5, 6)**. This arteriogram demonstrated that the extravasation had ceased. The degree of vasospasm was acceptable as the patient was not experiencing any abdominal symptoms that suggested mesenteric ischemia. The infusion was continued for 12 hours and then changed to normal saline for 6 hours. No further bleeding ensued and the catheter was removed. The patient was discharged and experienced no further bleeding.

Discussion

Interventional radiologists are frequently called upon to diagnose and treat small and large bowel hemorrhage. Recently, embolization has gained popularity while vasopressin therapy has lost favor. Embolization offers the benefit of an immediate result whereas vasopressin requires a relatively lengthy infusion. However, coil or particle embolization is irreversible and, should severe bowel ischemia occur, there is no nonsurgical recourse. On the other hand, the degree of ischemia induced by vasopressin can usually be well controlled. In this patient, embolization was not deemed possible because of the tortuosity of the vessels leading to the bleeding site. In addition, the focal traumatic nature of the injury, the normal coagulation status of the patient, and his overall good health made him an ideal candidate for vasopressin infusion.

For further information on this topic, please see Tutorial 15 and Teaching File Case 38.

Selected Readings

Gomes AS, Lois JF, McCoy RD. Angiographic treatment of gastrointestinal hemorrhage: comparison of vasopressin infusion and embolization. AJR 1986; 146:1031–1037.

Guy GE, Shetty PC, Sharma RP, Burke MW, Burke TH. Acute lower gastrointestinal hemorrhage: treatment by superselective embolization with polyvinyl alcohol particles. AJR 1992; 159:521–526.

Sebrechts C, Bookstein JJ. Embolization in the management of lower gastrointestinal hemorrhage. Semin Intervent Radiol 1988; 5:39–48.

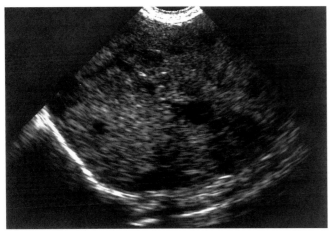

Figure 1. Transabdominal sonogram.

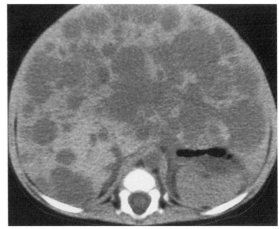

Figure 2. Precontrast image from a triple-phase CT study at a single level.

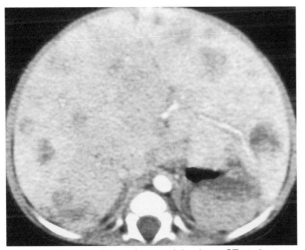

Figure 3. Mid phase image from a triple-phase CT study at a single level.

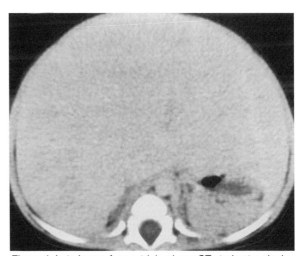

Figure 4. Late image from a triple-phase CT study at a single level.

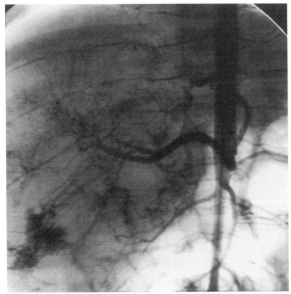

Figure 5. Abdominal aortogram.

TEACHING FILE CASE 40
Brian A. Solomon, M.D., and Ziv J. Haskal, M.D.

History
A 6-month-old boy was brought to the hospital with an enlarging abdominal mass and signs and symptoms of congestive heart failure. An abdominal ultrasound study was performed **(Fig. 1)**, followed by triple-phase contrast-enhanced computed tomography (CT) scanning **(Figs. 2–4)** and abdominal aortography **(Fig. 5)**.

What is your diagnosis?

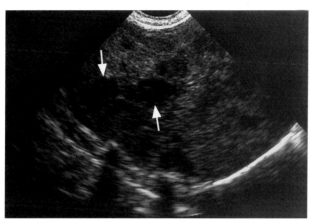

Figure 6. Transabdominal sonogram demonstrates an enlarged right lobe with multiple foci of low echogenicity (arrows).

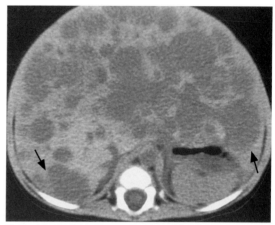

Figures 7. Earliest of a series of images from a triple-phase CT study obtained at a single axial level. Multiple low-density lesions (arrows) are present throughout the liver before the administration of intravenous (IV) contrast material.

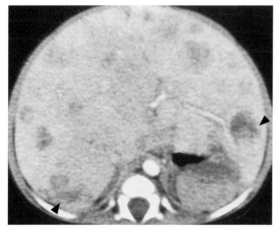

Figure 8. Image obtained during IV contrast material administration reveals centripetal enhancement of the low-density lesions (arrowheads).

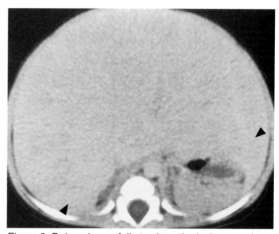

Figure 9. Delayed scan fails to show the lesions, as they have become isodense with the liver.

Radiographic Findings

The ultrasound scan demonstrates a diffusely enlarged right hepatic lobe with multiple ill-defined areas of low echogenicity **(Fig. 6)**. These findings are nonspecific and the differential diagnosis would include metastatic disease (especially neuroblastoma and Wilms' tumor), mesenchymal hamartoma, and primary hepatic neoplasms such as hepatoblastoma.

The triple-phase CT scan demonstrates a diffusely enlarged liver with multifocal areas of low attenuation on the noncontrast image **(Fig. 7)**. Of note, there is no evidence of parenchymal calcification. The dynamic contrast-enhanced phase shows a characteristic peripheral enhancement pattern **(Fig. 8)** with homogeneous parenchymal opacification on the delayed image **(Fig. 9)**. The abdominal aortogram demonstrates enlargement of the proximal abdominal aorta in response to the vascular demands of the mass. The aorta distal to the origin of the markedly enlarged hepatic artery appears narrow, but may simply be approaching its more normal caliber. There is venous pooling of contrast material in the hepatic parenchyma **(Fig. 10)**.

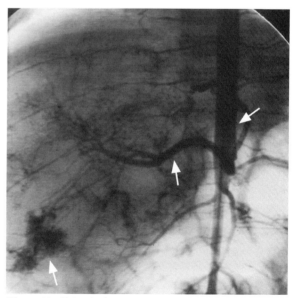

Figure 10. Abdominal aortogram. The proximal aorta and hepatic artery are enlarged. The aorta tapers just distal to the celiac axis. There are multiple foci of contrast material pooling in the large, slow flow venous channels (arrows).

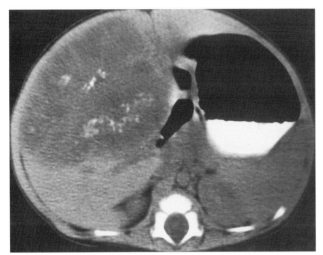

Figures 11. Hepatoblastoma in a pediatric patient. The precontrast image shows a low-density mass in the right and medial segments of the left lobe containing calcification.

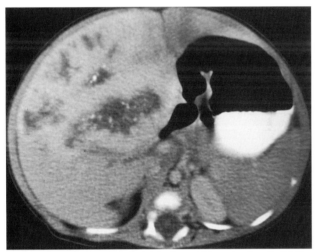

Figure 12. Following the administration of IV contrast material, the enhancement pattern is inhomogeneous.

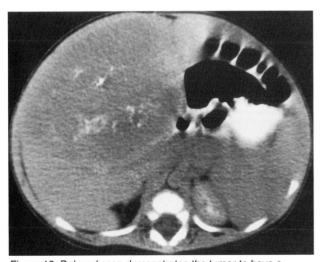

Figure 13. Delayed scan demonstrates the tumor to have a central area of necrosis and to be of lower attenuation than the surrounding liver.

Diagnosis
Infantile hemangioendothelioma.

Discussion
Infantile hemangioendothelioma is a benign tumor composed of multiple anastomosing vascular spaces lined by plump endothelial cells in single, or less often, multiple layers. The vascular spaces often contain both hematopoietic elements as well as scattered bile ducts. The tumor may vary in size from a few millimeters to 20 cm and occur either as a single mass or as multifocal lesions.

Hepatic tumors are relatively uncommon in children, representing 6% of childhood abdominal neoplasms. The majority of liver tumors in children are metastatic, primarily from Wilms' tumors and neuroblastoma. Primary liver tumors are classified on the basis of the cells of origin and most simply can be divided into mesenchymal and epithelial. Benign tumors, which represent 33% of neoplasms, are typically mesenchymal and include infantile hemangioendotheliomas and mesenchymal hamartomas. Conversely, most malignant tumors are epithelial and include hepatoblastomas **(Fig. 11)** and hepatocellular carcinoma. The diagnosis is made on the basis of imaging characteristics, age of presentation, and serum markers.

Infantile hemangioendotheliomas typically present between 1 and 6 months of life, with one third occurring in the first month of life. Fewer than 5% occur after 1 year. Most series report a slight female predominance, and there is no racial predilection. Initial presentation usually consists of an abdominal mass, and patients may have signs of congestive heart failure secondary to arteriovenous shunting through the tumor. Patients may also develop a bleeding diathesis due to platelet sequestration within the tumor, the so-called Kasabach-Merritt syndrome. Associated cutaneous hemangiomas have been reported and occur more often with the multifocal variety.

In the appropriate age group, the imaging findings on CT are diagnostic and consist of a hypoattenuating lesion on the noncontrast CT scan with centripetal contrast enhancement which becomes isodense to the liver on delayed images. CT scanning, ultrasound imaging, and arteriography demonstrate the characteristically enlarged proximal abdominal aorta and hepatic artery with tapering distal to the celiac axis. These findings are secondary to the hypervascular nature of the tumor. Of note, approximately 16% of the tumors demonstrate calcification on plain film radiographs. Compare these imaging findings to those of a hepatoblastoma **(Figs. 11–13)**.

The natural history of infantile hemangioendothelioma is similar to that of cutaneous hemangiomas of infancy. There is a proliferative phase with rapid growth in the first 6 months which is followed by spontaneous regression. Therefore, treatment is usually not required. If, however, the child is symptomatic, a therapeutic intervention may be necessary. Most children with congestive heart failure are effectively treated with digoxin and diuretics. Prednisone and interleukin-2 can also accelerate regression. If medical therapy fails, transcatheter embolization is an effective alternative therapy. The prognosis depends on the patient's symptoms, with a greater than 95% survival rate for asymptomatic patients. The survival rate in complicated cases is 32%–75%, with a poorer prognosis seen in patients with congestive heart failure and thrombocytopenia.

For further information on this topic, please see Tutorial 12 and Teaching File Case 41.

Selected Readings

Burke DR, Verstandig A, Edwards O, Meranze SG, McLean GK, Stein EJ. Infantile hemangioendothelioma: angiographic features and factors determining efficacy of hepatic artery embolization. Cardiovasc Intervent Radiol 1986; 9:154–157.

Dachman AH, Lichtenstein JE, Friedman AC, Hartman DS. Infantile hemangioendothelioma of the liver: a radiologic-pathologic-clinical correlation. AJR 1983; 140:1091–1096.

Davenport M, Hansen L, Heaton ND, Howard ER. Hemangioendothelioma of the liver in infants. J Pediatr Surg 1995; 30:44–48.

Klein MA, Slovis TL, Chang CH, Jacobs IG. Sonographic and Doppler features of infantile hepatic hemangiomas with pathologic correlation. J Ultrasound Med 1990; 9:619–624.

Mahboubi S, Sunaryo FP, Glassman MS, Patel K. Computed tomography, management, and follow-up in infantile hemangioendothelioma of the liver in infants and children. J Comput Tomogr 1987; 11:370–375.

McHugh K, Burrows PE. Infantile hepatic hemangioendotheliomas: significance of portal venous and systemic collateral arterial supply. J Vasc Interv Radiol 1992; 3:337–344.

Powers C, Ros PR, Stoupis C, Johnson WK, Segel KH. Primary liver neoplasms: MR imaging with pathologic correlation. Radiographics 1994; 14:459–482.

Stanley P, Geer GD, Miller JH, Glisanz V, Landing BH, Boechat IM. Infantile hepatic hemangiomas: clinical features, radiologic investigations and treatment of 20 patients. Cancer 1989; 64:936–949.

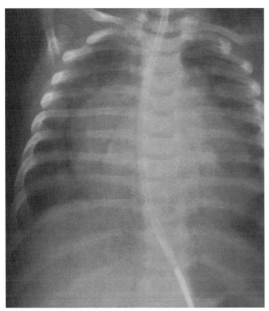
Figure 1. Supine chest radiograph.

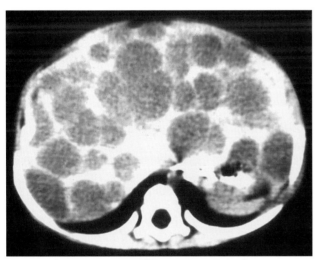
Figure 2. Contrast-enhanced CT scan through the liver.

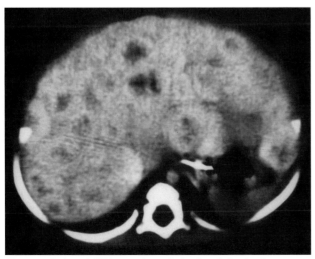
Figure 3. Delayed CT image through the liver following intravenous contrast.

TEACHING FILE CASE 41
Michael J. Flood, M.D., and
Richard R. Saxon, M.D.

History
A 3-month-old boy was brought to the hospital with progressive recurrent episodes of dyspnea since birth. The infant also had multiple raised purpuric lesions on the skin. Cardiac auscultation and echocardiography demonstrated no evidence of congenital heart disease. A chest radiograph was obtained **(Fig. 1)**, followed by a contrast-enhanced computed tomographic (CT) scan of the abdomen **(Figs. 2, 3)**.

What is your diagnosis?

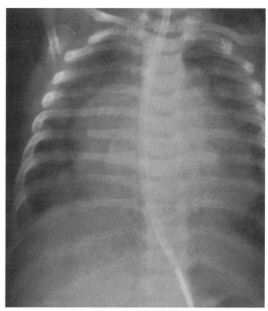

Figure 4. Chest radiograph demonstrates cardiomegaly and pulmonary vascular congestion.

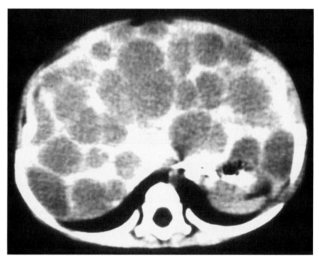

Figure 5. CT scan of the liver during intravenous contrast material infusion demonstrates hepatomegaly with multiple low-density nodules.

Radiographic Findings

The portable chest radiograph **(Fig. 4)** demonstrates moderate cardiomegaly with biventricular enlargement. There is pulmonary vascular congestion. Two equivalent CT images are shown. The image during infusion **(Fig. 5)** shows multiple low-density nodules with enhancing rims and there is diffuse hepatomegaly. The delayed image **(Fig. 6)** reveals contrast material filling in the nodules from the periphery.

Diagnoses

1. High-output cardiac failure.
2. Diffuse hepatic hemangioendothelioma.

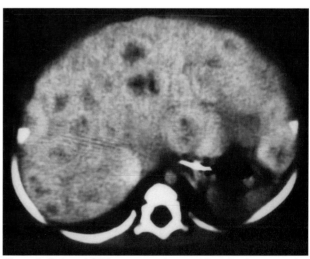

Figure 6. Delayed CT image reveals a centripetal enhancement pattern of these lesions.

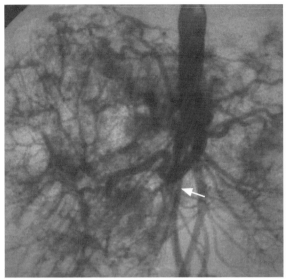

Figure 7. Abdominal aortogram demonstrates marked change in the caliber of the aorta below the celiac axis (arrow). A high-flow state to the liver is present.

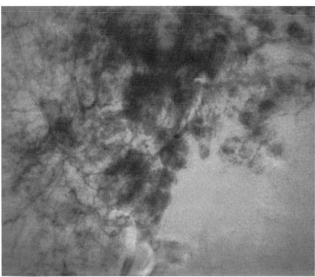

Figure 8. Hepatic arteriogram demonstrates multiple vascular lesions diffusely scattered throughout the liver.

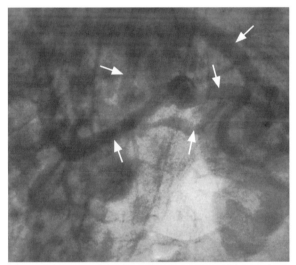

Figure 9. Large draining hepatic veins are noted (arrows) on the venous phase of the aortogram.

Management

Because of the patient's deteriorating condition, embolization was performed. The initial aortogram **(Fig. 7)** and selective hepatic arteriogram **(Fig. 8)** demonstrated diffuse involvement of the liver with multiple focal vascular lesions. The supraceliac aorta was approximately three times as large as the infraceliac aorta, indicative of the high-flow state of the liver. No significant arteriovenous shunting is present, but there are very large draining hepatic veins **(Fig. 9)**.

A 4-F end-hole catheter was used to selectively catheterize the proper hepatic artery, which was embolized using 250–750 micron particles of polyvinyl alcohol. Gelfoam pledgets (Upjohn, Kalamazoo, MI) were used after the polyvinyl alcohol to achieve complete hemostasis. The postembolization aortogram **(Fig. 10)** demonstrated marked diminution in blood flow to the liver. After the embolization, the patient's congestive heart failure resolved. No further therapy was needed.

Discussion

Infantile hemangioendothelioma is a benign liver tumor usually appearing before 6 months of age. Common presenting signs and symptoms are hepatomegaly, high-output cardiac failure, thrombocytopenia (Kasabach-Merritt syndrome), anemia, and cutaneous hemangiomas. The arteriographic appearance of the lesion is characterized by an abrupt decrease in the caliber of the aorta below the celiac artery. Typically, there are also large feeding hepatic and extrahepatic arteries, persistent pooling of contrast material in the vascular lesion, and large draining hepatic veins.

The natural history of the tumors is spontaneous regression. In a child with no serious symptoms, no therapy may be needed, but follow-up studies should be obtained to document regression.

For symptomatic children, supportive therapy with prednisone, digoxin, and furosemide is provided until the tumor regresses. If medical therapy is unsuccessful, further treatment is needed. Embolotherapy is probably the treatment of choice. Other therapies used are chemotherapy with cyclophosphamide or alpha-interferon, radiation therapy, hepatic artery ligation, or surgical excision for large solitary tumors.

For further information on this topic, please see Tutorials 12 and 13, and Teaching File Case 40.

Selected Readings

Keslar PJ, Buck JL, Selby DM. From the archives of the AFIP. Infantile hemangioendothelioma of the liver revisited. Radiographics 1993; 13:657–670.

Nguyen L, Shandling B, Ein S, Stephens C. Hepatic hemangioma in childhood: medical management or surgical management? J Pediatr Surg 1982; 17:576–579.

Stanley P, Geer GD, Miller JH, Gilsanz V, Landing BH, Boechat IM. Infantile hepatic hemangiomas: clinical features, radiologic investigations, and treatment of 20 patients. Cancer 1989; 64:936–949.

Stanley P, Grinnell VS, Stanton RE, Williams KO, Shore NA. Therapeutic embolization of infantile hepatic hemangioma with polyvinyl alcohol. AJR 1983; 141:1047–1051.

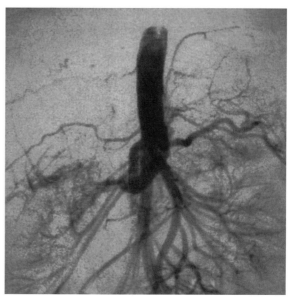

Figure 10. Postembolization aortogram. There is diminished flow to the liver with a dramatic decrease in the prominence of the hepatic vascular lesions. Note the improved filling of the infraceliac aorta, superior mesenteric artery, and splenic artery after tumor embolization.

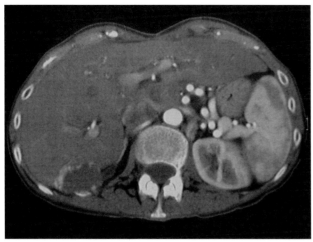

Figure 1. Contrast-enhanced hepatic CT scan.

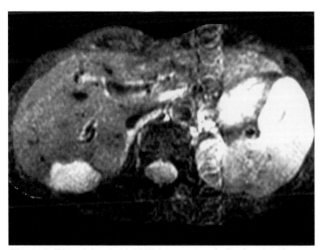

Figure 2. T2-weighted axial MR image at a similar level to that shown in Figure 1.

TEACHING FILE CASE 42
Robert K. Kerlan Jr., M.D., and
Mark W. Wilson, M.D.

History
A 50-year-old woman with newly diagnosed colon carcinoma underwent computed tomography (CT) scanning **(Fig. 1)** and magnetic resonance (MR) imaging **(Fig. 2)** as part of her preoperative evaluation.

What is your diagnosis?

Radiographic Findings

The contrast-enhanced CT scan **(Fig. 3)** reveals a 3-cm mass with peripheral lobular enhancement in the posterior segment of the right lobe of the liver. The T2-weighted MR image **(Fig. 4)** of this region reveals the mass to have a very high intensity.

Diagnosis

Cavernous hemangioma of the liver.

How would you manage this patient?

Management

Hepatic cavernous hemangiomas are benign tumors which seldom lead to clinical problems. Though surgical resection and transcatheter embolization have been used in patients with pain or bleeding attributable to these tumors, therapeutic intervention is seldom necessary. In this patient, the tumor was presumed to be incidental and no further work-up or therapy was provided. She subsequently underwent a sigmoid colectomy and no hepatic metastases were noted at surgery.

Discussion

Hemangioma is by far the most common benign hepatic tumor, being incidentally detected during unrelated imaging studies in 4%–7% of patients. This lesion has been identified in up to 20% of patients in a prospective autopsy series. The tumor has a 5:1 female to male predominance and is most common in the postmenopausal age group. The lesions are solitary in 90% of patients, and the majority are less than 3 cm in diameter. Hemangiomas larger than 10 cm in diameter are arbitrarily termed giant hemangiomas. There is an increased incidence of cavernous hemangiomas in patients who also have lesions of focal nodular hyperplasia.

The typical ultrasonographic appearance of a well-defined, homogeneous, hyperechoic lesion with slight posterior acoustic enhancement is seen in about 70% of patients **(Fig. 5)**. Doppler sonography usually demonstrates visible flow at the peripheral aspect of the lesion with no identifiable flow in the central area. Some lesions may contain cystic areas or have an atypical appearance secondary to fibrosis; these lesions require further evaluation to establish the diagnosis.

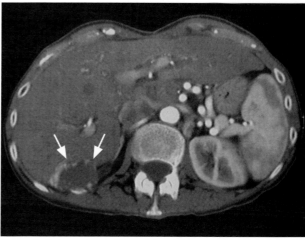

Figure 3. A 3-cm mass with peripheral lobular enhancement isodense with the aorta is present (arrows).

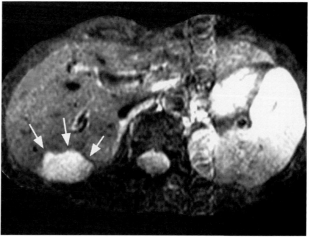

Figure 4. T2-weighted MR image shows this mass (arrows) to be hyperintense.

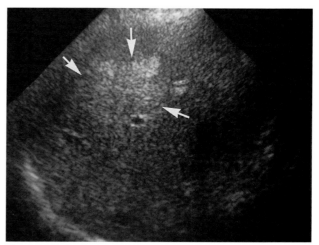

Figure 5. Abdominal ultrasound shows a sharply defined homogeneous hyperechoic lesion typical of cavernous hemangioma.

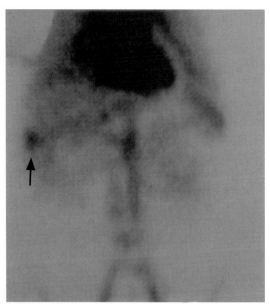

Figure 6. Technetium-99m labeled red blood cell study demonstrates a small cavernous hemangioma peripherally in the right lobe (arrow).

Further evaluation may merely involve a follow-up sonogram if clinical suspicion is low. When the lesion has a more worrisome appearance, further evaluation with one of a number of modalities may be conclusive. These modalities include nuclear scintigraphy, CT scanning, MR imaging, arteriography, or percutaneous biopsy.

Stability in the size of cavernous hemangiomas over time was documented by Mungovan et al in twenty-one patients whose diagnosis was biopsy-proven. Follow-up imaging studies were obtained from 5 to 84 months following the initial diagnosis. Nineteen of the twenty-one lesions (90%) did not change in size. Interval growth by 1 and 2 cm respectively was noted in the remaining two lesions. Therefore, lack of growth over time supports the diagnosis of cavernous hemangioma.

Nuclear scintigraphy with technetium-tagged pooled red blood cell imaging **(Fig. 6)** is a sensitive and cost-effective study that can confirm that a lesion represents a cavernous hemangioma. The typical scintigraphic features of this lesion include early hypoperfusion followed by an intense accumulation of radionuclide on images obtained 30 minutes after injection. While conventional planar imaging may be unreliable in detecting lesions smaller than 3 cm in diameter, dedicated single photon emission computed tomography (SPECT) can detect lesions as small as 5 mm in diameter. When the lesions are 1.4 cm and larger, the SPECT technique has been reported to have a 100% sensitivity. However, lesions located adjacent to the heart or major hepatic vascular structures may still be problematic.

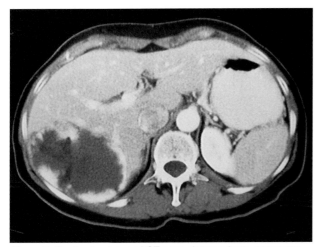

Figure 7. Contrast-enhanced CT scan shows a large cavernous hemangioma with peripheral nodular enhancement isodense with the aorta during the arterial phase.

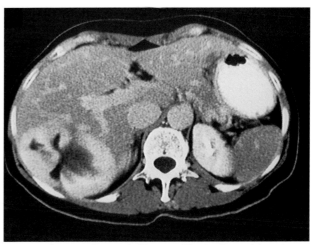

Figure 8. Same patient as in Figure 7. The 3-minute delayed image depicts centripetal filling. A hypodense central scar is present.

CT scanning (**Figs. 7–10**) is diagnostic for cavernous hemangioma when the appropriate criteria are satisfied. These criteria are: 1) hypodensity compared to the surrounding hepatic parenchyma on the precontrast images; 2) peripheral enhancement during the arterial phase of a bolus intravenous contrast material injection; and 3) centripetal filling with complete isodensity when compared to the surrounding hepatic parenchyma on 30-minute delayed images. Unfortunately, only 55%–62% of hemangiomas fulfill these criteria. Leslie et al have suggested that the pattern of globular enhancement coupled with isodensity to the abdominal aorta is 100% specific but only 67% sensitive in detecting cavernous hemangiomas with a single-pass dynamic CT scan (which does not require obtaining delayed images).

MR imaging is a highly accurate, though expensive, method of diagnosing hepatic cavernous hemangiomas. Typically these lesions demonstrate marked hyperintensity on heavily T2-weighted sequences. Moreover, a pattern of enhancement with gadolinium-DTPA on T1-weighted images may also differentiate this lesion from hepatic metastases. MR imaging has a greater sensitivity than radionuclide SPECT scintigraphy for assessment of lesions smaller than 2.5 cm in diameter. In addition, MR imaging is clearly superior for identifying hemangiomas that are adjacent to the heart or major hepatic vascular structures.

Because of the accuracy of the noninvasive imaging modalities, arteriography (**Figs. 11–16**) is seldom used to establish the diagnosis of cavernous hemangioma. However, these lesions may be encountered incidentally during arteriography performed for unrelated indications.

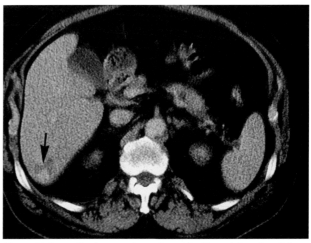

Figure 9. A smaller hemangioma (arrow) with peripheral nodular enhancement isodense with the aorta.

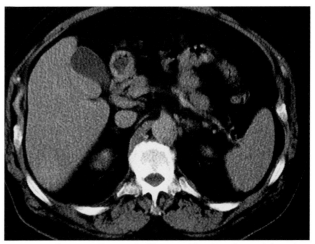

Figure 10. Same patient as in Figure 9. The 20-minute delayed image shows that the lesion has become isodense with the surrounding liver and is no longer visible.

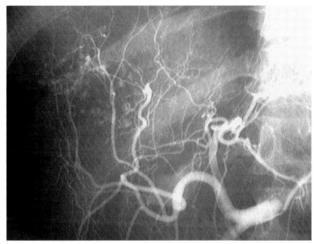

Figure 11. Selective common hepatic arteriogram, early arterial phase, shows typical the contrast material puddling of cavernous hemangioma.

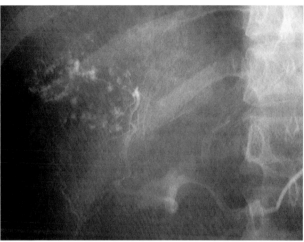

Figure 12. Same patient as in Figure 11. Delayed image reveals the typical cotton wool appearance of cavernous hemangioma.

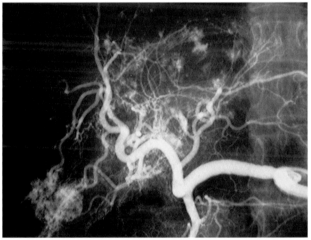

Figure 13. A more diffuse cavernous hemangioma during the late arterial phase of a common hepatic arteriogram.

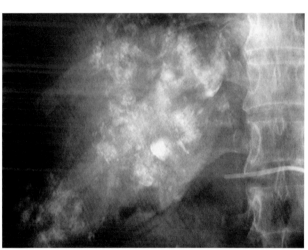

Figure 14. Same patient as in Figure 13. 30-second delayed image reveals the typical appearance of giant cavernous hemangioma.

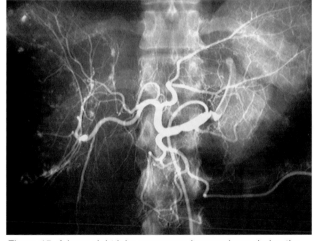

Figure 15. A large right lobe cavernous hemangioma during the early arterial phase of a common hepatic arteriogram.

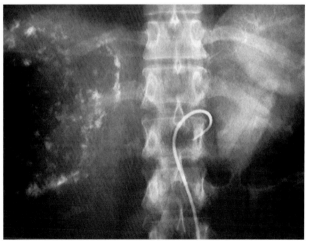

Figure 16. Same patient as in Figure 11. 30-second delayed film confirms the diagnosis.

Arteriography is often employed preoperatively if resection of a symptomatic giant cavernous hemangioma is being contemplated. The pathognomonic arteriographic feature is the "cotton-wool" stain which appears in the mid arterial phase and persists on films delayed 30–60 seconds from the time of injection. Arteriovenous shunting and enlargement of the hepatic artery are not typically observed.

Percutaneous biopsy is usually unnecessary and is very seldom performed to confirm the diagnosis of cavernous hemangioma. However, in patients with a normal coagulation profile, percutaneous biopsy can be performed safely with 20-gauge or smaller needles which traverse areas of normal liver prior to entering the tumor. Cytologic interpretation may be difficult; an experienced cytopathologist is required to make the diagnosis with confidence.

For further information on this topic, please see Tutorial 12.

Selected Readings

Birnbaum BA, Weinreb JC, Megibow AJ, et al. Definitive diagnosis of hepatic hemangiomas: MR imaging versus Tc-99m labeled red blood cell SPECT. Radiology 1990; 1776:95–101.

Freeny PC, Marks WM. Hepatic hemangioma: dynamic bolus CT. AJR 1986; 147:711–719.

Karhunen PJ. Benign hepatic tumors and tumor-like conditions in men. J Clin Pathol 1986; 39:183–188.

Leslie DF, Johnson CD, Johnson CM, Ilstrup DM, Harmsen WS. Distinction between cavernous hemangiomas of the liver and hepatic metastases on CT: value of contrast enhancement patterns. AJR 1995; 164:625–629.

Marn CS, Bree RL, Silver TM. Ultrasonography of liver: technique and focal and diffuse disease. Radiol Clin North Am 1991; 29:1151–1170.

Mungovan JA; Cronan JJ, Vacarro J. Hepatic cavernous hemangiomas: lack of enlargement over time. Radiology 1994; 191:111–113.

Rubin RA, Lichtenstein GR. Scintigraphic evaluation of liver masses: cavernous hepatic hemangioma. J Nucl Med 1993; 34:849–852.

Tung GA, Cronan JJ. Percutaneous needle biopsy of hepatic cavernous hemangioma. J Clin Gastroenterol 1993; 16:117–122.

Ziessman HA, Silverman PM, Patterson J, et al. Improved detection of small cavernous hemangiomas of the liver with high-resolution three-headed SPECT. J Nucl Med 1991; 32:2086–2091.

End Notes

Figures 7–10 courtesy of Judy Yee, M.D., University of California, San Francisco, CA.

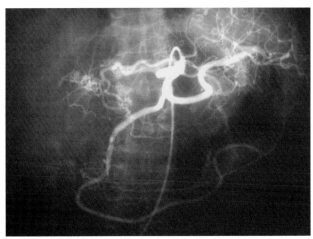

Figure 1. Celiac arteriogram, mid arterial phase.

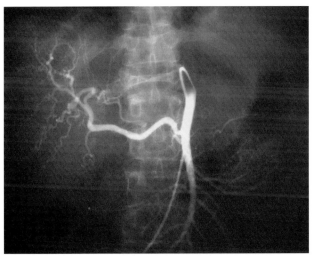

Figure 2. Superior mesenteric arteriogram, mid arterial phase.

TEACHING FILE CASE 43
Michael J. Flood, M.D., and
Richard R. Saxon, M.D.

History
A 73-year-old man complained of swelling of his feet and abdomen for 1 month. Laboratory data were significant for a serum albumin of 2.3, a moderately decreased prothrombin time, and mildly elevated serum bilirubin. A mesenteric arteriogram was obtained shortly after admission **(Figs. 1, 2)**.

What is your diagnosis?

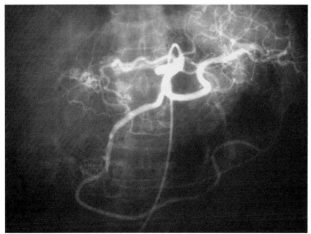

Figure 3. Celiac arteriogram shows a large left hepatic artery with tortuous branches. No right hepatic artery is identified.

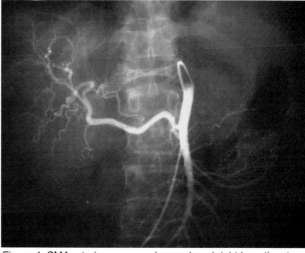

Figure 4. SMA arteriogram reveals a replaced right hepatic artery which is prominent in size. The intrahepatic branches are elongated, tortuous, and have the classic "corkscrew" appearance.

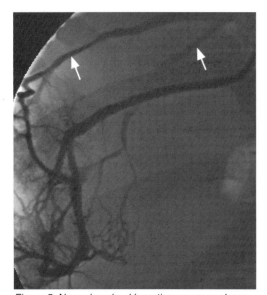

Figure 5. Normal wedged hepatic venogram shows prompt filling of other hepatic veins (arrows).

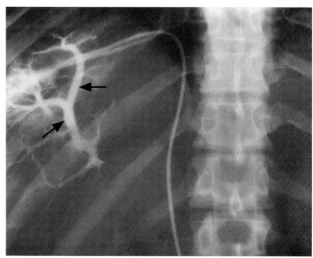

Figure 6. Portal venous filling (arrows) is present on this abnormal wedged hepatic venogram in a patient with cirrhosis.

Radiographic Findings

Selective celiac **(Fig. 3)** and superior mesenteric **(Fig. 4)** arteriograms demonstrate a replaced right hepatic artery. Both right and left hepatic arteries are prominent in size with tortuous intraparenchymal branches that have a "corkscrew" appearance.

Diagnosis

Hepatic cirrhosis.

Management

Wedged hepatic venography, often with hemodynamic evaluation, can be a useful adjunct in evaluating patients with suspected cirrhosis. A normal wedged hepatic venogram has a homogeneous parenchymal pattern with prompt filling of the hepatic veins **(Fig. 5)**. With cirrhosis, sinusoidal fibrosis develops and obstruction of venous outflow occurs. Wedged hepatic venography at this time shows preferential filling of portal vein radicles **(Fig. 6)**.

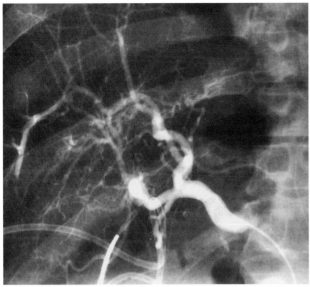

Figure 7. A prominent proper hepatic artery with corkscrewing of intrahepatic branches is noted in the arterial phase of this selective arteriogram.

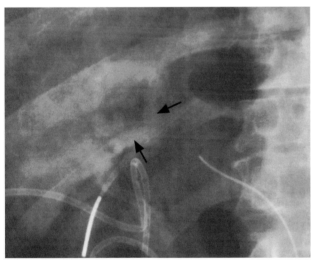

Figure 8. Venous phase of the same proper hepatic arteriogram as in Figure 7 reveals the portal vein acting as an outflow tract in this patient with severe cirrhosis (arrows).

As cirrhosis progresses, the portal vein becomes an outflow tract for the liver. Injection of the hepatic artery at this stage of disease will show contrast material entering the portal vein during the venous phase of the injection (**Figs. 7, 8**).

Discussion

Though the diagnosis of hepatic cirrhosis is usually established prior to arteriography, occasionally the initial diagnosis is made during mesenteric arteriography. The typical arteriographic findings of cirrhosis include mild enlargement of the supplying arteries with rapid flow and elongated, tortuous arteries within the hepatic parenchyma leading to the typical "corkscrew" appearance. The arterial enlargement and increased flow are likely compensatory for the diminished portal venous flow. The "corkscrew" appearance has been attributed to the redundancy created by diminished size of the liver and fibrosis.

Arteriograms are obtained in patients with cirrhosis for several reasons including the diagnosis of gastrointestinal bleeding, detection and treatment of hepatocellular carcinoma, and delineation of arterial and portal venous anatomy prior to surgery. Therefore, the arteriographic appearance of hepatic cirrhosis is frequently encountered.

In cases where the diagnosis of cirrhosis is suspected but not unequivocally established, hepatic venography with wedged hepatic pressure measurements can be extremely useful.

Selected Readings

Heeney DJ, Bookstein JJ, Bell RH, Orloff MJ, Miyai K. Correlation of hepatic and portal wedged venography and manometry with histology in alcoholic cirrhosis and periportal fibrosis. Radiology 1982; 142:591–597.

Kreel L, Gitlin N, Sherlock S. Hepatic artery angiography in portal hypertension. Am J Med 1970; 48:618–623.

Reuter SR, Redman HC, Cho KJ. Gastrointestinal angiography. 3rd edition. Philadelphia: W.B. Saunders Company, 1986; 382–445.

Viamonte M Jr, Warren WD, Fomon JJ. Liver panangiography in the assessment of portal hypertension in liver cirrhosis. Radiol Clin North Am 1970; 8:147–167.

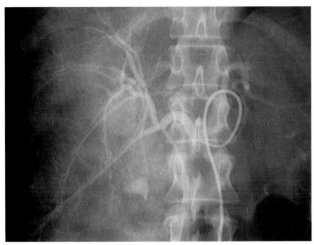

Figure 1. Common hepatic arteriogram, mid arterial phase.

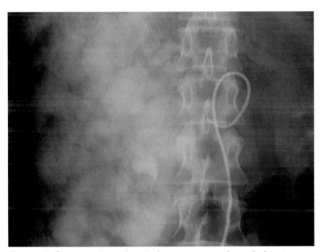

Figure 2. Common hepatic arteriogram, parenchymal phase.

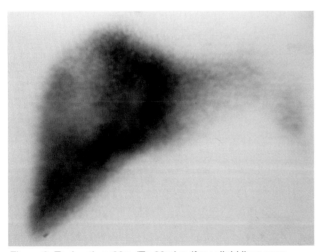

Figure 3. Technetium-99m (Tc-99m) sulfur colloid liver scan.

TEACHING FILE CASE 44
*Rajiv Sawhney, M.D., and
Susan D. Wall, M.D.*

History
The patient is a 45-year-old woman with a palpable
right-sided abdominal mass. Arteriography and
nuclear scintigraphy were performed **(Figs. 1–3)**.

What is your diagnosis?

Radiographic Findings

The arteriogram **(Fig. 4)** demonstrates hepatic arteries which are displaced and stretched by the mass. Though neovascularity is present, disorganized and irregular arteries are not identified. The parenchymal phase of the study **(Fig. 5)** shows increased contrast staining throughout the mass with an overall "lumpy" appearance. The nuclear scintigraphic image **(Fig. 6)** reveals a photopenic area in the right lobe. The differential diagnosis would include primary and metastatic neoplasm as well as hepatic adenoma.

Diagnosis

Vascular hepatic mass.

Management

Following the arteriogram, a biopsy was performed that was diagnostic of hepatic adenoma. The tumor was surgically excised.

Discussion

Hepatic adenoma is a benign tumor of the liver which is seen most often in women of childbearing age, especially those taking oral contraceptives. The tumor consists of normal hepatocytes arranged in sheets and cords without acinar structure. Reticuloendothelial (Kupffer) cells are not usually present. The lesions are usually solitary. Patients may be asymptomatic or have right upper quadrant pain. A palpable mass is often present. These tumors can bleed spontaneously or as a result of minor trauma, and occasionally patients may present with a subcapsular hematoma or intraperitoneal hemorrhage. Because there is a risk of life-threatening hemorrhage and potential for malignant degeneration, surgical resection of hepatic adenoma is the preferred treatment.

Arteriographically, hepatic adenomas are usually hypervascular. The hepatic artery branches are enlarged and appear to be displaced by the mass. Multiple small vessels emanating from the stretched arteries feed the tumor. Hepatic adenomas lack the "pooling" or "lakes" that are typical of hepatocellular carcinoma. Differentiation of hepatic adenoma from focal nodular hyperplasia can be difficult.

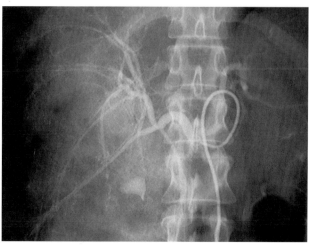

Figure 4. Right lobe hepatic arteries are stretched around a mass, but malignant-appearing neovascularity is absent.

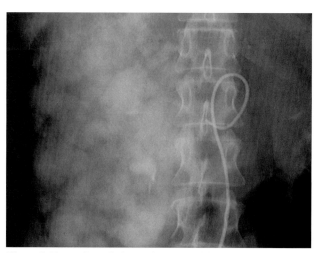

Figure 5. Parenchymal phase shows multilobulated dense staining indicative of a neoplasm.

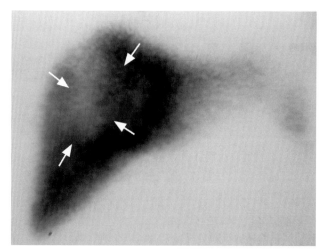

Figure 6. Tc-99m sulfur colloid scan demonstrates a photopenic area (arrows) in the right lobe of the liver.

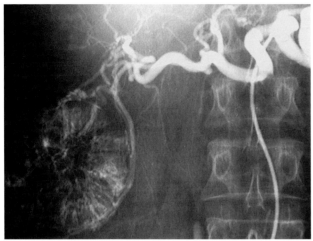

Figure 7. Celiac arteriogram. A pedunculated mass with a "spokewheel" arterial pattern is present in the right lobe of the liver.

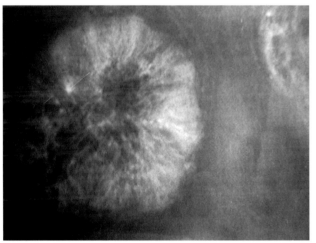

Figure 8. A magnification view of the same lesion shown in Figure 7, later in the arteriographic sequence. The appearance is typical for focal nodular hyperplasia.

Focal nodular hyperplasia (FNH) is a benign focal liver abnormality most commonly seen in young and middle-aged women. It is encountered with increased frequency in patients who are taking oral contraceptives, and often coexists with cavernous hemangiomas. Pathologically, it differs from hepatic adenoma in that the mass contains reticuloendothelial (Kupffer) cells. Therefore, if a lesion accumulates Tc-99m sulfur colloid, it is assumed to represent FNH rather than a hepatic adenoma. Unfortunately, uptake is present in only 65%–70% of cases and, rarely, hepatic adenomas will accumulate the radiopharmaceutical.

FNH often contains a central scar, a useful differential feature which can be recognized on both CT and MR imaging.

Angiographically FNH has a "spokewheel" appearance with arteries radiating from the central region **(Figs. 7, 8)**. It has been suggested that the major arterial feeding vessel extends to the central portion of the mass and then arborizes. Though this is true for smaller (<3 cm) lesions, larger lesions often appear to be supplied from the periphery. Despite a peripheral entry, the "spokewheel" pattern is usually maintained.

As FNH is usually not associated with spontaneous hemorrhage or malignant degeneration, these lesions are generally followed with observation rather than surgical resection.

For further information on this topic, please see Tutorial 12.

Selected Readings

Arrive L, Flejou JF, Vilgrain V, et al. Hepatic adenoma: MR findings in 51 pathologically proved lesions. Radiology 1994; 193:507–512.

Bernardino ME. Space-occupying lesions of the liver. In: Taveras JM, Ferrucci JT, eds. Radiology: diagnosis, imaging, intervention. Volume 4: Ferrucci JT, Newhouse, eds. Abdominal and pelvic genitourinary. Philadelphia: J.B. Lippincott Company, 1988; 9–10.

Kadir S. Angiography of the liver, spleen, and pancreas. In: Diagnostic angiography, Kadir S. Philadelphia: W.B. Saunders Company, 1986; 418.

Reuter SR, Redman HC, Cho KJ. Gastrointestinal angiography. 3rd edition. Philadelphia: W.B. Saunders Company, 1986; 132–139.

Shamsi K, De Schepper A, Degryse H, Deckers F. Focal nodular hyperplasia of the liver: radiologic findings. Abdom Imaging 1993; 18:32–38.

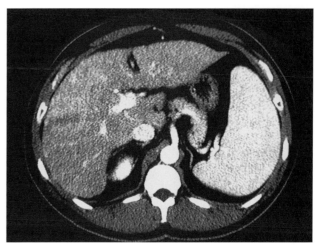

Figure 1. Contrast-enhanced CT scan through the upper abdomen.

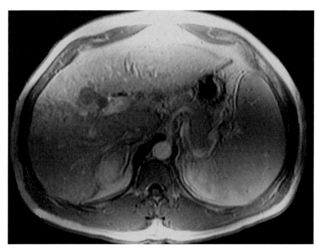

Figure 2. Magnetic resonance image through a similar region as depicted in Figure 1.

TEACHING FILE CASE 45
Mark W. Wilson, M.D., and
Robert K. Kerlan Jr., M.D.

History
A 54-year-old Asian man with a 1-month history of abdominal pain and weight loss has been referred for evaluation. He undergoes abdominal computed tomography (CT) **(Fig. 1)** and abdominal magnetic resonance (MR) imaging **(Fig. 2)**.

What is your diagnosis?

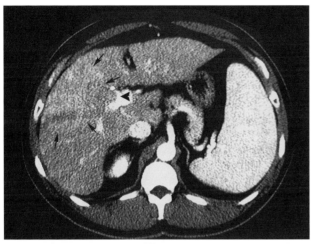

Figure 3. Contrast-enhanced CT scan shows a vague area of enhancement in the right lobe of the liver (arrows) with a soft-tissue nodule (arrowhead) extending into the right portal vein.

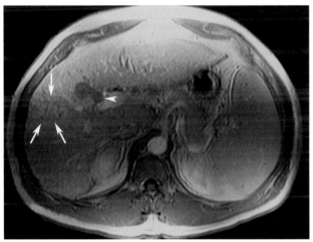

Figure 4. Magnetic resonance image through a similar region shows heterogeneous signal intensity in the right lobe of the liver (arrows) and confirms the presence of a soft tissue mass that extends into the right portal vein (arrowhead).

Radiographic Findings

The abdominal CT scan **(Fig. 3)** shows a subtle mass with contrast enhancement in the right lobe of the liver. MR imaging **(Fig. 4)** confirms the presence of a solid-appearing mass in the right lobe of the liver manifested as an area of diminished signal intensity. Both the CT and MR scans show a focal soft tissue density extending into the right portal vein.

Diagnosis

Hepatocellular carcinoma (hepatoma).

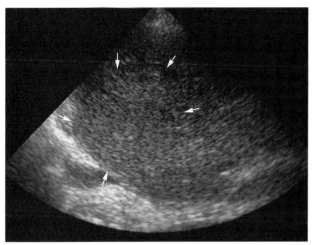

Figure 5. Ultrasound through the right lobe of the liver reveals a vague area of increased echogenicity which was biopsied and shown to be hepatocellular carcinoma (HCC).

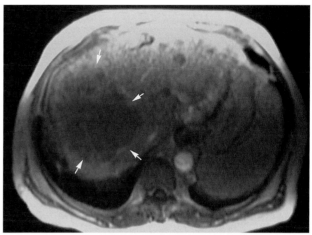

Figure 6. Gadolinium-enhanced T1-weighted MR image through the upper abdomen shows a large, hypointense HCC in the right lobe.

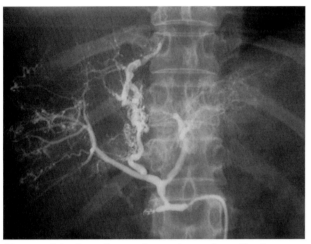

Figure 7. Selective celiac arteriogram in a patient with a large right lobe HCC.

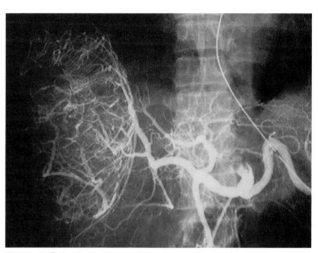

Figure 8. Selective common hepatic arteriogram in a patient with HCC. An occluding spring embolus has been placed in the gastroduodenal artery prior to intraarterial chemotherapy.

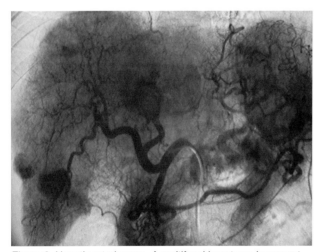

Figure 9. Hepatic arteriogram. A multifocal hepatoma is present.

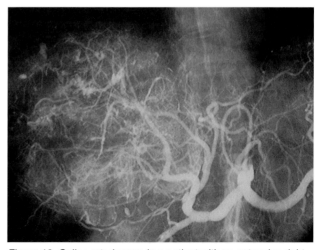

Figure 10. Celiac arteriogram in a patient with an extensive right lobe HCC.

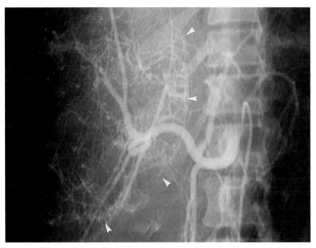

Figure 11. Common hepatic arteriogram in a patient with a large hepatoma (arrows) which is less hypervascular compared to previous examples.

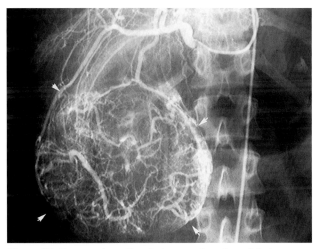

Figure 12. Common hepatic arteriogram. A pedunculated hepatoma simulates the appearance of a hepatic adenoma.

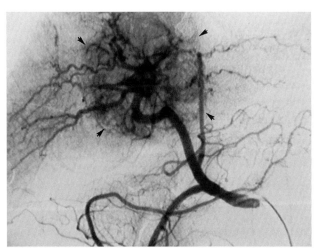

Figure 13. Common hepatic arteriogram. A right lobe HCC with a "spoke-wheel" configuration simulates the appearance of focal nodular hyperplasia (arrows).

Additional images from patients with hepatocellular carcinoma are shown in **Figures 5–13**.

Management

Treatment options for hepatocellular carcinoma (HCC) include surgical resection, orthotopic liver transplantation (OLT), systemic chemotherapy, regional chemotherapy, chemoembolization, and imaging-guided local ablation.

When it is technically feasible and the hepatic function is sufficient, surgical resection clearly offers the best chance of prolonged survival.

When the lesion cannot be curatively resected, OLT would seem to be the most attractive option, at least theoretically. Though there does appear to be a survival benefit with OLT, the incidence of recurrent tumor is relatively high and the utilization of this expensive and scarce resource in patients with advanced malignancy is usually not justified.

Systemic chemotherapy is an unattractive option because a favorable response can only be achieved in about 20% of patients.

Though regional chemotherapy through a hepatic arterial catheter has been attempted in many trials, this form of therapy has largely been replaced by transarterial chemoembolization (TACE). With TACE, chemotherapeutic agents are combined with an embolic material (usually gelatin sponge or iodized oil) and injected into an intrahepatic arterial branch supplying the tumor. With use of this method, the doses of chemotherapeutic agent delivered to the tumor may be as much as twenty times higher than can be achieved with intravenous injection. Moreover, the chemotherapeutic effect is enhanced by a prolongation of the dwell time and is combined with ischemic necrosis of the tumor induced by the arterial embolization. TACE trials have shown a much more consistent tumor response when compared to systemic chemotherapy, and TACE has been shown to offer significant palliation for right upper quadrant pain. Unfortunately, a survival benefit with this form of therapy has not been unequivocally established.

Imaging-guided ablation with percutaneous alcohol injections has also received recent attention as a potential therapeutic option for unresectable hepatocellular carcinoma. Percutaneous ethanol injection (PEI) is generally reserved for patients with four or fewer lesions, none of which are larger than 3 cm in maximal diameter. Multiple injections are usually required over several days to a few weeks to complete PEI. Though an extremely high immediate response rate has been reported, a prolongation of survival has not been clearly demonstrated. Regional therapies involving the application of laser energy as well as cryosurgery (which requires laparotomy) have also been used to treat hepatocellular carcinoma.

In this case, the patient declined therapy and died 4 months later.

Discussion

HCC is not a common tumor in the United States, ranking 22nd in frequency with an annual incidence of approximately four cases per 100,000. In contrast, this tumor is extremely common in eastern Asia and Africa with an incidence up to 150 per 100,000. This disparity almost certainly reflects the prevalence of chronic hepatitis B and C infections in both Asia and Africa.

Right upper quadrant pain is the most common presenting symptom in patients with HCC, and is observed in the majority of patients. Physical examination most often reveals tender hepatomegaly. Jaundice, splenomegaly, and ascites are also frequently observed. Laboratory evaluation may demonstrate anemia, hyperbilirubinemia, and elevations of the serum alkaline phosphatase, glutamic oxaloacetic transaminase, and lactic dehydrogenase. An elevation of the serum alpha-fetoprotein level is seen in 30%–40% of patients. An alpha-fetoprotein level above 500 ng/dL strongly suggests the presence of HCC.

Imaging studies including ultrasound, radiographic computed tomography, and MR imaging are usually abnormal but may be nonspecific due to the variable appearance of the tumor. Three major patterns of growth may be encountered: 1) solitary mass (often large); 2) multifocal HCC in which multiple distinct masses may simulate metastatic disease; and 3) diffuse or cirrhotomimetic HCC with widespread contiguous hepatic involvement.

In Western countries, HCC is more commonly encountered as a solitary mass in an elderly patient (70–80 years old) with a noncirrhotic liver. When HCC develops in Western patients with cirrhosis, the cirrhosis is most often secondary to alcoholic liver disease or hemochromatosis. In Asia and Africa, multifocal disease in younger patients (30–45 years old) is more common, with the disease almost always occurring against the background of hepatic cirrhosis secondary to long-standing viral hepatitis.

Percutaneous biopsy is required for diagnosis in nonendemic regions. In endemic areas, the detection of a mass with cross-sectional imaging combined with a marked elevation of the alpha-fetoprotein level is often accepted as diagnostic without pathologic confirmation. Arteriography is usually not required to establish the diagnosis, but it may be requested to delineate the vascular anatomy prior to surgical resection, or performed in conjunction with TACE.

The classic arteriographic features include enlargement of the hepatic artery associated with rapid flow into a hypervascular mass containing markedly irregular (malignant-appearing) neovascularity. Arteriovenous shunting into portal venous branches is not uncommon. Arteriovenous shunting into the hepatic venous system is observed less frequently. Portal vein occlusion with tumor thrombus is typical of advanced cases.

Once the diagnosis has been established, the natural history without treatment is quite grim, with an expected median survival of 4–6 months.

For further information on this topic, please see Tutorial 12.

Selected Readings

Haug CE, Jenkins RL, Rohrer RJ, et al. Liver transplantation for primary hepatic cancer. Transplantation 1992; 53:376–382.

Kanematsu T, Matsumata T, Furuta T, et al. Lipiodol drug targeting in the treatment of primary hepatocellular carcinoma. Hepatogastroenterology 1990; 37:442–444.

Livraghi T, Salmi A, Bolondi L, et al. Small hepatocellular carcinoma: percutaneous alcohol injection—results in 23 patients. Radiology 1988; 168:313–317.

Oberfield RA, Steele G Jr, Gollan JL, Sherman D. Liver cancer. CA Cancer J Clin 1989; 39:206–217.

Venook AP. Treatment of hepatocellular carcinoma: too many options? J Clin Oncol 1994; 12:1323–1334.

Venook AP, Stagg RJ, Lewis BJ, et al. Chemoembolization for hepatocellular carcinoma. J Clin Oncol 1990; 8:1108–1114.

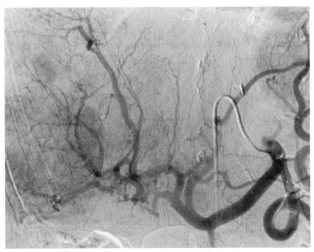

Figure 1. Celiac arteriogram, early arterial phase.

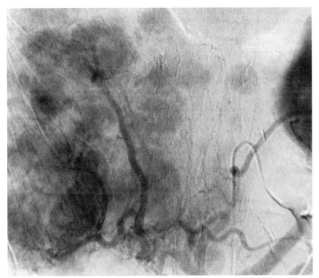

Figure 2. Celiac arteriogram, late arterial phase.

TEACHING FILE CASE 46
Joseph Krysl, M.D.

History

An 82-year-old woman with known hepatocellular carcinoma came to the hospital with a complaint of vague abdominal pain. She had no other medical problems. Hepatic arteriography was performed **(Figs. 1, 2)**.

What is your diagnosis?

Radiographic Findings

The arteriogram **(Figs. 3, 4)** demonstrates focal areas of abnormal blush in multiple locations in the right lobe of the liver. There is neovascularity but no arterioportal shunting.

Diagnosis

Hepatocellular carcinoma, multifocal.

The differential diagnosis includes hypervascular metastases, such as renal cell carcinoma, choriocarcinoma, islet cell tumors, and melanoma.

How would you manage this patient?

Management

Transcatheter chemoembolization of the hepatocellular carcinoma was chosen because the patient was not a candidate for surgical resection or cryotherapy.

A mixture of cisplatin, doxorubicin, and mitomycin mixed with Lipiodol (Laboratoire Guerbet, Aulnay-sous-Bois, France) was infused subselectively via a coaxial microcatheter system. Toward the end of the infusion, polyvinyl alcohol particles were added to the chemotherapy-Lipiodol mixture to effect embolization to stasis.

Figure 5 demonstrates the parenchymal stain in the liver from the Lipiodol in the embolization mixture. The primary feeding artery to this large area of tumor blush was embolized to stasis.

Discussion

The intraarterial administration of chemotherapeutic agents for the treatment of hepatocellular carcinoma has been attempted in an effort to provide therapies to those patients ineligible for tumor resection. Hepatic artery infusion systems have been used but require either prolonged percutaneous catheterization or the placement of an infusion pump at the time of laparotomy. Percutaneous transcatheter chemoembolization combines regional administration of chemotherapeutic agents with reduction of the arterial blood flow to the liver. The ischemia induced by embolotherapy has been shown to increase the concentration of the chemotherapeutic agents remaining in the liver.

A variety of embolic agents has been used for this purpose including Gelfoam (Upjohn, Kalamazoo, MI), Gelfoam powder, polyvinyl alcohol, and autologous blood clot. Lipiodol is added to the mixture because it tends to concentrate in neoplastic tissue in the liver.

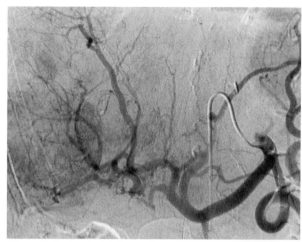

Figure 3. Early arterial phase of a celiac arteriogram demonstrates multiple focal areas of blush in the right lobe of the liver, indicative of multifocal malignancy.

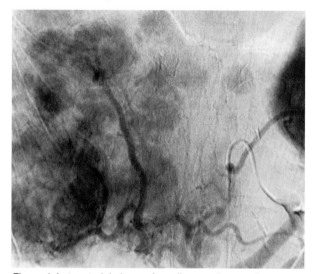

Figure 4. Late arterial phase of a celiac arteriogram demonstrates multiple areas of tumor blush in the liver with a large region of blush seen along the lateral margin of the right lobe.

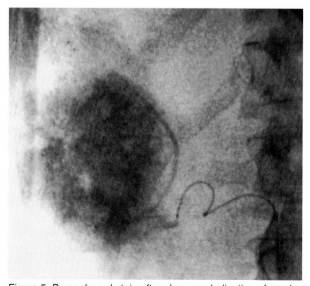

Figure 5. Parenchymal stain after chemoembolization of one large focal tumor (hepatocellular carcinoma) in the right lobe of the liver. A microcatheter is in the primary feeding artery to this region of tumor.

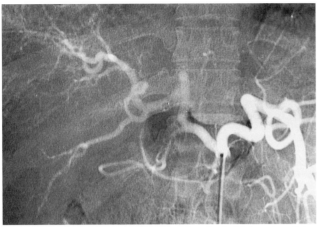

Figure 6. Celiac arteriogram of a second patient with hepatocellular carcinoma. The arterial phase shows tumor vessels in the superior portion of the right lobe of the liver.

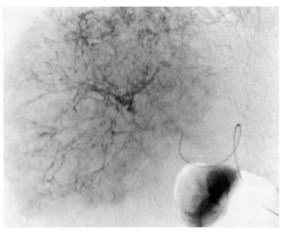

Figure 7. Same patient as in Figure 6. Parenchymal stain and static flow in the vessels in the region of the hepatocellular carcinoma after chemoembolization with a Lipiodol-chemotherapy mix.

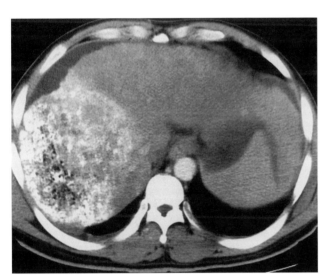

Figure 8. Same patient as in Figure 6. Axial CT scan of the liver approximately 1 week after chemoembolization of a hepatocellular carcinoma. Parenchymal staining with Lipiodol and areas of air bubbles indicate regions of tumor infarction.

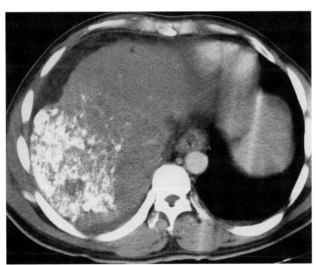

Figure 9. Same patient as in Figure 6. Axial CT scan of the liver approximately 6 weeks after chemoembolization of hepatocellular carcinoma. There is persistent staining of the tumor, which has decreased in size.

Response rates of up to 50% have been demonstrated with chemoembolization of hepatocellular carcinoma; however, the response tends not to last. Long-term survival following chemoembolization in patients with small hepatocellular carcinomas has been reported.

A second case of hepatoma embolized with a Lipiodol-chemotherapy mixture and polyvinyl alcohol particles is shown in **Figures 6–9**. Computed tomography (CT) scans obtained 2 weeks and 6 weeks after embolization **(Figs. 8, 9)** show reduction in the size of the tumor. There is relatively uniform staining of the hepatoma with the oily contrast material.

Chemoembolization has also been shown to be effective in the palliation of symptomatic carcinoid liver metastases as well as those from other hormone-secreting tumors (APUDomas). Response rates of 72%–90% have been reported, depending on the outcomes me1asured. Chemoembolization has also been used to treat other tumors, including ocular melanoma metastases and colorectal metastases, with varying degrees of success.

For further information on this topic, please see Tutorials 16 and 17, and Teaching File Cases 47, 50, and 51.

Selected Readings

Carrasco CH, Charnsangavej C, Ajani J, Samaan NA, Richli W, Wallace S. The carcinoid syndrome: palliation by hepatic artery embolization. AJR 1986; 147:149–154.

Pentecost MJ. Transcatheter treatment of hepatic metastases. AJR 1993; 160:1171–1175.

Venook AP. Treatment of hepatocellular carcinoma: too many options? J Clin Oncol 1994; 12:1323–1334.

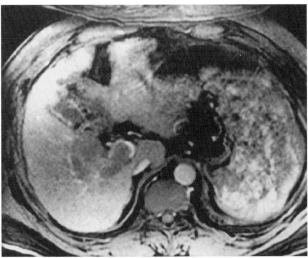

Figure 1. Axial T1-weighted magnetic resonance image through the upper abdomen.

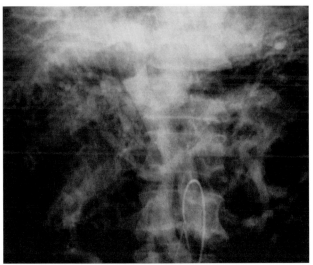

Figure 2. Superior mesenteric arteriogram, venous phase.

TEACHING FILE CASE 47
Kevin L. Sullivan, M.D.

History
This 51-year-old man with a history of hepatitis B was found to have an elevated alpha-fetoprotein. Magnetic resonance (MR) imaging and arterial portography were performed **(Figs. 1, 2)**.

What is your diagnosis?

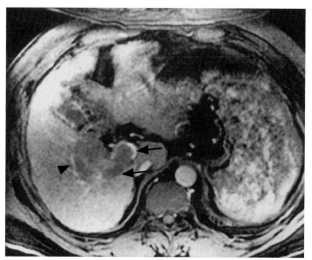

Figure 3. Axial MR image depicts a mass with diminished signal intensity in the right lobe (arrowhead). Tumor thrombus is present in the right portal vein (arrows).

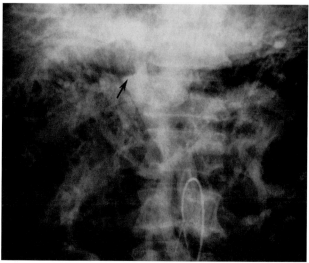

Figure 4. Arterial portogram confirms occlusion of the right portal vein (arrow).

Radiographic Findings

The MR image **(Fig. 3)** shows a mass of diminished signal intensity in the right hepatic lobe. Soft tissue is present in the right portal vein. The arterial portogram **(Fig. 4)** confirms occlusion of the right portal vein.

Diagnosis

Hepatocellular carcinoma with extension into the right portal vein.

How would you manage this patient?

Management

Although not done in this case, the portal vein filling defect could be needle biopsied to determine if there is tumor invasion. The size of the tumor precludes transplantation, and surgical resection is not an option due to portal vein invasion. Chemoembolization is the best treatment option.

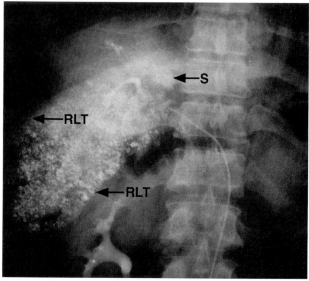

Figure 5. Abdominal radiograph performed immediately after chemoembolization. RLT=right lobe tumor; S=superior collection of Ethiodol.

The right hepatic artery was chemoembolized with an emulsion of Ethiodol (Savage Laboratories, Melville, NY) and doxorubicin. Following this, embolization with Gelfoam (Upjohn, Kalamazoo, MI) was performed until stasis was achieved. Immediately after chemoembolization, a radiograph of the abdomen demonstrated retention of Ethiodol in the right lobe tumor **(Fig. 5)**. In addition, superior and medial to this there is a separate, smaller area of Ethiodol retention.

What might this smaller area represent?

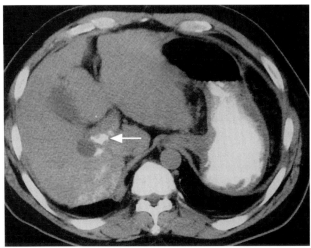

Figure 6. Noncontrast CT scan performed 1 month after chemoembolization. Ethiodol has been retained by tumor within the right portal vein (arrow).

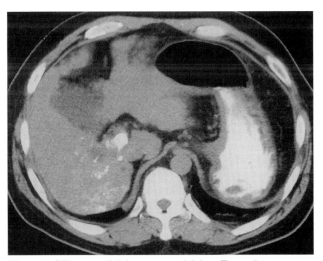

Figure 7. CT image slightly more caudal than Figure 6.

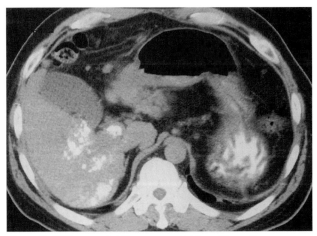

Figure 8. CT image slightly more caudal than Figure 7.

Discussion

Tumor in the portal vein can be supplied by the hepatic artery, and retain Ethiodol. The smaller collection of Ethiodol on this patient's abdominal radiograph is Ethiodol within the hepatoma invading the portal vein. **Figures 6**, **7**, and **8** demonstrate Ethiodol in the portal vein tumor on a 1-month follow-up CT scan performed without intravenous contrast material.

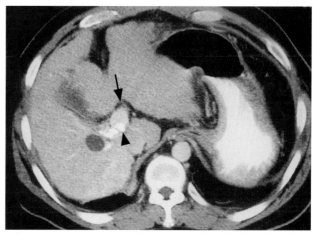

Figure 9. Contrast-enhanced CT scan 1 month following chemoembolization reveals partial patency of the portal vein (arrow) surrounding Ethiodol (arrowhead) within the portal vein tumor.

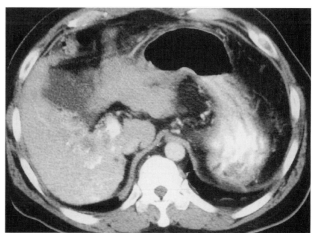

Figure 10. Contrast-enhanced CT scan slightly more caudal than Figure 9.

Intravenous contrast enhancement demonstrates flow around the Ethiodol-containing tumor within the portal vein **(Figs. 9–11)**. Portal vein invasion has a negative influence on survival. Retention of Ethiodol in a portal vein tumor is associated with tumor regression, which probably leads to improved survival if it is accompanied by a good response in the parenchymal tumor. Complete portal vein tumor regression and recanalization can occur in patients with dense, homogeneous retention of Ethiodol.

For further information on this topic, please see Tutorials 13, 16, and 17, and Teaching File Cases 46, 50, and 51.

Selected Readings

Chung JW, Park JH, Han JK, Choi BI, Han MC. Hepatocellular carcinoma and portal vein invasion: results of treatment with transcatheter oily chemoembolization. AJR 1995; 165:315–321.

Dodd GD, Carr BI. Percutaneous biopsy of portal vein thrombus: a new staging technique for hepatocellular carcinoma. AJR 1993; 161:229–233.

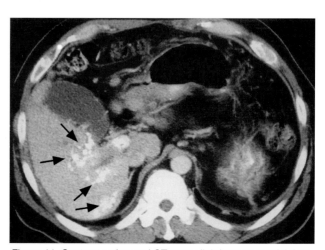

Figure 11. Contrast-enhanced CT scan slightly more caudal than Figure 10. Ethiodol is present (arrows) within the right lobe tumor.

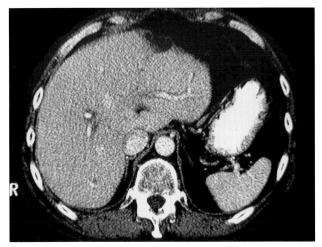

Figure 1. Contrast-enhanced CT scan through the upper abdomen.

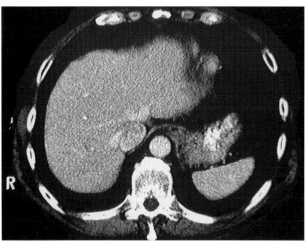

Figure 2. Contrast-enhanced CT scan at a slightly more cranial level.

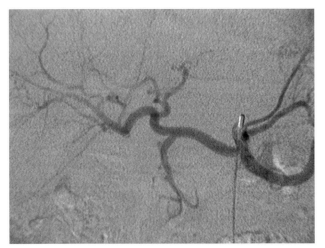

Figure 3. Celiac arteriogram.

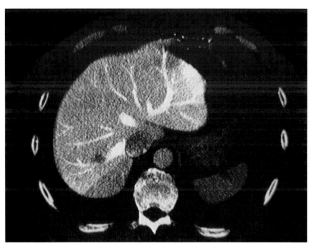

Figure 4. Computed tomographic arterial portography.

TEACHING FILE CASE 48
Robert K. Kerlan, Jr., M.D., and
Shelley R. Marder, M.D.

History
A 62-year-old asymptomatic man with a history of colon cancer resected 2 years earlier underwent an abdominal computed tomography (CT) scan **(Figs. 1, 2)** as part of a routine postoperative evaluation. Subsequently, arteriography **(Fig. 3)** and computed tomographic arterial portography (CTAP) **(Fig. 4)** were performed.

What is your diagnosis?

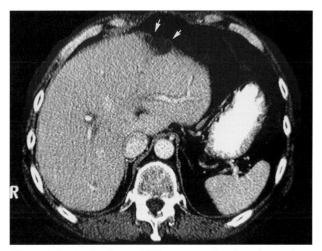

Figure 5. Contrast-enhanced CT scan reveals a 2-cm focus of diminished attenuation (arrows) along the ventral surface of the liver, within the lateral segment of the left lobe.

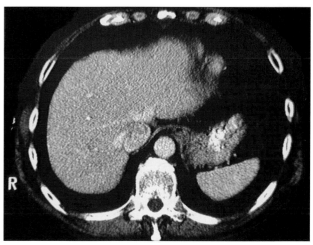

Figure 6. Image at a slightly more cephalic level shows no definite abnormality.

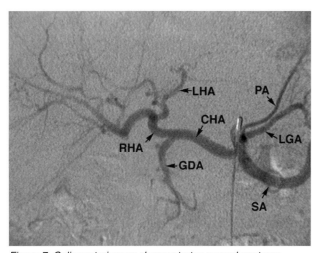

Figure 7. Celiac arteriogram demonstrates normal anatomy. CHA=common hepatic artery; GDA=gastroduodenal artery; LGA=left gastric artery; LHA=left hepatic artery; PA=left inferior phrenic artery; RHA=right hepatic artery; SA=splenic artery.

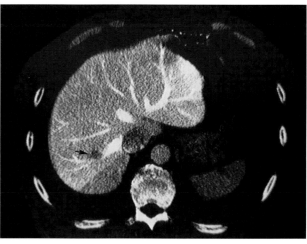

Figure 8. CTAP of the liver at a similar level to Figure 6 reveals a 1-cm area of diminished attenuation suspicious for metastasis adjacent to the right hepatic vein (arrow).

Radiographic Findings

The abdominal CT scan **(Fig. 5)** shows a 2-cm area of decreased attenuation in the lateral segment of the left lobe of the liver. The CT image from a slightly more cephalic level **(Fig. 6)** shows no definite abnormality. The celiac arteriogram **(Fig. 7)** demonstrates conventional hepatic arterial anatomy, without evidence of a parenchymal mass. The CTAP **(Fig. 8)** from a similar level to **Figure 6** reveals a suspicious low-density region adjacent to the right hepatic vein. This was subsequently proven to be metastatic adenocarcinoma.

Diagnosis

Metastatic adenocarcinoma to the liver, presumably from the previously resected primary tumor of the colon.

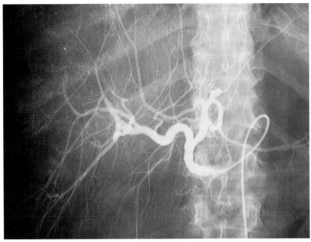

Figure 9. Common hepatic arteriogram demonstrates nonspecific arterial "stretching."

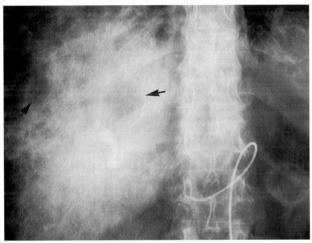

Figure 10. Parenchymal phase film from the same injection as in Figure 9 shows scattered hypovascular areas (arrows) suggesting metastases.

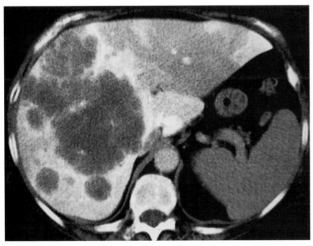

Figure 11. Same patient as in Figure 9. CTAP reveals massive metastatic deposits throughout the right lobe. A perfusion defect is evident in the left lobe.

Discussion

Metastases are the most common cause of malignant liver lesions by a margin of 18:1. Of all patients who die from cancer, 25%–50% have liver metastases. The liver ranks as the second most common site, behind regional lymph nodes, as a location for metastatic deposits.

The most common primary sites of metastatic carcinoma to the liver are the colon, pancreas, breast, and lung. Imaging modalities used in the detection of metastatic disease include computed tomography, ultrasound, magnetic resonance imaging, and nuclear scintigraphy. The precise modality used depends on the type of primary tumor, the importance of establishing the diagnosis, and the available medical and financial resources. In many patients, the presence or absence of hepatic metastases is moot because of the presence of metastatic disease in other locations. The vast majority of these patients are treated symptomatically or with systemic chemotherapy.

However, when the primary tumor is carcinoma of the colon and the liver is the only apparent site of tumor spread, surgical resection may be contemplated. Surgical resection of hepatic metastases is attempted when the number of metastatic deposits is small (four or fewer) and when the lesions exist in a location devoid of a major biliary or vascular structure, permitting complete resection. In this group of patients, the 5-year survival ranges from 25% to 40% compared to 0% for patients who do not undergo resection.

In this patient population, a highly accurate assessment of the number and location of metastatic deposits is essential. The most accurate way to evaluate the liver for metastases appears to be intraoperative ultrasound. However, currently the most precise way to make this determination preoperatively is with CTAP. Despite the fact that conventional arteriography is not sensitive for the detection of hypovascular metastases **(Figs. 9–11)**, transarterial portography performed during hepatic computed tomography is an excellent method to identify these tumors.

With CTAP **(Figs. 12, 13)**, an arterial catheter is placed either in the superior mesenteric artery (SMA) or the splenic artery, and the patient is taken to the CT scanner. Some evidence suggests that placement in the splenic artery is preferred. A number of different protocols have been assessed but the usual technique involves injection of 100–200 mL of contrast material at a rate of 2–5 mL/second through the arterial catheter followed by dynamic scanning of the liver after an initial delay of 30–60 seconds. The images obtained will usually reveal dramatic enhancement of the hepatic parenchyma. Metastatic deposits are usually identified as regions of diminished attenuation. This diminished attenuation has been attributed to the theory that primary and metastatic liver tumors derive most of their blood supply from hepatic arterial branches. Because the hepatic artery is not opacified during CTAP, metastatic lesions are revealed as areas of diminished attenuation.

More recent work suggests that the blood supply to metastatic tumors is more complex. Microangiographic studies have revealed that the portal venous radicles actually form the dominant supply to most tumors. However, due to flow dynamics at the precapillary arteriolar level, blood is shunted from the hepatic artery into the small portal venous radicles to supply the tumor. Therefore, though the tumor may be supplied anatomically from the portal venules, it is supplied functionally by the hepatic artery.

As with any technique, the performance of CTAP carries with it certain pitfalls, which can be either technical or physiologic.

Technical pitfalls include catheter dislodgment into the aorta or a small branch vessel **(Fig. 14)** during transfer of the patient from the angiographic suite to the CT scanner, and reflux of contrast material into a hepatic arterial branch. Reflux of contrast material may be caused by overinjection of the splenic artery or filling of the hepatic artery through inferior pancreaticoduodenal collaterals when the catheter has been positioned in the SMA. If an accessory hepatic artery from the SMA is present, the catheter must be placed either distal to this vessel or in the splenic artery.

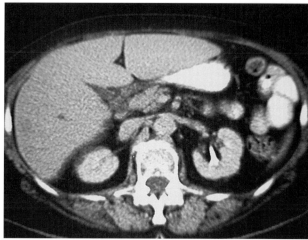

Figure 12. Intravenous (IV) contrast-enhanced hepatic CT scan shows a vague area of diminished density in the right lobe. The examination is inconclusive for the presence of a lesion.

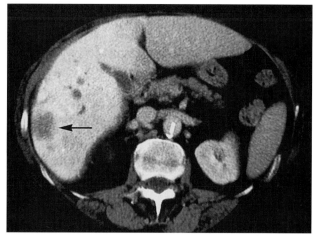

Figure 13. CTAP close to the level depicted in Figure 12 reveals a definite lesion in the right lobe (arrow).

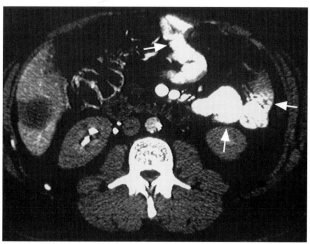

Figure 14. Attempted CTAP. The tip of the arterial catheter has dislodged into a jejunal branch leading to intense contrast staining of the small bowel (arrows).

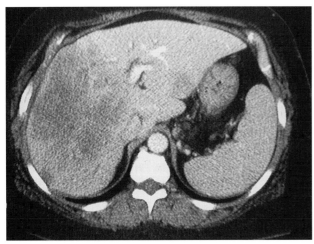

Figure 15. IV contrast-enhanced CT scan shows right lobe and probable lateral segment left lobe metastases.

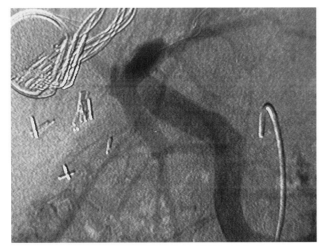

Figure 16. Same patient as in Figure 15. Transarterial (SMA) portogram prior to CTAP reveals right portal vein occlusion.

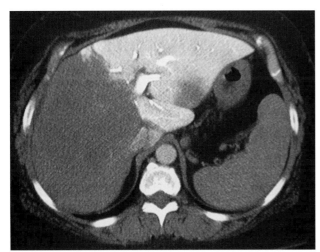

Figure 17. Same patient as in Figure 15. CTAP confirms the left lateral segment metastasis, but the right lobe of the liver is not opacified.

Physiologic problems encountered include laminar flow in the portal vein leading to perfusion defects, focal fatty infiltration of the hepatic parenchyma which may mimic metastases, and portal venous hypertension where portal vein flow may be diverted away from the liver. In addition, focal portal venous occlusion may prevent complete hepatic evaluation **(Figs. 15–17)**.

Overall, the sensitivity of CTAP for the detection of metastatic lesions 1 cm in diameter or larger is greater than 90%. Unfortunately, the sensitivity in detecting smaller lesions appears to be considerably less (40%–60%).

For further information on this topic, please see Tutorial 11.

Selected Readings

Bluemke DA, Fishman EK. Spiral CT arterial portography of the liver. Radiology 1993; 186:576–579.

Chezmar JL, Bernardino ME, Kaufman SH, Nelson RC. Combined CT arterial portography and CT hepatic angiography for evaluation of the hepatic resection candidate: work in progress. Radiology 1993; 189:407–410.

Hughes KS and participants of the Registry of Hepatic Metastases. Resection of the liver for colorectal carcinoma metastases: A multi-institutional study of indications for resection. Surgery 1988; 103:278–288.

Scheele J, Stangl R, Altendorf-Hofmann A. Hepatic metastases from colorectal carcinoma: impact of surgical resection on the natural history. Br J Surg 1990; 77:1241–1246.

Wagner JS, Adson MA, van Heerden JA, Adson MH, Ilstrup DM. The natural history of hepatic metastases from colorectal cancer: a comparison with resective treatment. Ann Surg 1984; 199:502–508.

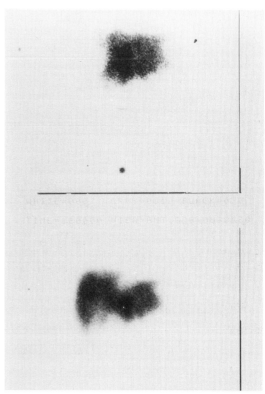

Figure 1. Tc MAA image (top) injected through an indwelling chemotherapeutic infusion pump, and technetium sulfur colloid image (bottom) injected intravenously.

TEACHING FILE CASE 49
Jeffrey L. Groffsky, M.D., and
Ziv J. Haskal, M.D.

History
A 63-year-old man with a history of colon carcinoma diffusely metastatic to the liver had undergone surgical placement of a hepatic arterial pump for chemotherapy. The distal portion of the pump catheter was positioned within the proximal gas-troduodenal artery, which had been ligated distally.

A nuclear medicine study was performed after pump placement to evaluate the distribution of the chemoinfusion **(Fig. 1)**. The upper image was obtained following injection of the pump itself with technetium macroaggregated albumin (Tc MAA). The lower image represents technetium sulfur colloid activity following intravenous administration.

What is your diagnosis?

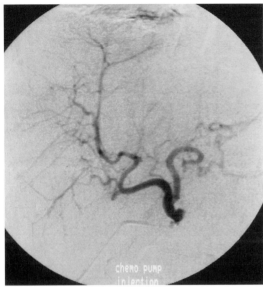

Figure 2. Digital subtraction hepatic arteriogram performed by injection of contrast material through the chemoinfusion pump catheter (arrow) shows right and left hepatic arterial branches.

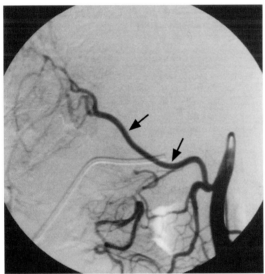

Figure 3. Superior mesenteric arteriogram reveals an accessory right hepatic artery (arrows).

Radiographic Findings

The technetium studies demonstrate a discrepancy in the distribution of activity. A large portion of the right hepatic lobe is unperfused during the chemoinfusion pump injection. Arteriography was performed to further evaluate the scintigraphic findings. Contrast material injection of the chemoinfusion pump confirms only partial perfusion of the right lobe **(Fig. 2)**. A superior mesenteric arteriogram demonstrates a large vessel coursing superolaterally **(Fig. 3)**.

Diagnosis

Accessory right hepatic artery arising from the proximal superior mesenteric artery (SMA).

In this setting, only a portion of the liver affected by metastatic disease will receive intraarterial chemotherapy via pump infusion.

What can be done for this patient?

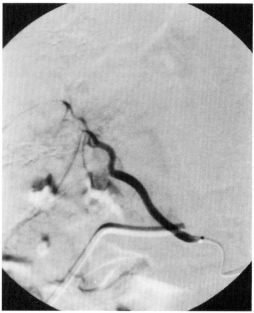

Figure 4. Accessory right hepatic artery is selectively catheterized and embolized.

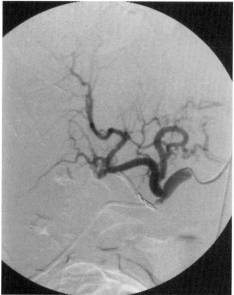

Figure 5. Postembolization arteriogram of the common hepatic artery, early arterial phase, shows a similar distribution to the pump injection shown in Figure 2.

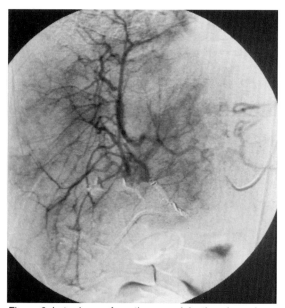

Figure 6. Later image from the same injection shown in Figure 5 demonstrates filling of the accessory right hepatic arterial distribution through intrahepatic collaterals.

Management

Selective embolization can be performed to redirect hepatic arterial flow. In this case, a microcatheter was passed coaxially and placed within the proximal aspect of the accessory right hepatic artery **(Fig. 4)**. The pump catheter can be seen in the mid inferior aspect of the image. Coils were deployed through the microcatheter, with successful embolization of the aberrant vessel **(Fig. 5)**. This early arterial image from the postembolization common hepatic arteriogram shows vascular opacification in the distribution of the original pump injection.

Later in the arterial phase, opacification is seen in the distribution of the embolized accessory right hepatic artery, with filling of vessels right up to the most distally placed coil **(Fig. 6)**. An early parenchymal image **(Fig. 7)** from the same study confirms perfusion of the entire right hepatic lobe. The final image **(Fig. 8)** superimposes the early and late arterial phases, shown in black and white, respectively.

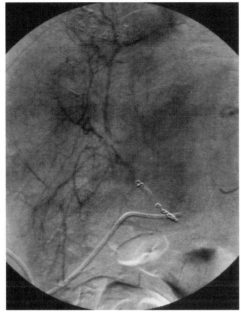

Figure 7. Parenchymal phase image from the common hepatic arterial injection shows opacification of the entire right lobe.

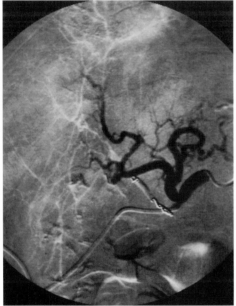

Figure 8. Superimposed early (black) and late (white) arterial phase images from the common hepatic arteriogram confirm perfusion of the entire liver.

Discussion

The anatomic variant of an accessory or replaced hepatic artery occurs in approximately 45% of the population. The most common variants are a replaced right hepatic artery from the SMA (~12%) or a replaced left hepatic artery from the left gastric artery (~10%).

In the clinical setting of intraarterial infusion for hepatic malignancy, an aberrant hepatic artery can result in incomplete distribution of the chemotherapeutic agents, as seen in this case. Selective embolization of the aberrant vessel to redirect flow is usually the simplest and most effective solution to this problem. Proximal occlusion using coils allows redistribution of the arterial supply from a single source. These collaterals are already present, and they enlarge almost instantaneously upon embolization of the aberrant artery. The efficacy of chemoinfusion via the collateral network has been confirmed clinically.

Selected Readings

Chuang VP, Wallace S. Hepatic arterial redistribution for intraarterial infusion of hepatic neoplasms. Radiology 1980; 135:295–299.

Koehler RE, Korobkin M, Lewis F. Arteriographic demonstration of collateral arterial supply to the liver after hepatic artery ligation. Radiology 1975; 117:49–54.

Wallace S, Carrasco CH, Charnsangavej C, Richli WR, Wright K, Gianturco C. Hepatic artery infusion and chemoembolization in the management of liver metastases. Cardiovasc Intervent Radiol 1990; 153–160.

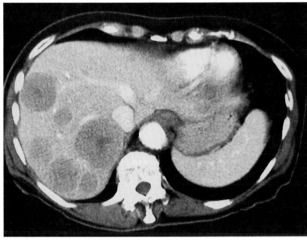

Figure 1. Contrast-enhanced CT scan through the cephalic aspect of the liver.

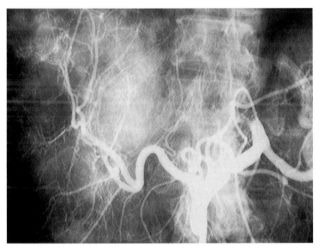

Figure 2. Celiac arteriogram.

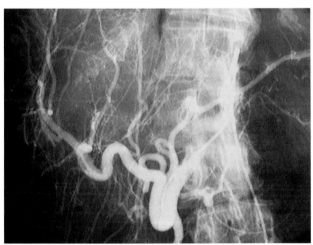

Figure 3. Common hepatic arteriogram.

TEACHING FILE CASE 50
Mark W. Wilson, M.D., and
Robert K. Kerlan Jr., M.D.

History
A 63-year-old woman came to the hospital with a 6-week history of episodic flushing and diarrhea. As part of her evaluation, an abdominal computed tomography (CT) scan **(Fig. 1)**, a celiac arteriogram **(Fig. 2)**, and a common hepatic arteriogram **(Fig. 3)** were obtained.

What is your diagnosis?

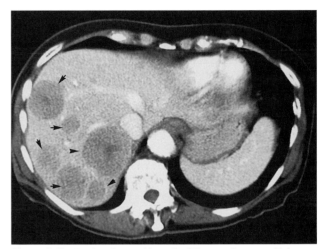

Figure 4. Contrast-enhanced hepatic CT scan shows multiple round lesions with diminished attenuation most compatible with metastatic deposits (arrows).

Radiographic Findings

The contrast-enhanced CT scan of the upper abdomen **(Fig. 4)** reveals multiple low-density hepatic parenchymal lesions predominantly in the right lobe of the liver. The lesions are round and sharply defined, and at least two of them contain central low-density regions suggesting necrosis. The selective celiac arteriogram **(Fig. 5)** and selective hepatic arteriogram **(Fig. 6)** show multiple hypervascular masses within the liver.

Diagnosis

Metastatic carcinoid tumor to the liver.

How would you manage this patient?

Management

When there are four or fewer metastatic deposits in the liver, a valid argument can be made for surgical resection of the primary tumor, usually in the small bowel or appendix, as well as of the hepatic meta-stases. When a larger number of hepatic meta-stases are present, surgical resection is not an option and other strategies must be employed. Systemic chemotherapy with interferon combined with symptomatic control with somatostatin has been successful in some cases.

Figure 5. Celiac arteriogram, mid arterial phase, reveals multiple ill-defined foci of increased vascularity (arrows).

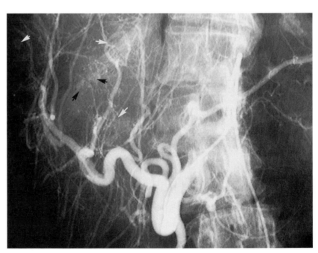

Figure 6. Common hepatic arteriogram, early to mid arterial phase, demonstrates early filling of multiple hypervascular lesions (arrows).

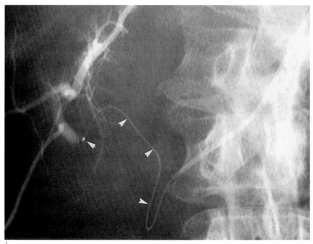

Figure 7. Embolization of the right lobe was performed through a 3-F coaxial catheter (arrowheads).

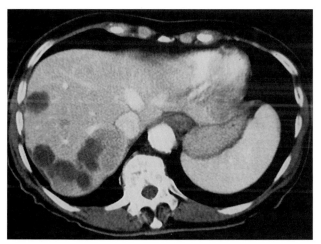

Figure 8. Contrast-enhanced hepatic CT scan 4 weeks after embolization demonstrates necrosis of multiple metastases.

Transcatheter embolization and chemoembolization have been applied to primary and a variety of secondary hepatic neoplasms with mixed results. However, metastatic carcinoid responds to hepatic embolotherapy in a high percentage of cases, and a symptom-free interval of 5 to 10 months can be achieved in more than 90% of patients. The procedure must be conducted with appropriate precautions, however, because the massive release of vasoactive amines can lead to a potentially life-threatening carcinoid crisis. Chemoprophylaxis with octreotide or somatostatin should be administered prior to the procedure. The patient's blood pressure must be closely monitored both during and after embolization.

This patient underwent transcatheter embolization **(Fig. 7)** which palliated her symptoms of flushing and diarrhea. A follow-up CT scan **(Fig. 8)** confirmed the therapeutic response.

Though both bland embolization and chemo-embolization have been applied to metastatic carcinoid tumor, it is unclear which type of therapy is most beneficial. An increase in the length of symptomatic palliation of up to 24 months can be achieved with the addition of the chemotherapeutic agent, but this benefit may be offset by an increased complication rate due to chemotherapeutic agent toxicity.

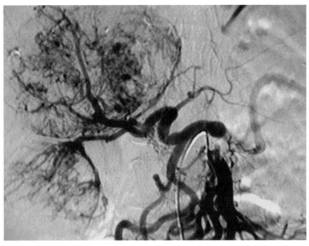

Figure 9. Metastatic hemangiopericytoma in a patient with an occluded celiac trunk origin. The hepatic arteries are opacified via the superior mesenteric arterial injection.

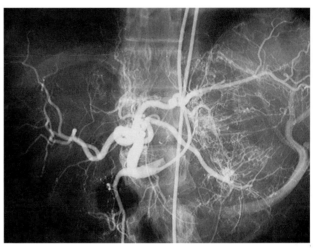

Figure 10. Common hepatic arteriogram shows metastatic leiomyosarcoma to the left lobe.

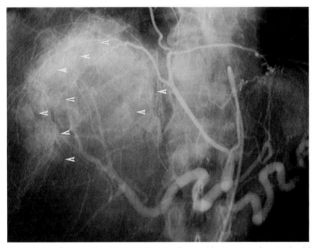

Figure 11. Celiac arteriogram in a patient with metastatic carcinoid tumor to the liver (arrowheads) with parasitization of a right inferior phrenic artery.

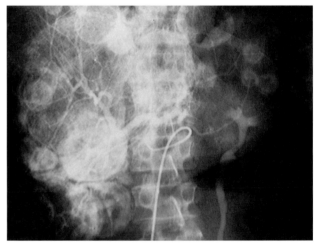

Figure 12. Proper hepatic arteriogram, parenchymal phase, reveals multiple metastases from leiomyosarcoma.

Discussion

Arteriographic examples of other patients with hypervascular metastases are shown in **Figures 9–13**. Hypervascular hepatic metastases are commonly observed with carcinoid tumor, islet cell adenocarcinoma, choriocarcinoma, renal cell carcinoma, thyroid carcinoma, melanoma, and metastatic sarcoma.

Although hepatic arteriography is no longer used to detect metastases, these lesions may be incidentally discovered during arteriography performed for other indications. More frequently, these findings are observed as part of therapeutic planning for either hepatic resection, long-term arterial chemoperfusion (via a surgically implanted pump), or prior to transcatheter embolization therapy.

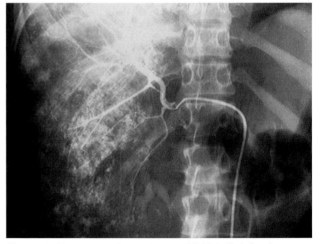

Figure 13. Proper hepatic arteriogram. Multiple ill-defined hypervascular metastases in the right lobe of the liver from choriocarcinoma are present.

Metastatic carcinoid tumor is one type of hypervascular metastasis that responds to transcatheter embolization and chemoembolization. Because of the encouraging response, embolization and chemoembolization have been applied to other types of hypervascular metastases including other neuroendocrine tumors, ocular melanoma, and leiomyosarcomas. The response rate has been mixed. A number of clinical trials with a variety of embolic and chemotherapeutic agents are currently in progress.

For further information on this topic, please see Tutorials 13, 16, and 17, and Teaching File Cases 46, 47, and 51.

Selected Readings

Hajarizadeh H, Ivancev K, Mueller CR, Fletcher WS, Woltering EA. Effective palliative treatment of metastatic carcinoid tumors with intraarterial chemotherapy/ chemoembolization combined with octreotide acetate. Am J Surg 1992; 163:479–483.

Soulen MC. Regional therapy of hepatic malignancies. Presented at the SCVIR 21st Annual Scientific Meeting, Seattle; 1996.

Stokes KR, Stuart K, Clouse ME. Hepatic arterial chemoembolization for metastatic endocrine tumors. J Vasc Interv Radiol 1993; 4:341–345.

Therasse E, Breittmayer F, Roche A, et al. Transcatheter chemoembolization of progressive carcinoid liver metastasis. Radiology 1993; 189:541–547.

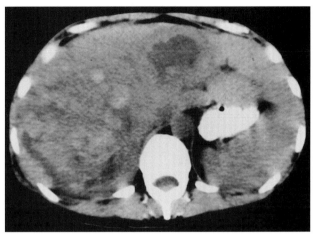

Figure 1. Noncontrast CT scan.

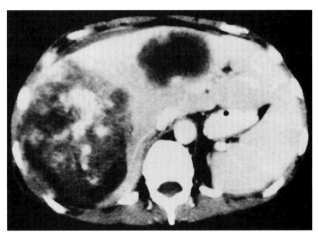

Figure 2. Dynamic contrast-enhanced CT scan.

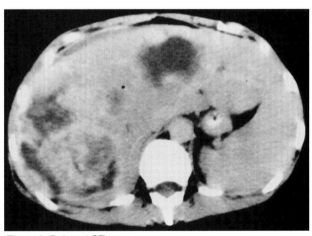

Figure 3. Delayed CT scan.

TEACHING FILE CASE 51
Anthony G. Verstandig, M.D.

History

A 33-year-old woman came to the hospital because of the sudden onset of upper abdominal pain. She was found to be in hypovolemic shock which improved with the administration of intravenous fluids. One year earlier, she had undergone left mastectomy for an angiosarcoma. Noncontrast and dynamic contrast-enhanced computed tomography (CT) scans were obtained **(Figs. 1, 2). Figure 3** is a scan obtained 6 minutes after injection of contrast material.

What is your diagnosis?

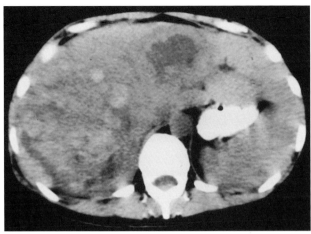

Figure 4. Noncontrast CT scan shows liver masses of mixed density. Hyperdense areas are compatible with acute hemorrhage.

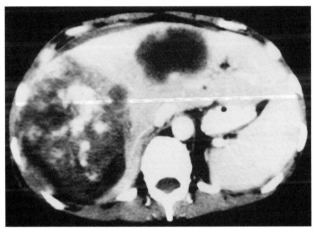

Figure 5. Dynamic contrast-enhanced CT scan reveals predominantly hypodense masses with areas of hyperdensity.

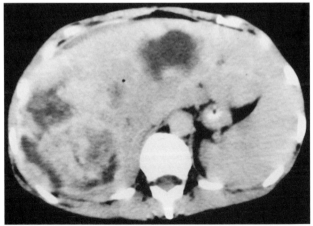

Figure 6. Delayed CT scan demonstrates partial filling in of the masses.

Radiographic Findings

On the unenhanced scan **(Fig. 4)**, large masses are seen in both lobes of the liver with areas of hypo- and isodensity relative to normal liver parenchyma. The larger right lobe mass also contains areas of hyperdensity representing fresh hematoma. Dynamic scanning after injection of contrast material **(Fig. 5)** shows the main part of the masses to be hypodense, with scattered areas of hyperdensity, particularly in the right lobe mass. Repeat scanning after 6 minutes **(Fig. 6)** shows partial filling in of both masses. The patient underwent arteriography.

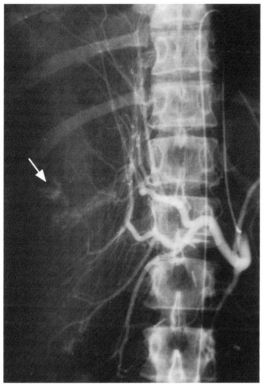

Figure 7. Hepatic arteriogram shows extravasation of contrast material into a right hepatic mass (arrow).

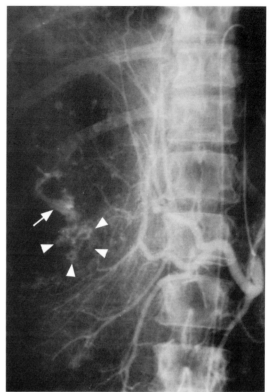

Figure 8. Later film from the arteriogram shows further extravasation (arrow) and filling of vascular lakes (arrowheads).

Selective hepatic arteriography **(Fig. 7)** demonstrates a large right lobe mass causing displacement and splaying of arterial branches. There is active extravasation of contrast material into the mass. A later film **(Fig. 8)** shows continued extravasation and filling of numerous small vascular lakes. A parenchymal phase film shows the mass as a hypodense defect in the right lobe **(Fig. 9)**.

Diagnosis
Spontaneous bleeding from hepatic metastases presumably secondary to breast angiosarcoma.

The right lobe mass on the CT scan represents tumor with fresh hematoma. The hyperdense areas on the post-contrast scan represent a combination of extravasated contrast material and vascular lakes. The arteriographic appearance is similar to that of the much more common hemangioma; however, spontaneous bleeding from hemangiomas is rare, and the history of breast angiosarcoma is key in establishing the correct diagnosis.

How would you manage this patient?

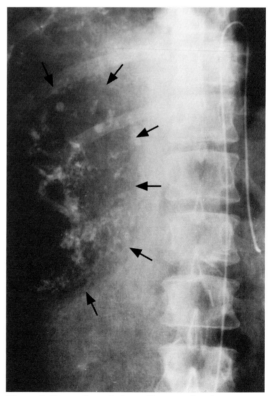

Figure 9. Parenchymal phase film reveals a hypovascular defect (arrows), indicative of the true mass size.

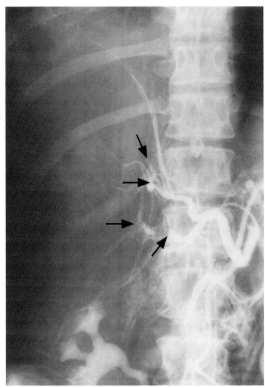

Figure 10. Postembolization hepatic arteriogram shows occlusion of multiple hepatic arterial branches (arrows) and no further extravasation of contrast material.

Management

It was elected to perform transcatheter embolization to achieve hemodynamic stability prior to surgical resection of the bleeding metastases. Before embolization, superior mesenteric arteriography was performed to confirm patency of the portal vein. The hepatic artery was subsequently embolized with small pieces of Gelfoam (Upjohn, Kalamazoo, MI). Postembolization selective hepatic arteriography **(Fig. 10)** demonstrates successful occlusion of multiple hepatic arterial branches and no extravasation of contrast material. The patient underwent resection of the right lobe of the liver with an uneventful postoperative course and died 5 months later from her disease.

Discussion

Transcatheter embolization can be life-saving in the treatment of acute bleeding. Arterial blockade can be achieved with gelatin sponge or polyvinyl alcohol particles. In the liver, a patent portal vein provides sufficient blood flow to prevent extensive necrosis of normal hepatic tissue.

Angiosarcoma of the liver is a rare malignancy that can be primary, often related to exposure to toxins such as vinyl chloride and thorotrast, or metastatic from a remote site. Both pathologically and radiologically it has similarities to cavernous hemangioma.

For further information on this topic, please see Tutorials 13, 16, and 17, and Teaching File Cases 46, 47, and 50.

Selected Readings

Whelan JG Jr, Creech JL, Tamburro CH. Angiographic and radionuclide characteristics of hepatic angiosarcoma found in vinyl chloride workers. Radiology 1976; 118:549–557.

White PG, Adams H, Smith PM. The computed tomographic appearances of angiosarcoma of the liver. Clin Radiol 1993; 48:321–325.

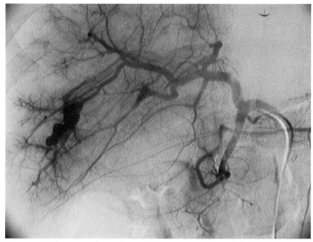

Figure 1. Common hepatic arteriogram, mid arterial phase.

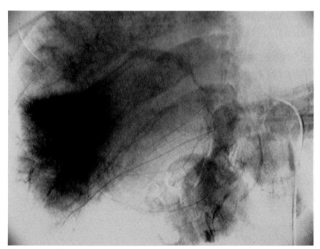

Figure 2. Common hepatic arteriogram, parenchymal phase.

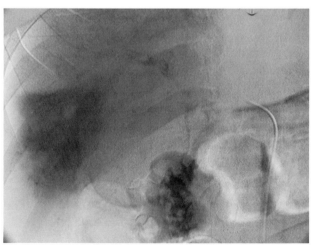

Figure 3. Common hepatic arteriogram, delayed film.

TEACHING FILE CASE 52
Robert K. Kerlan Jr., M.D., and
Shelley R. Marder, M.D.

History
A 28-year-old man underwent a percutaneous liver biopsy with a 15-gauge needle to evaluate acute hepatic dysfunction. Following the biopsy, the patient developed hematemesis and melena. An upper gastrointestinal endoscopy was performed and showed blood in the stomach and duodenum without evidence of a bleeding source. The patient underwent arteriography (Figs. 1–3).

What is your diagnosis?

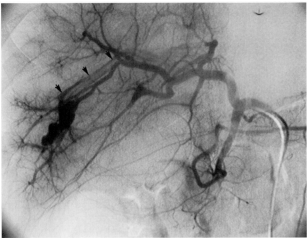

Figure 4. Common hepatic arteriogram, mid arterial phase, shows a complex pseudoaneurysm of a right hepatic arterial branch. Opacification of a linear structure (arrows) representing a bile duct adjacent to the artery is also seen.

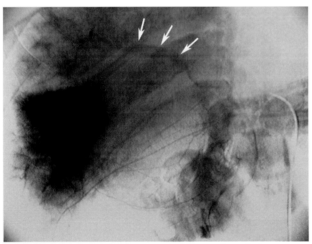

Figure 5. Common hepatic arteriogram, parenchymal phase, reveals contrast opacification of the right hepatic duct (arrows).

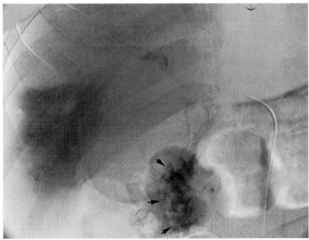

Figure 6. Delayed film from the hepatic arteriogram demonstrates contrast material outlining duodenal mucosal folds (arrows).

Radiographic Findings

The early arterial phase **(Fig. 4)** of the common hepatic arteriogram shows a focal abnormality of a right hepatic arterial branch. The mid arterial phase **(Fig. 5)** depicts a linear collection of contrast material that parallels the arterial branch in the liver then turns caudally as it extends more medially. A film obtained 20 seconds after the termination of the arterial injection **(Fig. 6)** shows contrast material in the duodenum.

Diagnosis

False aneurysm of a right hepatic arterial branch with extravasation into a biliary ductal radicle resulting in massive hemobilia.

How would you manage this patient?

Management

When a hepatic arterial injury leading to hemobilia is identified, selective embolization should be performed to occlude the damaged vessel. Embolization should be as selective as possible and ideally should occlude the vessel both proximal and distal to the area of injury. With this technique, recurrent hemorrhage from collateral arterial supply can be effectively avoided.

This patient underwent selective embolization with Gelfoam pledgets (Upjohn, Kalamazoo, MI) and stainless steel coils. A postembolization arteriogram **(Fig. 7)** confirms successful occlusion of the damaged artery. Arteriograms from other patients with hemobilia are shown in **Figures 8–14**.

Discussion

Hemobilia can be secondary to a number of etiologies including gallstone disease, primary vascular abnormalities, neoplasms, and trauma. Iatrogenic trauma is by far the most frequent cause, being observed in 4% of patients following percutaneous transhepatic cholangiography, 5% after percutaneous liver biopsy, and up to 25% subsequent to placement of a transhepatic biliary drain. Undoubtedly, the majority of these injuries are self-limited and have no significant clinical sequelae. On occasion, however, the injury is more serious and may even be life-threatening.

The classic clinical presentation of hemobilia includes the triad of right upper quadrant pain, jaundice, and gastrointestinal bleeding. Unfortunately, these classic features are present in fewer than 50% of patients. Yoshida et al reported a series of 103 patients with hemobilia due to a variety of causes in which the initial diagnosis of hemobilia was made intraoperatively in 34% of the patients, angiographically in 28%, and endoscopically in 12%. The remainder were related to percutaneous biliary drainage. In patients who have undergone percutaneous biliary drainage, significant hemobilia is usually apparent by inspection of the drainage tube effluent.

It should be noted that bleeding following percutaneous hepatic interventions is not always manifested as hemobilia. Intraperitoneal hemorrhage may result from injury to a hepatic, mesenteric, or intercostal artery branch. In the unstable patient with hemoperitoneum, prompt surgical exploration may be warranted.

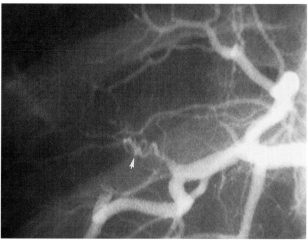

Figure 7. Gelfoam and coil embolization (arrow) were performed, successfully occluding the artery.

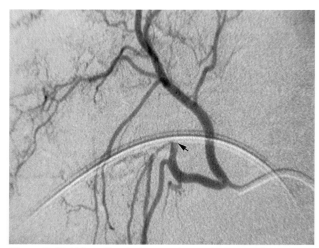

Figure 8. Right hepatic arteriogram demonstrates an abrupt cutoff (arrow) of a right hepatic arterial branch but no evidence of extravasation. This appearance is not infrequent when the tube is tamponading the arterial laceration.

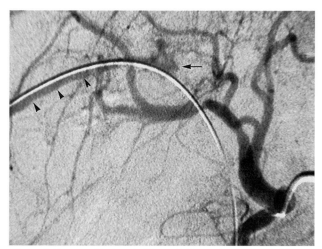

Figure 9. Same patient as in Figure 8. Repeat selective right hepatic arteriogram following removal of the biliary drainage tube over a guide wire shows parenchymal extravasation (arrow) as well as extravasation into the transhepatic track (arrowheads).

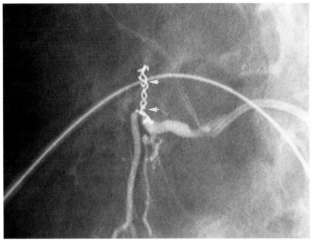

Figure 10. Same patient as in Figures 6 and 7. Subselective right hepatic arteriogram following embolization with platinum microcoils (arrows) confirms successful occlusion of the damaged arterial branch.

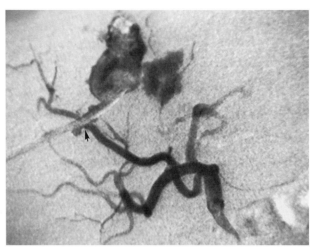

Figure 11. Right hepatic arteriogram demonstrates a laceration of a right hepatic arterial branch (arrow) caused by a percutaneous hepatic abscess drainage catheter.

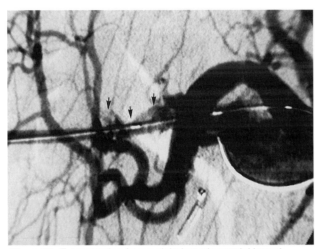

Figure 12. Extravasation from a right hepatic arterial branch (arrows) secondary to a transhepatic biliary drainage catheter.

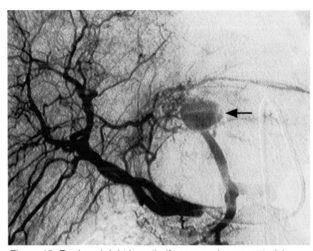

Figure 13. Replaced right hepatic (from superior mesenteric) arteriogram reveals a left hepatic artery pseudoaneurysm (arrow) secondary to blunt trauma. The aneurysm is filling via intrahepatic collaterals.

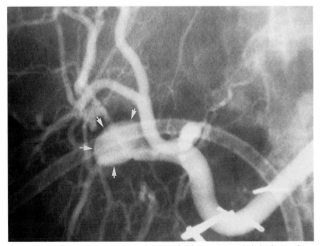

Figure 14. Pseudoaneurysm (arrows) of a proximal right hepatic arterial branch secondary to a transhepatic biliary drainage catheter.

In contrast, the source of hemobilia cannot always be easily identified and managed with open surgical techniques; in these cases, arteriography is the procedure of choice. If hemobilia has occurred after placement of a transhepatic drainage tube, it may be necessary to remove the tube temporarily over a guide wire in order to identify the site of bleeding. Only 25% of patients will have direct extravasation from the hepatic artery into the biliary system. Bleeding sites are more frequently manifested as a focus of ill-defined extravasation **(Fig. 12)**, a pseudoaneurysm **(Figs. 13, 14)**, or the presence of a hepatic artery to portal vein fistula. Fistulas extending from the hepatic artery to the hepatic vein are unusual.

When a potential arterial bleeding source is identified, embolization should be performed as selectively as possible. The embolization is most effective when the artery both proximal and distal to the arterial injury is occluded. A combination of metallic coils and Gelfoam pledgets is appropriate for most cases, and clinical as well as anatomic success can be achieved in up to 95% of patients.

A more problematic situation occurs when there is a high clinical suspicion of hemobilia but the source cannot be identified arteriographically. A significant percentage of these arteriograms are falsely negative. If a percutaneous drainage tube has been placed, the source is sometimes revealed by injection of contrast material into the percutaneous track. This is accomplished by removing the drainage tube over a guide wire and inserting a vascular access sheath. The side-arm of the sheath is injected with contrast material as the sheath is slowly retracted through the track. Digital subtraction imaging during this maneuver will often reveal the offending vessel. When hemobilia is secondary to iatrogenic trauma, empiric arterial embolization of the most likely anatomic site is sometimes performed.

For further information on this topic, please see Tutorials 13 and 18.

Selected Readings

D'Agostino RD, Josephs LG. Hemobilia. In: Pitt HA, Carr-Locke DL, Ferrucci JT, eds. Hepatobiliary and pancreatic disease: the team approach to management. 1st edition. Boston: Little, Brown and Company, 1995; 101.

Olcott EW, Saxon RR, Ring EJ, Gordon RL. Catheter tract hemorrhage during percutaneous biliary intervention: management with use of a retained transhepatic guide wire. J Vasc Interv Radiol 1995; 6:433–438.

Schwartz RA, Teitelbaum GP, Katz MD, Pentecost MJ. Effectiveness of transcatheter embolization in the control of hepatic vascular injuries. J Vasc Interv Radiol 1993; 4:359–365.

Yoshida J, Donahue PE, Nyhus LM. Hemobilia: review of recent experience with a worldwide problem. Am J Gastroenterol 1987; 82:448–453.

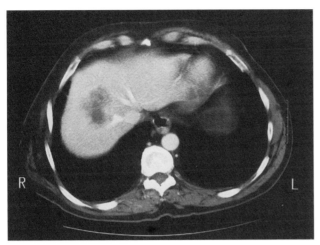

Figure 1. Contrast-enhanced CT image through the cephalic aspect of the liver.

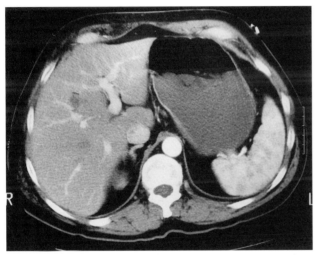

Figure 2. Contrast-enhanced CT image through the mid portion of the liver.

TEACHING FILE CASE 53
Sandra J. Althaus, M.D.

History
A 52-year-old man came to the hospital with metastatic colon cancer to the liver. The patient was being evaluated for a trisegmentectomy. A spiral abdominal computed tomography (CT) scan was obtained at 7-mm contiguous intervals during the administration of intravenous contrast material **(Figs. 1, 2)**.

What is your diagnosis?

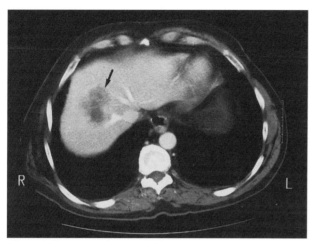

Figure 3. Contrast-enhanced CT image through the cephalic aspect of liver shows a 5-cm x 4-cm lesion (arrow) in the anterior segment of the right lobe.

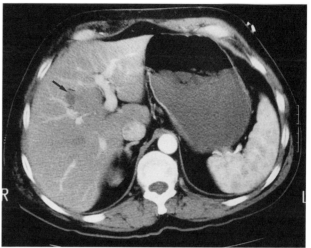

Figure 4. A 2-cm x 2-cm lesion (arrow) is present in the medial segment of the left lobe.

Radiographic Findings

A 5-cm x 4-cm lesion was identified in the anterior segment of the right lobe of the liver (Couinaud segment 8) **(Fig. 3)**. An additional lesion was seen in the medial segment of the left lobe of the liver (Couinaud segment 4) which measures approximately 2 cm x 2 cm **(Fig. 4)**.

Diagnosis

Metastatic colon carcinoma to the liver.

Management

Because the lateral segment of the left lobe showed no evidence of tumor, the patient was considered to be a candidate for trisegmentectomy. Preoperative selective right portal vein embolization was performed to stimulate hypertrophy of the left lobe.

With use of ultrasound guidance, a 21-gauge needle was advanced into the liver via a right mid axillary approach, and a right portal vein branch was punctured. A guide wire was advanced into the right portal vein, and a 5.5-F cobra catheter was placed **(Fig. 5)**. Portal venography was performed at an injection rate of 10 mL per second for 30 mL. The right portal vein branches were selectively catheterized. Embolization of the right portal vein branches was carried out with twelve 3-mm Gianturco coils (Cook, Bloomington, IN), eight 5-mm Gianturco coils, and two 8-mm Gianturco coils **(Fig. 6)**.

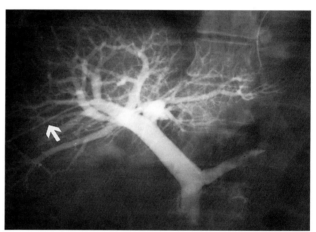

Figure 5. Portal venogram obtained through a transhepatic catheter (arrow) inserted through a right portal venous branch.

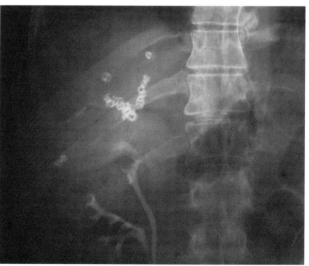

Figure 6. Multiple stainless steel coils have been deposited into right portal vein branches.

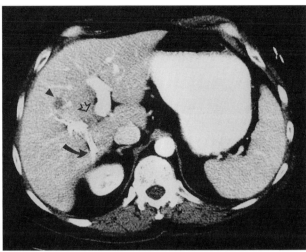

Figure 7. Contrast-enhanced CT scan reveals clot within the right portal vein (open arrow), a streak artifact from a stainless steel coil (curved arrow), and hepatic metastasis (arrowhead).

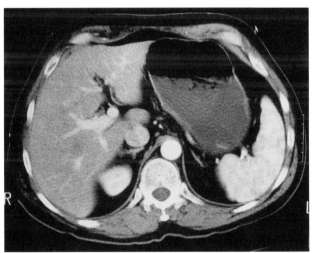

Figure 8. CT scan obtained before right portal venous embolization.

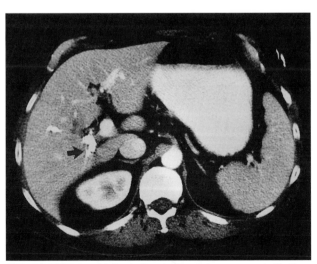

Figure 9. CT scan obtained after right portal venous embolization. Stainless steel coils (arrow) are present within right portal venous branches, and the lateral segment of the left lobe has enlarged slightly.

A follow-up CT scan was obtained 1 month after the embolization **(Fig. 7)**. Thrombus is visualized in the right portal vein. The left lateral segment of the liver has enlarged slightly. The general time span for liver hypertrophy after embolization is approximately 3 weeks. Comparable pre- and postprocedure scans at a lower level are shown in **Figures 8** and **9**.

Selected Readings

de Baere T, Roche A, Vavasseur D, et al. Portal vein embolization: utility for inducing left hepatic lobe hypertrophy before surgery. Radiology 1993; 188:73–77.

Elias D, Lasser P, Rougier P, Ducreux M, Bognel C, Roche A. Frequency, technical aspects, results, and indications of major hepatectomy after prolonged intraarterial hepatic chemotherapy for initially unresectable hepatic tumors. J Am Coll Surg 1995; 180:213–219.

Nagino M, Nimura Y, Kamiya J, et al. Changes in hepatic lobe volume in biliary tract cancer patients after right portal vein embolization. Hepatology 1995; 21:434–439.

Soyer P, Roche A, Elias D, Levesque M. Hepatic metastases from colorectal cancer: influence of hepatic volumetric analysis on surgical decision making. Radiology 1992; 184:695–697.

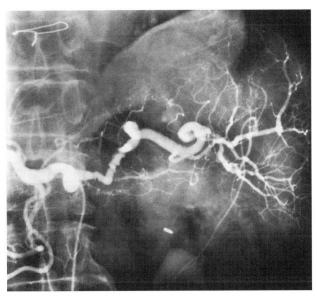

Figure 1. Celiac arteriogram.

TEACHING FILE CASE 54
J. Mark McKinney, M.D., and
James C. Andrews, M.D.

History

A 67-year-old man came to the hospital with abdominal pain that was clinically characteristic of mesenteric ischemia. A visceral arteriogram was obtained for further evaluation **(Fig. 1)**.

What is your diagnosis?

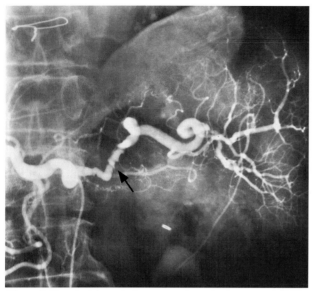

Figure 2. Serrated, irregularly narrowed proximal splenic artery (arrow).

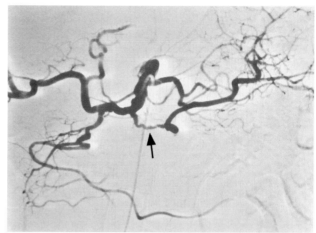

Figure 3. More severely stenotic and serrated splenic artery (arrow).

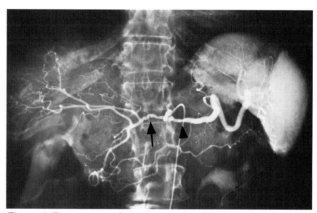

Figure 4. Encasement of the common hepatic (arrow) and splenic arteries (arrowhead).

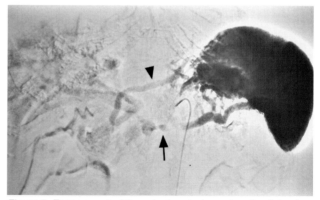

Figure 5. Encasement of the splenic vein (arrow) and collateral flow via the coronary vein (arrowhead).

Radiographic Findings

The celiac arteriogram (**Fig. 2**) demonstrates a segment of proximal splenic artery that is irregularly stenotic and serrated.

Diagnosis

Arterial encasement by pancreatic adenocarcinoma.

Discussion

With the availability of spiral computed tomography, magnetic resonance, and ultrasound imaging, arteriography is rarely performed for the diagnosis of pancreatic or abdominal neoplasms. However, as in this case, an unsuspected neoplasm may be discovered during the work-up of other diseases. It is important to recognize the characteristic findings of vascular encasement. The arterial narrowing is most often irregular and serrated. Arterial or venous occlusion may also occur. Correlation with other imaging modalities is helpful to confirm the presence of extravascular tumor. The appearance of neoplastic vascular encasement may be simulated by pancreatitis, vasculitis, or previous surgery.

Figures 3–5 are arteriograms from other patients with pancreatic carcinoma. **Figure 3** reveals isolated encasement of the proximal splenic artery. **Figure 4** displays involvement of both the common hepatic and splenic arteries. **Figure 5** is the venous phase of a celiac artery injection. The splenic vein is encased by tumor and the coronary vein is serving as a hepatopetal collateral.

For further information on this topic, please see Tutorial 12.

Selected Readings

Bookstein JJ, Reuter SR, Martel W. Angiographic evaluation of pancreatic carcinoma. Radiology 1969; 93:757–764.

Kadir S. Diagnostic angiography. Philadelphia: W.B. Saunders Company, 1986; 416–439.

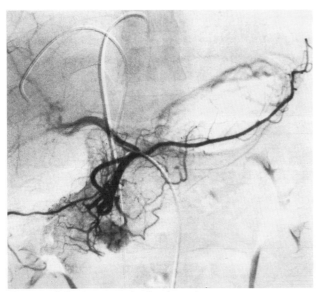

Figure 1. Selective gastroduodenal arteriogram.

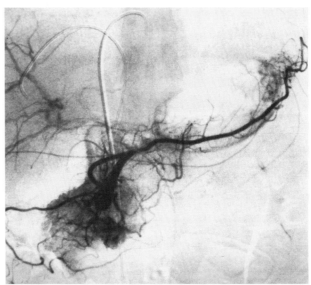

Figure 2. Selective gastroduodenal arteriogram, late arterial phase.

Time (secs)	GDA		SMA		Splenic Artery	
	RHV	LHV	RHV	LHV	RHV	LHV
0	43	36	32	36	51	39
30	200	140	44	48	84	68
60	650	276	52	50	92	75
120	324	203	48	38	93	82

Figure 3. Insulin levels obtained from the right and left hepatic veins following infusion of calcium gluconate into the GDA, the superior mesenteric artery, and the splenic artery.

TEACHING FILE CASE 55
Eric W. Olcott, M.D.

History
A 57-year-old man came to the hospital with intermittent fasting hypoglycemia. Laboratory studies disclosed elevated serum insulin levels. A beta cell tumor (insulinoma) was suspected.

Because preoperative localization of such tumors is of great help to the surgeon attempting resection, imaging studies were ordered. Ultrasound (US), computed tomography (CT) scanning, and magnetic resonance (MR) imaging, however, failed to demonstrate any definite lesion.

A visceral arteriogram including selective gastroduodenal artery (GDA) injections was obtained (Figs. 1, 2), and a calcium gluconate arterial infusion study with hepatic venous sampling (Fig. 3) was performed.

What is your diagnosis?

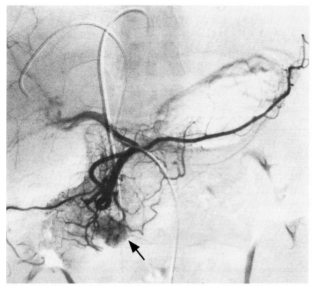

Figure 4. A hypervascular lesion is present in the pancreatic head (arrow).

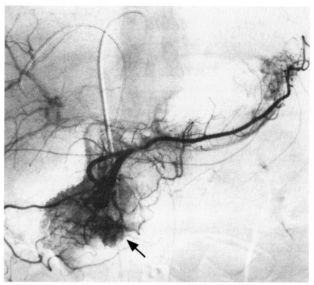

Figure 5. On later images, the hypervascular lesion becomes more conspicuous (arrow).

Radiographic Findings
Selective gastroduodenal arteriography shows a 15–20-mm area of hypervascularity in the pancreatic head **(Figs. 4, 5)**. The calcium gluconate infusion study indicates that the lesion is located in the distribution of the gastroduodenal artery.

Diagnosis
Insulinoma of the pancreatic head.

Discussion
Localization of occult islet cell tumors can be difficult. Arteriography of the pancreatic arterial supply is one option. Another is transhepatic portal venous sampling, in which the insulin concentrations in blood samples from multiple branches of the portal venous system are measured. This rather involved procedure is usually reserved for tumors not localized by other means. The location of the lesion is inferred from the portal branches carrying the highest hormone levels. A more recently reported approach is to stimulate insulin release with intraarterial calcium gluconate while conducting hepatic venous insulin sampling, usually in conjunction with pancreatic arteriography, as described by Doppman et al.

The pancreas is supplied by the splenic artery, the gastroduodenal artery, and the superior mesenteric artery (SMA). The GDA and SMA supply the head and the uncinate process of the pancreas; the splenic artery supplies the body and tail **(Fig 6)**.

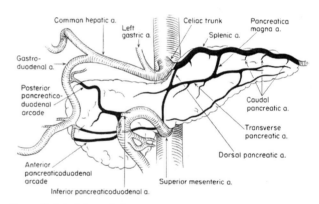

Figure 6. Arterial supply to pancreas.

Calcium gluconate injected into an artery feeding an insulinoma stimulates release of insulin. The hormone traverses the portal system, hepatic sinusoids, and hepatic veins. A rise in hepatic venous insulin in response to selective injection of a particular artery serves to localize the insulin source to the territory served by that artery.

In this patient, calcium gluconate was infused in conjunction with selective arteriography of the GDA, SMA, and splenic artery. Insulin sampling was conducted via catheters in the right and left hepatic veins. Venous samples were obtained at 0 seconds, 30 seconds, 60 seconds, and 120 seconds after infusion. Doppman et al consider a doubling of the venous insulin concentration from baseline to constitute a positive localizing result.

In this case, interventional biochemical provocation may have been unnecessary as the tumor was identified arteriographically. However, the calcium gluconate procedure is extremely helpful in cases where arteriography is unrevealing. Doppman et al report that arteriography with biochemical provocation has greater sensitivity than arteriography alone for the detection of insulinomas. This technique is an attractive alternative to transhepatic portal venous sampling. In the present case, surgery revealed a 14-mm diameter insulinoma in the head of the pancreas.

For further information on this topic, please see Tutorial 12.

Selected Readings

Doppman JL, Miller DL, Chang R, Gorden P, Eastman RC, Norton JA. Intraarterial calcium stimulation test for detection of insulinomas. World J Surg 1993; 17:439–443.

Doppman JL, Miller DL, Chang R, Shawker TH, Gorden P, Norton JA. Insulinomas: localization with selective intraarterial injection of calcium. Radiology 1991; 178:237–241.

King CM, Reznek RH, Dacie JE, Wass JA. Imaging islet cell tumors. Clin Radiol 1994; 49:295–303.

End Notes

Figure 6 from Reuter SR, Redman HC, Cho KJ. Gastrointestinal angiography. In: Saunders monographs in clinical radiology. 3rd edition. Philadelphia: W.B. Saunders Company, 1986. Used with permission.

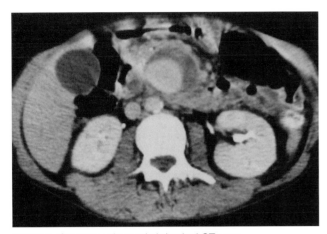

Figure 1. Contrast-enhanced abdominal CT scan.

TEACHING FILE CASE 56
Linda J. Bagley, M.D.,
Ziv J. Haskal, M.D., and
Roy L. Gordon, M.D.

History
A 58-year-old man with a history of alcohol abuse, pancreatitis, and a known pseudocyst came to the hospital with acute worsening of abdominal pain and hypotension.

An abdominal computed tomography (CT) scan was obtained **(Fig. 1)**.

What is your diagnosis?

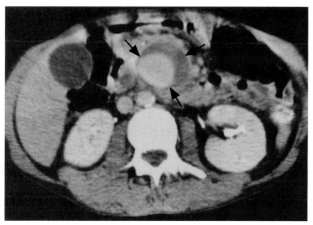

Figure 2. Contrast-enhanced abdominal CT scan shows an abnormal accumulation of contrast material (arrows) in the pancreas, most compatible with a pseudoaneurysm.

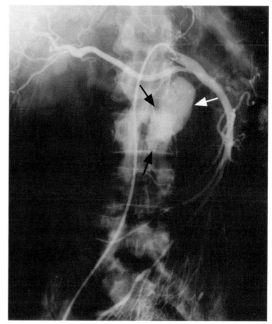

Figure 3. Superior mesenteric arteriogram reveals a pseudoaneurysm (arrows) medial to the SMA and caudal to the replaced right hepatic artery.

Radiographic Findings

The contrast-enhanced CT scan reveals an approximately 4-cm enhancing, round structure representing a partially thrombosed pseudoaneurysm in the region of the patient's known pseudocyst **(Fig. 2)**.

A visceral arteriogram was obtained **(Fig. 3)**. Injection of the superior mesenteric artery (SMA) reveals a large pseudoaneurysm arising from the inferior pancreaticoduodenal artery. There is leftward displacement of the superior mesenteric artery. The large thrombosed portion of the pseudoaneurysm accounts for the mass effect exceeding the opacified size of the aneurysm. The right hepatic artery arises from the superior mesenteric artery.

Diagnoses

1. Pancreatic pseudocyst with pseudoaneurysm of the inferior pancreaticoduodenal branch of the superior mesenteric artery.
2. Replaced right hepatic artery from the superior mesenteric artery.

What are the therapeutic options?

Management

A microcatheter was advanced coaxially through a cobra catheter, into the pseudoaneurysm **(Fig. 4)**. The pseudoaneurysm was occluded by the placement of a nest of platinum coils within the inferior pancreaticoduodenal artery proximal to the aneurysm.

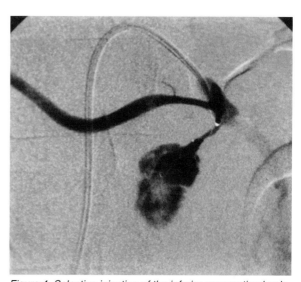

Figure 4. Selective injection of the inferior pancreaticoduodenal artery delineates the origin of the false aneurysm.

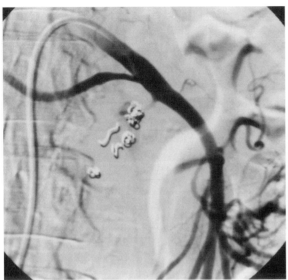

Figure 5. Postembolization superior mesenteric arteriogram confirms occlusion of the pseudoaneurysm.

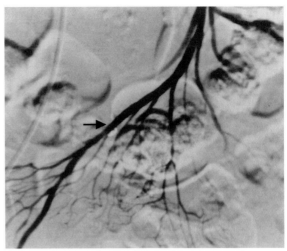

Figure 6. Postembolization digital subtraction superior mesenteric arteriogram reveals flow around the nonocclusive coil (arrow).

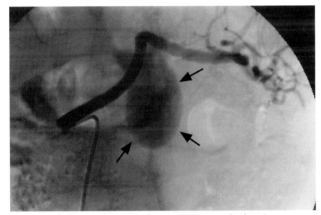

Figure 7. Celiac arteriogram demonstrates a splenic artery pseudoaneurysm (arrows).

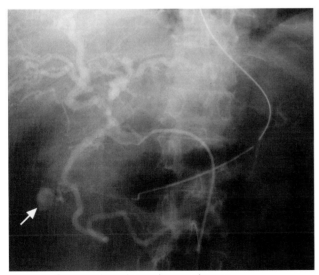

Figure 8. Common hepatic arteriogram shows a pseudoaneurysm (arrow) of the gastroduodenal artery.

The postembolization arteriogram (Fig. 5) demonstrates successful occlusion of the pseudoaneurysm. After embolization, the patient's abdominal pain resolved, and he became hemodynamically stable. At 1 month follow-up, he remained asymptomatic. A single coil had been inadvertently deposited into an ileal branch of the superior mesenteric artery. Repeat superior mesenteric angiography revealed flow around the nonocclusive coil (Fig. 6).

Discussion

While the incidence of hemorrhage of arterial origin complicating pancreatitis is low, occurring in only 1%–10% of patients, it can lead to significant morbidity and mortality. Patients with acute pancreatitis or pseudocysts can release intensely lytic enzymes that may erode into pancreatic vessels or adjacent visceral arteries, leading to pseudoaneurysm formation or frank bleeding. Intracystic, gastrointestinal, pancreatic ductal, intraperitoneal, or retroperitoneal hemorrhage may ensue.

The splenic and gastroduodenal arteries are the vessels most commonly affected in pancreatitis. Celiac arteriograms (Figs. 7, 8) obtained in two other patients with chronic pancreatitis demonstrate pseudoaneurysms of the splenic and gastroduodenal arteries, respectively.

Surgical Therapy

Surgical therapy for bleeding pseudocysts may entail resection of the involved pancreatic segment and/or ligation of the bleeding vessels accompanied by pseudocyst drainage. Estimates of mortality following operative management range from 12% to 56%, with the higher rates accompanying treatment of pancreatic head lesions.

Arteriography

Endoscopy, barium studies, and scintigraphy may fail to reveal the etiology of hemorrhage in the actively bleeding patient with chronic pancreatitis. Selective visceral arteriography during such active bleeding may demonstrate extravasation and/or pseudoaneurysm formation. Additional complications, such as venous thromboses, may also be detected. The venous phase of a celiac arteriogram from a patient with chronic pancreatitis is shown in **Figure 9**. It demonstrates splenic vein occlusion, multiple splenic hilar varices, retrograde flow in the coronary vein, and collateral splenic drainage through the gastroepiploic vein.

Percutaneous Embolization

Embolic materials used in the successful treatment of vascular lesions secondary to pancreatitis have included coils, thrombin, Gelfoam (Upjohn, Kalamazoo, MI), autologous clot, and detachable balloons. Such embolotherapy may be complicated by errant embolization, ischemia, and recurrent hemorrhage but is associated with lower morbidity and mortality than comparable open surgical procedures. Percutaneous therapy may serve as a temporizing, preoperative measure in the acutely unstable patient, or it may provide definitive therapy.

For further information on this topic, please see Tutorial 13 and Teaching File Case 57.

Selected Readings

Boudghene F, L'Hermine C, Bigot J. Arterial complications of pancreatitis: diagnostic and therapeutic aspects in 104 cases. J Vasc Interv Radiol 1993; 4:551–558.

el Hamel A, Parc R, Adda G, Bouteloup PY, Huguet C, Malafosse M. Bleeding pseudocysts and pseudo-aneurysms in chronic pancreatitis. Br J Surg 1991; 78:1059–1063.

Gadacz TR, Trunkey D, Kieffer RF. Visceral vessel erosion associated with pancreatitis: case reports and a review of the literature. Arch Surg 1978; 113:1438–1440.

Steckman ML, Dooley MC, Jaques PF, Powell DW. Major gastrointestinal hemorrhage from peripancreatic blood vessels in pancreatitis: treatment by embolotherapy. Dig Dis Sci 1984; 29:486–497.

Vujic I. Vascular complications of pancreatitis. Radiol Clin North Am 1989; 27:81–91.

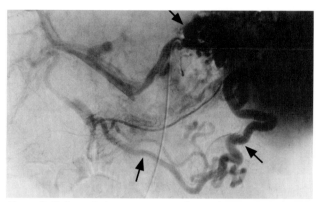

Figure 9. Celiac arteriogram, venous phase, demonstrates splenic vein occlusion. Collateral veins (arrows) are present.

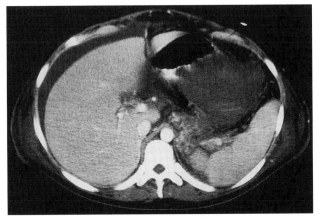

Figure 1. Contrast-enhanced abdominal CT scan.

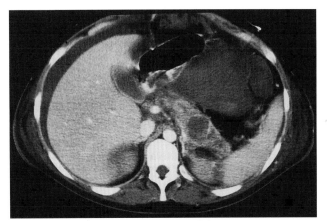

Figure 2. Contrast-enhanced abdominal CT scan.

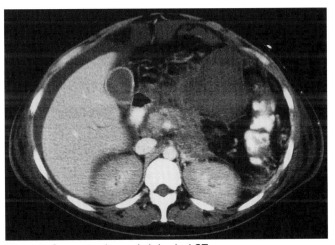

Figure 3. Contrast-enhanced abdominal CT scan.

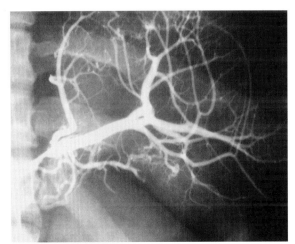

Figure 4. Splenic arteriogram.

TEACHING FILE CASE 57
Jeet Sandhu, M.D.

History
A patient experiencing an acute episode of chronic relapsing pancreatitis secondary to excessive alcohol consumption came to the hospital because of increasing abdominal pain. Abdominal computed tomography (CT) scanning **(Figs. 1–3)** and visceral arteriography were performed. The splenic injection is shown in **Figure 4**.

What is your diagnosis?

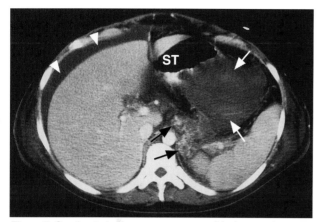

Figure 5. Swollen heterogeneous pancreas (black arrows) contiguous with a lesser sac fluid collection behind the stomach (ST). Fluid in the lesser sac (white arrows) is slightly higher in density than ascites (white arrowheads).

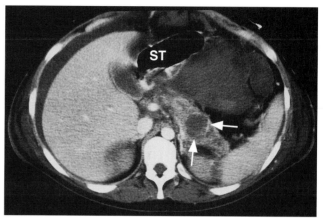

Figure 6. Higher-density fluid in the lesser sac is again demonstrated. An evolving pseudocyst (arrows) is present in the pancreas.

Radiographic Findings

Selected transaxial CT images of the abdomen **(Figs. 5–7)** demonstrate a heterogeneous pancreas with swelling of the gland and loss of the normal fatty interdigitation that should be present in older patients. The fluid in the lesser sac has a higher density than the ascites around the liver. The higher density of the lesser sac fluid should suggest the possibility of acute hemorrhage or contrast material extravasation. There is contiguity of the pancreas with the lesser sac fluid collection. An evolving pseudocyst is seen on **Figure 6**. Infiltration of the peripancreatic fat and the space of the gastrohepatic ligament is seen on **Figure 7**. These findings are consistent with the patient's history of acute pancreatitis.

Because of the history of abrupt onset of abdominal pain and the suggestion of hemorrhage in the lesser sac fluid collection, an arteriogram was obtained to exclude pancreatic pseudoaneurysm. The splenic arteriogram **(Fig. 8)** demonstrates a small pseudo-aneurysm arising from a pancreatic branch artery originating from the left gastroepiploic artery.

Diagnosis

Pancreatitis-induced pancreatic pseudoaneurysm which had bled into a lesser sac fluid collection.

Management

A 3-F coaxial microcatheter was advanced selectively into the pancreatic artery **(Fig. 9)**. A straight Hilal coil (Cook, Bloomington, IN) was deposited across the mouth of the pseudoaneurysm and no filling was noted on the hand injection. However, a follow-up arteriogram **(Fig. 10)** still demonstrated filling of the pseudoaneurysm through pancreatica magna collaterals.

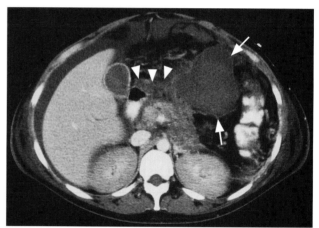

Figure 7. Caudal extent of the lesser sac fluid collection (arrows). Infiltration (arrowheads) of the prepancreatic fat and space of the gastrohepatic ligament is indicative of pancreatitis.

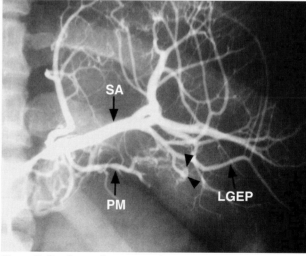

Figure 8. Small pseudoaneurysm (arrowheads) of a pancreatic tail branch. SA=splenic artery; PM=pancreatica magna; LGEP=left gastroepiploic artery.

586

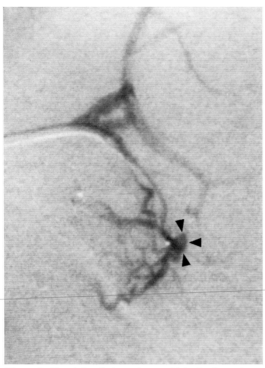

Figure 9. Coaxial catheter advanced into the branch with the pseudoaneurysm (arrowheads).

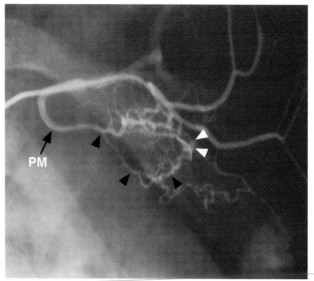

Figure 10. Splenic arteriogram demonstrates a coil in place across the orifice of the pseudoaneurysm with persistent filling of the pseudoaneurysm (white arrowheads). There is collateral flow (black arrowheads) from the pancreatica magna (PM).

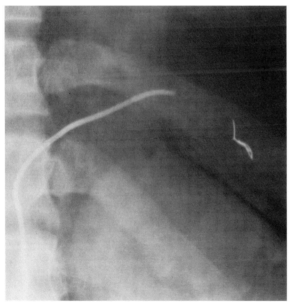

Figure 11. Plain film shows placement of additional coils.

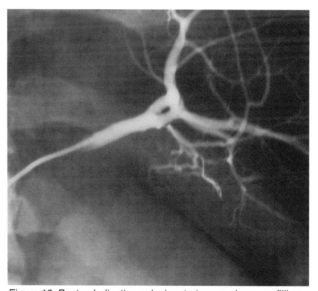

Figure 12. Postembolization splenic arteriogram shows no filling of the pseudoaneurysm.

This arteriogram delineates a critical technical point. Because of the rich collateral network of blood vessels in the pancreas, hemostatic control must be obtained on both sides of the pseudoaneurysm to prevent its reconstitution from collaterals.

The microcatheter was re-advanced past the mouth of the pseudoaneurysm and more coils were deposited **(Fig. 11)**. Completion arteriography demonstrated no filling of the pseudoaneurysm **(Fig. 12)**. The patient remained hemodynamically stable after the embolization and was discharged without any further episodes of bleeding. The pseudocyst in the lesser sac was marsupialized once the wall had matured.

Discussion

Pseudoaneurysms may occur in up to 10% of individuals with severe acute or recurrent pancreatitis. Bleeding, which is one of the most significant complications of pancreatitis, may occur in 2%–10% of cases. With pancreatitis, proteolytic enzymes seep into the surrounding tissues. These enzymes induce a severe inflammatory response which can cause stenosis and occlusions of adjacent vessels. Occasionally these enzymes will produce autodigestion of the vascular wall, resulting in pseudoaneurysms. Because of the proximity of the splenic artery to the pancreas, it is the vessel most commonly involved, followed by the gastroduodenal artery and the pancreaticoduodenal arcades.

The symptoms and clinical presentation attributable to the pseudoaneurysms will depend on the location and site of the rupture. The most common symptom of pancreatic pseudoaneurysm rupture is acute gastrointestinal bleeding caused by erosion into the alimentary tract. Rupture into the biliary tree or the pancreatic duct will also result in gastrointestinal bleeding.

Because these patients are usually quite sick and can have a variety of symptoms and alternative explanations for their pain or gastrointestinal bleeding, a high clinical and radiographic suspicion should be maintained. Any patient with recurrent or unexplainable hemorrhage who has pancreatitis should be considered for arteriography to exclude a pseudoaneurysm.

Pseudoaneurysms are occasionally detected with cross-sectional imaging. On CT scanning, the lesion will be demonstrated as an area of contrast enhancement. With ultrasonography, the aneurysm appears as a cystic structure that has arterial blood flow by Doppler analysis. The size of these pseudoaneurysms will vary from 2–3 mm to 10 cm or more **(Figs. 13–15)**. However, 30% of pancreatic pseudoaneurysms are smaller than 5 mm in diameter, making cross-sectional imaging unlikely. Arteriography remains the only modality that can diagnose lesions of this size.

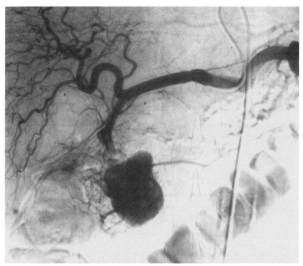

Figure 13. Large pseudoaneurysm of the gastroduodenal artery secondary to pancreatitis.

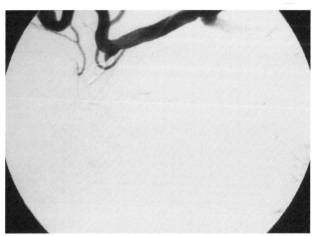

Figure 14. After embolization of the gastroduodenal artery with coils, the pseudoaneurysm no longer fills.

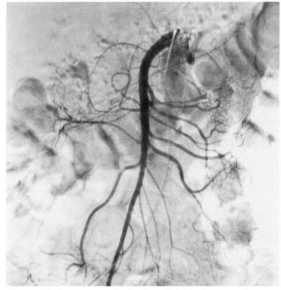

Figure 15. Because embolization distal to the pseudoaneurysm could not be obtained, a superior mesenteric arteriogram was done to exclude filling from the inferior pancreaticoduodenal arcade. No filling of the pseudoaneurysm is noted.

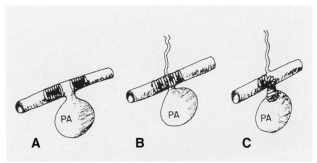

Figure 16. Proper embolization technique for pseudoaneurysms. Coils should be placed: (A) on either side of the pseudoaneurysm; (B) extending across the region of the arterial defect; or (C) extending through the vessel defect.

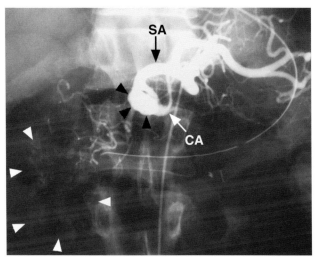

Figure 17. Celiac arteriogram in a patient with a long history of pancreatitis displays a pseudoaneurysm at the origin of the hepatic artery (white arrowheads), with occlusion of the vessel distally. SA=splenic artery; CA=origin of the celiac axis.

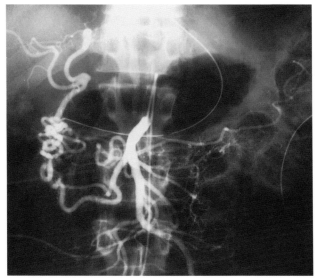

Figure 18. Same patient as in Figure 17. Superior mesenteric arteriogram shows reconstitution of the gastroduodenal and hepatic arteries from the inferior pancreaticoduodenal arcade.

Once a pancreatic pseudoaneurysm is diagnosed, it should be treated promptly. Historically, these pseudoaneurysms have been treated with surgical resection; however, the surgery is technically difficult and carries a mortality rate of 16%–50%. Because of these problems, arteriography with embolization has become the standard treatment for pancreatic pseudoaneurysms.

Selective arteriograms of the hepatic, gastroduodenal, splenic, and superior mesenteric arteries should be obtained. When a pseudoaneurysm is identified, embolization with a permanent agent should be performed. Steel or platinum coils are the preferred agents. The most crucial issue in embolization is to exclude the pseudoaneurysms from the vascular system **(Fig. 16)**.

If the pseudoaneurysm is not excluded from the vascular system, collateral flow will preclude thrombosis. This is the most common reason for embolization failure. The pseudoaneurysm can be excluded by depositing coils on both sides of the arterial defect or across the orifice of the pseudoaneurysm. If the pseudoaneurysm can be selectively catheterized, a coil can be placed within the neck.

Procedural mortality due to the embolization is extremely low. Follow-up studies have confirmed the durability of the procedure. Recurrent bleeding is extremely unusual following a technically successful embolization. In more than 80% of cases, embolization is the only procedure required. In the remaining 20%, ancillary surgical procedures such as pseudocyst drainage or splenectomy are performed.

In addition to pseudoaneurysms, pancreatitis can produce other significant complications in the vascular system. Pancreatitis can cause arterial occlusion, as shown in **Figure 17**. This patient had a pseudoaneurysm of the hepatic artery associated with distal arterial occlusion. Hepatic arterial reconstitution via the inferior pancreaticoduodenal arcade to the gastroduodenal artery is present **(Fig. 18)**.

Although arterial occlusions can occur, venous occlusions are more common. Splenic vein thrombosis may occur in up to 45% of patients with pancreatitis (**Figs. 19, 20**).

Collateral venous drainage in the presence of splenic vein occlusion is shown in **Figure 20**. Short gastric veins drain into the coronary vein, which flows into the portal vein. The gastroepiploic vein runs along the greater curve of the stomach and drains into the gastrocolic trunk. In some patients, a large vein is present in the greater omentum that parallels the gastroepiploic vein and is termed the arc of Barkow.

Splenectomy is the procedure of choice for splenic vein occlusion. However, due to dense adhesions from pancreatitis and numerous varices from the splenic vein occlusion, the surgery may be difficult. Preoperative embolization of the spleen can be performed to facilitate the surgical procedure.

For further information on this topic, please see Tutorial 13 and Teaching File Case 56.

Selected Readings

Burke JW, Erickson SJ, Kellum CD, Tegtmeyer CJ, Williamson BR, Hansen MF. Pseudoaneurysms complicating pancreatitis: detection by CT. Radiology 1986; 161:447–450.

Mandel SR, Jaques PF, Sanofsky S, Mauro MA. Nonoperative management of peripancreatic arterial aneurysms: a 10-year experience. Ann Surg 1987; 205:126–128.

Mauro MA, Jaques PF. Transcatheter management of pseudoaneurysms complicating pancreatitis. J Vasc Interv Radiol 1991; 2:527–532.

Savastano S, Feltrin GP, Antonio T, Miotto D, Chiesura-Corona M, Castellan L. Arterial complications of pancreatitis: diagnostic and therapeutic role of radiology. Pancreas 1993; 8:687–692.

Stabile BE, Wilson SE, Debas HT. Reduced mortality from bleeding pseudocysts and pseudoaneurysms caused by pancreatitis. Arch Surg 1983; 118:45–51.

Vujic I. Vascular complications of pancreatitis. Radiol Clin North Am 1989; 27:81–91.

Walter JF, Chuang VP, Bookstein JJ, Reuter SR, Cho KJ, Pulmano CM. Angiography of massive hemorrhage secondary to pancreatic disease. Radiology 1977; 124:337–342.

White AF, Baum S, Buranasiri S. Aneurysms secondary to pancreatitis. AJR 1976; 127:393–396.

End Notes

Figure 16 from Kadir S, ed. Current practice of interventional radiology. St. Louis: Mosby Year Book, 1991; 595. Used with permission.

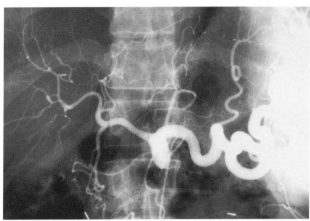

Figure 19. Celiac arteriogram in another patient with a long history of pancreatitis reveals normal arterial morphology.

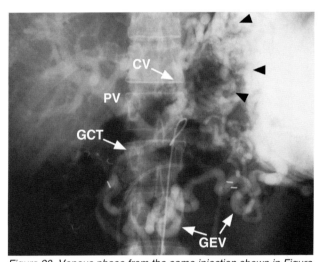

Figure 20. Venous phase from the same injection shown in Figure 19. The splenic vein is occluded. Venous drainage of the spleen is via short gastric veins (arrowheads) which outline the fundus of the stomach, and via the gastroepiploic vein (GEV). PV=portal vein; CV=coronary vein; GCT=gastrocolic trunk.

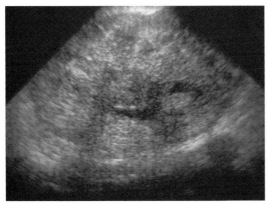

Figure 1. Coronal ultrasonographic image through the left kidney.

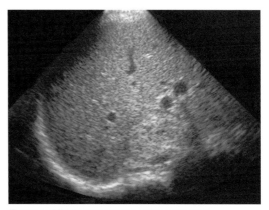

Figure 2. Mid liver transverse ultrasonogram.

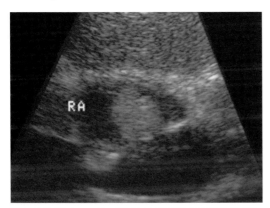

Figure 3. Transverse ultrasonographic image through the base of the right atrium (RA).

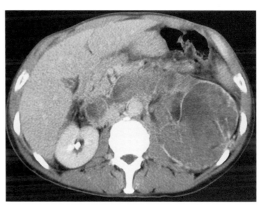

Figure 4. Contrast-enhanced CT scan through the upper abdomen.

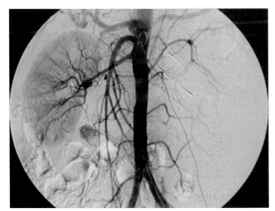

Figure 5. Abdominal aortogram.

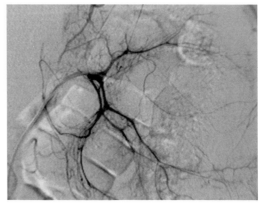

Figure 6. Left renal arteriogram.

TEACHING FILE CASE 58
**Robert K. Kerlan Jr., M.D., and
Mark J. Sands, M.D.**

History
A 56-year-old man came to the hospital with a 2-month history of vague left flank pain and a 1-week history of intermittent gross hematuria. The patient's imaging evaluation included a renal and abdominal ultrasound **(Figs. 1–3)**, abdominal computed tomography (CT) **(Fig. 4)**, and arteriography **(Figs. 5, 6)**.

What is your diagnosis?

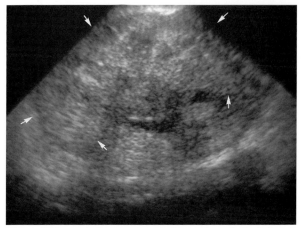

Figure 7. Coronal ultrasonographic image through the left kidney shows a heterogeneous soft tissue mass (arrows) replacing the majority of the left renal parenchyma.

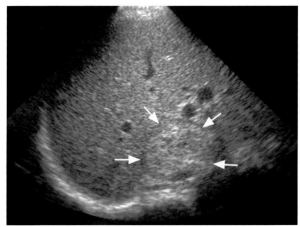

Figure 8. Transverse ultrasonogram through the mid liver reveals the inferior vena cava to be filled and expanded with echogenic materials (arrows).

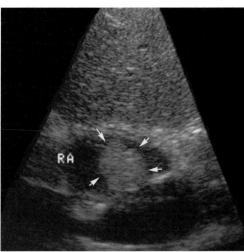

Figure 9. Transverse ultrasonographic image through the base of the right atrium (RA) shows that this echogenic material (arrows) extends into the heart.

Radiographic Findings

The left renal ultrasound **(Fig. 7)** demonstrates a solid mass of mixed echogenicity originating from the parenchyma of the left kidney. The sonographic image through the liver **(Fig. 8)** shows an echogenic mass in the anticipated position of the inferior vena cava. Ultrasound through the caudal aspect of the heart **(Fig. 9)** reveals tumor or thrombus within the right atrium. The CT study **(Fig. 10)** depicts the mass more clearly and reveals enlargement and heterogeneous density within the left renal vein. Abdominal aortography **(Fig. 11)** shows a single left renal artery. Selective left renal arteriography **(Fig. 12)** demonstrates minimal irregular hypervascularity with heterogeneous staining. The majority of the tumor is hypovascular.

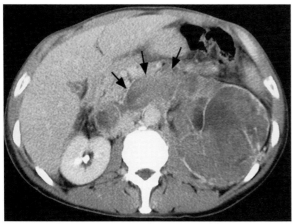

Figure 10. Contrast-enhanced CT scan through the mid abdomen. A large mixed-density tumor replaces the paren-chyma of the left kidney. The mass extends along the course and position of the left renal vein (arrows) which indicates that the vein is filled with tumor thrombus.

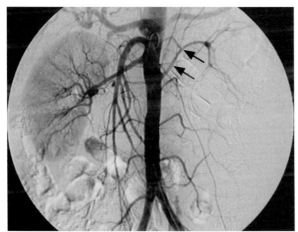

Figure 11. Abdominal aortogram demonstrates single renal arteries bilaterally. Though the left renal artery (arrowheads) is patent, it is reduced in size and no left nephrogram is seen.

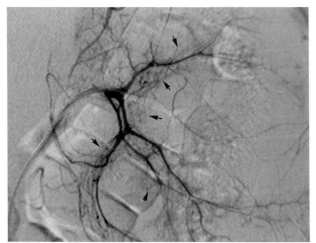

Figure 12. Left renal arteriogram shows that the majority of the tumor is hypovascular, with scattered areas of neovascularity (arrows).

Diagnosis

Renal cell carcinoma with extension into the left renal vein.

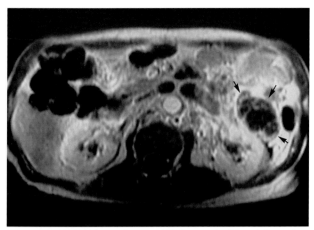

Figure 13. Gadolinium-enhanced MR image depicts a left renal cell carcinoma (arrows) with decreased signal intensity.

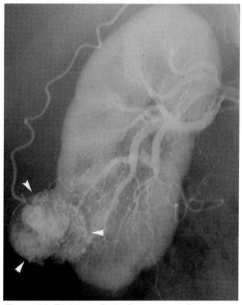

Figure 14. Right renal arteriogram reveals a hypervascular renal cell carcinoma (arrows) extending from the cortex of the right kidney.

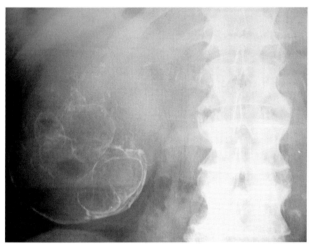

Figure 15. Abdominal radiograph shows a curvilinear calcification in the right mid abdomen subsequently proven to contain renal cell carcinoma.

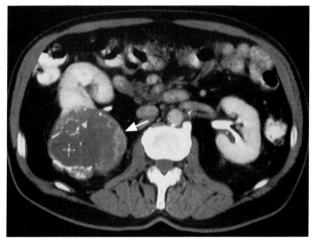

Figure 16. Same patient as in Figure 15. Contrast-enhanced CT scan shows that the mass is low density, compatible with cystic change. An area of higher density soft tissue (arrow) is seen along the medial wall.

Discussion

Additional images from patients with renal cell carcinoma are shown in **Figures 13–23**. Renal cell carcinoma is known by several other names including renal cell adenocarcinoma, hypernephroma, clear-cell carcinoma, and Grawitz's tumor. It is the most common primary renal malignancy, with an annual incidence of 15,000 new cases per year and 7,500 deaths per year in the United States. This tumor is most common in men (2.5:1) with a median age of 55 years at the time of diagnosis. Risk factors for developing this tumor include smoking and a high fat diet. In addition, patients on dialysis with acquired renal cystic disease are seven times more likely to develop renal cell carcinoma when compared to the general population.

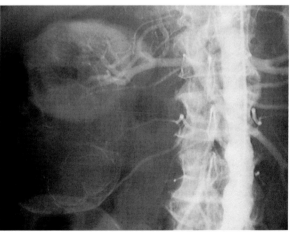

Figure 17. Same patient as in Figure 15. The abdominal aortogram reveals no definite tumor vascularity within the mass. Renal cell carcinoma with extensive metastatic disease to the lungs was found at autopsy.

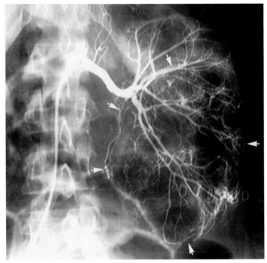

Figure 18. Left renal arteriogram from a patient with a large, hypovascular, renal cell carcinoma (arrows).

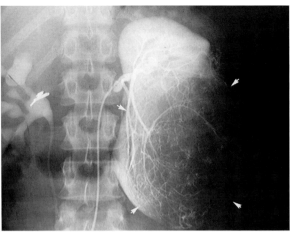

Figure 19. Left renal arteriogram from another patient shows a renal cell carcinoma (arrows) of intermediate vascularity replacing the mid and lower pole of the left kidney.

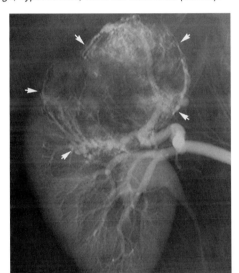

Figure 20. Right renal arteriogram shows a hypovascular carcinoma (arrows) in the upper pole of the right kidney.

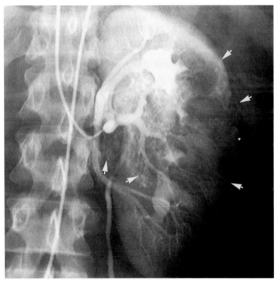

Figure 21. Left renal arteriogram shows a subtle hypovascular carcinoma (arrows) in the mid pole of the left kidney.

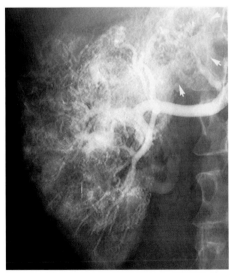

Figure 22. Right renal arteriogram. A hypervascular renal cell carcinoma is present extending medially (arrows) indicating either spread to regional lymph nodes or extension into the right renal vein and inferior vena cava.

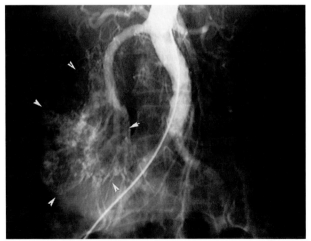

Figure 23. Abdominal aortogram depicts a hypervascular renal cell carcinoma (arrows) in the lower pole of the right kidney.

A hereditary form of renal cell carcinoma is found in patients with von Hippel-Lindau disease. This disease, inherited as an autosomal dominant trait with a variable degree of penetration, consists of retinal angiomas, central nervous system hemangioblastomas, and both cystic and solid tumors of the abdominal viscera. Thirty-five percent of these patients will develop renal cell carcinoma between the ages of 20 and 50, and bilateral involvement occurs in up to 75% of patients.

Renal cell carcinoma may be asymptomatic until it reaches a considerable size, often greater than 6 cm in diameter. The classic clinical triad of flank pain, hematuria, and flank mass is encountered in less than 10% of patients, and usually heralds the presence of advanced disease. However, with the increasing utilization of cross-sectional imaging modalities, many asymptomatic small renal cell carcinomas are discovered incidentally during evaluation for unrelated complaints.

Most of the typical imaging findings are present in this case with a solid renal mass which is heterogeneous on both ultrasound and contrast-enhanced CT. It should be noted, however, that 5%–7% of renal cell carcinomas are cystic, with four patterns recognized: 1) multilocular cystic type; 2) unilocular cystic type (cystadenocarcinoma); 3) cystic necrosis type; and 4) carcinoma arising within a simple renal cyst.

Though arteriography and venography were once used to evaluate the presence or absence of venous invasion, magnetic resonance angiography and spiral CT scanning have made invasive evaluations unnecessary. However, the arteriographic appearance should be familiar to the interventional radiologist.

The majority of renal cell carcinomas are hypervascular with obvious malignant neovascularity. Arteriovenous shunting and parasitization of nonrenal arteries such as the adrenal, phrenic, and lumbar arteries are commonly observed. Parasitized vessels do not necessarily indicate extrarenal tumor extension, but may merely reflect the diminished vascular resistance and flow requirements of the tumor. Approximately 22% of renal cell carcinomas are hypovascular and up to one quarter of these are avascular. Tumors with diminished vascularity are frequently associated with papillary histology.

The prognosis of renal cell carcinoma is greatly dependent upon its stage at the time of discovery. The most common staging system is that of Robson **(Fig. 24)**.

The prognosis for stage I and II disease is excellent with surgical resection. The prognosis for stage III disease is intermediate; for stage IV disease the prognosis is dismal.

Robson Staging System

Stage I—Tumor contained within renal capsule
Stage II—Tumor spread into perinephric fat
Stage III-A—Venous tumor thrombus in renal vein, inferior vena cava, or right atrium
Stage III-B—Regional lymph node metastases
Stage III-C—Venous tumor thrombus and regional nodal metastases
Stage IV-A—Direct invasion of organs outside Gerota's fascia
Stage IV-B—Distant metastases

Figure 24.

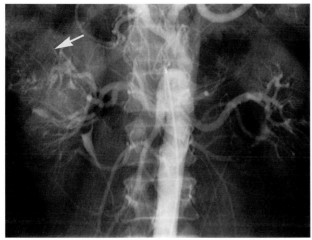

Figure 25. Abdominal aortogram shows a single right renal artery and a right renal cell carcinoma (arrow).

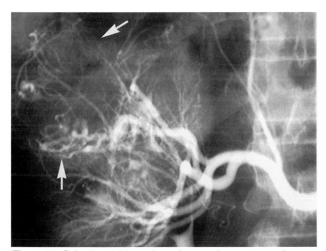

Figure 26. Selective right renal arteriogram demonstrates the tumor (arrows) in more detail.

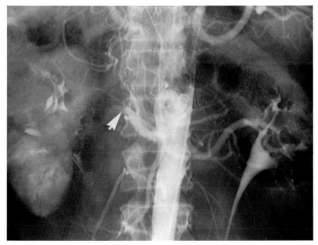

Figure 27. Following instillation of 12 mL of dehydrated ethanol, there is cessation of arterial flow (arrow). Note that the right inferior adrenal artery was not embolized.

The differential diagnoses of vascular renal parenchymal masses include angiomyolipoma, oncocytoma, and metastatic disease from hypervascular primary tumors.

Arteriography is no longer used to diagnose renal cell carcinoma, being replaced by a combination of CT, ultrasound, and magnetic resonance imaging. However, arteriograms are still obtained in patients in whom a partial nephrectomy is being considered (including patients with single kidneys and congenital anomalies), and in patients in whom embolization is desired. Transcatheter embolization is used preoperatively to diminish blood loss and facilitate surgical resection. Moreover, in patients who are poor surgical candidates, transcatheter embolization may be used as the sole form of therapy.

The technique of preoperative renal embolization **(Figs. 25–27)** is variable. Dehydrated ethanol has been used by many investigators and has been shown to reduce transfusion requirements during nephrectomy when compared to nonembolized patients. It should be recognized that this cytotoxic agent can be associated with complications such as bowel infarction and nerve injury. As an unequivocal benefit from using alcohol has never been established, many investigators prefer using particulate agents such as Gelfoam (Upjohn, Kalamazoo, MI) or polyvinyl alcohol.

Renal arterial embolization is often performed through an occlusion balloon to prevent reflux of embolic material into the aorta. The inflated occlusion balloon, however, does not ensure that non-target embolization will be prevented. Renal arterial hemodynamics change when the proximal artery is occluded. Parasitized vessels may serve as undesirable egress routes for embolic material during embolization through an occlusion balloon. Careful fluoroscopic monitoring with admixture of the embolic material with contrast material is recommended to guard against non-target embolization.

The use of occluding spring emboli (coils) for preoperative renal artery embolization is controversial. Arterial clamping during nephrectomy can potentially dislodge these coils into the aorta, leading to non-target embolization.

For further information on this topic, please see Tutorials 12 and 13, and Teaching File Cases 59 and 60.

Selected Readings

Bakal CW, Cynamon J, Lakritz PS, Sprayregen S. Value of preoperative renal artery embolization in reducing blood transfusion requirements during nephrectomy for renal cell carcinoma. J Vasc Interv Radiol 1993; 4:727–731.

Bracken RB. Renal carcinoma: clinical aspects and therapy. Semin Roentgenol 1987; 22:241–247.

Buist TA. Parasitic arterial supply to intracapsular renal cell carcinoma. Am J Roentgenol Radium Ther Nucl Med 1974; 120:653–659.

Jennings CM, Gaines PA. The abdominal manifestation of von Hippel-Lindau disease and a radiological screening protocol for an affected family. Clin Radiol 1988; 39:363–367.

Johnson CD, Dunnick NR, Cohan RH, Illescas FF. Renal adenocarcinoma: CT staging of 100 tumors. AJR 1987; 148:59–63.

Levine E, Hartman DS, Smirniotopoulos JG. Renal cystic diseases associated with renal neoplasms. In: Hartman DS. Renal cystic disease. Philadelphia: W.B. Saunders Company, 1989; 38–73.

Smith SJ, Bosniak MA, Megibow AJ, Hulnick DH, Horii SC, Raghavendra BN. Renal cell carcinoma: earlier discovery and increased detection. Radiology 1989; 170:699–703.

Watson RC, Fleming RJ, Evans JA. Arteriography in the diagnosis of renal carcinoma: review of 100 cases. Radiology 1968; 91:888–897.

Yamashita Y, Miyazaki T, Ishii A, Watanabe O, Takahashi M. Multilocular cystic renal cell carcinoma presenting as a solid mass: radiologic evaluation. Abdom Imaging 1995; 20:164–168.

Yamashita Y, Watanabe O, Miyazaki T, Yamamoto H, Harada M, Takahashi M. Cystic renal cell carcinoma: imaging findings with pathologic correlation. Acta Radiol 1994; 35:19–24.

End Notes

Figures 15–17 courtesy of Dr. Edward Baker, California Pacific Medical Center, San Francisco, CA.

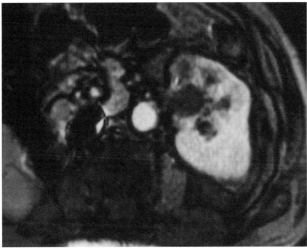
Figure 1. Axial MR image through the mid abdomen.

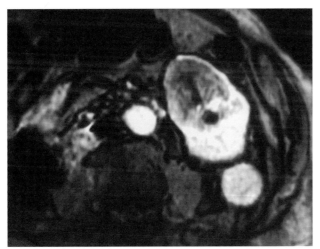
Figure 2. Axial MR image slightly more caudal than in Figure 1.

TEACHING FILE CASE 59
Donald J. Ponec, M.D.

History

A 77-year-old man who is status post right nephrectomy came to the hospital with severe hematuria necessitating multiple transfusions. The patient had renal insufficiency with a creatinine of 3.5. In addition, he had biopsy-proven renal cell carcinoma involving the left kidney for which he refused surgery and dialysis. A magnetic resonance (MR) scan of the left kidney was obtained **(Figs. 1, 2)**.

What is your diagnosis?

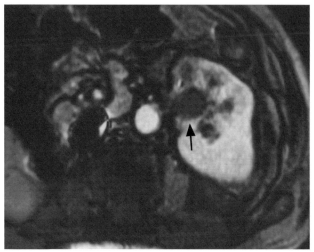

Figure 3. MR image shows a dilated renal pelvis (arrow) containing thrombus.

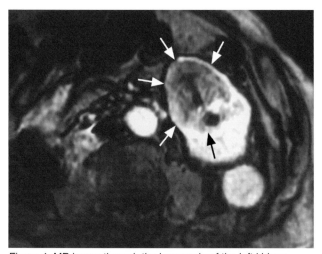

Figure 4. MR image through the lower pole of the left kidney reveals a low signal intensity mass (arrows) indicative of renal cell carcinoma.

Radiographic Findings

The MR study revealed a large renal tumor replacing the lower pole of the left kidney, along with a clot in the renal collecting system **(Figs. 3, 4)**. Other images revealed a smaller upper pole lesion. No perinephric bleeding was noted. Tumor thrombus in the renal vein was also suggested.

Diagnosis

Renal cell carcinoma in a solitary kidney causing hematuria.

How would you manage this patient?

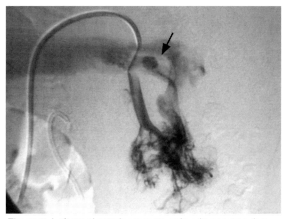

Figure 5. Left renal arteriogram reveals a hypervascular mass and arteriovenous shunting. Tumor thrombus in the renal vein is seen as a filling defect (arrow).

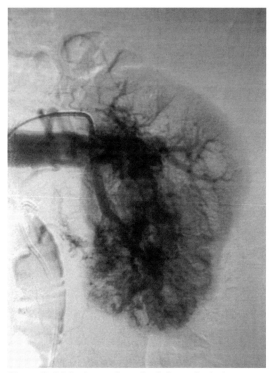

Figure 6. A later image from the left renal arteriogram demonstrates normal remaining upper pole parenchyma.

Management

Selective renal arteriography of the left kidney was performed **(Figs. 5, 6)**. Care was exercised to minimize the volume of contrast material used. The hypervascular tumor mass in the lower pole was selectively embolized with ethanol, polyvinyl alcohol particles and Gelfoam pledgets (Upjohn, Kalamazoo, MI). No additional contrast material injections were performed and the total dye load was kept below 20 mL. The patient's bleeding stopped and his creatinine level decreased from 3.5 to 1.8 over the following week. He experienced recurrent hematuria after 3 months and repeat embolization was performed in a similar fashion. He required no further blood transfusions and his creatinine remained below 2.0. He was alive 11 months after the procedure with a good quality of life and no further bleeding.

Discussion

Selective therapeutic embolization of renal cell carcinoma in solitary kidneys has been previously reported. The primary indications were massive hematuria (as in this patient) or control of paraneoplastic symptoms in patients who could not (or would not) undergo partial or complete nephrectomy. Selective tumor embolization and preservation of the remaining normal parenchyma is of obvious importance. This patient's renal function improved after embolization. It was postulated that the patient's improved renal function was related in part to improved perfusion of normal tissue following embolization of the tumor and the consequent reduction in arteriovenous shunting. In addition, a ureteral stent was placed at the time of treatment, which also may have had a beneficial effect.

For further information on this topic, please see Tutorials 12 and 13, and Teaching File Cases 58 and 60.

Selected Readings

Cos LR, Gutierrez O. Repeat selective embolization of a solitary kidney with renal cell carcinoma: case report. J Urol 1989; 141:115–116.

Kozak BE, Keller FS, Rösch J, Barry J. Selective therapeutic embolization of renal cell carcinoma in solitary kidneys. J Urol 1987; 137:1223–1225.

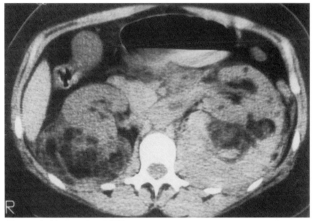

Figure 1. Noncontrast CT scan.

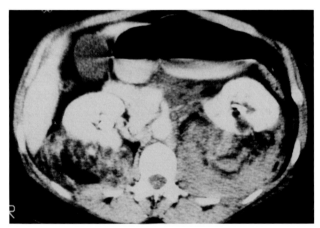

Figure 2. Contrast-enhanced CT scan.

TEACHING FILE CASE 60
Jeffrey L. Groffsky, M.D., and
Ziv J. Haskal, M.D.

History
A 42-year-old woman came to the emergency department complaining of the acute onset of severe left flank pain and hematuria. She reported no history of trauma. On examination, bilateral renal masses were suspected.

The patient initially underwent computed tomography (CT) scanning of the abdomen. Noncontrast and contrast-enhanced images are shown (**Figs. 1, 2**).

What is your diagnosis?

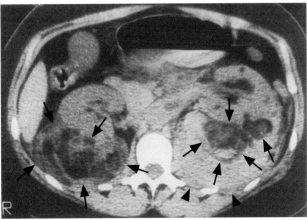

Figure 3. CT scan through the upper abdomen without intravenous contrast material shows bilateral masses containing fat posterior to both kidneys (arrows). A crescentic soft tissue density (arrowheads) compatible with hematoma is present on the left side.

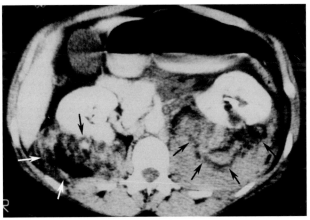

Figure 4. Following the administration of intravenous contrast material, the CT scan demonstrates the renal masses more clearly (arrows).

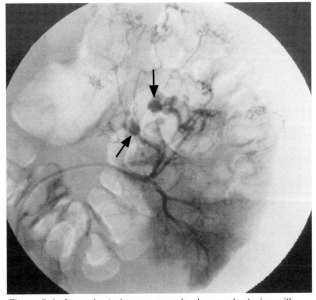

Figure 5. Left renal arteriogram reveals abnormal arteries with aneurysms (arrows) in the left renal mass.

Radiographic Findings
The CT images **(Figs. 3, 4)** demonstrate anterior displacement of both kidneys by large masses arising from the kidney margins. Portions of these masses are of fatty attenuation. In addition, on the left, a large crescent-shaped collection of high attenuation is seen in association with the mass.

Diagnosis
Large, bilateral renal angiomyolipomas with associated acute hemorrhage on the left side.

What are the treatment options for this patient?

Management
Treatment options consist primarily of surgical resection or embolotherapy. In this case, the patient was hemodynamically stable upon presentation. She underwent staged, selective embolization of the tumors, with treatment first directed toward the symptomatic left side. The arterial phase from a left renal arteriogram is shown **(Fig. 5)**. Abnormal vasculature with tangles of vessels and multiple aneurysms are seen associated with the upper pole mass. No arteriovenous shunting is identified.

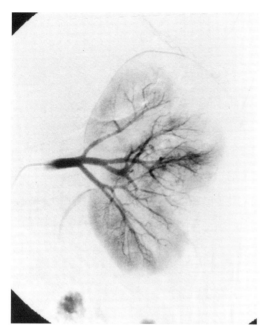

Figure 6. Left renal arteriogram following embolization of the angiomyolipoma shows preservation of the normal renal parenchyma and no opacification of the abnormal vessels.

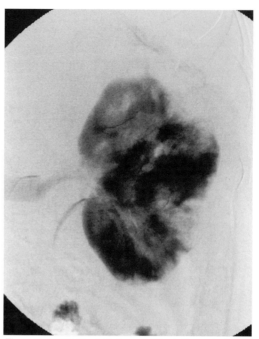

Figure 7. Parenchymal phase of the left renal arteriogram shown in Figure 6.

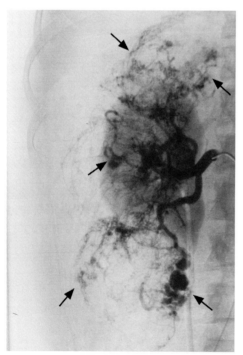

Figure 8. Right renal arteriogram shows abnormal arteries (arrows) secondary to multifocal angiomyolipomas.

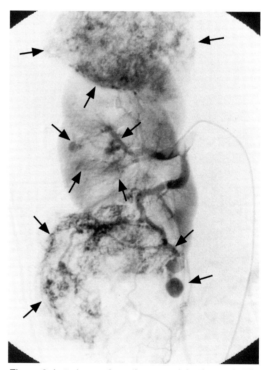

Figure 9. Late image from the same injection as in Figure 8 shows the angiomyolipomas to better advantage (arrows).

Selective embolization of the primary feeding vessels was performed, using polyvinyl alcohol particles ranging in size from 150 to 500 microns. The arterial and parenchymal phases of the postembolization study demonstrate absence of flow to the tumor and preservation of normal renal parenchyma **(Figs. 6, 7)**. At a later date, the patient underwent prophylactic embolization of the right-sided angiomyolipomas **(Figs. 8–11)**. Postembolization images document successful treatment, again with preservation of normal portions of the kidney **(Figs. 12, 13)**.

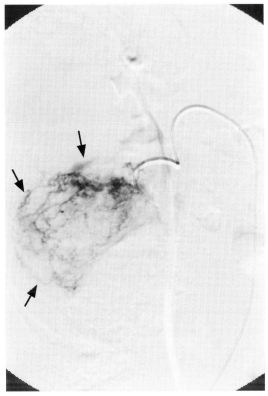

Figure 10. Superselective right renal arteriogram obtained during embolization shows abnormal arterial structures compatible with angiomyolipoma (arrows) in the lower pole.

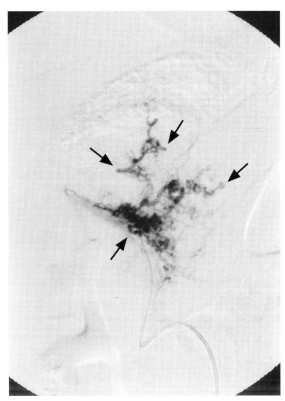

Figure 11. Superselective right upper pole arteriogram depicts similar pathologic arterial morphology (arrows).

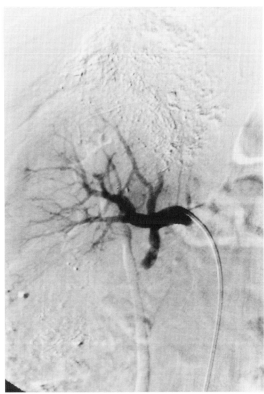

Figure 12. Right renal arteriogram following embolization confirms preservation of normal arteries.

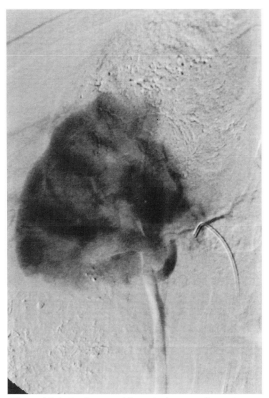

Figure 13. Later image of the arteriogram shown in Figure 12 demonstrates preserved renal parenchyma.

Discussion

Angiomyolipomas are benign tumors of the kidney which consist of vascular, fatty, and smooth muscle elements. Approximately 80% are sporadic; the remainder occur in patients with tuberous sclerosis. The majority are asymptomatic. However, when they are 4 cm or greater in size, approximately 90% are symptomatic and 50%–60% of them spontaneously bleed. Bleeding is occasionally massive and may be life-threatening.

Treatment options include surgical resection or embolotherapy. Embolization may be performed both for acute hemorrhage or as a prophylactic measure. Superselective catheterization is often required to maximize preservation of normal renal tissue. The choice of embolic agents varies among institutions. At our institution, absolute ethanol or polyvinyl alcohol particles are used, with or without Ethiodol (Savage Laboratories, Melville, NY). With alcohol embolization, a balloon occlusion catheter is used whenever the feeding vessel is of adequate size.

Most patients develop a postembolization syndrome, manifested as pain, fever, and nausea. Postprocedure care includes treatment of these symptoms and follow-up monitoring of renal status.

For further information on this topic, please see Tutorials 12 and 13, and Teaching File Cases 58 and 59.

Selected Readings

Earthman WJ, Mazer MJ, Winfield AC. Angiomyolipomas in tuberous sclerosis: subselective embolotherapy with alcohol, with long-term follow-up study. Radiology 1986; 160:437–441.

Soulen MC, Faykus MH, Shlansky-Goldberg RD, Wein AJ, Cope C. Elective embolization for prevention of hemorrhage from renal angiomyolipomas. J Vasc Interv Radiol 1994; 5:587–591.

Zerhouni EA, Schellhammer P, Schaefer JC, et al. Management of bleeding renal angiomyolipomas by transcatheter embolization following CT diagnosis. Urol Radiol 1984; 6:205–209.

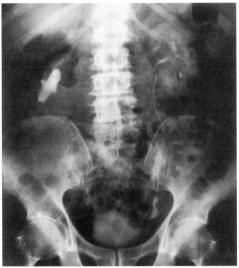
Figure 1. 5-minute film from an intravenous pyelogram.

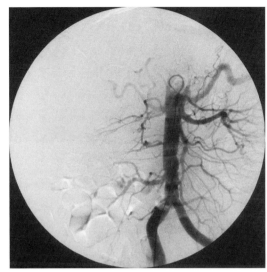
Figure 2. Abdominal aortogram, early arterial phase.

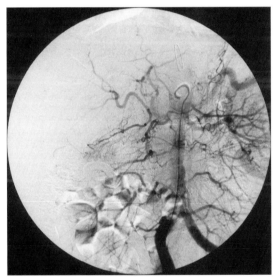
Figure 3. Abdominal aortogram, late arterial phase.

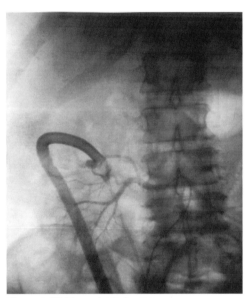
Figure 4. Right renal arteriogram.

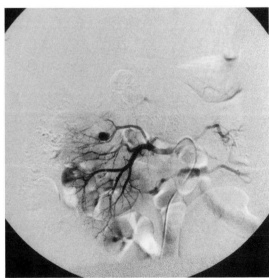
Figure 5. Right renal arteriogram, subtracted image.

TEACHING FILE CASE 61
Matthew S. Johnson, M.D.

History

A 75-year-old man underwent right percutaneous nephrolithotomy for a large lower pole calculus **(Fig. 1)**. Percutaneous access into the right upper pole was achieved with some difficulty, but the stone was completely removed through this track. After the procedure, a 22-F Malecot re-entry catheter was left in place. The patient had intermittent hematuria over the next several days, requiring transfusion of 2 units of packed red blood cells, but his urine gradually cleared and his hemoglobin stabilized, permitting discharge 10 days after the procedure. He came to the emergency department 4 days later, hypotensive, with grossly bloody urine. Emergency arteriography was performed **(Figs. 2–5)**.

What is your diagnosis?

607

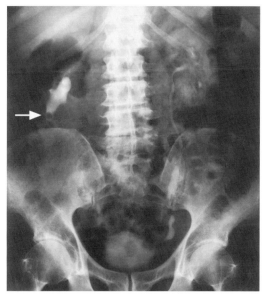

Figure 6. A radiolucent stone (arrow) is present in a right lower pole calyx projected en face.

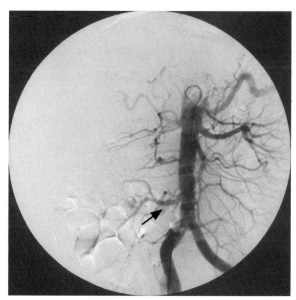

Figure 7. Right renal artery (arrow) arises from the distal aorta just proximal to the bifurcation.

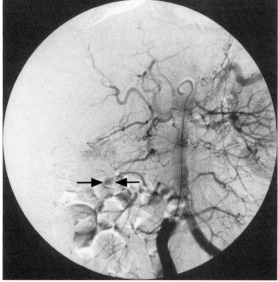

Figure 8. A faintly opacified collection of contrast material (arrows) is present in the superior aspect of the right kidney, almost obscured by bowel gas.

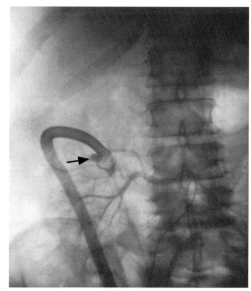

Figure 9. Unsubtracted image from selective right renal artery injection shows a small pseudoaneurysm (arrow).

Radiographic Findings

The 5-minute delayed film from the IVP demonstrates a malrotated right kidney, with a filling defect in the lower pole collecting system **(Fig. 6)**. The abdominal aortogram demonstrates a very low origin of the right renal artery **(Fig. 7)**. Bowel gas obscures the right kidney, but late images suggest the presence of an abnormal collection of contrast material **(Fig. 8)**. Selective injection of the right renal artery better demonstrates the abnormal collection adjacent to the re-entry catheter **(Figs. 9, 10)**.

Diagnosis

Traumatic pseudoaneurysm.

How would you manage this patient?

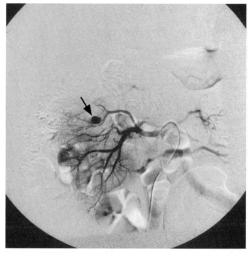

Figure 10. Subtracted image from the selective right renal artery injection depicts this pseudoaneurysm (arrow) more clearly.

608

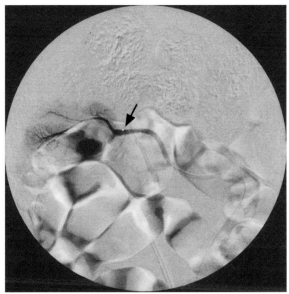

Figure 11. Coaxial microcatheter (arrow) is used to super-selectively catheterize the interlobar artery immediately proximal to the pseudoaneurysm.

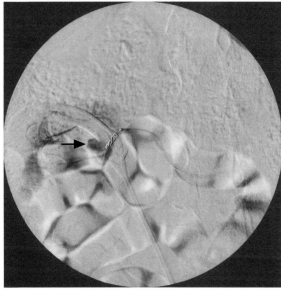

Figure 12. Despite the deposition of two microcoils, there is persistent filling of the pseudoaneurysm (arrow).

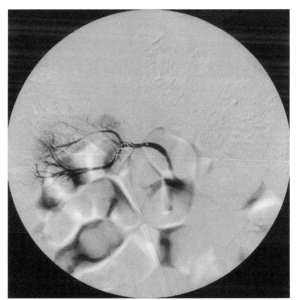

Figure 13. Following placement of additional coils, no filling of the pseudoaneurysm is present.

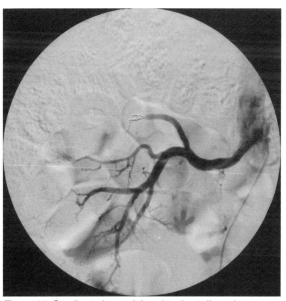

Figure 14. Small arteries peripheral to the coils no longer opacify.

Management

A cobra catheter had been used to select the main right renal artery. This catheter was removed over a guide wire and replaced with a Simmons catheter, which was guided into the origin of the upper pole lobar branch. A coaxial microcatheter was advanced through the Simmons catheter into the interlobar branch supplying the pseudoaneurysm **(Fig. 11)**. Two complex helical microcoils were introduced into this vessel at the base of the arterial defect; however, there was persistent opacification of the pseudoaneurysm **(Fig. 12)**. Therefore, additional coils were introduced **(Fig. 13)**. Completion arteriography demonstrated no further filling of the pseudoaneurysm **(Fig. 14)**. The patient's hematuria resolved, and his creatinine remained stable. He was discharged in good condition 3 days after the procedure.

Discussion

Injury to the renal vasculature may result from blunt or penetrating abdominal trauma, surgery, or percutaneous intervention, including percutaneous nephrostomy, biopsy, and angioplasty. The most common manifestation of renal injury is hematuria; however, hypotension due to blood loss, or hypertension due to renal artery occlusion, stenosis, or perirenal hematoma may also be observed. Persistent hematuria following percutaneous intervention warrants imaging of the affected kidney. Though noninvasive imaging such as ultrasound may demonstrate an arteriovenous fistula, pseudoaneurysm, or hematoma, arteriography is usually required. Arteriography may demonstrate arterial occlusion, extravasation, intimal injury, arteriovenous fistula or pseudoaneurysm. Both arteriovenous fistulas and pseudoaneurysms should be embolized. Superselective techniques permit preservation of the majority of normal renal parenchyma, although a small portion of the kidney will be lost due to occlusion of the feeding vessel. Embolization is successful in stopping the hemorrhage in over 80% of cases.

For further information on this topic, please see Tutorials 13 and 18, and Teaching File Case 62.

Selected Readings

Kadir S. Angiography of the kidneys. In: Kadir S. Diagnostic angiography. Philadephia: W.B. Saunders Company, 1986; 468–469.

Uflacker R. Interventional management of visceral aneurysms. In: Strandness DE Jr, van Breda A, eds. Vascular diseases: surgical and interventional therapy. New York: Churchill Livingstone, 1994; 840.

Uflacker R, Paolini RM, Lima S. Management of traumatic hematuria by selective renal artery embolization. J Urol 1984; 132:662–667.

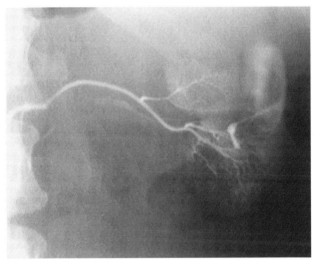
Figure 1. Left renal arteriogram.

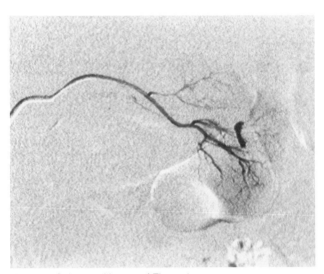
Figure 2. Subtracted image of Figure 1.

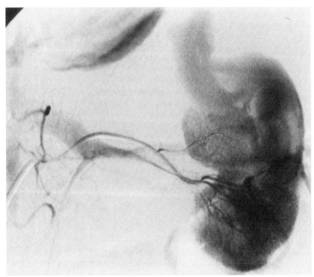
Figure 3. Left renal arteriogram, late arterial phase.

TEACHING FILE CASE 62
*Richard Duszak, Jr., M.D., and
Ziv J. Haskal, M.D.*

History
A 45-year-old man with suspected glomerulonephritis underwent biopsy of his left kidney. Shortly after the procedure, he developed gross hematuria and profound hypotension. Vigorous fluid resuscitation was initiated and selective arteriography of the left renal artery was performed **(Figs. 1–3)**.

What is your diagnosis?

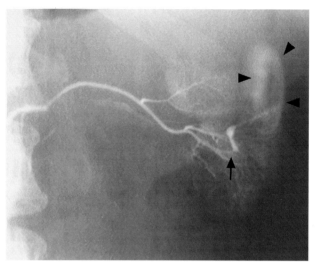

Figure 4. Left renal arteriogram shows a crescentic collection of contrast material (arrow) contiguous with a segmental branch artery. An amorphous collection of contrast material (arrowheads) is present adjacent to the kidney.

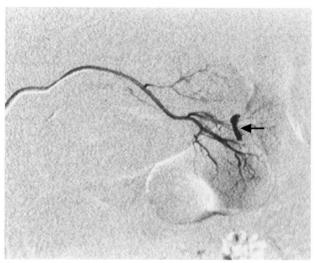

Figure 5. Subtracted image shows the crescentic collection (arrow) to better advantage.

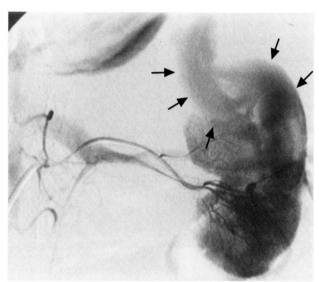

Figure 6. Delayed subtracted image reveals contrast material extravasation into the perinephric space (arrows).

Radiographic Findings

Selective arteriography of the left renal artery demonstrates a crescentic collection of contrast material in the interpolar region, contiguous with the segmental branches **(Fig. 4)**. There is an amorphous collection of contrast material adjacent to the upper pole. This central crescentic collection is more easily identified on the subtracted image **(Fig. 5)**. A delayed image demonstrates contrast material in the perinephric space surrounding the mid and upper kidney **(Fig. 6)**.

Diagnosis

Post-biopsy pseudoaneurysm of a segmental branch of the left renal artery, with active extravasation into the perinephric space.

What intervention could you offer?

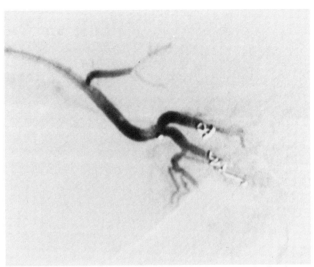

Figure 7. Left renal arteriogram obtained following embolization with stainless steel coils confirms successful control of the hemorrhage.

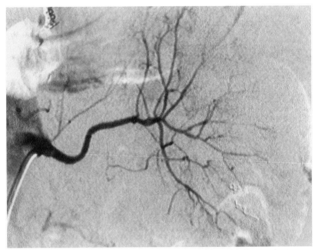

Figure 8. Selective arteriogram into an additional left renal artery shows no visible extravasation.

Management

Subselective catheterization of segmental renal artery branches adjacent to the visualized pseudoaneurysm was performed with use of a 5-F cobra catheter. Several Gianturco coils (Cook, Bloomington, IN) were deployed through an 0.035-inch lumen.

The postembolization arteriogram, with coils now in place, demonstrates cessation of the extravasation and no further filling of the pseudoaneurysm **(Fig. 7)**.

Did you notice that on the diagnostic pre-embolization arteriograms **(Figs. 1, 2)** an upper pole nephrogram is not seen?

This should lead you to suspect multiple renal arteries and search for additional vascular lesions. Indeed, after a brief search, a second left renal artery was identified, but no vascular abnormalities were demonstrated **(Fig. 8)**.

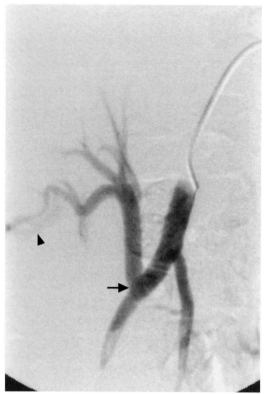

Figure 9. Right common iliac arteriogram shows a renal allograft in the right pelvis with an end-to-side anastomosis (arrow) to the external iliac artery. A faint collection of contrast material (arrowhead) is noted in the lower pole of the kidney.

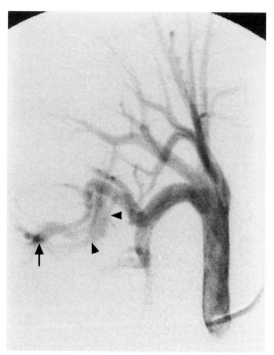

Figure 10. Selective renal allograft arteriogram shows a small pseudoaneurysm (arrow) associated with an early draining vein (arrowheads).

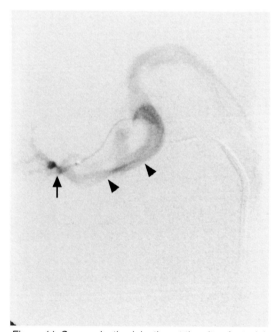

Figure 11. Superselective injection at the site of arterial injury (arrow) through a coaxially placed 3-F microcatheter. The early draining vein (arrowheads) is well visualized.

Discussion

An additional case of renal artery embolization for biopsy-induced bleeding is shown in **Figures 9–13**. This patient had a renal transplant. Common iliac arteriography was performed after biopsy of the transplanted kidney resulted in gross hematuria **(Fig. 9)**. An end-to-side anastomosis of the donor renal artery to the native external iliac artery is present. A faint linear stain of contrast material is noted in the lower pole.

Further selective arteriography, first of the donor renal artery **(Fig. 10)** and then through a 3-F coaxial microcatheter system **(Fig. 11)**, demonstrates a traumatic arteriovenous fistula with early venous filling. Subselective embolization was performed with platinum coils **(Fig. 12)**, and the arteriovenous fistula was successfully occluded. The small defect in the nephrographic phase **(Fig. 13)** serves as a reminder that embolization in the kidney involves end arteries and should be as selective as possible to minimize parenchymal loss.

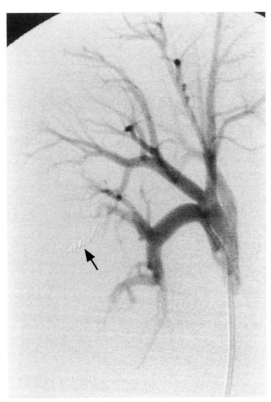

Figure 12. Selective renal allograft arteriogram obtained following selective deposition of platinum coils (arrow) confirms occlusion of the traumatic arteriovenous fistula.

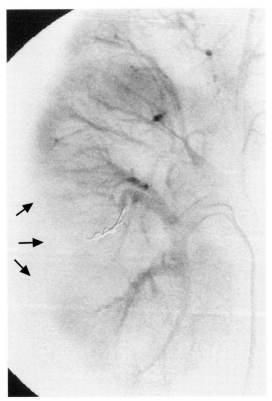

Figure 13. Late arterial phase image reveals a defect in the nephrogram (arrows) peripheral to the embolized branch.

Clinically significant renal vascular injuries, such as pseudoaneurysm and arteriovenous fistula formation, are uncommon complications of renal biopsy. Almost all of these patients will have persistent or recurrent hematuria. Other reported complications of renal biopsy include self-limited hematuria, perinephric hematoma, ileus, septicemia, pneumothorax, and inadvertent puncture of adjacent organs.

Patients with significant or persistent hematuria should undergo diagnostic arteriography. Arterial injuries are usually identified without difficulty by selective renal arteriography. An initially negative study, however, should prompt a diligent search, including additional selective injections in multiple projections. The search for multiple renal arteries may include abdominal aortography.

Percutaneous biopsy is the most common cause of penetrating vascular injury to the kidney. Percutaneous nephrostomy or noniatrogenic penetrating trauma may also lead to similar arterial damage. Subselective embolization has been shown to be a safe and effective treatment for such injuries.

For further information on this topic, please see Tutorials 13 and 18, and Teaching File Case 61.

Selected Readings

Baquero A, Morris MC, Cope C, Raja R, Bannett AD. Selective embolization of vascular complications following renal biopsy of the transplant kidney. Transplant Proc 1985; 17:1751–1754.

Fisher RG, Ben-Menachem Y, Whigham C. Stab wounds of the renal artery branches: angiographic diagnosis and treatment by embolization. AJR 1989; 152:1231–1235.

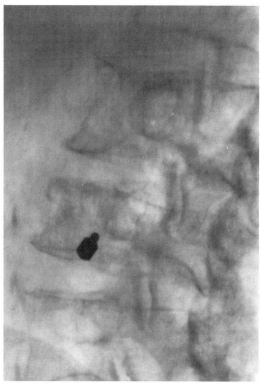

Figure 1. Oblique spot film obtained during percutaneous needle biopsy of L3.

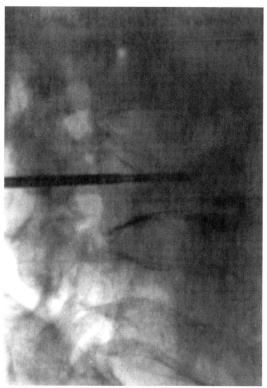

Figure 2. Oblique spot film obtained with the biopsy needle positioned into the ventral-cephalic aspect of the L3 vertebral body.

TEACHING FILE CASE 63
David Sacks, M.D.

History

An 81-year-old man underwent percutaneous biopsy of L3 with an Ackerman needle after a computed tomography (CT) scan showed lytic lesions of the vertebral body **(Figs. 1, 2)**. After the biopsy, the patient became hypotensive. There was palpable fullness in the left lower quadrant. The patient was stabilized with intravenous fluids, and an abdominal CT scan **(Figs. 3, 4)** and an arteriogram were obtained **(Fig. 5)**.

What is your diagnosis?

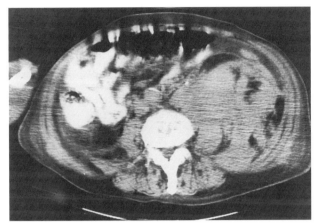

Figure 3. CT scan of the mid abdomen.

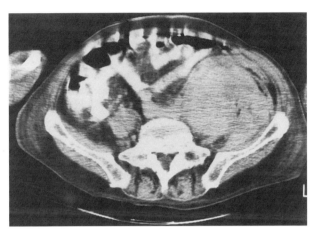

Figure 4. CT scan of the lower abdomen.

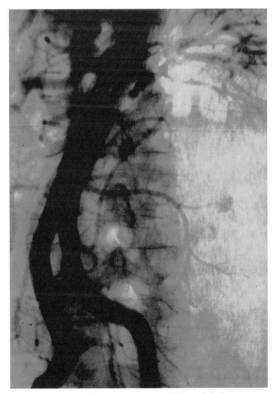

Figure 5. Abdominal aortogram, mid arterial phase.

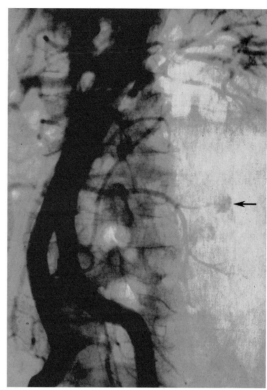

Figure 6. Abdominal aortogram reveals extravasation (arrow) from a branch of the left L3 lumbar artery.

Radiographic Findings
The CT images show a large left retroperitoneal hematoma. The aortogram shows extravasation from the left L3 lumbar artery **(Fig. 6)**.

Diagnosis
Lumbar artery injury following percutaneous biopsy.

What treatment would you recommend?

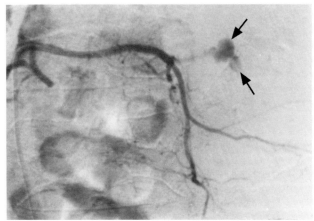

Figure 7. Selective left L3 lumbar arteriography shows the area of extravasation (arrows).

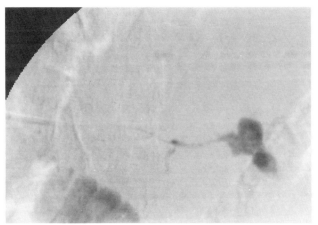

Figure 8. The damaged arterial branch is superselectively catheterized with a coaxial catheter.

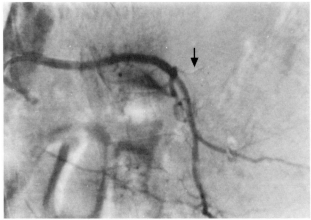

Figure 9. Postembolization selective lumbar arteriogram confirms control of the hemorrhage. The occluding spring embolus can be faintly visualized (arrow).

Management

The lumbar artery was selectively catheterized and arteriography was repeated **(Fig. 7)**. Superselective catheterization was then performed with use of a 3-F catheter **(Fig. 8)**, and a single microcoil was deposited in the lacerated branch. A follow-up selective lumbar arteriogram showed no further extravasation **(Fig. 9)**. A subtraction artifact shows the location of the coil. Clinically, the bleeding stopped.

Discussion

Percutaneous bone biopsy, including spinal biopsy, is considered a safe procedure. The overall accuracy of biopsy is as high as 95% with a complication rate of under 1%. The complication of large vessel laceration causing major hemorrhage is rare. In this case, arteriography was necessary to diagnose and treat the arterial injury. Had the pseudoaneurysm not been visible on the flush aortogram, selective lumbar arteriography would still be necessary because the abnormal vessel may not opacify optimally on the aortogram due to spasm or tamponade from adjacent hematoma.

Subselective embolization of the bleeding vessel is necessary to prevent continued hemorrhage through collateral pathways. Embolization both proximal and distal to the bleeding site is ideal, although proximal embolization is usually sufficient to reduce the perfusion pressure enough to stop bleeding. A follow-up aortogram is necessary to ensure that the hemorrhage has been controlled.

For further information on this topic, please see Tutorials 13 and 18.

Selected Readings

Mink J. Percutaneous bone biopsy in the patient with known or suspected osseous metastases. Radiology 1986; 161:191–194.

Young AT, Tadavarthy SM, Yedlicka JW Jr, et al. Embolotherapy: agents, equipment, and techniques. In: Castaneda-Zuniga WR, Tadavarthy SM, eds. Interventional radiology. 2nd edition. Baltimore: Williams and Wilkins, 1992.

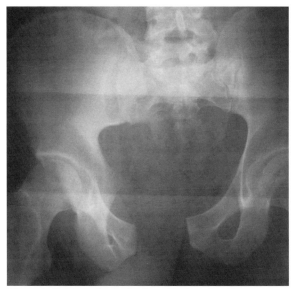

Figure 1. Pelvic radiograph of a patient involved in a motorcycle accident.

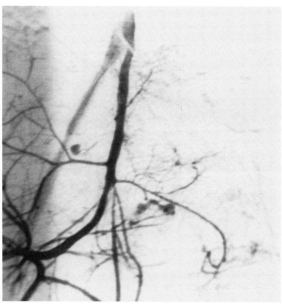

Figure 2. Right internal iliac arteriogram, mid arterial phase.

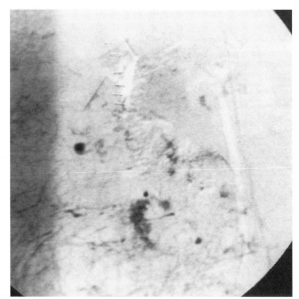

Figure 3. Right internal iliac arteriogram, 30 seconds after injection.

TEACHING FILE CASE 64
Jeet Sandhu, M.D.

History
A 30-year-old man was involved in a motorcycle accident and came to the hospital with continuously decreasing hematocrit and persistent hypotension (systolic blood pressure of 100 mm Hg) despite volume re-expansion. A pelvic radiograph **(Fig. 1)** and a pelvic arteriogram were obtained **(Figs. 2, 3)**.

What is your diagnosis?

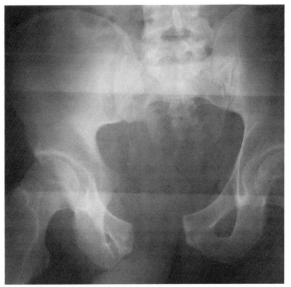

Figure 4. Type 2 anterior posterior compression pelvic fracture.

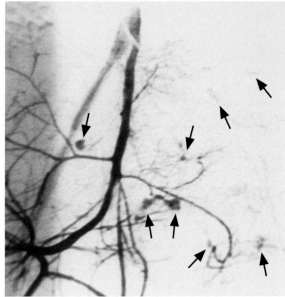

Figure 5. Multiple areas of contrast material extravasation (arrows) from several branches of the internal iliac artery.

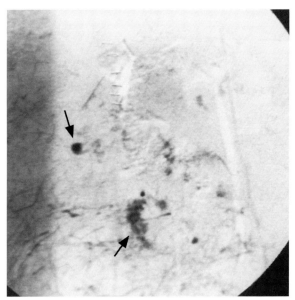

Figure 6. Areas of extravasation are better visualized on the delayed image (arrows).

Radiographic Findings

The plain film of the pelvis **(Fig. 4)** demonstrates an anterior posterior compression (APC) type 2 injury with diastasis of the pubic symphysis and widening of the right sacroiliac (SI) joint. The posterior portion of the right SI joint appears to be intact. If the posterior portion were also disrupted, this would be classified as an APC type 3 injury. Because of the patient's clinical status and need for continuous blood replacement, an arteriogram was obtained **(Figs. 5, 6)**. Multifocal areas of contrast material extravasation indicative of arterial injury are delineated on both the early and late phases of the arteriogram.

Diagnosis

Pelvic hemorrhage secondary to traumatic injury to internal iliac arterial branches.

How would you manage this patient?

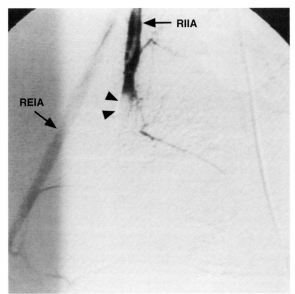

Figure 7. Postembolization arteriogram of the right internal iliac artery demonstrates Gelfoam particles (arrowheads) in the artery with stagnant flow and no evidence of extravasation. REIA=right external iliac artery; RIIA=right internal iliac artery.

Management

It was decided to proceed with embolization. Because of the multiple sites of bleeding involving numerous vessels, the internal iliac artery was nonselectively embolized with Gelfoam pledgets (Upjohn, Kalamazoo, MI). The postembolization arteriogram **(Fig. 7)** showed no further extravasation. The contralateral left internal iliac artery also had multiple areas of extravasation and was similarly embolized.

Discussion

Despite improved transport networks and treatment algorithms, morbidity and mortality from pelvic trauma remain a significant problem. Most pelvic fractures can be managed conservatively or with simple orthopedic fixation. However, over one third are complex fractures associated with severe pelvic hemorrhage or injuries to other body organs. With complex fractures, the mortality rates may be as high as 50% due to exsanguination, associated injuries, multiple organ failure, or sepsis. In order to maximize the chances of survival, treatment of complex pelvic fractures requires a committed multidisciplinary effort with contributions from traumatologists, surgeons, orthopedists, and interventional radiologists.

Complex pelvic fractures result from the high-energy interactions associated with motor vehicle accidents, falls from heights, or crush injuries. In addition to the bony fractures, there may be disruption of the stabilizing pelvic ligaments, including the sacroiliac, sacrospinous, and sacrotuberous ligaments. As will be discussed later, ligamentous disruption contributes significantly to the incidence and etiology of pelvic hemorrhage.

There are several mechanisms by which the vessels can be injured. Vessels can be directly lacerated by the sharp ends of the fractured bones. They can also be disrupted by the significant shear forces caused by diastasis that results from ligamentous injury.

Despite the presence of associated hematomas, contrast material extravasation is seen in only 20%–30% of arteriograms performed for pelvic trauma. In the majority of cases, the bleeding results from small-caliber veins or from the richly vascularized pelvic bones. Because of this, the role of pelvic arteriography and embolization remains unsettled.

Before performing a pelvic arteriogram, it is necessary to ascertain that the bleeding is indeed from the pelvic injury. In the traumatized patient, associated intraabdominal injury occurs in 50% of cases. Intraabdominal sources should be eliminated as an etiology of hemodynamic instability with a diagnostic peritoneal lavage or abdominal computed tomography (CT) scanning. If both intraabdominal and pelvic sources of significant hemorrhage are present, a laparotomy should be performed expeditiously followed by immediate postoperative pelvic arteriography.

The role of external fixation in ameliorating pelvic hemorrhage continues to evolve. In the past, external fixators have been large, bulky devices that were difficult to apply and that interfered with subsequent therapeutic maneuvers such as laparotomy and arteriography. Because of these drawbacks, external fixation was not extensively utilized. With the development of the C-clamp, many of these concerns have been eliminated. Because of its design, it can be rotated out of the way for other procedures and can be rapidly applied in the emergency department.

There are numerous advantages to prompt stabilization of pelvic fractures with an external device. The most significant is reduction of the pelvic volume, which promotes more effective tamponade. Ligamentous disruption has a dramatic impact on pelvic geometry. Because of the spherical configuration of the pelvis, small increases in the radius induced by diastasis produce marked increases in the pelvic volume. Because volume is a function of the cube of the radius, a 2-cm increase in radius enlarges the pelvic volume from 1.5 L to 4.5 L. External fixation can normalize the pelvic volume and thereby limit the amount of bleeding. External fixation also creates apposition of the bony fragments.

Reapposing the fractures compresses the hemorrhaging osseus surfaces and allows clot formation to occur. Because most pelvic bleeding is osseus or venous in nature, temporary external fixation may obviate the need for arteriography in a large number of cases. An important caveat concerning the use of external C-clamps or fixators is that they must be deployed rapidly and expertly. If experienced personnel are not available to apply the fixators, the patient should immediately proceed to arteriography, provided that other sources of hemorrhage have been excluded.

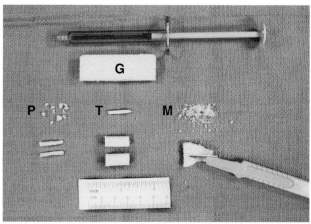

Figure 8. Gelfoam sponge (G) can be tailored in a number of ways for delivery, including pledgets (P), torpedoes (T), and microparticles (M). Microparticles are admixed with contrast material and injected as a slurry.

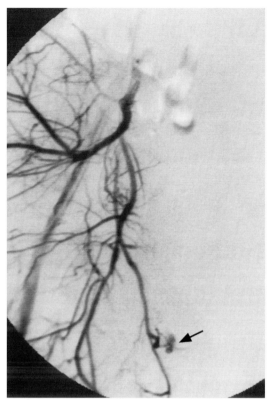

Figure 9. Right internal iliac arteriogram shows extravasation (arrows) from the internal pudendal artery.

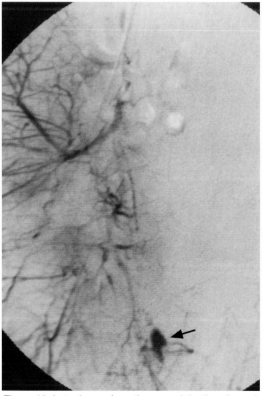

Figure 10. Later image from the same injection shown in Figure 9. The extravasation (arrows) is more apparent.

Open surgical management of bleeding pelvic fractures is extremely difficult. If the pelvic hematoma is incised, all effects from the tamponade are lost and the patient may exsanguinate before vascular control can be obtained. If a large retroperitoneal hematoma is identified during exploratory laparotomy, open drainage should not be attempted and the patient should be transferred to the angiography suite for possible embolization.

The importance of a rapid coordinated approach to pelvic hemorrhage cannot be overemphasized. Patients who arrive at the emergency department hemodynamically unstable and can not be stabilized have a mortality rate of 42%, while those who are hemodynamically stable or can be stabilized have a mortality rate of 3%. Embolization can play a critical role in stabilizing and treating the patient. The patient who is persistently hypotensive (systolic blood pressure <90 mm Hg) and does not have an intraabdominal source of bleeding should proceed directly to angiography (instead of undergoing external fixation) because the chances of a significant arterial injury are increased.

Any patient who continues to require transfusion support or does not stabilize hemodynamically despite external fixation should undergo arteriography. The transfemoral approach is preferred but if both groins are inaccessible, an axillary approach can be utilized. The study should commence with an abdominal aortogram to exclude lumbar artery injuries and to identify the site of maximal pelvic contrast material extravasation.

If extravasation is noted on the aortogram, that vessel should be embolized initially. Gelfoam **(Fig. 8)** and coil spring emboli are the agents of choice. These agents are inexpensive, readily available, and easily delivered. Microvascular occluding agents (Gelfoam powder, polyvinyl alcohol microparticles) and liquid embolic agents are contraindicated because of the risk of nerve, bladder, and bowel infarction.

On arteriography, extravasation appears as a collection of contrast material outside the normal confines of the vessel which persists and may increase in size on later images **(Figs. 9, 10)**.

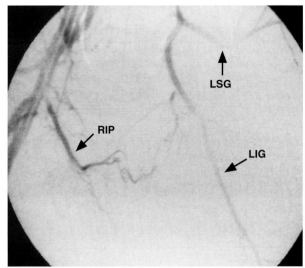

Figure 11. Pelvic arteriogram, early arterial phase. RIP=right internal pudendal artery; LSG=left superior gluteal artery; LIG=left inferior gluteal artery.

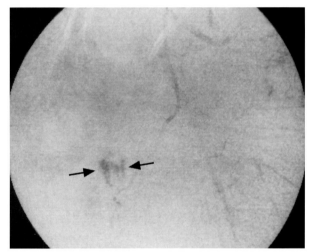

Figure 12. Pelvic arteriogram, late arterial phase. A prominent cavernosal blush is present (arrows), which could simulate extravasation.

There are several entities that can mimic contrast material extravasation in the pelvis. The most common of these is a cavernosal blush (Figs. 11, 12), which can be differentiated from contrast material extravasation by its location and lack of persistence. A uterine blush, ureteral peristalsis, or retained contrast material in a diverticulum can all mimic extravasation on occasion. Once contrast material extravasation, pseudoaneurysm, or vessel transection is identified, embolization should be performed.

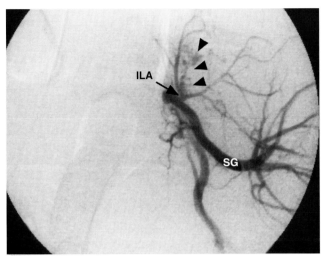

Figure 13. Left internal iliac arteriogram shows extravasation (arrowheads) from the iliolumbar artery (ILA). SG=superior gluteal artery.

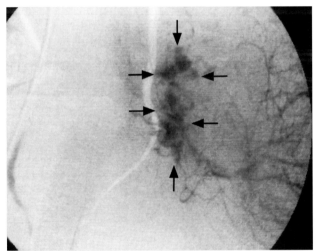

Figure 14. Late arterial phase of the arteriogram shown in Figure 13. Extravasation (arrows) from the iliolumbar artery has become more prominent.

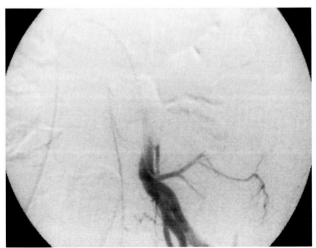

Figure 15. Internal iliac arteriogram after embolization with Gelfoam slurry and pledgets. No extravasation is present.

Figures 13–15 review the case of a patient who was struck by an automobile. On the initial arteriogram, there is contrast material extravasation from the iliolumbar artery. This vessel was successfully embolized with Gelfoam slurry and pledgets. In most cases, there is multifocal vessel involvement. In these cases, nonselective embolization is performed. If massive extravasation is present and the patient is hemodynamically unstable, an expeditious embolization of the entire internal iliac artery should be performed. If the proximal portions of the internal iliac artery are being embolized, forceful injections of the Gelfoam or contrast material should be avoided to prevent refluxing embolic material into the external iliac artery.

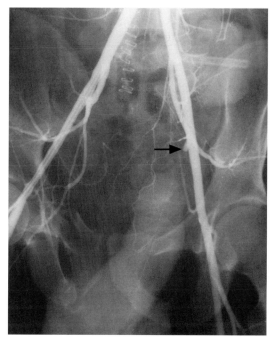

Figure 16. Pelvic arteriogram from a patient who was struck by a car demonstrates abrupt termination of the anterior division (arrow) of the left internal iliac artery. Note fractures through both inferior and superior pubic rami with widening of the left sacroiliac joint.

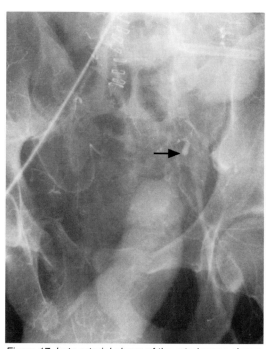

Figure 17. Late arterial phase of the arteriogram shown in Figure 16. Contrast material opacifies the origin of the occluded anterior division but extravasation is not seen.

Rarely, a transected vessel that is not actively bleeding will be identified **(Figs. 16–18)**. The patient shown in **Figures 16–20** became hemodynamically unstable during the examination. Additional contrast material injections while the patient was hypotensive showed active extravasation from the transected anterior division of the left internal iliac artery. The bleeding artery was then successfully embolized. Fortunately, the bleeding occurred during the procedure; transected vessels can have delayed hemorrhage. Vessel transection is most commonly noted in the superior gluteal artery where it impacts against the sciatic notch in patients who have fallen and landed on their feet.

If extravasation is not identified but the patient has a large pelvic hematoma and evidence of continued blood loss, empiric embolization should be considered. Bilateral internal iliac artery embolization is generally performed because cross-pelvic collaterals usually make unilateral embolization ineffective.

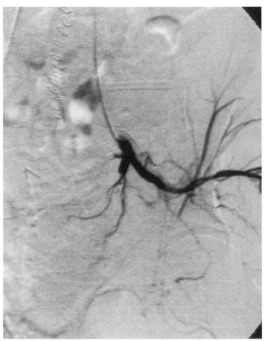

Figure 18. Left internal iliac arteriogram confirms the absence of extravasation.

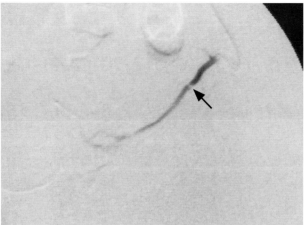

Figure 19. Injection into the anterior division after the patient became hemodynamically unstable shows flow past the site of previous termination with an area of intimal injury at the site of transection (arrow).

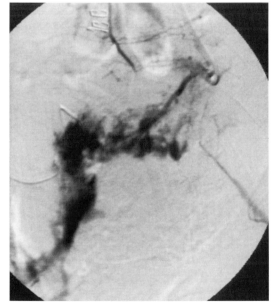

Figure 20. Gross extravasation from the transected branch is evident on later images. The artery was successfully embolized.

Complications related to pelvic embolization are very uncommon. Bilateral occlusion of the internal iliac arteries seldom results in bladder or rectal ischemia. The question of impotence induced by a pelvic embolization always arises. Because of the associated urologic injuries and damage to the lumbosacral plexus, it is difficult to know whether to ascribe impotence to the embolization itself or to the underlying trauma. As noted by Ben-Menachem, "most of us would rather have the patient alive and impotent, than dead."

Complex pelvic fractures result in serious morbidity and mortality and require a rapid integrated multispecialty approach to minimize deaths. Interventional radiologists are an integral part of this team, providing recommendations regarding the appropriate timing of diagnostic and therapeutic arteriographic procedures.

For further information on this topic, please see Tutorials 13 and 18, and Teaching File Case 65.

Selected Readings

Agnew SG. Hemodynamically unstable pelvic fractures. Orth Clin North Am 1994; 25:715–721.

Ben-Menachem Y, Coldwell DM, Young JW, Burgess AR. Hemorrhage associated with pelvic fractures: causes, diagnosis, and emergent management. AJR 1991; 157:1005–1014.

Berger JJ, Britt LD. Pelvic fracture hemorrhage: current strategies in diagnosis and management. Surg Annu 1995; 27:107–112.

Burgess AR, Eastridge BJ, Young JW, et al. Pelvic ring disruptions: effective classification system and treatment protocols. J Trauma 1990; 30:848–856.

Ghanayem AJ, Stover MD, Goldstein JA, Bellon E, Wilber JH. Emergent treatment of pelvic fractures: comparison of methods for stabilization. Clin Orthop 1995; 318:75–80.

Moreno C, Moore EE, Rosenberger A, Cleveland HC. Hemorrhage associated with major pelvic fracture: a multispecialty challenge. J Trauma 1986; 26:987–994.

Mucha P, Farnell MB. Analysis of pelvic fracture management. J Trauma 1984; 24:379–386.

Panetta TM, Sclafani SJ, Goldstein AS, Phillips TF, Shaftan GW. Percutaneous transcatheter embolization for massive bleeding from pelvic fractures. J Trauma 1985; 25:1021–1029.

Yellin AE, Lundell CJ, Finck EJ. Diagnosis and control of post-traumatic pelvic hemorrhage: transcatheter angiographic embolization techniques. Arch Surg 1983; 118:1378–1383.

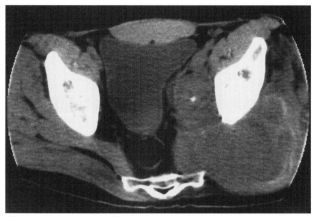

Figure 1. Noncontrast CT scan.

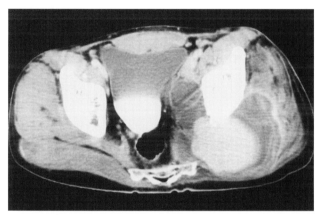

Figure 2. Contrast-enhanced CT scan.

TEACHING FILE CASE 65
Anthony G. Verstandig, M.D.

History

A 25-year-old man came to the hospital with a painful pulsatile left buttock mass and progressive left leg weakness. Two months earlier he had suffered a gun shot wound to the left buttock with an exit wound close to the spinous process of L4. At that time, radiographs demonstrated a fracture of the left side of the first sacral vertebra. Exploratory surgery had revealed no damage to major organs or the sciatic nerve, and the patient had been discharged with no neurologic deficit. Pre- and post-contrast computed tomography (CT) scans of the pelvis were performed **(Figs. 1, 2)**.

What is your diagnosis?

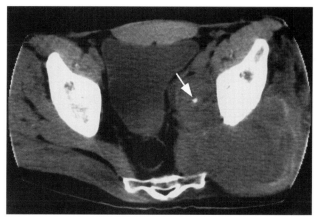

Figure 3. Noncontrast CT scan demonstrates a bilobed mass straddling the left sciatic notch and containing a small bone fragment (arrow).

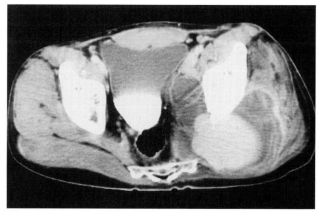

Figure 4. Contrast-enhanced CT scan shows intense homogeneous enhancement most compatible with a large pseudoaneurysm.

Radiographic Findings

The unenhanced scan **(Fig. 3)** demonstrates a bilobed mass measuring 12 x 9 x 8 cm and straddling the sciatic notch on the left. The intrapelvic component of the mass contains a small bone fragment and displaces the bladder to the right. The post-contrast scan **(Fig. 4)** demonstrates rim enhancement and, in addition, marked enhancement of an oval-shaped 7.5 x 6-cm area in the center of the mass.

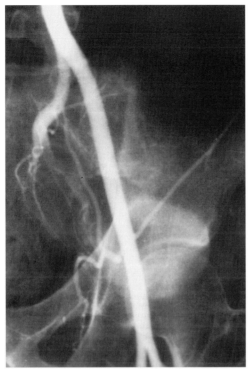

Figure 5. Left common iliac arteriogram shows a pseudoaneurysm extending from the left sciatic notch.

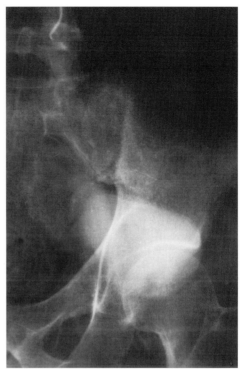

Figure 6. Later film from the arteriogram shown in Figure 5 demonstrates the full extent of the pseudoaneurysm.

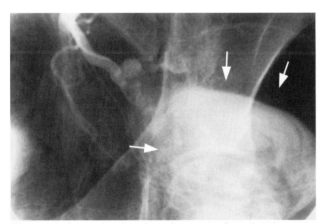

Figure 7. Left superior gluteal arteriogram confirms that the pseudoaneurysm (arrows) is supplied by this vessel.

Diagnosis
Post-traumatic pseudoaneurysm causing sciatic nerve compression.

An arteriogram was obtained to evaluate the pseudoaneurysm and its arterial supply. Left common iliac arteriography **(Figs. 5, 6)** and selective superior gluteal arteriography **(Fig. 7)** demonstrate an 8-cm x 6-cm pseudoaneurysm arising from the superior gluteal branch of the internal iliac artery.

What treatment would you recommend?

Management
The superior gluteal artery was occluded with Gianturco coil spring emboli (Cook, Bloomington, IN). The first two coils were placed too distally within the superior gluteal artery (SGA) and migrated into the pseudoaneurysm. Repeat left common iliac arteriography **(Figs. 8, 9)** shows occlusion of the SGA with no filling of the pseudoaneurysm. A right common iliac arteriogram was also obtained which demonstrated no filling of the pseudoaneurysm from cross-pelvic collaterals. Within minutes the buttock mass became non-pulsatile and less painful.

A contrast-enhanced CT scan obtained 6 weeks later **(Fig. 10)** showed that the size of the mass had decreased to 9 x 7.5 x 6 cm with no central enhancement. Both the mass and the leg weakness secondary to sciatic nerve compression resolved.

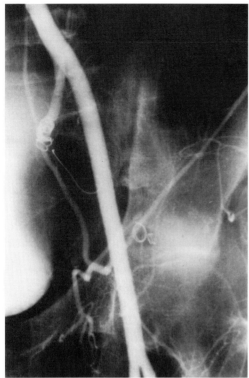

Figure 8. Left common iliac arteriogram following embolization shows successful occlusion of the superior gluteal artery.

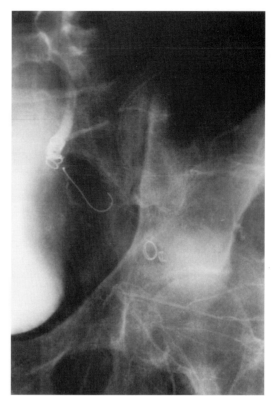

Figure 9. Later film from the same injection shown in Figure 8 confirms successful arterial occlusion. Residual contrast material from the previous injection persists within the pseudoaneurysm.

Discussion

Pseudoaneurysm of the gluteal artery is a rare sequela of penetrating or severe blunt pelvic trauma. Surgical treatment is difficult because it requires a combined anterior and posterior approach to control the internal iliac artery and obliterate the aneurysm. Post-traumatic pseudoaneurysms are nearly always supplied by a single artery and are therefore ideally suited for transcatheter embolotherapy.

In cases where there is continuation of the damaged vessel beyond the origin of the aneurysm, it is necessary to occlude the artery both proximal and distal to the aneurysm neck to prevent retrograde filling. In all cases, *complete* postembolization arteriography is essential to ensure that there is no filling of the aneurysm via collateral vessels. Because there is good collateral supply in the pelvis, occlusion of a single artery rarely causes ischemic complications.

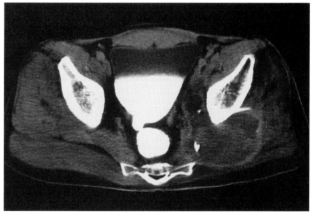

Figure 10. Contrast-enhanced CT scan 6 weeks after embolization shows a decrease in the size of the mass with no central enhancement.

For further information on this topic, please see Tutorials 13 and 18, and Teaching File Case 64.

Selected Readings

Hultborn KA, Kjellman TH. Gluteal aneurysm: report of three cases and review of the literature. Acta Chir Scand 1963; 125:318–328.

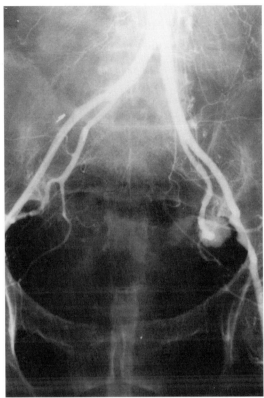

Figure 1. Pelvic arteriogram, mid arterial phase.

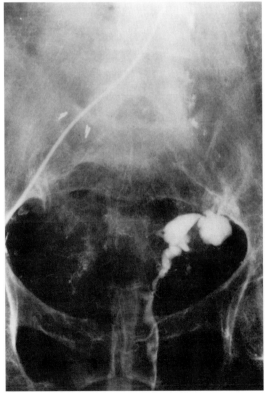

Figure 2. Pelvic arteriogram, delayed film.

TEACHING FILE CASE 66
Anthony G. Verstandig, M.D.

History

A 56-year-old woman came to the emergency department with massive vaginal bleeding and hemodynamic instability. She was known to have ovarian carcinoma with extensive pelvic spread. A pelvic arteriogram was obtained **(Figs. 1, 2)**.

What is your diagnosis?

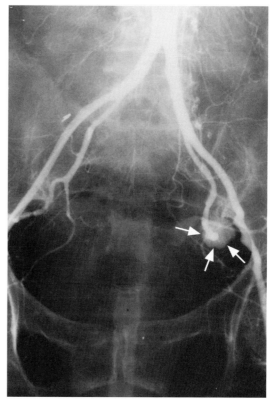

Figure 3. Pelvic arteriogram shows massive contrast material extravasation on the left with filling of a pseudoaneurysm (arrows). There is marked irregularity of the medial border of the external iliac artery.

Radiographic Findings

Pelvic arteriography was performed via a pigtail catheter placed in the distal abdominal aorta from a right common femoral artery puncture. An early film **(Fig. 3)** demonstrates marked extravasation of contrast material into a pseudoaneurysm that was thought to arise from the left internal iliac artery. Marked irregularity of the medial wall of the external iliac artery at the same level is also noted. A delayed film **(Fig. 4)** shows contrast material from the pseudoaneurysm streaming out through the vagina.

Diagnosis

Massive vaginal hemorrhage secondary to malignant neoplastic arterial invasion.

How would you manage this patient?

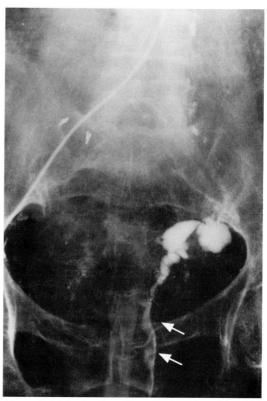

Figure 4. A later film from the same injection shown in Figure 3 reveals contrast material leaking from the pseudoaneurysm into the vagina (arrows).

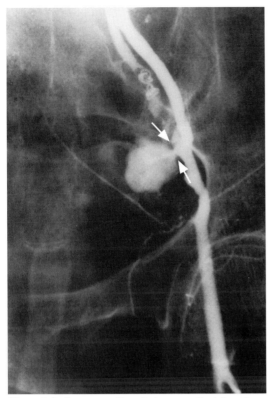

Figure 5. Left common iliac ateriogram after internal iliac artery embolization continues to show massive extravasation, with contrast material jetting out from the external iliac artery (arrows).

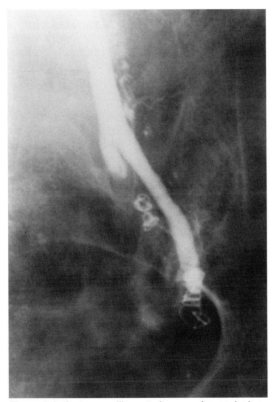

Figure 6. Left common iliac arteriogram after occlusion of the internal and external iliac arteries shows no further extravasation.

Management

The left internal iliac artery was embolized with pieces of Gelfoam (Upjohn, Kalamazoo, MI) and stainless steel coils. A postembolization arteriogram **(Fig. 5)** demonstrates that the site of extravasation was in fact the invaded external iliac artery; a jet of contrast material from this area could be seen filling the pseudoaneurysm. Stainless steel coils were used to occlude the external iliac artery at the level of the extravasation **(Fig. 6)**, and a cross-femoral bypass graft was subsequently performed to revascularize the left leg. The patient initially stabilized but died several days later from complications of the surgery.

Discussion

Pelvic arterial bleeding usually arises from branches of the internal iliac artery which can be occluded with a very low risk of complications. External iliac artery embolization will cause acute lower limb ischemia. In this case, because the bleeding was life-threatening and operating on a tumor-filled pelvis would be difficult, it was decided to occlude the artery and then revascularize the leg with a bypass graft. The external iliac artery was therefore occluded with stainless steel coils. Coils with a diameter larger than the diameter of the vessel being occluded should be used. The coils will then lodge in the vessel at the site of deployment without migrating distally.

As an alternative, a covered stent-graft could have been used to maintain vascular continuity and exclude the false aneurysm. Unfortunately, stent-grafts are not readily available and the rate of blood loss in this patient demanded prompt intervention.

For further information on this topic, please see Tutorial 13.

Selected Readings

Murphy KD, Richter GM, Henry M, Encarnacion CE, Le VA, Palmaz JC. Aortoiliac aneurysms: management with endovascular stent-graft placement. Radiology 1996; 198:473–480.

Yamashita Y, Harada M, Yamamoto H, et al. Transcatheter arterial embolization of obstetric and gynaecological bleeding: efficacy and clinical outcome. Br J Radiol 1994; 67:530–534.

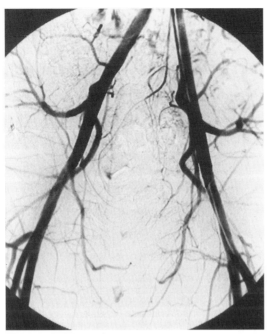
Figure 1. Pelvic arteriogram.

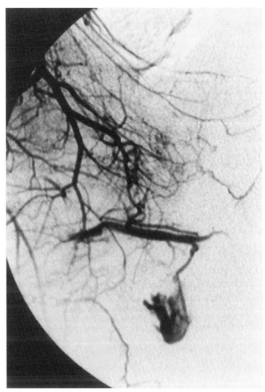
Figure 2. Right internal iliac arteriogram.

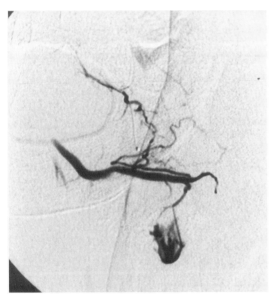
Figure 3. Right internal pudendal arteriogram.

TEACHING FILE CASE 67
Richard Duszak, Jr., M.D., and
Ziv J. Haskal, M.D.

History

A 17-year-old male came to the hospital with several weeks of painless priapism, which began shortly after he sustained a straddle injury while climbing over a fence. There was no history of sickle cell disease or hypercoagulable state. Examination by the referring urologist demonstrated strong corporeal arterial pulsations by Doppler sonography and bright red blood with high oxygen tension at corporeal aspiration. Nonselective digital arteriography of the pelvis was performed **(Fig. 1)**, followed by selective and subselective arteriography of the right internal iliac artery **(Figs. 2, 3)**.

What is your diagnosis?

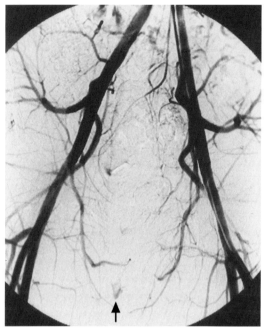

Figure 4. Pelvic arteriogram shows an amorphous blush (arrow) in the inferior right pelvis.

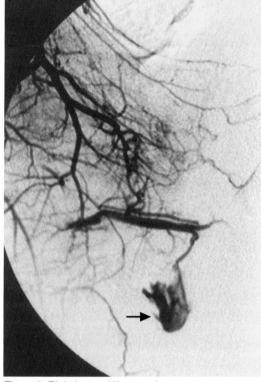

Figure 5. Right internal iliac arteriogram demonstrates intravasation of contrast material (arrow) from the right cavernosal artery into the right corpus cavernosum.

Figure 6. An early draining vein (arrows) is identified following a superselective right internal pudendal arteriogram.

Radiographic Findings

Nonselective digital arteriography of the pelvis demonstrates an amorphous blush of contrast material just to the right of midline in the lower pelvis **(Fig. 4)**. Selective arteriography of the right internal iliac artery reveals intravasation of contrast material from the proximal right cavernosal artery into the right corpus cavernosum **(Fig. 5)**. Early venous filling is also present **(Fig. 6)** on pudendal arteriography.

Diagnosis

High-flow arterial priapism, secondary to injury of the cavernosal artery, with arterial-corporeal and arterio-venous fistulas.

What intervention could you offer?

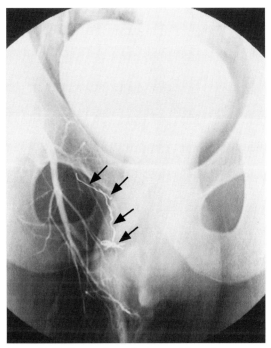

Figure 7. Platinum microcoils (arrows) have been deposited into the internal pudendal artery proximal to the damaged right cavernosal artery.

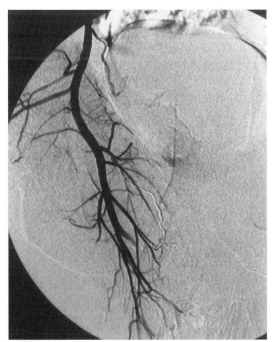

Figure 8. Right internal iliac arteriogram obtained following embolization shows no extravasation from the damaged artery.

Management

Subselective catheterization of the right pudendal artery was performed using a 7-F cobra catheter and a 3-F coaxial microcatheter system. Embolization was performed with platinum coils, resulting in occlusion of the arteriovenous fistula and cessation of corporeal intravasation **(Figs. 7, 8)**. Partial detumescence occurred moments later.

Discussion

Based upon the underlying pathophysiology, priapism has been classified into two types:
1) low-flow veno-occlusive priapism;
2) high-flow arterial priapism.

The veno-occlusive type is considerably more common and is characterized by pain, absence of arterial flow by Doppler, and dark hypoxic corporeal blood aspirates. Venous outflow is impeded by intravascular obstruction at the venular level, often related to hematological syndromes (such as sickle cell disease), hypercoagulable states, fat emboli, or metastatic tumor.

The less common high-flow form of priapism is typically related to a traumatic insult and is characterized by the relative absence of pain, and by the presence of corporeal arterial pulsations by Doppler sonography and oxygenated red blood at aspiration. Laceration of an intracavernosal artery produces unregulated arterial flow into the corpora cavernosa. In contrast to veno-occlusive priapism, venous outflow remains unimpeded.

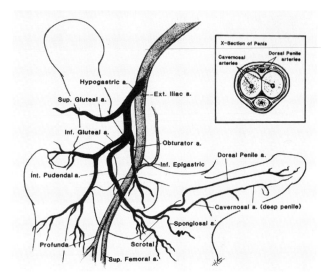

Figure 9. Diagram of right internal iliac arterial anatomy.

In cases of high-flow priapism, intravasation of contrast material into the corpora is usually demonstrable at arteriography. Familiarity with normal angiographic anatomy will facilitate diagnosis and aid in planning embolization **(Fig. 9)**.

Surgical options for the treatment of this condition include ligation of the internal pudendal artery or ligation of the cavernosal artery, if it can be localized at dissection. Surgical ligation, particularly of the pudendal artery, can be complicated by impotence and gangrene.

Recently, transcatheter embolization has been used effectively. Embolization was previously performed nonselectively with autologous clot; however, the technique has since evolved into superselective coil embolization.

For further information on this topic, please see Tutorials 13 and 18.

Selected Readings

Brock G, Breza J, Lue TF, Tanagho EA. High-flow priapism: a spectrum of disease. J Urol 1993; 150:968–971.

Crummy AB, Ishizuka H, Madsen PO. Post-traumatic priapism: successful treatment with autologous clot embolization. AJR 1979; 133:329–330.

Walker TG, Grant PW, Goldstein I, Krane RJ, Greenfield AJ. High-flow priapism: treatment with superselective transcatheter embolization. Radiology 1990; 174:1053–1054.

Witt MA, Goldstein I, Saenz de Tejada I, Greenfield A, Krane RJ. Traumatic laceration of intracavernosal arteries: the pathophysiology of nonischemic, high-flow, arterial priapism. J Urol 1990; 143:129–132.

End Notes

Figure 9 from Rosen MP, Walker TG, Greenfield AJ. Arteriography and radiology of impotence. Urol Radiol 1988; 10:136–143. Used with permission.

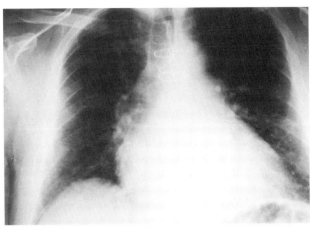

Figure 1. Initial chest radiograph.

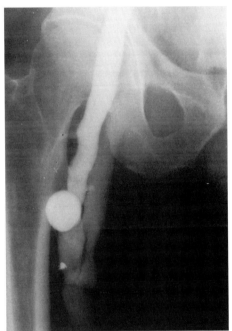

Figure 2. Right femoral arteriogram.

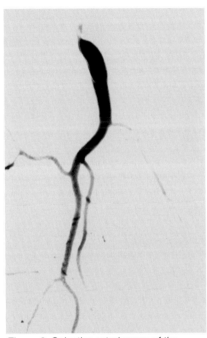

Figure 3. Selective arteriogram of the distal profunda femoral artery.

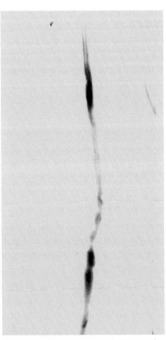

Figure 4. Selective arteriogram of the superficial femoral artery.

TEACHING FILE CASE 68
David Sacks, M.D.

History

A 67-year-old man was admitted to the hospital for evaluation of shortness of breath and was found to be in high-output congestive heart failure **(Fig. 1)**. Forty years earlier he had been hit by shrapnel in the right groin and recalls having been told that some of the pieces were too deep to remove. He had a bruit over the right groin with normal pedal pulses. An arteriogram was obtained **(Figs. 2–4)**.

What is your diagnosis?

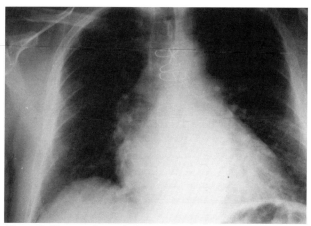

Figure 5. Chest radiograph demonstrates cardiomegaly and pulmonary vascular engorgement.

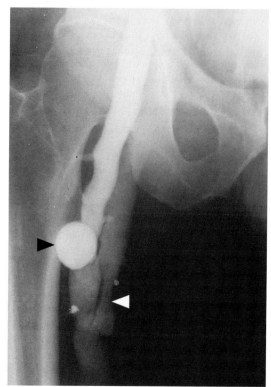

Figure 6. Right common femoral arteriogram reveals an aneurysm in the PFA (black arrowhead) and a mild stenosis of the PFV (white arrowhead).

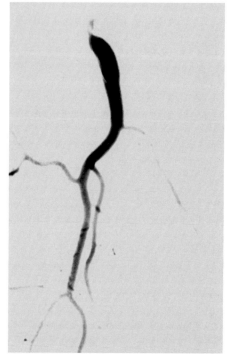

Figure 7. Selective profunda femoris arteriogram beyond the arteriovenous fistula shows a normal distal artery.

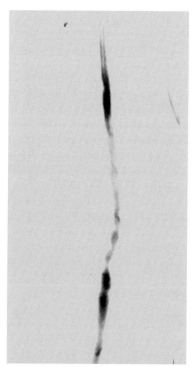

Figure 8. Selective superficial femoral arteriogram reveals moderate atherosclerotic irregularity.

Radiographic Findings

The chest radiograph **(Fig. 5)** shows cardiomegaly and pulmonary vascular engorgement compatible with congestive heart failure. The right leg arteriogram **(Fig. 6)** shows huge common femoral and profunda femoral arteries with rapid filling of enlarged profunda femoral and common femoral veins. There is an aneurysm in the profunda femoral artery (PFA) and a mild stenosis of the profunda femoral vein (PFV). There is no filling of the more distal PFA or of the superficial femoral artery (SFA). A small piece of metal shrapnel is present adjacent to the distal PFV. Selective injection of the PFA beyond the arteriovenous communication **(Fig. 7)** shows a normal-sized vessel with antegrade flow. Selective injection into the SFA **(Fig. 8)** shows moderate atherosclerosis with no filling of the PFA or PFV.

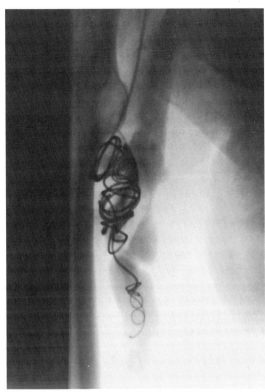

Figure 9. Coils are deposited in the PFA both proximal and distal to the arteriovenous communication.

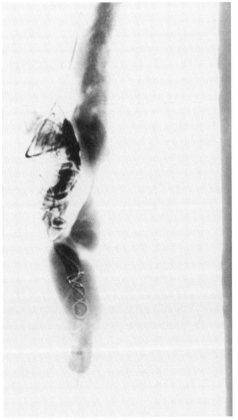

Figure 10. Persistent flow in the AV fistula is present following the embolization despite inflation of an occlusion balloon in the PFA for 1 hour.

Diagnosis

Congestive heart failure due to a chronic traumatic arteriovenous (AV) fistula from the profunda femoral artery to vein.

What treatment would you recommend?

Management

Embolization of the fistula was performed using Gianturco stainless steel coils (Cook, Bloomington, IN) soaked in thrombin. A 5-mm coil was placed into the distal PFA. A second coil was draped from the distal to the proximal PFA across the fistula to prevent systemic venous embolization by subsequent coils. Twenty additional thrombin-soaked coils were then placed into the proximal PFA **(Fig. 9)**. Flow continued to be present across the coils. A latex occlusion balloon was then inflated in the proximal PFA for 1 hour, following which flow was still present **(Fig. 10)**, although slowed.

What would you do next?

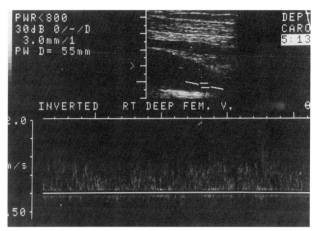

Figure 11. Duplex sonogram shows persistent flow in the PFV 1 day after embolization.

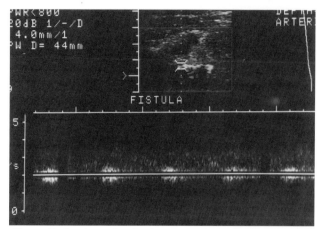

Figure 12. Persistent flow is also present in the fistula 1 day after embolization.

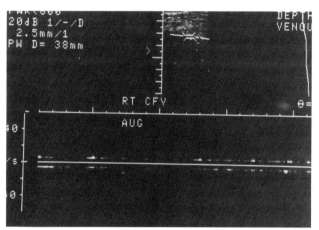

Figure 13. There is no flow in the common femoral vein 2 weeks after embolization.

The catheter was removed, and the patient was studied with duplex sonography the next day. This showed persistent arterialized flow in the PFV **(Fig. 11)** and flow in the fistula **(Fig. 12)**. The patient was discharged and advised to stop taking the aspirin he had been taking for his coronary artery disease. The patient was readmitted 2 weeks later with an acutely swollen right leg. Duplex sonography showed no flow in the profunda femoral vein, common femoral vein **(Fig. 13)**, or superficial femoral vein **(Fig. 14)**. He was treated with anticoagulants for acute deep venous thrombosis with resolution of his leg swelling. A follow-up chest radiograph **(Fig. 15)** showed reduction of cardiac size and resolution of the pulmonary vascular congestion. Clinically, the congestive heart failure had resolved.

Discussion
Acute traumatic arteriovenous fistulas (AVF), particularly those due to arterial catheterization injuries, may resolve spontaneously. Although the acute fistula is usually fed by a single artery, the chronic traumatic AVF can recruit additional feeding vessels so that the angiographic appearance mimics a congenital arteriovenous malformation. Surgical repair of an acute traumatic AVF is usually not technically difficult. Ligation of a chronic arteriovenous fistula can be extremely difficult due to the presence of innumerable large veins under arterial pressure.

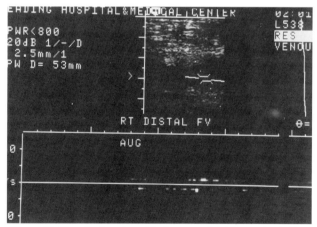

Figure 14. Flow is also absent in the superficial femoral vein 2 weeks after embolization.

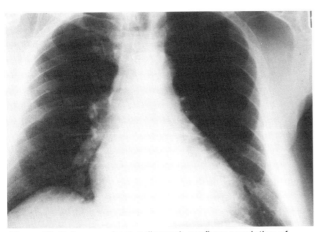

Figure 15. Follow-up chest radiograph confirms resolution of congestive heart failure.

It is essential to visualize all potential feeding vessels prior to embolization. In this case it was also essential to confirm the patency of the SFA in order to ascertain that occlusion of the PFA would not render the leg ischemic. Because of the sump effect of the arteriovenous connection, it is necessary to occlude the feeding artery both proximal and distal to the fistula to prevent retrograde filling of the fistula. An alternative treatment is to attempt to occlude the fistula directly, but this increases the risk of losing emboli into the lungs. In this case the risk of embolizing to the lungs was reduced because of the stricture of the PFV.

Coils were chosen in this case because of their availability and ease of placement. In the presence of rapid flow coils may not be sufficiently thrombogenic to occlude the vessel. Thrombogenicity can be enhanced by soaking the coils in thrombin prior to use. Detachable balloons could have been used but were not available. Covered endovascular stents are ideal for traumatic arterial injuries but are not yet approved for use. The difference in size between the proximal and distal PFA in this case would make placement of a covered stent difficult.

Other treatment options were placement of additional coils or injection of large particulate emboli or glue in an attempt to occlude the fistula during the initial procedure. Large pieces of Gelfoam (Upjohn, Kalamazoo, MI) might pass through the coils and go to the lungs, and glue is not readily available. In this case additional time off aspirin was all that was necessary to complete the occlusion.

Deep venous thrombosis is not a surprising complication of chronic AV fistula occlusion. Markedly dilated veins are suddenly converted from high-flow to low-flow vessels while the patient is immobile recovering from the procedure. There is little information currently available on the best way to avoid this complication.

Selected Readings

Clark RA, Gallant TE, Alexander ES. Angiographic management of traumatic arteriovenous fistulas: clinical results. Radiology 1983; 147:9–13.

Harman JT, Becker GJ. Thrombin-soaked coils: estimation of thrombin dose. J Vasc Interv Radiol 1991; 2:166–168.

Lawdahl RB, Routh WD, Vitek JJ, McDowell HA, Gross GM, Keller FS. Chronic arteriovenous fistulas masquerading as arteriovenous malformations: diagnostic considerations and therapeutic implications. Radiology 1989; 170:1011–1015.

McLean GK, Stein EJ, Burke DR, Meranze SG. Steel occlusion coils: pretreatment with thrombin. Radiology 1986; 158:549–550.

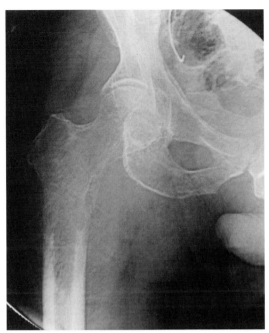

Figure 1. Digital hip radiograph.

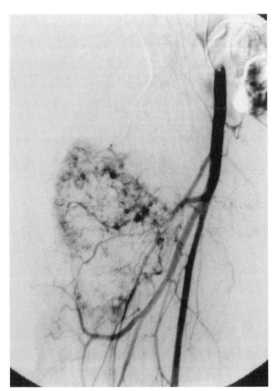

Figure 2. External iliac arteriogram.

TEACHING FILE CASE 69
Michael A. Amygdalos, M.D., and Ziv J. Haskal, M.D.

History

A 69-year-old man with a history of renal cell carcinoma came to the hospital with right hip pain. A radiograph of the hip was obtained **(Fig. 1)**. Subsequent work-up confirmed the diagnosis of metastatic renal cell carcinoma to the right femur. A surgical resection and hip replacement was planned. A preoperative arteriogram was obtained **(Fig. 2)**.

What is your diagnosis?

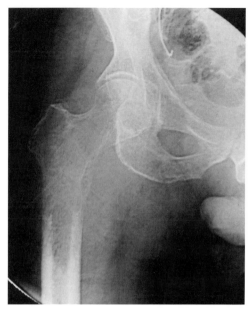

Figure 3. Digital hip radiograph reveals lytic destruction of the femoral neck and proximal femoral shaft.

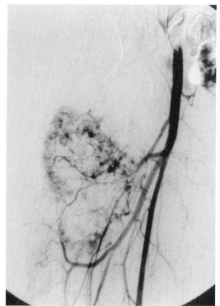

Figure 4. External iliac arteriogram. Malignant neovascularity is present within the metastatic deposit.

Radiographic Findings

The radiograph of the right hip **(Fig. 3)** demonstrates a lytic lesion involving the proximal femur. The arteriogram **(Fig. 4)** demonstrates a hypervascular mass involving the right femoral metadiaphysis.

Diagnosis

Hypervascular renal cell metastasis to the femur.

What preoperative treatment would you recommend?

Management

The metastasis was embolized preoperatively to reduce blood loss during surgery. Arterial branches supplying the tumor were superselectively catheterized. **Figure 5** demonstrates a selective medial femoral circumflex arteriogram. Gianturco coils (Cook, Bloomington, IN) 2 cm long by 3 mm in diameter were placed in branches distal to those supplying the lesion. The lesion was then embolized using a Gelfoam slurry (Upjohn, Kalamazoo, MI) **(Fig. 6)**. A repeat arteriogram **(Fig. 7)** shows continued filling of tumor vessels. The lateral circumflex femoral artery was then superselectively catheterized **(Fig. 8)**. This vessel was embolized using a Gelfoam slurry. The final arteriogram **(Fig. 9)** demonstrates marked reduction in tumor vascularity. The patient did well at surgery.

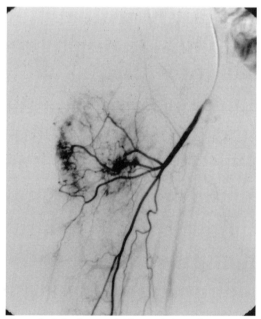

Figure 5. Selective medial femoral circumflex arteriogram shows several branches supplying the tumor.

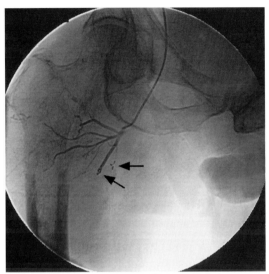

Figure 6. Postembolization arteriogram. Coils have been placed (arrow) to prevent particulate embolization of normal muscular branches.

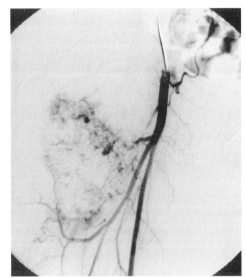

Figure 7. External iliac arteriogram after the initial embolization demonstrates continued flow to the tumor.

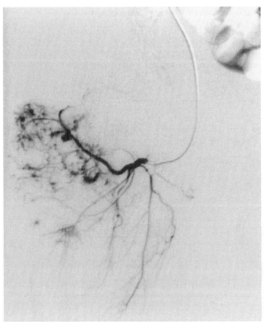

Figure 8. Selective lateral circumflex arteriogram reveals additional branches supplying the tumor.

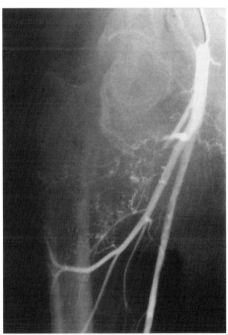

Figure 9. Completion external iliac arteriogram shows a marked decrease in the tumor vascularity.

Discussion

This case demonstrates the value of preoperative embolization of hypervascular lesions. The risk of non-target embolization is reduced when vessels are superselectively catheterized. The use of coils distal to the branches supplying the lesion (distal blockade) allows for preferential filling of tumor vessels with Gelfoam slurry. Nonselective postembolization arteriograms should be obtained to locate other vessels feeding the lesion.

For further information on this topic, please see Tutorial 13.

Selected Readings

Chuang VP, Wallace S, Swanson D, et al. Arterial occlusion in the management of pain from metastatic renal carcinoma. Radiology 1979; 133:611–614.

Feldman F, Casarella WJ, Dick HM, Hollander BA. Selective intraarterial embolization of bone tumors. Am J Roentgenol Radium Ther Nucl Med 1975; 123:130–139.

McLean G, Freiman DB. Angiography of skeletal disease. Orthop Clin North Am 1983; 14:257–270.

CME QUIZZES

Tutorial 1: Anatomy of the Thoracic Aorta

1. The familiar pattern of branching of the normal aortic arch is seen in what percentage of the population?
      a. 50%
      b. 60%
      c. 70%
      d. 80%
      e. 90%

2. The most common anomaly of the branching pattern of the innominate, carotid, and subclavian arteries is?
      a. common origin of the BCA and the right CCA
      b. left CCA originates from the BCA
      c. right and left brachiocephalic trunks
      d. left SCA originates from a bicarotid trunk
      e. bicarotid trunk

3. The left vertebral artery arises directly from the aorta in what percentage of the population?
      a. 1%
      b. 2%
      c. 4%
      d. 6%
      e. 8%

4. An aberrant right subclavian artery with a left aortic arch usually crosses between the trachea and esophagus, potentially causing a condition termed dysphagia lusoria.
      a. true
      b. false

5. The right aortic arch with an aberrant left subclavian artery is often associated with congenital heart diseases.
      a. true
      b. false

Tutorial 2: Thoracic Aneurysms

1. The normal aorta:
1) is widest at the sinotubular junction.
2) gets progressively smaller further from the valve.
3) is generally smaller in females than in males.
4) increases in diameter with age.
      a. 1, 2, and 3
      b. 1 and 3 only
      c. 2 and 4 only
      d. 4 only
      e. All of the above

2. Match the following terms with their corresponding definitions:
1) Diffuse increase in diameter of a vessel larger than 1.5 times expected diameter.
2) Focal dilatation of a vessel, but less than 50% increase in normal expected diameter.
3) A focal enlargement of vessel diameter, over 50% more than expected diameter.
      a. ectasia
      b. aneurysm
      c. arteriomegaly

3. Atherosclerosis tends to worsen with distance from the aortic valve.
      a. true
      b. false

4. Atherosclerosis has a predilection for branch points and vessel ostia.
      a. true
      b. false

5. True aneurysms always show evidence of athero-sclerotic change.
      a. true
      b. false

6. Atherosclerosis can be detected at birth.
      a. true
      b. false

7. Obesity is not a risk factor for atherosclerosis.
      a. true
      b. false

8. Which of the following is/are true?
1) Atherosclerotic plaques are prominent in aneurysms of the arch and ascending thoracic aorta.
2) Atherosclerotic plaques are prominent in aneurysms of the abdominal aorta.
3) The risk of rupture over 5 years for abdominal aneurysms smaller than 5 cm in diameter is high.
4) The protease collagenase may be in part responsible for aneurysm growth.
      a. 1, 2, and 3
      b. 1 and 3 only
      c. 2 and 4 onlly
      d. 4 only
      e. All of the above

9. Aneurysms can erode adjacent osseous structures.
      a. true
      b. false

10. Aneurysm is part of the differential diagnosis of a mass in the retrosternal space.
      a. true
      b. false

11. Aortography accurately depicts aneurysm diameter.
      a. true
      b. false

12. Calcification can lead to artifacts on spiral CT that can be mistaken for dissection.
      a. true
      b. false

13. TEE is the current ACR standard diagnostic exam for detection of descending thoracic aneurysms.
      a. true
      b. false

14. Which one of the following factors complicate aneurysm repair in the descending thoracic aorta:
1) renal failure
2) MI
3) paralysis/paraplegia
4) stroke
      a. 1, 2, and 3
      b. 1 and 3 only
      c. 2 and 4 only
      d. 4 only
      e. all of the above

15. Which of the following is/are true?
1) Penetrating aortic ulcer and dissection tend to occur in the same age group.
2) Penetrating ulcer can mimic the symptoms of dissection.
3) Severe atherosclerosis promotes propagation of a dissection.
4) Penetrating ulcer can progress to pseudoaneurysm formation.
      a. 1, 2, and 3
      b. 1 and 3 only
      c. 2 and 4 only
      d. 4 only
      e. all of the above

16. Penetrating aortic ulcer can cause an atypical dissection.
      a. true
      b. false

17. Erdheim's cystic medial necrosis is so named because of the presence of areas of smooth muscle cell necrosis and the resultant cystic spaces in the media of the aortic wall.
      a. true
      b. false

18. Effacement of the sinotubular junction can occur in annuloaortic ectasia.
      a. true
      b. false

19. The following are features of Marfan's syndrome:
1) hyperflexible joints
2) thoracic aortic aneurysms
3) blue sclerae
4) dolichocephaly
      a. 1, 2, and 3
      b. 1 and 3 only
      c. 2 and 4 only
      d. 4 only
      e. all of the above

20. Regarding Ehlers-Danlos syndrome:
1) Patients typically present at a young age with arterial catastrophes.
2) It is an inherited disorder of connective tissue.
3) Patients may have hypermobile joints.
4) Conventional arteriography should be avoided if possible.
      a. 1, 2, and 3
      b. 1 and 3 only
      c. 2 and 4 only
      d. 4 only
      e. all of the above

Tutorial 3: Aortic Dissection

More than one correct answer may apply

1. Which of these aortic catastrophes has the highest incidence?
   - a. traumatic aortic rupture
   - b. abdominal aortic aneurysm rupture
   - c. aortic dissection
   - d. thoracic aortic aneurysm rupture

2. An aortic dissection has an entry tear at the level of the left subclavian artery and propagates antegrade to the level of the celiac artery and retrograde to the mid ascending aorta. What type is this lesion?
   - a. Debakey type I
   - b. Debakey type II
   - c. Debakey type III
   - d. none of the above

3. The most crucial feature of an aortic dissection to be determined in the imaging work-up is:
   - a. the presence of aortic insufficiency
   - b. involvement of the ascending aorta
   - c. location of the entry tear
   - d. involvement of the brachiocephalic arteries

4. Intramural hemorrhage (dissection) can accompany the following:
   - a. ruptured aortic aneurysm
   - b. penetrating ulcer
   - c. classical type I aortic dissection

5. In classical aortic dissection, common features of the false lumen include:
   - a. larger in cross section than the true lumen
   - b. pressure exceeds or is equal to pressure in the true lumen
   - c. aortic branches arising exclusively from the false lumen have uncompromised flow
   - d. has a thicker outer wall compared to that of the true lumen

6. In aortic dissection, modes of branch vessel compromise include:
   - a. the dissecting hematoma extends into the branch artery
   - b. the dissecting hematoma spares the branch artery, but the dissection flap acts as an obstructing curtain across the origin
   - c. the dissecting hematoma spares the branch artery, but the true lumen is compressed above the branch origin

7. Fenestration of the mural flap between the true and false lumens:
   - a. is indicated to help relieve ischemic complications of aortic dissection
   - b. by decompressing the false lumen, reduces false lumen pressure and thereby reduces the risk of later false lumen expansion and eventual rupture

Tutorial 4: Thoracic Aortic Trauma

1. Plain film findings helpful in suggesting aortic rupture include all of the following except:
   - a. tracheal deviation
   - b. aortic knob obscuration
   - c. mediastinal widening
   - d. left lower lobe consolidation

2. Conventional computed tomography for the diagnosis of aortic injury in the setting of blunt aortic trauma:
   - a. should be used routinely as a screening tool
   - b. relies primarily on identification of second ary signs (ie, mediastinal hematoma)
   - c. is superior to spiral CT
   - d. none of the above

3. The mechanism causing aortic rupture includes
   - a. compressive forces
   - b. shearing forces
   - c. hydrostatic forces
   - d. all of the above

4. Concerning arteriography for suspected aortic injury:
   - a. the pigtail catheter should be positioned in the ascending aorta proximal to the innominate artery
   - b. inclusion of the proximal great vessels and aorta at the level of the diaphragm are essential
   - c. if resistance to catheter passage is met the exam should be cancelled immediately

5. Regarding types of acute injury:
   - a. the most common injury occurs just distal to the left subclavian artery
   - b. overall, ascending aortic injuries are most common
   - c. great vessel injury is usually an isolated injury
   - d. ascending aortic injury has the lowest associated mortality

6. Acute post-traumatic aortic coarctation syndrome:
   - a. is commonly seen
   - b. may be diagnosed on clinical findings
   - c. may be caused by an intimal flap or adjacent pseudoaneurysm compressing the true lumen
   - d. is universally fatal

7. Chronic pseudoaneurysms
   - a. may involve the entire circumference of the aorta
   - b. occur in areas where mediastinal structures contain aortic rupture
   - c. are most frequently identified within one year of injury
   - d. a and b
   - e. all of the above
   - f. none of the above

Tutorial 5: Pulmonary Arteriovenous Malformations

1. Pulmonary arteriovenous malformation most commonly occurs:
    a. in association with pulmonary sequestration
    b. in association with congenital heart disease
    c. in association with hereditary hemorrhagic telangiectasia
    d. in association with the scimitar (pulmonary venolobar) syndrome
    e. sporadically

2. In pulmonary arteriovenous malformation, there is generally an abnormal connection between:
    a. systemic artery and pulmonary vein
    b. pulmonary artery and pulmonary vein
    c. pulmonary artery and systemic vein

3. Common sequelae of pulmonary arteriovenous malformation include:
    a. dyspnea and fatigue
    b. high-output heart failure
    c. stroke
    d. a and c
    e. a, b, and c

4. Patients with pulmonary arteriovenous malformation should be treated:
    a. only if they have symptoms
    b. for prophylaxis against paradoxical emboli
    c. conservatively if asymptomatic
    d. a and c
    e. a, b, and c

5. The definitive modality for diagnosing pulmonary arteriovenous malformation is:
    a. plain chest radiograph
    b. contrast echocardiography
    c. computed tomography
    d. pulmonary angiography
    e. arterial blood gases on room air and 100% oxygen

6. Advantages of embolotherapy for pulmonary arteriovenous malformation over surgery are:
    a. less invasive
    b. treatment of multiple and bilateral lesions at one time
    c. easy repeatability
    d. less loss of normal lung
    e. all of the above

7. Principles of transcatheter occlusion of pulmonary arteriovenous malformation include:
    a. avoidance of air emboli
    b. occlusion of the nidus or connecting aneurysm
    c. the use of detachable balloons or coil emboli
    d. a and c
    e. a, b, and c

8. Advantages of detachable balloons include:
    a. flow directionality
    b. test occlusion
    c. cross-sectional occlusion
    d. all of the above

9. Potential complications of embolotherapy are:
    a. paradoxical embolization
    b. angina and bradycardia
    c. pleurisy
    d. a and c
    e. a, b, and c

10. After treatment, most patients with pulmonary arteriovenous malformation require:
    a. follow-up assessment every 3 to 5 years
    b. anticoagulation
    c. antibiotics before dental work
    d. a and c
    e. a, b, and c

11. Acquired pulmonary arteriovenous fistulas can be due to:
    a. trauma
    b. cirrhosis
    c. Glenn shunt
    d. metastatic cancer
    e. all of the above

12. True statements concerning pulmonary artery aneurysms include:
    a. iatrogenic trauma is a relatively common cause
    b. embolization is contraindicated for peripherally located aneurysms
    c. embolization is the preferred treatment for centrally located aneurysms
    d. a and c
    e. a, b, and c

Tutorial 6: Bronchial Artery Embolization

1. The *least* likely cause of massive hemoptysis is:
    a. tuberculosis
    b. acute pulmonary embolism
    c. bronchiectasis
    d. aspergillosis

2. The *least* acceptable indication for bronchial artery embolization is:
    a. single massive episode of hemoptysis from pulmonary arteriovenous fistula
    b. single massive episode of hemoptysis in patient with tuberculosis
    c. recurrent minor hemoptysis in cystic fibrosis patient that interferes with physiotherapy

3. The artery *least* likely to have branches supplying the spinal cord is:
    a. an intercostal artery
    b. right intercostobronchial trunk
    c. left bronchial artery
    d. costocervical trunk

4. The most important reason to use nonionic contrast material for selective bronchial artery injections is:
    a. decrease patient coughing
    b. prevent allergic reaction
    c. decrease cost
    d. minimize chance of spinal cord injury

5. The embolic agent of choice in a patient with cystic fibrosis and massive hemoptysis is:
    a. absolute alcohol
    b. autologous clot
    c. polyvinyl alcohol particles
    d. Gianturco coil

6. Pulmonary infarction is most likely to occur following bronchial embolization for massive hemoptysis due to:
    a. chronic pulmonary embolism
    b. cystic fibrosis
    c. tuberculosis
    d. aspergillosis

7. The method of treatment for massive hemoptysis associated with the highest mortality is:
    a. bronchial embolization
    b. surgical resection
    c. conservative medical management

8. The most appropriate therapy for recurrent massive hemoptysis in a young, otherwise healthy patient with a focal lung abscess is:
    a. bronchial embolization
    b. antibiotic therapy and observation
    c. surgical resection of the involved area

Tutorial 7: Supra-Aortic Percutaneous Transluminal Angioplasty and Stents

1. The current treatment of choice for symptomatic carotid artery disease is:
   a. ticlopidine
   b. ASA
   c. endarterectomy
   d. stenting

2. Patients undergoing carotid angioplasty should be premedicated with:
   a. nifedipine
   b. nitroglycerine
   c. verapamil
   d. atropine

3. Clinical indications for subclavian artery angioplasty include:
   a. claudication
   b. subclavian steal
   c. atheroemboli
   d. all of the above

4. Subclavian occlusions are:
   a. not suitable for percutaneous intervention
   b. should not be stented
   c. should always be stented from the axillary approach
   d. none of the above

5. Transcranial Doppler has revealed cerebral emboli during:
   a. carotid angioplasty
   b. carotid endarterectomy
   c. neither
   d. both

6. Carotid angioplasty/stenting in symptomatic patients:
   a. is an acceptable alternative to endarterectomy
   b. should be performed on high-risk patients only
   c. should only be performed under an IRB-approved protocol

7. Completion of an accredited vascular/ interventional radiology fellowship:
   a. provides adequate training in cerebrovascular angioplasty
   b. does not necessarily provides adequate training in cerebrovascular angioplasty
   c. provides the basis for additional training in cerebrovascular angioplasty

8. The intrathoracic brachiocephalic artery most frequently atherosclerotic is:
   a. innominate artery
   b. right common carotid artery
   c. left common carotid artery
   d. left subclavian artery

9. The balloon diameter for a cerebrovascular PTA should:
   a. be 20% smaller than the normal diameter of the vessel
   b. be the same size as the corrected normal diameter of the vessel
   c. be up to 20% larger than the corrected normal diameter
   d. be up to 50% larger than the corrected normal diameter

10. Upon completion of a cerebrovascular angioplasty procedure, the following should be done:
   a. reverse 50% of the heparin with protamine
   b. remove the access sheath as soon as reversal is complete
   c. both of the above
   d. neither of the above

Tutorial 8: Intraarterial Thrombolysis for Acute Cerebral Infarction

1. The mechanism underlying the majority of strokes (60%–75%) is:
   a. vasculitis
   b. thromboembolic occlusion of large intracranial vessels
   c. subarachnoid hemorrhage
   d. small vessel occlusive disease

2. Thrombotic occlusion of small perforating brain vessels (<200 microns in diameter) is termed:
   a. amyloid angiopathy
   b. "lacunar" infarction
   c. hemorrhagic infarction
   d. moyamoya phenomenon

3. The most common site of extracranial atherosclerotic involvement of vessels to the brain is:
   a. the bifurcation of the common carotid artery
   b. the bifurcation of the internal carotid artery
   c. the cavernous internal carotid artery
   d. the cervical vertebral artery

4. The "ischemic penumbra" refers to areas of brain which are:
   a. irreversibly infarcted
   b. affected with potentially reversible ischemia
   c. involved by significant amounts of edema
   d. affected by herniation or mass effect

5. Mechanisms which may operate to decrease the severity and duration of cerebral ischemia and thereby limit the development of infarction include:
   a. physiological fibrinolytic mechanisms
   b. febrile response to cerebral ischemia
   c. collateral routes of blood supply
   d. a and c
   e. all of the above

6. Most transient ischemic attacks last:
   a. more than 24 hours
   b. 4–6 hours
   c. less than 1 hour
   d. more than 2 hours

7. Intraarterial thrombolysis in cerebral ischemia, analogous to experience in the peripheral and coronary circulations, is based on the assumption that thrombolytic reopening of an occluded vessel can restore function to areas of surviving tissue (ie, the ischemic penumbra).
   a. true
   b. false

8. Small amounts of red cell extravasation within an infarcted area, known as "hemorrhagic transformation":
   a. predominantly affects gray matter
   b. occurs commonly after untreated embolic infarcts
   c. is uncommonly symptomatic
   d. all of the above

9. Unenhanced CT scan within 6 hours of the onset of cerebral ischemia:
   a. is never normal
   b. is often normal
   c. usually demonstrates marked mass effect
   d. usually shows hemorrhage

1. What is a celiacomesenteric trunk (one answer)?
    a. a single common origin of both the celiac artery and the superior mesenteric artery.
    b. it is identical to the arc of Buhler
    c. an arteriovenous malformation of the celiac and SMA
    d. a collateral which develops in cases of SMA occlusion and mesenteric ischemia.

2. What is the arc of Buhler (one answer)?
    a. A common origin of the SMA and left gastric artery
    b. A collateral venous pathway in cases of splenic vein occlusion
    c. An embryonic remnant artery that connects the celiac and SMA, while they maintain separate origins off the abdominal aorta
    d. an arterial collateral arcade that courses throughout the transverse mesocolon

3. What percentage of left hepatic arteries partially or completely arise from the left gastric artery?
    a. 6%
    b. 42%
    c. 23%
    d. 36%

4. What is the second most common artery of origin of the left gastric artery, after the celiac artery?
    a. mesenterogastric trunk (SMA and left gastric artery) in 7%
    b. lienogastric trunk (splenic artery and left gastric artery) in 4%
    c. abdominal aorta, 16%
    d. left gastrophrenic trunk (phrenic artery and left gastric artery) in 4%

5. Choose the common arterial branches of the splenic artery (several answers):
    a. dorsal pancreatic
    b. right gastric
    c. short gastrics
    d. accessory left hepatic
    e. pancreatica magna
    f. transverse pancreatic
    g. superior polar splenic
    h. left gastroepiploic

6. What is the most common arterial supply (name, number, origin) to the gallbladder (one answer)?
    a. accessory right hepatic, single, originating from proper hepatic artery
    b. cystic artery, single in number, originating from the right hepatic artery
    c. cystic arteries, paired, originating from common hepatic artery
    d. cystic artery, single, originating from proper hepatic artery

7. What is the arc of Barkow (one or more answers)?
    a. an epiploic omental arc which parallels the right and left gastroepiploic arc
    b. a collateral arterial or venous pathway for splenic artery or vein occlusion
    c. a collateral pathway between the middle and left colic arteries
    d. an embryonic arcade between the superior and inferior mesenteric arteries

8. Which is the more proximal branch of the gastroduodenal artery:
    a. posterior branch of the superior pancreaticoduodenal artery
    b. anterior branch of the superior pancreaticoduodenal artery

9. What is most commonly the first major branch off the SMA?
    a. inferior pancreaticoduodenal artery
    b. first jejunal branch
    c. accessory right hepatic artery
    d. arc of Riolan

10. What two eponymous vessels serve as collaterals between the SMA and IMA?
    a. marginal artery of Drummond
    b. artery of Casinari
    c. arc of Riolan
    d. arc of Galen

11. What are the three major arterial branches of the IMA?
    a. right colic
    b. middle colic
    c. sigmoid
    d. superior hemorrhoidal
    e. left colic

Tutorial 10: Mesenteric Ischemia

1. The most frequent clinical finding on physical exam in patients with mesenteric ischemia is abdominal pain which is proportional to the physical exam.
    a. true
    b. false

2. Acute mesenteric ischemia is classified into occlusive and nonocclusive causes.
    a. true
    b. false

3. The mortality rate for mesenteric ischemia is less than 50%.
    a. true
    b. false

4. Infarction due to complete arterial occlusion occurs after 18 hours.
    a. true
    b. false

5. Thrombotic occlusion of main visceral vessels is gradual.
    a. true
    b. false

6. Classic peritoneal findings and shock are early clinical findings indicating the onset of mesenteric ischemia.
    a. true
    b. false

7. Bowel viability is at risk in acute mesenteric ischemia.
    a. true
    b. false

8. Causes of nonocclusive mesenteric ischemia include:
    a. myocardial infarction
    b. sepsis
    c. hypotension
    d. shock
    e. all of the above

9. In patients with chronic mesenteric ischemia, which percentage of patients had occlusion of the celiac axis and the superior mesenteric artery:
    a. 20%–25%
    b. 40%–50%
    c. 70%–75%
    d. 80%–85%
    e. 98%–99%

Tutorial 11: Computed Tomography- Arterial Portography

1. What are three ways to improve liver-to-lesion detection?
    a. limit the contrast material used during the DSA.
    b. ensure the catheter is well seated within SMA or SA.
    c. insert the catheter beyond the take-off of replaced right HA or other anatomic variants if present

2. How can you limit the amount of contrast material used during the preliminary arteriogram?
    a. use saline instead of contrast to insure that the catheter is secure.
    b. perform a DSA instead of using cut film.
    c. forego lesion detection. Concentrate only on catheter positioning and detection of arterial variants such as a replaced right hepatic artery.

3. What is the optimal scan delay for non-spiral CT?
    a. 5–10 sec
    b. 15–20 sec
    c. 20–40 sec

4. What is the optimal scan delay for spiral CT?
    a. 5–10 sec
    b. 20 sec
    c. 30 sec

5. What are three typical sites of perfusion abnormalities?
    a. Adjacent to the gallbladder fossa
    b. Anteromedial to the fissure separating the medial and lateral segments of the left hepatic lobe.
    c. Anterior to the porta hepatis in the medial segment of the left hepatic lobe.

1. Which of the following is *not* an angiographic manifestation of visceral tumors?
   a. vascular invasion
   b. displacement of vessels
   c. tumor blush/contrast hyperaccumulation
   d. arterial dissection
   e. neovascularity
   f. arterial-venous shunting

2. True/False? The following tumors often extend intraluminally within veins:
   a. hepatoma
   b. cholangiocarcinoma
   c. leiomyosarcoma
   d. renal cell carcinoma
   e. pancreatic carcinoma

3. True/False? Encasement of arteries and veins is a prominent feature in the following tumors:
   a. pancreatic Carcinoma
   b. cholangiocarcinoma
   c. hepatoma
   d. gastric carcinoma
   e. insulinoma

4. Which feature(s) is/are typical of functional islet cell tumors?
   a. dense tumor blush
   b. ill-defined borders
   c. rapid .washout of contrast material
   d. early arterial opacification
   e. hypervascularity
   f. benign tumor easily distinguished from malignancy

5. True/False?
   a. hemangiomas are the most common hepatic tumor
   b. hemangioendotheliomas require surgical resection
   c. arterial to hepatic vein shunting is common with hemangioendotheliomas
   d. FNH is a premalignant lesion

6. Which of the following is a feature of hepatic adenomas?
   a. arterial-venous shunting
   b. pooling of contrast material
   c. metastases
   d. hypervascular mass with neovascularity
   e. major artery encasement

7. True/False concerning renal cell carcinoma:
   a. preoperative embolization may be helpful
   b. angiography is sensitive for tumor detection
   c. angiography is the first choice for tumor detection
   d. bilateral tumor occurs in approximately 10%
   e. 1 microgram intraarterial epinephrine may aid in angiographic diagnosis
   f. it may be mimicked by several other renal tumors/processes

8. True/False features of hepatoma:
   a. enlarged draining hepatic veins
   b. neovascularity
   c. dense parenchymal enhancement
   d. portal vein invasion
   e. mimicked by some metastases and regenerating nodules

9. All are features of carcinoid *except*:
   a. markedly enlarged feeding artery
   b. vessel displacement toward the tumor
   c. mesenteric shortening
   d. ulcerations/GI bleeding
   e. "arteritis"

10. True/False features of myomatous tumors:
   a. only occur below the ligament of Treitz
   b. hemorrhage
   c. tumor blush
   d. dense venous drainage
   e. vascular encasement signifies malignancy

Tutorial 13: Embolization—General Principles and Techniques

More than one correct answer may apply.

1. In a patient scheduled for possible embolization for bleeding:

    a. blood pressure should first be completely normalized

    b. oxygen saturation need not be monitored when the patient is on nasal oxygen

    c. deep sedation is contraindicated

    d. an absolute limit on the volume of contrast material administered should be set at 250 mL

2. In a patient with daily intermittent hemobilia for 5 days after biliary drain placement:

    a. the proximal drain holes are malpositioned

    b. a larger caliber drain should be inserted

    c. celiac arteriography is performed to diagnose and treat possible arterial laceration

    d. visceral arteriography is performed during temporary removal of the biliary drain over a safety guide wire

3. Site of bleeding can be manifested by which of the following?

    a. contrast stain

    b. local vessel spasm

    c. pseudoaneurysm

    d. localized dissection

    e. isolated occlusion of the inferior mesenteric artery with well-developed collaterals

4. In a patient with pelvic hemorrhage:

    a. subselective arteriography is not necessary to identify the bleeding site

    b. contralateral hypogastric arteriography is unnecessary, post-embolization

    c. ipsilateral arteriography of the pro funda femoris is indicated pre- and post-embolization

    d. Gelfoam powder is safe and effective for embolization

5. Which of the following statements is/are true?

    a. severe coagulopathy can affect the efficacy of particulate and coil embolization

    b. the GDA is often embolized for endoscopically demonstrated upper GI bleeding even when visceral arteriography is normal

    c. concomitant administration of vasopressin and emboli is safe and effective for arresting poorly controlled GI bleeding

    d. Partial splenic embolization is effective for managing severe hyper-splenism

6. Which of the following statements is/are false?

    a. pseudoaneurysms can be safely occluded with intraluminal coils

    b. vascular malformations are best managed by periodic embolization with coils

    c. small peripheral feeding vessels can prevent aneurysmal thrombosis

    d. an aneurysm can usually be throm-bosed by embolizing its main afferent artery

7. Reflux of embolic particles is minimized by:

    a. distal superselective injections

    b. balloon occlusion

    c. wedging of catheter in distal vessel

    d. achieving complete stasis of blood flow

    e. slow, continuous infusion

8. Which of the following factors are true for hepatic chemoembolization?

    a. Pre-embolization assessment of portal vein patency is usually unnecessary

    b. Infusion catheter tip should be distal to the cystic artery origin

    c. Embolization end-point is complete distal hepatic arterial stasis

    d. Internal mammary and phrenic arteries may be important tumor feeders

    e. Presence of gas in the tumor after embolization usually represents a serious septic complication

Tutorial 14: Upper Gastrointestinal Bleeding

More than one correct answer may apply.

1. Gastroduodenal artery embolization can be safely performed with the following agents:
   a. Gelfoam pledgets
   b. Gelfoam powder
   c. absolute alcohol
   d. coils
   e. acrylate glues

2. Left gastric artery embolization is useful for treatment of:
   a. Mallory-Weiss tears
   b. antral gastric ulcers
   c. left hepatic pseudoaneurysm
   d. hemorrhagic gastritis

3. The complications of intraarterial vasopressin infusion include:
   a. myocardial infarction
   b. marked diuresis
   c. reperfusion injury
   d. visceral infarction

4. The intact left gastric artery anastomosis with the left gastroepiploic artery allows safe embolization of one of these arteries.
   a. true
   b. false

5. Intraarterial infusion of vasopressin provides emergency control of variceal hemorrhage.
   a. true
   b. false

Tutorial 15: Lower Gastrointestinal Bleeding

More than one correct answer may apply.

1. Published literature has shown that after other diagnostic measures have failed, angiography can define the cause of chronic lower GI bleeding in:
   a. 2% of patients
   b. 10% of patients
   c. 30% of patients
   d. 85% of patients

2. Diverticular hemorrhage is most often caused by diverticula within the:
   a. ascending colon
   b. descending colon
   c. sigmoid colon

3. Angiodysplasia (choose all that apply):
   a. most commonly affects the sigmoid colon
   b. bleeding may be controlled by embolization
   c. is characterized by visualization of an early draining vein
   d. can be present at multiple sites
   e. is often seen in young men

4. Vasopressin infusion (choose all that apply):
   a. can cause cerebral hemorrhage
   b. can cause hyponatremia
   c. is infused intraarterially for control of bleeding esophageal varices

5. Regarding embolization of lower GI bleeding (choose all that apply):
   a. alcohol is the most useful agent
   b. rectal lesions are amenable to therapy
   c. should be performed as proximally as possible
   d. Gelfoam pledgets or microcoils are useful agents

Tutorial 16: Chemoembolization of Hepatic Malignancies

More than one correct answer may apply.

1. Tumors typically amenable to hepatic chemo-embolization include:
   - a. hepatoma
   - b. metastatic colon cancer
   - c. metastatic breast cancer
   - d. carcinoid
   - e. metastatic GI sarcomas

2. Chemoembolization can generally be performed safely with:
   - a. portal vein thrombosis
   - b. serum bilirubin of 2.0
   - c. dilated ducts, but serum bilirubin >2.0
   - d. encephalopathy
   - e. LDH >425, AST >100, bilirubin >2, 50% liver replacement by tumor

3. Non-target chemoembolization of the gut typically occurs through the:
   - a. left gastric artery
   - b. right gastric artery
   - c. cystic artery
   - d. supraduodenal artery
   - e. gastroduodenal artery

4. Theoretical advantages of chemoembolization over infusion chemotherapy include:
   - a. increased drug concentration in tumor
   - b. increased exposure time of tumor to drug
   - c. decreased extrahepatic spread of tumor
   - d. decreased tumor drug resistance
   - e. decreased systemic toxicity

5. Predictable side effects of chemoembolization include:
   - a. pain
   - b. nausea
   - c. neutropenia
   - d. alopecia
   - e. diarrhea

6. Major complications of chemoembolization include:
   - a. cholecystitis
   - b. hepatic abscess
   - c. peptic ulcer
   - d. biloma
   - e. liver failure

7. The preprocedure work-up for chemo-embolization includes:
   - a. creatinine clearance
   - b. bone marrow biopsy
   - c. head CT scan
   - d. bleeding time
   - e. abdominal CT or MR scan

1. Portal vein occlusion:
    a. is an absolute contraindication to chemoembolization
    b. does not preclude chemoembolization if there is adequate portal vein flow via collaterals
    c. is unimportant with respect to chemoembolization
    d. can lead to hepatic necrosis if there is inadequate portal vein flow
    e. can recanalize after chemoembolization

2. Origin of the left hepatic artery from a left gastric-left hepatic artery trunk:
    a. is very rare and not of importance during chemoembolization
    b. can be associated with gastric necrosis if the left gastric artery is inadvertently chemoembolized
    c. is always easy to identify on celiac or hepatic arteriography because either all or none of the left hepatic artery arises from the left gastric-left hepatic artery trunk
    d. can be clarified in ambiguous cases by carbon dioxide gastric distention.
    e. can be safely chemoembolized with superselective catheterization

3. Superior mesenteric arteriography should be performed prior to hepatic chemoembolization because:
    a. total or partial origin of the right hepatic artery from the superior mesenteric artery is possible
    b. the gastroduodenal artery may not be identified on a celiac arteriogram due to "sumping," but may be identified on a superior mesenteric arteriogram, permitting placement of the chemoembolization distal to the gastroduodenal artery
    c. this is the only way to opacify the portal vein via an arterial injection

4. Regarding the dose of Ethiodol:
    a. it should be the same in every patient, about 20 mL
    b. it should be varied with the size of hypervascular tumors
    c. if excess is given, it will be harmlessly eliminated, and is of no clinical consequence
    d. if given in excess, it will opacify central portal vein branches, and can lead to hepatic necrosis
    e. is hepatotoxic at doses at or above 0.2 mL/kg

5. Gas formation within the tumor after chemo-embolization only occurs with the presence of an abscess.
    a. true
    b. false

6. Abscess formation within the tumor after chemoembolization can only be managed by surgical debridement or resection.
    a. true
    b. false

7. Biliary strictures after chemoembolization:
    a. occur because of compromise of portal vein flow due to passage of Ethiodol into the portal vein
    b. resolve spontaneously and do not produce clinical symptoms
    c. only occur in patients with elevated serum bilirubin
    d. are refractory to percutaneous management
    e. may occur more often in patients with prior hepatic artery chemotherapy infusions

8. Ablation of hepatic tumors with percutaneous infiltration of ethanol:
    a. generally requires conscious sedation, but can be performed upon outpatients
    b. must be visible on a cross-sectional imaging modality which can be used to guide a needle into the tumor
    c. is ideal for large tumors, generally larger than 5 cm in diameter
    d. is less suited for colorectal metastases
    e. can be performed easily under CT or US guidance

9. Regarding liver CT 1 month after chemoembolization of a hepatoma that takes up Ethiodol:

    a. normal liver will generally not have lost
    much Ethiodol compared to immediately
    post-chemoembolization

    b. the tumor will generally still be opacified
    with Ethiodol

    c. portions of the tumor not retaining oil are
    necrotic

    d. the more homogeneous the retention of
    Ethiodol by tumor, the greater will be the
    degree of tumor necrosis

    e. enhancement with intravenous contrast
    material is generally due to viable tumor

10. Following multiple chemoembolizations:

    a. arterial narrowing can occur, probably due
    to an arteritis

    b. If further chemoembolization of recurrent
    or new neoplasm cannot be performed due
    to arterial occlusion or stenosis, options
    include alcohol ablation or
    chemoembolization via collaterals

    c. most new hepatomas are due to
    recurrence of treated lesions rather than
    new lesions

    d. Recurrent tumors are less likely to
    respond than the originally treated ones

11. Collateral blood supply to hepatic neoplasms can
occur through the:

    a. inferior phrenic artery

    b. intercostal artery

    c. inferior mesenteric artery

    d. internal mammary artery

    e. inferior pancreaticoduodenal artery

12. Pitfalls in the performance of chemoembolization
include:

    a. patient belongs to an HMO

    b. sumping to hypervascular tumors

    c. catheter too small

    d. catheter too large

    e. too much stasis

Tutorial 18: Embolization of Abdominal Trauma

More than one correct answer may apply.

1. Potential benefits of embolization therapy in the abdominal trauma patient include:
   - a. angiography may allow more precise identification of bleeding points than surgical exploration
   - b. embolization is often a less risky option than surgical exploration
   - c. embolization generally allows greater preservation of tissue than surgical repair
   - d. all of the above

2. A "stable" patient is generally one who:
   - a. has a systolic blood pressure greater than 100 with a pulse rate of less than 110 mm Hg
   - b. has a systolic blood pressure greater than 80 with a pulse rate of less than 150 mm Hg
   - c. is alert and oriented
   - d. does not require endotracheal intubation

3. Concerning the initial evaluation of the abdominal trauma patient:
   - a. unstable trauma patients should always be taken to the operating room for exploration before arteriography is contemplated
   - b. a negative peritoneal lavage confidently excludes both intraperitoneal and retroperitoneal bleeding
   - c. in the stable patient, CT scanning is useful to detect abdominal injury as well as highlight which areas need to be evaluated arteriographically

4. Angiographic sheaths:
   - a. are usually not needed for embolization cases
   - b. should be used in all embolization cases to maintain arterial access should embolic material occlude the catheter
   - c. should not be used in trauma cases since this increases the size of the arterial hole in a potentially coagulopathic patient

5. Which of the following embolic agents is least likely to be used for pelvic trauma?
   - a. Gianturco coils
   - b. Gelfoam
   - c. microcoils
   - d. alcohol

6. Embolization of the splenic artery:
   - a. is not indicated in splenic trauma and splenectomy is the preferred therapy
   - b. should be undertaken if the diagnostic arteriogram demonstrates the mass effect of a splenic hematoma even if there is no active extravasation
   - c. can be done in the proximal splenic artery which decreases arterial pressure to the spleen without causing infarction

7. Regarding trauma to the lumbar arteries:
   - a. lumbar arteries are well seen on aorto graphy and selective lumbar injections are not necessary
   - b. one must look carefully for the artery of Adamkiewicz arising from the upper lumbar arteries
   - c. after embolizing an injured lumbar artery there is little risk of collateral perfusion to the injury due to poor connections between lumbar vessels

8. Concerning retroperitoneal hemorrhage related to pelvic fractures:
   - a. even unstable patients with retroperitoneal hematomas should be considered for prompt embolization therapy
   - b. internal iliac artery ligation is somewhat riskier but more effective than embolization
   - c. significant arterial injury is most common with anterior disruptions of the pelvic ring
   - d. orthopedic fixators should be placed to stabilize the pelvis before taking the patient to the angiography suite

More than one correct answer may apply.

1. Pediatric hemangiomas:
     a. are congenital lesions
     b. all require immediate therapy
     c. are tumors of infancy that exhibit a
     proliferative phase and then an involutive
     phase to complete regression
     d. require treatment only with strong
     indications
     e. none of the above.

2. Pediatric hemangiomas:
     a. usually manifest within the first month
     of life
     b. can be treated with embolization and
     surgical excision
     c. can be treated with intravenous
     corticosteroids
     d. can be treated with alpha interferon
     therapy
     e. none of the above

3. Arteriovenous malformations are characterized by:
     a. abnormal arteries and veins without
     AV shunting
     b. abnormal arteries and veins with AV
     shunting
     c. absence of an intervening capillary
     bed
     d. a high-flow lesion
     e. none of the above

4. Arteriovenous malformations:
     a. are high-flow malformations
     b. can involve multiple tissue planes
     c. always need to be treated
     d. in the body can be treated with
     radiation therapy
     e. none of the above

5. Color Doppler imaging:
     a. is useless in the work-up of AVMs
     b. can calculate flow volumes in feeding
     arteries to the AVM
     c. can calculate resistive indexes in
     addition to spectral analysis
     d. is an important noninvasive tool for
     follow-up of AVMs
     e. none of the above

6. Management of AVMs includes:
     a. surgery
     b. embolization followed by surger.
     c. embolotherapy alone
     d. alpha interferon therapy
     e. none of the above

7. Because nerves parallel arteries:
     a. ethanol should never be used to treat
     AVMs
     b. with superselective catheterization
     and direct puncture techniques, ethanol
     can be used to treat AVMs
     c. if the nerve injury occurs, it will always
     be permanent
     d. only motor nerves can expect to be
     injured if a neuropathy occurs
     e. oone of the above

8. In ethanol embolotherapy of AVMs:
     a. proximal catheter position, which can
     be used with PVA embolization, is
     mandatory
     b. in-flow vascular occlusion may be
     helpful to induce thrombosis
     c. volumes of 10 mL per kilogram per
     total dose are safe
     d. anesthesia is optional
     e. none of the above

1. Which of the following are medium- to small-vessel arteritides?
1) Buerger's disease
2) Polyarteritis nodosa
3) Kawasaki's disease
4) Takayasu's arteritis
    a. 1 and 2
    b. 1 and 3
    c. 1, 2, and 3
    d. 4 only

2. Takayasu's arteritis principally affects:
    a. old men
    b. young women
    c. small arteries
    d. the lower extremities

3. Temporal arteritis can be distinguished from Takayasu's arteritis by the following criteria:
1) age
2) gender
3) pattern of affected arteries
4) histology
    a. 1 and 2
    b. 1 and 3
    c. 1, 2, and 3
    d. all of the above

4. The innominate artery is the most commonly involved vessel in patients with Takayasu's arteritis.
    a. true
    b. false

5. All of the following are true of infection-related arteritis except:
    a. emboli tend to lodge at vessel branch points
    b. 50% of patients with arteritis due to hematogenous seeding from blood-borne microbes have no obvious source of infection
    c. affected large vessels tend to develop aneurysms or perforate
    d. arteritis due to contiguous extension of infection usually results in stenosis or occlusion

6. Which of the following statements regarding Buerger's disease is false:
    a. the internal elastic lamina is destroyed by the disease process
    b. the arteries proximal to the knee and elbow are normal
    c. previously occluded arterial segments may recanalize
    d. in the lower extremity, the differential diagnosis includes popliteal entrapment syndrome

7. A specific diagnosis of polyarteritis nodosa can be made when the typical arteriographic and histologic findings are present.
    a. true
    b. false

8. In polyarteritis nodosa, the most commonly affected arteries are in the territories of the:
1) hepatic artery
2) renal artery
3) mesenteric arteries
4) internal carotid arteries
    a. 1 and 2
    b. 2 and 3
    c. 1, 2, and 3
    d. 4 only

9. Which of the following statements regarding substance-abuse vasculitis is false?
    a. intracranial arteries are most commonly affected
    b. symptoms may be delayed for days after drug use
    c. the arteriographic appearance may mimic polyarteritis nodosa
    d. it only occurs following use of illicit drugs

10. Pulmonary artery involvement may be seen with which of the following arteritides?
1) Takayasu's arteritis
2) polyarteritis nodosa
3) Behçet's disease
4) systemic lupus erythematosus
    a. 1 and 2
    b. 1 and 3
    c. 1, 2, and 3
    d. 4 only

INDEX

Tutorials

Teaching File Cases